BEHAVIORAL HEALTHCARE AND TECHNOLOGY

BEHAVIORAL HEALTHCARE AND TECHNOLOGY

Using Science-Based Innovations to Transform Practice

EDITED BY

LISA A. MARSCH, PhD

SARAH E. LORD, PhD

JESSE DALLERY, PhD

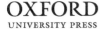

OXFORD
UNIVERSITY PRESS

Oxford University Press is a department of the University of
Oxford. It furthers the University's objective of excellence in research,
scholarship, and education by publishing worldwide.

Oxford   New York
Auckland   Cape Town   Dar es Salaam   Hong Kong   Karachi
Kuala Lumpur   Madrid   Melbourne   Mexico City   Nairobi
New Delhi   Shanghai   Taipei   Toronto

With offices in
Argentina   Austria   Brazil   Chile   Czech Republic   France   Greece
Guatemala   Hungary   Italy   Japan   Poland   Portugal   Singapore
South Korea   Switzerland   Thailand   Turkey   Ukraine   Vietnam

Oxford is a registered trademark of Oxford University Press
in the UK and certain other countries.

Published in the United States of America by
Oxford University Press
198 Madison Avenue, New York, NY 10016

Library of Congress Cataloging-in-Publication Data

Behavioral healthcare and technology : using science-based innovations to transform practice / edited by Lisa A. Marsch,
Sarah E. Lord, Jesse Dallery.
p. ; cm.
Includes bibliographical references.
ISBN 978–0–19–931402–7 (alk. paper)
I. Marsch, Lisa A., editor.   II. Lord, Sarah E. (Sarah Elizabeth), editor.   III. Dallery, Jesse, editor.
[DNLM: 1. Biomedical Technology.   2. Mental Disorders—therapy.   3. Mental Health Services—organization &
administration. WM 400]
RC455.2.D38
616.8900285—dc23
2014028147

This material is not intended to be, and should not be considered, a substitute for medical or other professional advice.
Treatment for the conditions described in this material is highly dependent on the individual circumstances. And, while this
material is designed to offer accurate information with respect to the subject matter covered and to be current as of the time it
was written, research and knowledge about medical and health issues is constantly evolving and dose schedules for medications
are being revised continually, with new side effects recognized and accounted for regularly. Readers must therefore always
check the product information and clinical procedures with the most up-to-date published product information and data sheets
provided by the manufacturers and the most recent codes of conduct and safety regulation. The publisher and the authors
make no representations or warranties to readers, express or implied, as to the accuracy or completeness of this material.
Without limiting the foregoing, the publisher and the authors make no representations or warranties as to the accuracy or
efficacy of the drug dosages mentioned in the material. The authors and the publisher do not accept, and expressly disclaim,
any responsibility for any liability, loss or risk that may be claimed or incurred as a consequence of the use and/or application of
any of the contents of this material.

9 8 7 6 5 4 3 2
Printed in the United States of America
on acid-free paper

CONTENTS

ACKNOWLEDGMENTS

The editors thank Sonia Oren, Operations Coordinator at the Dartmouth Center for Technology and Behavioral Health, for her exceptional partnership with the editors on the preparation of this book. The book has benefited tremendously from her endless energy, great ideas, and excellent organizational skills.

With deepest sympathies to her family and friends, we gratefully acknowledge the excellent chapter contribution by co-author Dr. Varda Shoham, who passed away before the publication of this book.

CONTRIBUTORS

Mustafa al'Absi, PhD
Department of Behavioral Sciences
University of Minnesota
Minneapolis, MN, USA

Lola Awoyinka, MPH
Center for Health Enhancement Systems
  Studies (CHESS)
Department of Industrial and Systems
  Engineering
University of Wisconsin—Madison
Madison, WI, USA

Amanda N. Baraldi, MA
Department of Psychology
Arizona State University
Tempe, AZ, USA

J. Gayle Beck, PhD
Department of Psychology
University of Memphis
Memphis, TN, USA

Dror Ben-Zeev, PhD
Dartmouth Psychiatric Research Center
Geisel School of Medicine
Dartmouth College
Lebanon, NH, USA

Matt Berg, MBA
Ona Systems, Kenya

Timothy Bickmore, PhD
College of Computer and Information Science
Northeastern University
Boston, MA, USA

Hayden B. Bosworth, PhD
Center for Health Services Research
  in Primary Care
Durham Veterans Affairs Medical Center
Department of Medicine
Division of General Internal Medicine
School of Nursing
Department of Psychiatry and
  Behavioral Sciences
Duke University
Durham, NC, USA

Rachel M. Brian, MPH
Dartmouth Psychiatric Research Center
Geisel School of Medicine
Dartmouth College
Lebanon, NH, USA

Aimee N.C. Campbell, PhD
New York State Psychiatric Institute
Department of Psychiatry
Columbia University
New York, NY, USA

Miraj Chokshi, MS
Northwestern University
Feinberg School of Medicine
Center for Behavioral Intervention Technologies
Chicago, IL, USA

Jesse Dallery, PhD
Director, Scientific Core
Center for Technology and Behavioral Health

Professor
Department of Psychology
University of Florida
Gainesville, FL, USA

ROBERT E. DRAKE, MD, PhD
Dartmouth Psychiatric Research Center
Geisel School of Medicine
Dartmouth College
Lebanon, NH, USA

EMRE ERTIN, PhD
Department of Electrical Engineering
The Ohio State University
Columbus, OH, USA

DEBORAH ESTRIN, PhD
Department of Computer Science
Cornell Tech
Department of Public Health
Weill Cornell Medical College
New York, NY, USA

MICHAEL CHRISTOPHER GIBBONS, MD, MPH
Johns Hopkins Urban Health Institute
Department of Medicine
Public Health and Health Informatics
Johns Hopkins University
Baltimore, MD, USA

WENDY J. NILSEN, PhD
Office of Behavioral and Social Sciences Research
National Institutes of Health
Bethesda, MD

MELISSA M. GOLDSTEIN, JD
Milken Institute School of Public Health
at the George Washington University
Washington, DC, USA

LIANNE GONSALVES, MSPH
Department of Reproductive Health and
Research
World Health Organization
Geneva, Switzerland

DAVID H. GUSTAFSON, PhD
Center for Health Enhancement Systems
Studies (CHESS)
Department of Industrial and Systems
Engineering
University of Wisconsin
Madison, WI, USA

JULIA E. HOFFMAN, PsyD
Mobile Health, Mental Health Services
US Department of Veterans Affairs
National Center for PTSD
Dissemination & Training Division
Menlo Park, CA, USA

PENELOPE P. HUGHES, JD, MPH
Office of the National Coordinator for Health
Information Technology
U.S. Department of Health and Human
Services
Washington, DC, USA

ROBERTA JOHNSON, MA, MEd
Center for Health Enhancement Systems
Studies (CHESS)
Department of Industrial and Systems
Engineering
University of Wisconsin–Madison
Madison, WI, USA

SANTOSH KUMAR, PhD
Department of Computer Science
University of Memphis
Memphis, TN, USA

ALLISON KURTI, PhD
Department of Psychology
University of Florida
Gainesville, FL, USA

ALAIN LABRIQUE, PhD
Johns Hopkins University Global mHealth
Initiative
Department of International Health
Johns Hopkins Bloomberg School of
Public Health
Baltimore, MD, USA

GINGER LOCKHART, PhD
Department of Psychology
Utah State University
Logan, UT, USA

SARAH E. LORD, PhD
Dissemination and Implementation Core,
Center for Technology and Behavioral
Health
Center for Supported Employment
Technology
Department of Psychiatry
Geisel School of Medicine
Dartmouth College
Hanover, NH, USA

DAVID P. MACKINNON, PhD
Department of Psychology
Arizona State University
Tempe, AZ, USA

LISA A. MARSCH, PhD
Center for Technology and Behavioral Health
Dartmouth Psychiatric Research Center
Department of Psychiatry
Geisel School of Medicine
Dartmouth College
Hanover, NH, USA

SARAH MARTNER, BS
Department of Psychology
University of Florida
Gainesville, FL, USA

GARRETT MEHL, PhD, MHS
Department of Reproductive Health and
    Research
World Health Organization
Geneva, Switzerland

DAVID C. MOHR, PhD
Northwestern University
Feinberg School of Medicine
Center for Behavioral Intervention Technologies
Chicago, IL, USA

FREDERICK MUENCH, PhD
Department of Psychiatry
Columbia University Medical Center
New York, NY, USA

INBAL NAHUM-SHANI, PhD
Survey Research Center
Institute for Social Research
University of Michigan
Ann Arbor, MI, USA

WENDY J. NILSEN, PhD
Office of Behavioral and Social Sciences
    Research
National Institutes of Health
Bethesda, MD, USA

EDWARD V. NUNES, PhD
New York State Psychiatric Institute
Department of Psychiatry
Columbia University
New York, NY, USA

LISA S. ONKEN, PhD
National Institute on Drug Abuse
Bethesda, MD, USA

MISHA PAVEL, PhD
College of Computer and Information Science
Bouvé College of Health Sciences
Northeastern University
Boston, MA, USA

DANIEL POLSKY, PhD
Leonard Davis Institute of Health Economics
Perelman School of Medicine and the Wharton
    School
University of Pennsylvania
Philadelphia, PA, USA

KELLY M. RAMSEY, BA
Mobile Behavior Design Lab
National Center for PTSD Dissemination &
    Training Division
Menlo Park, CA, USA

WILLIAM T. RILEY, PhD
Science of Research and Technology Branch
Behavioral Research Program
Division of Cancer Control and Population
    Sciences
National Cancer Institute
Rockville, MD, USA

STEPHEN M. SCHUELLER, PhD
Northwestern University
Feinberg School of Medicine
Center for Behavioral Intervention Technologies
Chicago, IL, USA

MARCIA S. SCOTT, PhD
National Institute on Alcohol Abuse and
    Alcoholism (NIAAA)
National Institutes of Health
Bethesda, MD, USA

TAMSYN SEIMON, MHS
Consultant, Switzerland

RYAN J. SHAW, PhD, RN
Center for Health Services Research in
    Primary Care
Durham Veterans Affairs Medical Center
School of Nursing
Duke University
Durham, NC, USA

VARDA SHOHAM, PhD
National Institute of Mental Health
Bethesda, MD, USA

DANIEL M. SMITH, MS
Department of Psychology
University of Rhode Island
Kingston, RI, USA

DEBORAH F. TATE, PhD
Department of Health Behavior
Department of Nutrition
Communication for Health Applications and
    Interventions Core
Lineberger Comprehensive Cancer Center
Nutrition Obesity Research Center
UNC Weight Research Program
University of North Carolina at Chapel Hill
Chapel Hill, NC, USA

MARLEEN TEMMERMAN, MD, MPH, PhD
Department of Reproductive Health and
    Research
World Health Organization
Geneva, Switzerland

CARMINA G. VALLE, PhD, MPH
Cancer Health Disparities Training Program
UNC Weight Research Program
University of North Carolina at Chapel Hill
Chapel Hill, NC, USA

LAVANYA VASUDEVAN, PhD, MPH, CPH
Duke Global Health Institute
Duke University
Durham, NC, USA
Johns Hopkins University Global mHealth
    Initiative
Department of International Health
Johns Hopkins Bloomberg School of Public
    Health
Baltimore, MD, USA

THEODORE A. WALLS, PhD
Department of Psychology
University of Rhode Island
Kingston, RI, USA

INGRID C. WURPTS, MA
Department of Psychology
Arizona State University
Tempe, AZ, USA

LEAH L. ZULLIG, PhD, MPH
Center for Health Services Research in
    Primary Care
Durham Veterans Affairs Medical Center
Durham, NC, USA

INTRODUCTION

LISA A. MARSCH, SARAH E. LORD, AND JESSE DALLERY

TRANSFORMING BEHAVIORAL HEALTHCARE WITH TECHNOLOGY

Internet and mobile technologies have radically changed countless sectors of our society. We can now conduct financial and retail transactions, arrange travel, and engage in social communications online remotely, securely, and conveniently. Digital technologies are also increasingly changing the way in which we manage our health and health behavior.

In recent years, there has been an explosion of research and development focused on using technology to promote health and wellness. These include Web and mobile health assessment and intervention tools—such as tools for tracking and providing therapeutic support for issues ranging from activity levels, medication taking, mood states, and medical conditions.

This work has shown that scientifically informed, technology-based tools offer considerable promise for monitoring and responding to individuals' health behavior in real time. They may extend the reach of clinicians or serve as stand-alone tools. They offer endless opportunities for tailoring behavioral interventions that are optimally responsive to the needs and preferences of each individual. They additionally offer an unprecedented opportunity for individuals (and an extended support network of their choosing) to play leading roles in the management of their own health and wellness. When implementation of technology-based therapeutic tools is scaled up to a population level, they may enable entirely new models of healthcare—both within and outside formal systems of care—enabling improved quality of care, health outcomes, and cost-effectiveness.

This book defines the state of scientific research related to the development, experimental evaluation, and effective dissemination of technology-based therapeutic tools targeting behavioral health (e.g., in areas of management of substance use, mental health, diet and exercise, medication adherence, as well as chronic disease management). The content has a priority focus on behavioral health, given that all health conditions require health behavior change, and the course and treatment of chronic diseases are frequently complicated by behavioral health problems.

This volume reflects outstanding contributions from an interdisciplinary group of authors who are leaders in fields of paramount importance to the arena of technology and behavioral health—including leaders in the science of behavior change, emerging technologies, health economics, novel methodologies and analytics, implementation science, regulation, privacy and security, and public policy.

At a time when there has been a rapidly growing interest in leveraging digital media in health promotion, this book is distinct in that it is grounded in science. The content reflects a comprehensive overview of the state of what is known from scientific research in this arena and what gaps remain in our scientific understanding of how to harness technology to provide evidence-based behavioral healthcare.

Although this book focuses on science, it is not intended only for an audience of scientists. Rather, it was prepared for a diverse stakeholder audience, including researchers, clinicians, program administrators, and persons in policy and regulatory arenas, and a wide array of audiences interested in innovative strategies for improving population health.

SECTION I: OPTIMAL MODELS FOR DEVELOPING TECHNOLOGY-BASED THERAPEUTIC TOOLS TARGETING BEHAVIORAL HEALTH

The book begins with an overview of optimal models for developing technology-based therapeutic tools. In the first chapter, Onken and Shoham provide an excellent overview of how the stage model of behavioral intervention development can be applied to the development and refinement of technology-based therapeutic approaches, and highlight the utility of this framework to guide development.

Effective technology-based interventions either begin with or contribute to theories of behavior change. Riley reviews the critical role of theory in developing interventions, and how advances in technology provide unique opportunities—due to the ability of technology to intensively measure behavior over time—to refine existing theories of behavior change.

SECTION II: EVIDENCE-BASED APPROACHES TO HARNESSING TECHNOLOGY TO PROMOTE BEHAVIORAL HEALTH

The second section of the book summarizes empirically supported approaches to harnessing technology across a broad behavioral health spectrum.

Kumar and colleagues start off this section with an overview of how mobile sensing technologies may be used to obtain continuous measures of health, behavior, and the environment in naturalistic settings. They provide a broad overview of recent advancements in converting wearable physiological sensor data into measures of behavior and highlight several examples to illustrate this approach—with applications to stress, conversation, and smoking. They also provide a summary of their research team's innovative work with a suite of sensors and mobile software as an excellent example of innovative work in this area.

Campbell and co-authors review the state of the science in applying technology to the prevention, treatment, and recovery support from substance use disorders. They provide a thoughtful discussion of the empirical support to date for this approach in targeting substance use disorders and consider various models for improving addiction treatment service delivery systems through the harnessing of technology-based therapeutic tools.

Schueller, Choksi, and Mohr cogently describe the evidence base for technology approaches to depression and anxiety and highlight the critical role of target end-user involvement in the development of these therapeutic tools for promoting end-user engagement and successful outcomes.

Ben-Zeev, Drake, and Brian present a compelling narrative for harnessing the powerful potential of mobile phones to promote real-time symptom self-management among individuals with serious mental illness. These authors highlight the potential of mobile technologies for both empowering traditionally underserved populations and for promoting patient-centered models of care.

Medication non-adherence represents a costly public health issue, and technology-based methods afford unique opportunities to promote adherence. Zullig, Shaw, and Bosworth review how technology can aid patients, providers, and even healthcare systems in promoting adherence. The authors discuss a range of advances, including pill-monitoring systems, mobile health technology, online resources and social media, and advances in electronic health records.

The subsequent chapter, by Dallery and colleagues, provides a theoretically and empirically grounded review of both technology-based assessment and treatment of cigarette smoking. This excellent overview provides a summary of the state of the science in this ever-growing area of research, including the promise of this approach for a wide variety of smoking populations.

Valle and Tate provide an excellent overview of how technology has been used to promote diet, exercise, and weight control. They focus on 21 illustrative examples of technology-based interventions that have been evaluated in the scientific literature, and they critically evaluate key dimensions across these interventions that may have impacted outcomes (e.g. self-monitoring, social support, tailoring, reminders, goal setting).

Bickmore provides a compelling case for the potential of virtual avatars to provide both social and emotional support in healthcare service delivery. The work described in this chapter high-lights the potential of these virtual avatars to serve as on-demand support "coaches" across a variety of health service needs, allowing human providers to potentially serve more clients and to work at their highest levels of expertise.

SECTION III: METHODS FOR THE EVALUATION OF TECHNOLOGY-BASED BEHAVIORAL HEALTHCARE

The third section of the book reviews best practices in methodologies for evaluating technology-based systems of behavioral healthcare.

As mobile devices are increasingly being used to capture information about individuals' behavior, enormous volumes of data are being generated on an ongoing basis. Understanding how to mean-ingfully interpret and apply these data streams is an important area of research. Smith and Walls provide an overview of best practices in research designs and analytic models available to meet this challenge. They also envision how the field of mobile data analytics may evolve over time and how this approach may inform clinical applica-tions of mobile health tools.

Dallery, Riley, and Nahum-Shani provide an excellent overview of research designs for both the development and evaluation of technology-based therapeutic approaches. This overview highlights how both traditional and innovative designs and methodologies can be used to elucidate not only mechanisms of behavior change associated with technology-based care approaches, but also opti-mal implementation of these approaches within diverse systems of care.

Baraldi, Wurpts, and MacKinnon examine mediation analysis in technology-based interven-tions. Mediation analysis seeks to identify the potential mechanisms of behavior change and thus go beyond documenting merely that a change in behavior has occurred to address why the change has occurred. They introduce the basics of the mediation model, and how it can be integrated with advances in intensive longitudinal data col-lection methods. Addressing generalizable, dura-ble, and parsimonious mechanisms of behavior change is critical in the face of rapid changes in technological tools.

The final chapter in the section on methods is prepared by health economist Daniel Polsky.

Given the economic constraints in healthcare systems, broad adoption of empirically sup-ported technology-based service delivery models will not be based on their effectiveness alone but rather will require a strong economic argument. Polsky's chapter reviews many important consid-erations when conducting economic analyses of technology-based therapeutic systems.

SECTION IV: EFFECTIVE DISSEMINATION AND IMPLEMENTATION

The fourth section of the book defines the state of implementation research examining models for integrating technology-based behavioral health-care systems into various care settings to increase the quality and reach of evidence-based and cost-effective behavioral healthcare.

The chapter by Lord starts off this section by detailing the importance of implementation research designed to understand factors that facili-tate or function as barriers to adoption and sus-tained use of technology in care settings in ways that bring value to an array of stakeholders. As part of this overview, she highlights important lessons learned from research in implementation of tech-nology-based innovations.

Hughes and Goldstein address the critically important issues of privacy and security with regard to use of technology-based therapeutic approaches in healthcare delivery. These authors provide an excellent overview of the regulatory issues that can impact use of these approaches to care.

A particularly important implication of tech-nology is its ability to impact health globally. Mehl and colleagues discuss how mobile health approaches can be harnessed in low-income settings to provide universal access to health interventions. The challenges faced in these envi-ronments are formidable and include staff short-ages, poor health literacy, lack of access to care, antiquated methods of record keeping, and access, to name a few. The authors provide data-based and concrete, real-world examples of how technology may circumvent (and have circumvented) these obstacles, and provide a framework for how future work should continue to break down barriers to health interventions.

Hoffman, Ramsey, and Estrin present a thought-provoking chapter on the potential benefits of open-source software development (including open standards and open architecture) to create efficiencies and new levels of innovation in the deploying technologies.

SECTION V: PUBLIC HEALTH AND POLICY IMPLICATIONS

The fifth and final section of this volume discusses important public health and policy implications of this work.

This section opens with an important discussion by Awoyinka, Gustafson, and Johnson on leveraging technology to promote the integration of behavioral healthcare into medical care settings. Given that the management of any physical health condition requires important behavioral management (e.g., medication taking, managing depression that may interfere with one's ability to manage illness), an integrated model of care holds great promise for improving the scope and quality of care delivered as well as health outcomes.

Gibbons addresses the potential of technology to address disparities in behavioral healthcare. He notes that although disparities have been recognized for quite some time, little progress has been made in reducing, not to mention eliminating, disparities in health or healthcare. Gibbons illustrates how technology may not only help us understand how disparities happen, but also how new technologies may help overcome these disparities.

Nilsen and Pavel provide an excellent overview of the adoption of behavioral health technologies in the context of a changing healthcare landscape. Using recent U.S. healthcare reform as an example, these authors provide an insightful view of how technology may be integrated into healthcare systems and healthcare policies.

Finally, Marsch envisions the future about how technology may transform healthcare systems. She highlights the scientific foundations of such a transformation and the tremendous capability of technology to usher in entirely new systems of healthcare. However, Marsch also notes the challenges ahead in "scaling up" science-based technology, as well as key strategies to address these challenges, such as engaging consumers, breaking down disciplinary boundaries that may hinder comprehensive approaches, increasing our understanding of the mechanisms of behavior change, and developing partnerships between science, government, and industry.

Overall, this book presents a compelling set of scientific research findings that inform optimal models for developing, testing, and implementing technology-based strategies to promote behavioral health. Collectively, these data underscore the tremendous promise of harnessing technology in transforming the delivery of behavioral healthcare.

Preparation of this editorial was supported in part by Center Grant #P30DA029926 from the National Institute on Drug Abuse, National Institutes of Health (www.c4tbh.org).

SECTION I

Models for Developing
Technology-Based Therapeutic
Tools Targeting Behavioral Health

1

Technology and the Stage Model of Behavioral Intervention Development

LISA S. ONKEN AND VARDA SHOHAM

INTRODUCTION

Technology can facilitate the development of behavioral interventions in a number of ways. There are computer-assisted modules of empirically supported treatments for mood and anxiety disorders (1–4) and for addiction (5,6). There are also exposure-based interventions that utilize virtual reality to help patients experience threatening situations safely that might be difficult to experience in real life (7,8). And there are delivery modes (e.g., iPhone) that make interventions far more accessible to certain populations, such as children and adolescents (9,10). Technology can also be used to measure what an individual is experiencing in objective, nonreactive ways (11–14), and in turn can provide tailored feedback in real time about emotions, cognitions, and behaviors (15) or help to decrease craving with neurofeedback (16). There are even soap-opera videos that have been used for HIV prevention (17). These are just a few examples of ways in which technology can be incorporated into behavioral interventions and intervention development research.

The goal of this chapter is to discuss how technology can be used to facilitate the process of behavioral intervention development research. For the purposes of this chapter, we will focus on technology-based behavioral *treatments*, leaving the important discussion of technology-assisted prevention interventions for other authors. Our discussion could include, for example, incorporating a virtual reality component into a treatment or computerizing part or all of a treatment. It could involve administering a technology-based treatment within a clinician's office. It could mean administering a technology-based treatment using a technology-based delivery system such as the Internet, a tablet, or a smartphone. Or the treatment could be administered partly through technology and partly through traditional in-person therapeutic strategies. Technology-assisted measurement of relevant behavioral and/or physiological information is often a part of technology-based interventions, and these interventions sometimes involve therapeutic feedback of these data to the patient or to the therapist (18–21).

To provide a context for how technology might benefit behavioral treatment development, we first will briefly summarize some possible benefits of technology to patients and clinicians.[1] Next, we review the stages of behavioral intervention development research and discuss how technology can enhance the treatment development process at each stage. Finally, we will discuss some challenges and unintended consequences of technology-based behavioral treatments.

WHAT'S IN IT FOR PATIENTS?

The potential benefits of technology-based interventions for people who struggle with emotional and behavioral problems are extensive. To name a few:

1. *Increasing reach and availability of treatment.* One thing technology promises to help with is the reach and availability of treatment. Much has been written about the paucity of available treatments, especially those that are empirically supported (22). Moreover, treatment for mental disorders begins on average 11 years after problem onset (23). It is patently obvious that if interventions can be delivered through the use of technology, such as through the Internet, telephone, or mobile phones, many more

people will be able to access treatments and do so earlier in the course of problem development (24) .

2. *Increasing the similarity between treatments that patients receive and treatments that were experimentally tested.* Even where patients think they are receiving empirically supported treatment, such treatments are not always delivered in the same manner or fidelity that is typical in controlled efficacy studies (25–27). Technology-based treatments have "built-in" fidelity, and patients can expect to receive the same treatment that patients in research studies receive. Some of these treatments are, in fact, encapsulated in an app.

3. *Increasing the affordability of treatment.* Technologically based treatments may not cost as much as traditional treatments. Although it may be costly to produce a computerized treatment, computerized intervention requires far less expert therapist time. So once produced, the administrative costs per patient could go down as the number of patients a treatment can reach goes up (28,29). Even when used in addition to treatment as usual, computer-based treatment can be cost-effective (30).

4. *Increasing individuals' sense of anonymity.* Some people might opt not to risk being seen at a mental health or substance abuse treatment clinic or even a traditional healthcare setting. Such people may prefer the sense of confidentiality that technology-based interventions might be able to offer. Given urgent needs of more than 2 million servicemen and women returning from war, the Veteran Health Administration has embarked on a large-scale implementation project, using anonymous Internet-based interventions (31).

5. *Improving the chance of alleviating a person's symptoms and problems.* For people who would not otherwise seek traditional treatments, having accesses to an experimentally supported technology-based treatment could substantially improve the likelihood of improvement.

But technology-based interventions could also be used in conjunction with traditional treatment to boost outcomes, as has been pursued with technology-based cognitive remediation strategies in conjunction with behavioral treatment for schizophrenia (32).

WHAT'S IN IT FOR CLINICIANS?

Technology-based interventions offer many attractive benefits for practitioners as well, including:

1. *Increasing the potency of treatment.* As in the example given regarding cognitive remediation for schizophrenia (32), technology-based treatments could be administered in addition to an intervention already provided by the clinician and could reinforce or add to what the clinician is already administering. Another example is "CBT4CBT," a computer-based version of cognitive behavioral therapy for substance abuse that is used in conjunction with standard treatment (5,33).

2. *Increasing reach and availability of training.* Technology holds promise for increasing the reach and availability of therapist training. It is entirely possible that the same technology-based treatments that patients receive could assist in training therapists to use the intervention. Alternatively, one could develop technology-based therapist training interventions. Rose et al. (34) administered to primary care providers computer-assisted training as part of a comprehensive training program to treat anxiety. Sholomskas and Carroll (35) randomized community-based drug abuse treatment providers to receive computer-assisted training (plus the treatment manual) in twelve step facilitation (TSF) or to receive training with the manual only. They found that the therapists who received the computer-assisted training in addition to the manual were able to implement TSF better than those who were trained with the manual only. Given that this training

is technology based, it may not require the effort to receive the training that traditional training requires.

3. *Increasing the affordability of training.* Technology-based training could be less costly than traditional training. Just as technology-based treatment as part of traditional treatment could decrease the amount of time required for costly face-to-face therapy, technology-based training has the potential to decrease the amount of time needed for expert clinicians to train front-line providers.

4. *Increasing the amount of time available to the clinician.* Technology-based treatments could supplant some of what the clinician already does that lends itself toward technological innovation (e.g., skills training) and could thereby free up clinicians' time to be used in a variety of other ways. For example, with increased time per patient, a clinician could devote more time to strengthening the therapeutic alliance.

As described throughout this compendium, the benefits of technology-based interventions for patients, therapists, and mental health clinics are apparent and well documented. The main aim of this chapter is to explore the potential benefits of technology-based interventions for researchers, particularly researchers interested in the development and testing of behavioral treatments.

BENEFITS OF TECHNOLOGY FOR STAGE-BASED INTERVENTION DEVELOPMENT RESEARCH

The National Institutes of Health (NIH) stage model is an iterative, recursive model of behavioral intervention development (36). The primary goal of the NIH stage model of behavioral intervention development is to go beyond developing efficacious behavioral interventions to continuously improve upon efficacious behavioral interventions by boosting their potency, broadening their impact, and enhancing their portability or "implementability" and "community friendliness." The benefits to those using the interventions, be it

patients or providers, is a critically important factor in intervention development.

Using technology as a basis for treatment or a treatment component enables a focus on implementability and portability factors early in the treatment development process. Technology also allows for the possibility of modifying elements in traditional empirically supported interventions to make them more implementable. The delivery format of the intervention may be changed without detriment to efficacy if one knows the essential ingredients or if one knows the "mechanism of action" of an intervention (i.e., how and why the intervention works). For a variety of reasons (e.g., inherent fidelity, ability to add or remove parts of an intervention easily, ability to measure outcomes in real time), technology-based interventions may help us get a better grasp on mechanisms of action. Technology may be utilized where appropriate not only to make an intervention more efficient, less costly, and more portable but also to potentially boost its effects—two of the major goals of the NIH stage model of intervention development. In the next section, we examine the potential for technology-based interventions at each stage of the stage model.

TECHNOLOGY AND THE EARLY STAGES (0–I) OF INTERVENTION DEVELOPMENT

Stage 0 in the stage model refers to basic research. It could be basic research (e.g., experimental psychopathology) that is conducted outside of the intervention development process. Or it could be basic research that is conducted within any other stage (I through V) to determine basic processes of behavior maintenance and change, that is, research on "mechanism of action" of behavioral interventions.

Stage I research involves generating an intervention that engages an identified target or targets (Stage IA) and pilot testing of the effect of such target engagement on initial efficacy as well as the intervention's feasibility (Stage IB). Ideally, intervention generation is based on a theory-derived putative mechanism of action. In Stage IA, when generating a novel behavioral intervention, it is essential to identify behavioral targets for that intervention. *Target* refers to a problem-maintaining process, which the intervention seeks to modify. *Target engagement* occurs when the intervention in fact modifies this process. *Target validation* occurs when target engagement leads to (or at least correlates with) symptom reduction outcomes. And finally, *mechanisms of action* (how the intervention works) encompasses both target engagement and target validation.

For example, the ultimate outcome of a specific treatment may be drug use, but the target that is hypothesized to have an effect on drug using behavior is approach bias to drug-related cues. Wiers, Eberl, Rinck, Becker, and Lindenmeyer (37) have developed the alcohol approach/avoidance task, in which they attempted to shift approach bias to alcohol-related cues by training a person to pull a joystick to enlarge (zoom in) the picture size, thus enhancing patients' sense of approach, and push the joystick to decrease (zoom out) the picture size, thus enhancing patients' sense of avoidance[37]. These researchers experimentally induced an avoidance bias to alcoholic drinks and an approach bias to nonalcoholic drinks, and found that people trained this way not only generalized their newly trained avoidance bias to untrained pictures but also shifted their bias for alcohol to an avoidance approach. Participants continued to show improved treatment outcomes 1 year later (37). This is an example of how changing a target (approach bias for alcohol) can improve ultimate treatment outcome (alcohol use).

Accurate measurement of behavioral and cognitive processes targeted by the intervention is important in all stages of treatment development and especially in Stages 0 and I. Technology can enable the measurement of processes that might not otherwise be measurable, and it can do so in a way that minimizes the reactivity and maximizes the reliability of the measure. It is difficult to imagine how constructs, such as attention bias[1] approach bias (37), and physiological processes relevant to emotional state, such as pupillary dilation (38), could be measured as reliably and validly without a technology-based assessment. Other examples of technology-based assessment include ecological momentary assessment (39), mobile eye-tracking applications (40), and wearable (41) and mobile sensors (42). Not only can technology-based measures help researchers identify, operationally define, and improve assessments of targets and outcomes, but many of these

very same measures can become incorporated into the treatment itself. Cohn, Hunter-Reel, Hagman, and Mitchel (43) have identified the measurement of alcohol use behavior and the incorporation of this measurement into treatment applications as a direction for future research. Drug craving has been linked to relapse in substance abusers, and drug craving can be measured in real time, using ecological momentary assessment (44). This opens up the possibility of developing an application that is specifically linked to the assessment of drug craving in real time, with the goal of preventing relapse.

Of course, targets are identified in Stage IA based on hypothesized factors that cause or at least maintain the problem behavior. Once a target is identified and operationally defined, the intervention needs to be designed to maximize target engagement in a way that produces the desired behavior change; that is, the intervention's presumed effects need to be consistent with the putative mechanism of that intervention. For example, if increasing working memory is hypothesized to be helpful when added to empirically supported treatment for schizophrenia, then working memory needs to be operationally defined and measurable, and the intervention being generated needs to be designed to increase working memory. Not only can technology be useful in measuring working memory (e.g., computerized tests can be developed to reliably assess memory), it can also be useful in generating an intervention to improve working memory and compensate for other social and neurocognitive deficits. For example, Eack et al. (45) administered cognitive enhancement therapy to individuals with early schizophrenia, and it was shown to effectively improve cognitive deficits. The intervention requires "45 social-cognitive group sessions," but it also includes a substantial component of computer-assisted training (about 60 hours) that targets problem-solving, attention, and memory.

After operationally defining a target and developing an intervention to engage that target in Stage IA, getting an initial signal that the intervention has some impact on the target behavior is an important Stage IB activity. Depending on the intervention being studied and the questions being asked, this could occur in a variety of forms, for example, a pilot randomized clinical trial, a within-subjects design, or a multiple-baseline design. In all of these cases, however, it is important that the target behavioral outcome be accurately measured at multiple points and in a way that can determined if the intervention, when administered with fidelity, is related to changes in that target. With traditional psychotherapy, it is not always so easy to measure a presumed target in real time, to deliver an intervention competently and with fidelity, and to determine if the intervention is having an effect on the presumed mechanism. With technology-assisted behavioral treatment, the interventions will not always be akin to traditional psychotherapy, but the measurement of target engagement in real time may be infinitely simpler, the integrity and fidelity of the intervention may be infinitely greater, and the ability to determine mechanism may fall within our grasp.

Once it is determined if the target was sufficiently engaged and the intervention is working the way it was intended, the intervention can be further defined or redefined on the basis of these initial Stage I findings. Next steps could potentially involve going back to Stage 0 to better understand hypothesized mechanisms, going back to Stage IA to further strengthen the intervention based on findings, going back to Stage IA to redefine targets and the presumed mechanisms of those targets, or proceeding forward to Stages II, III, or IV to conduct large-scale testing.

TECHNOLOGY-BASED INTERVENTIONS AND THE MIDDLE STAGES (II–IV) OF BEHAVIORAL INTERVENTION DEVELOPMENT RESEARCH

In Stages II and III, the efficacy of behavioral interventions is investigated. These stages involve controlled testing with maximal *internal* validity. In Stage II, interventions are delivered by research therapists or providers in research ("laboratory-based") settings, whereas in Stage III interventions are delivered by community therapists or practitioners in community settings. Stage IV is effectiveness research and it involves the testing of behavioral interventions with maximal *external* validity. Because technology-based behavioral interventions are inherently easier to implement with a high degree of fidelity, the distinctions between Stages II, III, and IV are blurred. For example, if an intervention is almost entirely

technology based, does it matter less in an efficacy trial if the intervention is delivered by a research therapist in a research setting (Stage II), or a community therapist in a community setting (Stage III)? To the extent that the intervention relies on the therapist it could matter whether the study is carried out in the investigator's laboratory or in a community setting. But many technology-based interventions rely less on the skill of a therapist than do traditional treatments. Suffice it to say that the less technology-based an intervention is, the more of a distinction there is between Stage II and Stage III, and the greater the need for Stage III research when an intervention is heavily dependent on therapist delivery. There may also be less of a distinction between Stage II and Stage III for technology-based interventions that one does apart from a therapist (e.g., at home on a PC, Internet-based, handheld device), and more of a distinction between Stage II and Stage III for technology-based interventions that are administered in the clinician's office.

What about the distinction between highly controlled, high internal validity efficacy research (Stages II and III) and less highly controlled, high external validity effectiveness research (Stage IV)? Again, these same points hold. That is, the less an intervention relies on therapist delivery, the less of a distinction there is between effectiveness (Stage IV) research and efficacy (Stages II and III) research. It is risky to take a traditional complex, difficult-to-train, behavioral intervention, dependent on faithful delivery by a treatment provider, directly from Stage I to Stage IV. However, some technology-based interventions, those that are more easily implementable with higher fidelity than traditional treatments, arguably may be ready for Stage IV research immediately following Stage I research. Hence, the translational pace from the laboratory to the community may be significantly accelerated.

The benefits noted in the early stages of intervention development lay the foundation for and parallel the benefits in the middle stages of intervention development research. Again, due to the inherently higher fidelity of most technology-based interventions, and due to the relative ease of measuring the purported mechanisms or targets, the outcome variable, and the parameters of the intervention itself, testing the effects of a focused intervention becomes much simpler. In addition, the sample size to test the treatment and the mechanisms of behavior change might be significantly increased without incurring additional costs if the technology-based treatment decreases therapist training time, decreases the cost of therapist time, and diminishes the need to take measures to ensure the fidelity of the intervention.

LATE-STAGE (V) BEHAVIORAL INTERVENTION DEVELOPMENT RESEARCH AND TECHNOLOGY-BASED INTERVENTIONS

Dissemination and implementation of empirically supported behavioral interventions—an enormous problem for traditional behavioral intervention research—has become a foreseeable goal for many technology-based interventions. Technological aids that help to administer technology-based interventions have become prevalent, and certain devices like cell phones are abundant even in low–socioeconomic status populations (46). Just as in the other stages of behavioral intervention development research, research on the implementation and dissemination of technology-based interventions is facilitated by the ease of administration of these interventions, and the degree to which they can be administered as they had been during the earlier stages of intervention development.

The challenge of technology-based interventions may not lie in getting them implemented and disseminated. Ironically, the challenge may be how to *not* get too many interventions implemented and disseminated; that is, there may be difficulties that arise from technology-based interventions that do get disseminated that do not have sufficient experimental support. Without experimental support, we will not be able to determine which interventions might be helpful, which are neutral, and which cause harm. It is a tautology to say that a harmful intervention causes harm. But the harm could extend beyond any direct harmful effects of the intervention; it could also potentially prevent individuals from seeking out other experimentally supported interventions shown to be helpful. This can also be a side effect of neutral interventions. So, even a neutral intervention could ultimately have negative ramifications. Carroll and Rounsaville (47) argue for "the need to more thoroughly assess

possible adverse effects, recognizing that even a modestly effective computer-assisted intervention could have enormous impact" (p. 436).

CHALLENGES AND UNINTENDED CONSEQUENCES OF TECHNOLOGY-BASED TREATMENT

Although technology-assisted treatments are game changers, they may also have some unintended consequences. As Verghese (48) pointed out, the complaints we hear from patients, family, and friends are rarely about the paucity of technology but about its excesses, turning patients into "i-patients." Shoham and Insel (49) suggested that technology-based interventions proceed with caution because there is still much to be learned about the treatments for which, and the patients for whom, a human relationship or therapeutic alliance is essential to behavior change. Without such knowledge, even in a best-case scenario, technology-based interventions will to some extent require shooting in the dark. A worst-case scenario is that "e-Health interventions could 'spend out' some of our most effective techniques, rendering them less amenable to subsequent, face-to-face intervention" (p. 481).

Some technology-based interventions necessitate a simplification or abbreviation of treatments that were empirically supported in their original form. It is troublesome in this regard that the field does not know enough about how psychosocial interventions work (49,50). Without knowledge of how interventions work, abbreviated—albeit more accessible—interventions may sacrifice essential mechanisms of change. Therefore, pared-down technology-based interventions could yield rather small effect sizes (51). On the other hand, the use of technology does not necessarily require that an intervention be pared down. It is entirely possible to add a technology-based intervention to supplement and boost the effects of a traditional treatment. For example, 60 hours of computer-assisted neurocognitive training in attention, memory, and problem-solving were successfully added to group therapy for people with psychotic spectrum disorders to improve outcome (45).

Technology-based interventions also lend themselves to commercialization, and with commercialization comes a risk of conflict of interest. If interventions are promoted on the basis that more money can be made to the exclusion of the ability of the intervention to help with a problem, then the potential of proliferation of technology-based interventions without empirical support could become a reality. No one doubts that it would be an obvious success if the market were flooded with highly effective commercialized products. But what if the market was flooded with highly advertised products of varying effectiveness, competing with non-commercialized empirically supported treatments? Even in the absence of commercial issues, determining which psychosocial interventions work best can be complex (52). The additional challenge of ensuring that consumers are able to ascertain the scientific support of a treatment is daunting. The Substance Abuse and Mental Health Services Administration (SAMHSA) has made an effort to do this with the National Registry of Evidence-Based Services and Practices (http://www.nrepp.samhsa.gov/). But with abundant and rapidly developed interventions, some with commercial backing and promotion, and with little known about how, why, and for whom they work, it remains unclear how well consumers can be advised which interventions work effectively, and for whom it works best.

Another unintended consequence of easier implementation might be that technology-based interventions could become the standard of care, risking the loss of the "therapeutic hour," even when technology-based interventions may not be capable of solving all mental health and addiction problems, and may not always be the best course of action for everyone. For example, imagine a mental health practitioner delivering cognitive behavioral therapy who now sees seven patients in seven 50-minute sessions. This is a heavy caseload, considering that the practitioner also needs to attend case conferences, enter electronic medical records notes, make phone calls, etc. Now imagine that a community clinic adopts a computerized CBT module that patients can access in cubbies in the waiting room before and after each session, and also has homework modules that work on the patient's phone or home computer. This frees up several extra therapist hours per day. It is not hard to foresee a scenario in which the clinic decides to double or triple a therapist's caseload, and fails to see that the paperwork and calls per

patient are also doubled or tripled. Doubling or tripling therapists' caseloads has obvious benefits in terms of treating more patients, and decreasing costs to the service delivery system, so the possibility of increased therapist workloads is not so far-fetched. But do we know what happens if the "therapeutic hour" is essentially lost? What happens to the therapist's ability to form a therapeutic alliance when there are so many patients with whom to form an alliance? And what happens when patients have crises and really need substantially more face-to-face interaction? Will that become impossible in the future? Science can help to answer questions to help understand why and how much "face time" is needed when treating certain people and problems, and why, when, and how much of treatment can be technology assisted. To be sure, the answer to this question will depend on the person and his or her relational context, the problem, the technology developed, and a variety of other factors. Research is needed to determine the optimal combinations of technology-based interventions and traditionally administered behavioral therapies. Treatment researchers need to understand when and how technology can boost treatment effects and at the same time ease the burden on therapists and decrease cost, and if and when technology-based treatment can diminish effects or even be iatrogenic.

Finally, another major challenge is the myriad legal and ethical problems that are introduced with technology-based interventions. What happens when a therapist in one state uses technology-based treatment to help a patient who is 5 miles away but located in another state? Are there ethical and legal ramifications, particularly if a problem arises in the treatment? The answer is that there is no simple answer, and legal issues can vary by state. The ethical and legal challenges of technology-based therapeutic approaches, including privacy and security concerns, are considered in Chapter 16 of this compendium and will not be addressed here. Suffice it to say that the challenges are real and need to be carefully addressed before technology-based approaches can safely proliferate throughout systems of care. But these challenges need to be considered in context, with full awareness of the benefits that technology can offer, and decision-making that is informed by science.

CONCLUSIONS

In this chapter, we have identified some benefits of technology-based interventions, some of the challenges, and how technology figures in treatment development research. There is no turning back the clock, as technology is here to stay. It may be helpful to remind ourselves that technology is a tool to be used when useful, and only when it is useful. The advantages of its use also bring questions about possible challenges and unintended consequences.

In terms of the research process, however, technology offers many opportunities to advance knowledge, and these could outweigh the challenges. And although in practice pared-down technology-based interventions currently may yield small effect sizes, potent components of technology-based interventions might be easier to identify than components of traditional treatments. With technology-assisted methods we can better address questions of how and why a treatment works, and test hypotheses of what to do next to improve the treatment under development. Such questions need to be included in all stages of treatment development research, from 0 through V. At the same time that technology can help us answer questions of mechanisms, it can increase the rapidity with which treatments are developed, tested, and disseminated. We have officially entered the next generation of behavioral treatment research, one that is heading toward behavioral treatment research as a dynamic, nimble, and progressive science that contributes to our basic knowledge of behavior, and to our goal of treating behavioral and emotional problems with effective treatments.

DISCLAIMER

These are the opinions of the authors, and not necessarily those of the NIDA, NIMH, NIH or Federal Government.

NOTE

1. This topic is addressed throughout the text in more depth.

REFERENCES

1. Amir N, Taylor CT. Combining computerized home-based treatments for generalized anxiety disorder: An attention modification program and cognitive behavioral therapy. *Behavior Therapy* 2012; 4:546–559.

2. Williams AD, Blackwell SE, Mackenzie A, Holmes EA, Andrews G. Combining imagination and reason in the treatment of depression: A randomized controlled trial of Internet-based cognitive-bias modification and Internet-CBT for depression. *Journal of Consulting and Clinical Psychology* 2013; 81:793–799.

3. Craske MG, Rose RD, Lang A, Welch SS, Campbell-Sills L, Sullivan G, et al. Computer-assisted delivery of cognitive behavioral therapy for anxiety disorders in primary-care settings. *Depression and Anxiety* 2009; 26:235–242.

4. Hallion LS, Ruscio AM. A meta-analysis of the effect of cognitive bias modification on anxiety and depression. *Psychological Bulletin* 2011; 137, 940–958.

5. Carroll KM, Ball SA, Martino S, Nich C, Babuscio TA, Nuro KF, et al. Computer-assisted delivery of cognitive-behavioral therapy for addiction: A randomized trial of CBT4CBT. *American Journal of Psychiatry* 2008; 165, 881–888.

6. Bickel WK, Marsch LA, Buchhalter AR, Badger GJ. Computerized behavior therapy for opioid-dependent outpatients: A randomized controlled trial. *Experimental and Clinical Psychopharmacology* 2008; 16:132–143.

7. Bordnick PS, Traylor A, Copp HL, Graap KM, Carter B, Ferrer M, et al. Assessing reactivity to virtual reality alcohol based cues. *Addictive Behaviors* 2008; 33:743–756.

8. Rothbaum BO, Garcia-Palacios A, Rothbaum AO. Treating anxiety disorders with virtual reality exposure therapy. *Revista de Psiquiatria y Salud Mental* 2012; 5:67–70.

9. Sheehan B, Lee Y, Rodriguez M, Tiase V, Schnall R. A comparison of usability factors of four mobile devices for accessing healthcare information by adolescents. *Applied Clinical Informatics* 2012; 3:356–366.

10. Dennison L, Morrison L, Conway G, Yardley L. Opportunities and challenges for smartphone applications in supporting health behavior change: Qualitative study. *Journal of Medical Internet Research* 2013; 15:e86.

11. Chen AC, Etkin A. Hippocampal network connectivity and activation differentiates post-traumaticstress disorder from generalized anxiety disorder. *Neuropsychopharmacology* 2013; 38:1889–1898.

12. Etkin A, Wager TD. Functional neuroimaging of anxiety: A meta-analysis of emotional processing in PTSD, social anxiety disorder, and specific phobia. *American Journal of Psychiatry* 2007; 164:1476–1488.

13. Hamilton JP, Etkin A, Furman DJ, Lemus MG, Johnson RF, Gotlib IH. Functional neuroimaging

of major depressive disorder: A meta-analysis and new integration of base line activation and neural response data. *American Journal of Psychiatry* 2012; 169:693–703.

14. Conner, T. S. & Mehl, M. R. (in press). Ambulatory assessment: Methods for studying everyday life. In: R. A. Scott & S. M. Kosslyn, Stephen M. (Eds.) *Emerging Trends in the Social and Behavioral Sciences.* Thousand Oaks, CA: SAGE Publications.

15. Ebner-Priemer UW, Trull T. Ecological momentary assessment of mood disorders and mood dysregulation. *Psychological Assessment* 2009; 21:463–475.

16. Canterberry M, Hanlon CA, Hartwell KJ, Li X, Owens M, Lematty T, et al. Sustained reduction of nicotine craving with real-time neurofeedback: Exploring the role of severity of dependence. *Nicotine & Tobacco Research* 2013; 15:2120–2124.

17. Jones R, Hoover DR, Lacroix LJ. (2013). A randomized controlled trial of soap opera videos streamed to smartphones to reduce risk of sexually transmitted human immunodeficiency virus (HIV) in young urban African American women. *Nursing Outlook* 2013; 61:205–215.

18. Rizvi SL, Dimeff LA, Skutch J, Carroll D, Linehan MM. A pilot study of the DBT coach: An interactive mobile phone application for individuals with borderline personality disorder and substance use disorder. *Behavior Therapy* 2011; 42:589–600.

19. Lappalainen P, Kaipainen K, Lappalainen R, Hoffrén H, Tero Myllymäki T, Marja-Liisa Kinnunen ML, et al. Feasibility of a personal health technology-based psychological intervention for men with stress and mood problems: Randomized controlled pilot trial. *Journal of Medical Internet Research* 2013; 2:e1.

20. Beard C, Amir N. A multi-session interpretation modification program: Changes in interpretation and social anxiety symptoms. *Behavior Research and Therapy* 2008; 46:1135–1141.

21. Smith B, Harms WD, Burres S, Korda H, Rosen H, Davis J. Enhancing behavioral health treatment and crisis management through mobile ecological momentary assessment and SMS messaging. *Health Informatics Journal* 2012; 18:294–308.

22. Institute of Medicine. *Improving the Quality of Health Care for Mental and Substance-Use Conditions: Quality Chasm Series.* Washington, DC: National Academies Press; 2006.

23. Wang PS, Berglund P, Olfson M, Pincus HA, Wells KB, Kessler RC. Failure and delay in initial treatment contact after first onset of mental disorders in the National Comorbidity Survey Replication. *Archives of General Psychiatry* 2005; 62(6):603–613.

24. Kazdin AE, Blase SL. Rebooting psychotherapy research and practice to reduce the burden of mental illness. *Perspectives on Psychological Science* 2011; 6:21–37.

25. Beidas RS, Kendall PC. Training therapists in evidence based practice: A critical review of studies from a systems-contextual perspective. *Clinical Psychology: Science and Practice* 2010; 17:1–30.

26. Olmstead TA, Abraham AJ, Martino S, Roman PM. Counselor training in several evidence-based psychosocial addiction treatments in private US substance abuse treatment centers. *Drug and Alcohol Dependence* 2012; 120:149–154.

27. Santa Ana E, Martino S, Ball SA, Nich C, Carroll KM. What is usual about 'treatment as usual': Audiotaped ratings of standard treatment in the Clinical Trials Network. *Journal of Substance Abuse Treatment* 2008; 35:369–379.

28. Yates B. Delivery systems can determine therapy costs and effectiveness, more than type of therapy. *Perspectives on Psychological Science* 2011; 6:498–502.

29. Lind C, Boschen MJ, Morrissey S. Technological advances in psychotherapy: Implications for the assessment and treatment of obsessive compulsive disorder. *Journal of Anxiety Disorders* 2013; 27, 47–55.

30. Olmstead TA, Ostrow CD, Carroll KM. Cost-effectiveness of computer-assisted training in cognitive-behavioral therapy as an adjunct to standard care for addiction. *Drug and Alcohol Dependence* 2010; 110:200–207.

31. Sloan DM, Marx BP, Keane TM. Reducing the burden of mental illness in military veterans: Commentary on Kazdin and Blase (2011). *Perspectives on Psychological Science* 2011; 6:503.

32. Wykes T, Huddy V, Cellard C, McGurk SR, Czobor P. A meta-analysis of cognitive remediation for schizophrenia: Methodology and effect sizes. *American Journal of Psychiatry* 2011; 168:472–485.

33. Carroll KM, Ball SA, Martino S, Nich C, Babuscio TA, Rounsaville BJ. (2009). Enduring effects of a computer-assisted training program for cognitive behavioral therapy: A 6-month follow-up of CBT4CBT. *Drug and Alcohol Dependence* 2009; 100:178–181.

34. Rose RD, Lang AJ, Welch SS, Campbell-Sills L, Chavira DA, Sullivan G. et al. (2011). Training primary care staff to deliver a computer-assisted cognitive-behavioral therapy program for anxiety disorders. *General Hospital Psychiatry* 2011; 33:336–342.

35. Sholomskas DE, Carroll KM. One small step for manuals: Computer-assisted training in twelve-step facilitation. *Journal of Studies on Alcohol* 2006; 67:939–945.

36. Onken LS, Carroll KM, Shoham V, Cuthbert BN, Riddle M. Reenvisioning clinical science: Unifying the discipline to improve the public health. *Clinical Psychological Science* 2014; 2:22–34.

37. Wiers RW, Eberl C, Rinck M, Becker ES, Lindenmeyer J. Retraining automatic action tendencies changes alcoholic patients' approach bias for alcohol and improves treatment outcome. *Psychological Science* 2011; 22:490–497.

38. Silk JS, Stroud LR, Siegle GJ, Dahl RE, Lee KH, Nelson EE. Peer acceptance and ejection through the eyes of youth: Pupillary, eyetracking and ecological data from the Chatroom Interact Task. *Social Cognitive and Affective Neuroscience* 2012; 7:93–105.

39. Phillips KA, Epstein DH, Preston KL. Daily temporal patterns of heroin and cocaine use and craving: Relationship with business hours regardless of actual employment status. *Addictive Behaviors* 2013; 38:2485–2491.

40. Mele ML, Federici S. (2012). Gaze and eye-tracking solutions for psychological research. *Cognitive Processing* 13(Suppl 1):S261–S265.

41. Sazonov E, Lopez-Meyer P, Tiffany S. A wearable sensor system for monitoring cigarette smoking. *Journal of Studies on Alcohol and Drugs* 2013; 74:956–964.

42. Dobkin BH. Wearable motion sensors to continuously measure real-world physical activities. *Current Opinion in Neurology* 2013; 26:602–608.

43. Cohn AM, Hunter-Reel D, Hagman BT, Mitchell J. Promoting behavior change from alcohol use through mobile technology: The future of ecological momentary assessment. *Alcoholism: Clinical and Experimental Research* 2011; 35:2209–2215.

44. Moore TM, Seavey A, Ritter K, McNulty JK, Gordon KC, Stuart GL. Ecological momentary assessment of the effects of craving and affect on risk for relapse during substance abuse treatment. *Psychology of Addictive Behaviors* 2014; 28(2):619–624.

45. Eack SM, Greenwald DP, Hogarty SS, Cooley SJ, DiBarry AL, Montrose DM, Keshavan MS. Cognitive enhancement therapy for early-course schizophrenia: Effects of a two-year randomized controlled trial. *Psychiatric Services* 2009; 60:1468–1476.

46. Chambers DA, Haim A, Mullican CA, Stirratt M. Health information technology and mental health services research: A path forward. *General Hospital Psychiatry* 2013; 35:329–331.

47. Carroll KM, Rounsaville BJ. Computer-assisted therapy in psychiatry: Be brave, its a new world. *Current Psychiatry Reports* 2010; 12:426–432.

48. Verghese A. Treat the patient, not the CT scan. *The New York Times*, February 26, 2011. Retrieved from http://www.nytimes.com/2011/02/27/opinion/27verghese.html?pagewanted=all.

49. Shoham V, Insel TR. Rebooting for whom? Portfolios, technology, and personalized intervention. *Perspectives on Psychological Science* 2011; 6:478–482.

50. Kazdin AE. Mediators and mechanisms of change in psychotherapy research. *Annual Review of Clinical Psychology* 2007; 3:1–27.

51. Baker T, McFall R, Shoham V. (2008). The current status and future of clinical psychology: Towards a scientifically principled approach. *Psychological Science in the Public Interest* 2008; 9:67–103.

52. De Los Reyes A, Kazdin AE. When the evidence says, "yes, no, and maybe so": Attending to and interpreting inconsistent findings among evidence-based interventions. *Current Directions in Psychological Science* 2008; 17:47–51.

2

Theoretical Models to Inform Technology-Based Health Behavior Interventions

WILLIAM T. RILEY

INTRODUCTION

"In theory, there is no difference between theory and practice, but in practice, there is" (1). Yogi Berra sayings are notoriously confusing, but in the field of technology-based health behavior interventions, there is some truth to the observation that a disconnect exists between theory and practice. Many technology-based applications, especially commercial applications, seem to have been developed without regard for theory or accepted treatment guidelines, (2) and even some technology-based interventions in the published research literature fail to acknowledge a theoretical basis (3,4).

There are myriad factors that contribute to this disconnect of theory and practice. Behavioral researchers are increasingly involved in the design and development of technology-based interventions, but most commercially available interventions have been designed and developed by engineers, computer programmers, and others who have limited exposure to these theories. Conversely, the health behavior theories most commonly used as the basis for "low-tech" behavioral interventions (e.g., in-person individual or group counseling, print materials, traditional mass media campaigns) were developed decades ago and may of limited use for designing behavioral interventions using current technologies (e.g., interactive Web, mobile phones, wireless sensors) that can deliver these interventions with much greater frequency, in the context of the behavior, and adaptively based on real-time inputs (3). Therefore, one goal of this chapter is to provide a guide to applying health behavior theory to technology-based interventions.

Applying theory to advance technology-based health behavior interventions, however, is only half of story. Technology-based interventions also provide a unique platform that can be leveraged to advance health behavior theory. Technology-based interventions allow us to better isolate intervention components associated with specific theoretical mediators of change. Mobile and wireless applications also provide us with a stream of intensive longitudinal data to model and test theoretical concepts and their interrelationships over time. Therefore, a second goal of this chapter is to demonstrate how theory can benefit from the recent advances in technology to assess and change behavior.

A BRIEF HISTORY OF HEALTH BEHAVIOR THEORIES

A comprehensive review of health behavior theories is beyond the scope of this chapter, but a brief summary of the major theories seems appropriate, particularly for those from outside the health behavior field who are applying technology to health behavior problems. Regardless of scientific field, a theory is a systematic set of concepts, definitions, and propositions that specify the relationship among concepts for the purposes of explaining or predicting phenomena (5). Theories are derived from observational data and hypotheses but also serve as the basis for determining what to observe and hypothesize. Some of the health behavior theories described later in the chapter are consistent with the general definition of a theory while others (e.g., transtheoretical model) are useful conceptual models for intervention development but were not intended to be explanatory or predictive.

In the 1950s, the U.S. Public Health Service began offering mobile tuberculosis (TB) screenings. Like many of our current technology-delivered behavioral interventions, it was assumed that greater convenience and access would result in everyone getting screened, but screening rates did not increase appreciably (6). Studies to understand why these screenings were not more effective led to the development of the health belief model (HBM). The HBM posits that an individual's perceived susceptibility and perceived severity of the illness (e.g., TB) interact with the perceived benefits and barriers of engaging in the health behavior (e.g., chest x-ray screening) and with cues to action to increase or decrease the likelihood of engaging in the behavior (7) (see Figure 2.1). Even though mobile TB screenings had removed an important barrier to obtain these screenings, increasing TB screenings also required that people (a) believe that they were susceptible to getting TB and that getting TB had severe consequences, (b) believe that that there were benefits to screening that outweighed the barriers to getting screened, and (c) be cued or reminded to engage in the screening. Many theories have been developed since the HBM, and it is an incomplete model of behavior, but it continues to be the basis for many health behavior interventions, particularly those that address screening behaviors.

The theory of reasoned action and its subsequent revision as the theory of planned behavior (TPB) incorporated some HBM concepts within its conceptualization of "attitude toward the behavior," but TPB also added social influences such as the perception of what is normative (8). TPB also placed an intermediate conceptual step, behavioral intention (i.e., readiness to perform a given behavior), between these theoretical mechanisms and the actual behavior. While the concept of behavioral intentions may have some explanatory value, its inclusion has often resulted in studies that use reported behavioral intentions, not actual behavior, as the dependent variable. Although both HBM and TPB have been useful for developing behavior change interventions, they have been criticized for their reliance on subjective cognitive influences that are difficult to measure (9).

Social cognitive theory (SCT) shares communalities with HBM and TPB but was developed from a different tradition more aligned with the behavioral learning principles of classical (or respondent or Pavlovian) and operant conditioning. Social learning theory expanded on the experiential learning of classical and operant

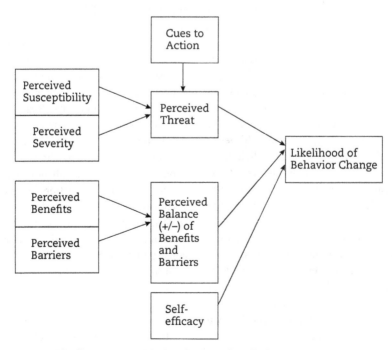

Note: Self-efficacy later added to the health belief model

FIGURE 2.1: Schematic representation of the health belief model.

conditioning to include observational or vicarious learning or modeling (10). A subsequent reformulation to what is now known as social cognitive theory included internal cognitive constructs such as self-efficacy and other perceived phenomena (11). SCT also makes explicit the bidirectional relationship of behavior and the environment via the concept of reciprocal determinism (11).

The transtheoretical model (TTM), or stages of change (12), is more heuristic model than theory, but the value of this model is in the organization of intervention components based on the stage of change (precontemplation, contemplation, preparation, action, or maintenance) and the ability to tailor interventions to these stages. This model has been the basis for numerous Web-based expert systems that tailor interventions to the stage of change (13).

The theories and models described above are the predominant theories in health behavior intervention development. Glanz and Bishop (14) summarized a number of systematic reviews and found that SCT, TTM, HBM, and TPB to be among the most commonly used theories in the health behavior intervention literature. These theories are also among the most commonly cited as the basis for mobile (3) and Internet (13) based interventions. While these theories are widely used for health behavior intervention development, they also have significant weaknesses. The application of these theories far exceeds rigorous testing and revision of these theories, and the lack of evidence for some of these constructs and their interrelationships is well documented (14). Moreover, these intrapersonal theories of behavior have predominated the behavioral intervention literature while higher level factors (e.g., interpersonal, community, organizational, policy) and their related theories and models are underutilized in intervention development (15).

APPLYING HEALTH BEHAVIOR THEORIES TO TECHNOLOGY-BASED INTERVENTIONS

Despite the weaknesses and limitations of current health behavior theories, there is strong evidence that interventions based on theory are more effective than those that are not (14,16), including technology-based interventions (13). This finding

may reflect positively on the validity of these theories, but it also may be the result of a more thoughtful and comprehensive approach to intervention development irrespective of theory.

While theories can be a useful heuristic, applying theory to an intervention requires more than simply addressing the constructs that the theory posits affect behavior. It is also important to distinguish between explanatory theories (or theories of the problem) and change theories (or theories of action) (17). For illustration, consider a core construct of SCT and other health behavior theories, self-efficacy, from an explanatory vs. change theory perspective. The explanatory aspect is that self-efficacy is one of the factors posited to explain and predict behavior, and there is long-standing research to support this relationship (18). Developing a robust intervention requires identifying these conceptual mediators of behavior change such as self-efficacy that have been shown to explain or predict the target behavior of interest.

But how should the intervention seek to change self-efficacy? This is the change theory aspect of theory-based intervention development. SCT posits a number of factors that contribute to self-efficacy, including social persuasion, modeling influences, and prior experiences engaging in the behavior. Therefore, an intervention that targets self-efficacy from an explanatory perspective will need to influence self-efficacy via skills training, social support, modeling of others successfully engaging in the behavior, and setting up successful experiences for the individual engaging in the behavior (19,20). This combination of explanatory and change aspects of theory is critical to developing a robust intervention. Regardless of how well the intervention strategies may affect the targeted mediator, the intervention will be ineffective if the mediator is not strongly associated with the targeted behavior. And regardless of how strongly the targeted mediator affects the behavior of interest, if there is little guidance on how to change the targeted mediator, then the intervention will be ineffective. Therefore, a theory-based intervention does not necessarily need to address all of the factors posited to influence behavior, but it does need to focus on the mediators that are most strongly associated with the behavior (explanatory theory) and the intervention components that are most likely to change those mediators (change theory).

For the developers of technology-based interventions, there are numerous intervention components from which to choose. Michie and colleagues have developed a comprehensive taxonomy of 93 distinct behavior change strategies hierarchically clustered into 16 groups (21), providing a rich array of potential intervention strategies for technology-based interventions. This taxonomy was not designed, however, to serve as a Chinese menu of intervention strategies in which an intervention developer selects two from column A, one from column B, etc. Instead, these behavioral strategies should be considered from the perspective of change theories and selected on the basis of their theoretical and empirical support to affect the targeted mediator or factor that is theorized to impact the target behavior.

EXAMPLES OF APPLYING THEORY TO TECHNOLOGY-BASED INTERVENTIONS

Web-based or eHealth interventions have evolved over time from simple, unidirectional provision of information to interactive and tailored Web applications. Even early Internet interventions provided information that was theoretically based (22), but the ability to automate the tailoring of Internet interventions increased the need for theoretical guidance on how to personalize interventions. This need led to the predominant use of the transtheoretical model's stages of change to develop tailored or personalized eHealth interventions (23).

While many have utilized health behavior theories to develop and tailor eHealth interventions, the research of Strecher, Kreuter, and colleagues is illustrative of the sophisticated use of theory for tailored eHealth interventions. Before the advent of eHealth, this group had developed and evaluated theory-based computer-tailored messaging delivered via print media (24–26). The theoretical case for tailoring itself is based in part on the value of personal relevancy from the elaboration likelihood model, and a number of health behavior theories, including the transtheoretical model, the health belief model, and social cognitive theory, serve as the basis for selecting tailoring variables and delivering unique intervention components based on these variables (27). Web-based delivery of these tailored materials not only further automated the tailoring of these interventions but also provided a vehicle from which to test the moderators and mediators of a tailored eHealth approach (28).

To illustrate the use of theory to inform eHealth intervention development, Kreuter and Strecher (25) noted that most health risk appraisal programs focus predominately on the perceived threat from smoking and other health risk behaviors, but that these programs did not address the perceived benefits and barriers of quitting smoking, which the health belief model posits is critical to health behavior change. They developed an enhanced health risk appraisal program that assessed not only perceived health risks from smoking but also (a) perceived benefits and barriers to quitting as per HBM, (b) readiness to quit as per TTM, and (c) relapse history as per the relapse prevention model. They then generated tailored message feedback based on assessments of these theoretically based constructs, resulting in over 4,500 different combinations of messages.

In much the same way as the capabilities of Web-based applications (eHealth) led to the application of theoretical models to guide tailoring algorithms, mobile and wireless health applications (mHealth) have challenged health behavior theories to guide interventions that tailor interventions not only initially but in real time and adaptively throughout the intervention process (3). Mobile and wireless health interventions have proliferated in recent years, and for good reason. Mobile technologies are ubiquitous, with more cell phones than people worldwide and with smartphone users now representing over half of current cell phone users in the United States (29). The widespread use of these powerful communication and computation devices provides a platform from which to assess and deliver interventions in real time and in the context of the behavior in ways not previously possible. Extending on the work in ecological momentary assessment (EMA), the ability to deliver interventions based on real-time data has been termed "ecological momentary interventions" (EMI) (30,31).

Although mHealth interventions are an exciting advance in technology-based interventions, this technology also introduces significant challenges in applying current theories to mobile interventions. In order to leverage the adaptive capabilities of mHealth interventions, theories that can guide these adaptative algorithms are needed. Unfortunately, current health behavior theories were developed primarily to explain differences between individuals, not within an individual (32). As a result, these theories provide reasonable conceptual models for why one would intervene differently from one person to another, but often provide little guidance on how to intervene differently in the same person at one time point vs. another. Additionally, health behavior theories are essentially moot on the timing, frequency, or dose of an intervention, much less the adaptation of dose over time. Therefore, while developers of smoking cessation applications, for example, have tended to wax and wane the frequency of text messages around the time of the quit date (33), these changes in intervention frequency are rationally determined, not based on any theoretical guidance on how timing and frequency of interventions impact different individuals at different times in the behavior change trajectory.

Although there are limitations of health behavior theories for the development of mHealth interventions, these theories do provide considerable guidance on the content and components of these interventions. One excellent illustration of theory applied to mHealth intervention is the work of Brendryen and colleagues on a smoking cessation text messaging program. The "Happy Ending" program is a text messaging program for smoking cessation that adjusts the frequency and content of messages based on stage of change (preparation, action, maintenance) for quitting that has been found effective in two randomized trials (34,35). In a subsequent paper (36), this research group described the intervention mapping process used to develop an intervention that was based on self-regulation theory, social cognitive theory, cognitive behavioral therapy, motivational interviewing, and relapse prevention. Using a stepwise approach, they devised proximal change objectives based on the self-observation, self-evaluation, and self-reaction processes of self-regulation theory and the behavioral determinants posited by social cognitive theory. They generated theory-based methods and strategies to address these change objectives and developed the text messaging intervention to deliver each of these strategies. For example, to address

the proximal program objective of coping adaptively with cravings, subobjectives such as coping self-efficacy and emotion-regulation skills were organized on the basis of SCT determinants (e.g., self-efficacy, skills). Practical and theory-based methods to achieve these subobjectives (e.g., for coping self-efficacy, increase salience of mastery experiences by encouraging imagining and writing down prior mastery experiences, use vicarious mastery by providing mastery stories from other quitters) were then developed. This study provides a useful framework for the process of applying health behavior theories to the development of a mobile health intervention.

Health behavior theories can and have been successfully applied to the development of technology-based health behavior interventions. The work of Strecher and colleagues in tailored Internet interventions and of Brendryen and colleagues in adaptive mobile interventions provide two illustrative examples of a rigorous and systematic application of theory to technology-delivered intervention development. Many have utilized theory to guide the development of these interventions, and the evidence to date indicates that theory-based, technology-delivered interventions produce better outcomes than those that are not theory based (13). As technology allows us to deliver these interventions in ways previously not possible, the ability of current theories to guide intervention development, however, becomes strained (3). Fortunately, the same technological advances that expose the limits of current health behavior theories also provide methods to advance theory.

USING TECHNOLOGY TO ADVANCE THEORY

Technology-based interventions present challenges to the current behavior theories and models, but these technologies also provide new platforms for improving behavior theory and better understanding human behavior. In an 1871 address to the British Association for the Advancement of Science, Lord Kelvin stated, "Accurate and minute measurement seems to the non-scientific imagination, a less lofty and dignified work than looking for something new. But nearly all the grandest discoveries of science have been but the rewards of accurate measurement and patient long-continued labor in the minute sifting of numerical results" (37). There is little question that for the behavioral sciences to advance, the measurement of behavior and the putative causal influences of behavior must improve. Three significant advances in technology and measurement science have provided a platform from which the next "grand discoveries" in behavioral science will be possible.

1. *Computer adaptive testing via item response theory.* Item response theory (IRT) has been used in the educational field for decades but has only recently been applied to health and health behavior constructs. The Patient-Reported Outcomes Measurement Information System (PROMIS) is perhaps the most well-known of these efforts (38). IRT-developed item banks have the potential to precisely estimate the underlying latent trait efficiently. While computerized administration of self-report measures has been available for some time, the combination of computerized administration and IRT psychometric calibrations provides the basis for computerized adaptive testing (CAT) in which items are flexibly administered based on prior responses from items in the bank, resulting in maximum precision for minimum respondent burden (39). CAT is agnostic to mode of administration and can be performed via desktop program, Web-based application, interactive voice response (IVR), or mobile device. Self-report measures are not without critics, but as long as constructs of interest in the behavioral sciences include phenomena known only to the person, including many of the constructs in current health behavior theories, behavioral sciences will continue to need self-report, and it is imperative that these measurements are performed in as efficient and precise a manner as possible (40).

2. *Ecological momentary assessment (EMA).* A valid criticism of retrospective self-report is recall bias, but by prompting self-reports in real time throughout the day, EMA or experience sampling minimizes recall bias, increases ecological validity, and allows for an intensive longitudinal analysis of the processes that influence behavior over time (41). EMA was initially implemented on PDA (personal digital assistant) platforms, but the advent and rapid penetration of smartphone use, especially in the United States, has provided a ubiquitous platform for EMA administration. The potential to combine EMA with CAT could allow for frequent and precise self-report while also minimizing habitual responding by varying the items administered (42). When further integrated with the sensor technologies described next, event-based reporting can be performed without relying on the individual to identify the event.

3. *Sensor technologies.* Perhaps the most exciting and most recent measurement advance in the behavioral sciences is the use of automated sensor technologies for measuring behaviors and the environments in which these behaviors occur. Accelerometers (43) and psychophysiological sensors (44) (heart rate, electrodermal activity, etc.) have been used for a number of years to measure behaviors and their associated physiology, but advances in computing miniaturization, wireless connectivity, and robust pattern recognition software have greatly improved the sensing of these parameters and expanded the number of parameters that can be passively and nearly continually assessed (45).

These technology-based measurement advances are transforming how we approach understanding and theorizing about human behavior. The traditional theoretical approach has been to understand the differences between individuals, and this approach was consistent with the predominantly cross-sectional "snapshots" of behavior derived almost exclusively from retrospective self-report instruments. With these more longitudinally intensive and prospective measurement capabilities, health behavior theories can and must be adapted to explain differences not only between individuals but also within any given individual over time (32). This shift from between-person to within-person theories is consistent with personalized medicine approaches occurring throughout the biomedical and behavioral research communities (46).

Fully utilizing intensive longitudinal data to develop, test, and revise and/or refute health behavior theories requires new data analytic capabilities. The emergence and application of "big data" techniques from statistics, engineering, and computer sciences to behavioral research provide these analytic capabilities. Hierarchical mixed models (47) and latent curve models (48) provide methods for analyzing these data, and various time series methods can be applied to longitudinal data (49). Pattern recognition and machine learning approaches are being used to identify patterns of longitudinal data and predict future outcomes (50).

Computational modeling provides a robust method for understanding the interrelationship of theoretical constructs over time. For example, the theory of planned behavior has been modeled and simulated via control systems engineering approaches (51,52). Control systems engineering has traditionally been used to model dynamic systems with inputs in the physical world (e.g., electrical, mechanical), to control or stabilize outputs, but this approach is particularly appropriate for modeling human behavior. We have argued that behavior is inherently regulatory in nature, that various brain functions have been modeled using control systems, and that control system engineering approaches provide a comprehensive and robust set of modeling approaches that are consistent with most theories (3).

The concept of applying control systems models to the understanding of behavior is not new. In the 1950s, Wiener conceptualized behavior from a control system perspective for robotic applications (53). A quarter century ago, Hanneman proposed "computer assisted theory building" using dynamic systems models (54), and Carver and Scheier proposed the use of dynamic models for understanding behavior from a self-regulation perspective (55). What is new, however, is that the behavioral sciences now have the ability to collect the intensive longitudinal data over extended time periods required to move beyond simulations to test and iterate these models with actual data. Use of dynamic systems models forces the additional

theoretical rigor of not only defining constructs and their interrelationships but also postulating specific mathematical relationships between constructs and changes to these relationships over time. With sufficient data and testing, these models can be used to predict future behavior, both in natural settings and in response to specific interventions, making health behavior theories truly explanatory in nature.

Technology can be used to advance theory not only by improving measurement precision but also by improving intervention precision. Much of our current theory testing occurs in the context of interventions and involves mediation analyses (56). These approaches are useful correlative analyses to assess the degree to which the outcomes observed are mediated by more proximal changes in the theoretical mechanisms of change targeted by the intervention. Although mediation analyses can be conducted with every behavioral intervention, these analyses are underutilized for various reasons. Mediator assessments must be planned a priori and may require additional assessment points if the timing of the mediator effect does not coincide with the primary outcome assessment points. In low-tech behavioral interventions, these additional mediator assessments are usually resource intensive. With technology-delivered interventions, however, these mediator assessments can be embedded within an automated intervention. Not only can these mediator assessments be timed to when each individual is expected to show maximal mediator change from the intervention (i.e., when the intervention component targeting this mediator is delivered plus the lag time for the mediator to be affected), but the adaptive, just-in-time nature of high-tech interventions allows for the intervention to adapt to the magnitude of mediator change observed over time.

Although an important tool for understanding behavior change, mediation analyses are correlative by nature and cannot be used to make a causal inference either that a specific intervention component caused the change in the mediator or that the mediator caused the change in the outcome. To infer causation, we need to isolate and compare the effects of intervention components hypothesized to target specific theoretical mediators. This is difficult to achieve with many low-tech interventions because it requires exceptional treatment fidelity by interventionists. In contrast, technology-delivered interventions are capable of isolating each intervention component and, assuming no technical glitches, delivering each intervention component with 100% treatment fidelity.

To isolate theoretically derived intervention components in a technology-based intervention, software modules must be created to isolate these intervention components. Object-oriented and modular software development is the current standard for most software development and allows for each module to be easily added or removed from the system (57). If these software modules isolate the theoretically derived intervention components, then these intervention components can then also be easily added or removed from the intervention, allowing researchers to test the efficacy of each component.

How should these intervention component software modules be organized? As noted previously, Michie and colleagues have developed a behavioral strategies taxonomy that can serve as a guide for isolating intervention components (21). The current taxonomy, however, is quite granular and includes 96 different behavior change strategies. Even if a given intervention used only a third of these strategies, it would result in far too many software modules to develop and far too many intervention components to compare.

The ultimate goal of the Michie work, however, is to map these behavioral strategies back to their theoretical basis. Not surprisingly, this is difficult work because there is not a one-to-one relationship between a behavior strategy and theory. Not only can a theory generate multiple behavior change strategies, but a single strategy can be claimed by multiple theories (58). This makes the grouping of theoretically derived and distinct intervention components quite difficult. Considering the putative mediator that these strategies are theorized to target is a helpful rubric for organizing intervention components within a software module. For instance, if videos of others successfully engaging in the behavior and mini-goal setting and monitoring are the two strategies hypothesized to change behavior by improving self-efficacy, then these strategies can be isolated as an intervention component within a software module or set of modules. This module can then be added or removed from the full technology-based intervention to compare the effects, not only on the behavioral

outcome but also on the mediator the intervention component targets.

Multiphase optimization strategy (MOST) is a useful set of methods to test these theoretically derived intervention components (59). MOST methods are derived from engineering and can answer two important questions for technology-based behavioral intervention developers:

1. Which combination of intervention components produces the optimal outcome?
2. Which sequence of these intervention components produces the optimal outcome?

The first question can be addressed via factorial designs, but since a full factorial design of three or more intervention components quickly becomes unwieldy, Collins, Murphy, and Strecher (59) have proposed the use of fractional factorial designs which focus on the more salient comparisons of interest. The second question can be addressed via sequential multiple assignment randomized trials (SMART) in which, after an initial randomization, participants are re-randomized at some later point based on a priori criteria for response to the initial randomization phase. SMART designs are particularly useful for determining what intervention component should occur next depending on the response of the participant to the first intervention component delivered.

If the intervention components tested via these methods are theoretically based such that each intervention component consists of a set a strategies hypothesized to target a specific mediator of behavior change, then the intervention optimization approaches described earlier not only produce more optimal interventions but also provide an experimental test of the theoretical basis of these intervention components. For example, if the addition of the self-efficacy intervention module described earlier (video modeling, mini-goals) produced improvements in self-efficacy and in the behavioral outcome compared to the intervention without this component, this would provide support for the inclusion of self-efficacy in health behavior theories. However, if the behavioral outcome improved but the targeted mediator did not, then it is reasonable to conclude that the strategies in this intervention component improve outcomes, but not via improvements in self-efficacy, which would necessitate a search for other mechanisms of action. The opposite result, an improvement in self-efficacy but no improvement in outcomes from adding this intervention component, could lead to the conclusion that self-efficacy does not have a significant influence on the behavior change of interest, and that other theoretical mechanisms may be more important to changing the behavior in question. By organizing intervention components based on their targeted theoretical mediators of change, MOST approaches to intervention optimization can provide important tests of theoretical constructs and their relationships to behavior for technology-delivered behavioral interventions.

It is also important to note in this context that the dynamic systems modeling approaches described earlier have the potential to answer similar questions of intervention optimization and theory. For example, Rivera, Pew, and Collins have shown how a control systems model can be used to optimize intervention intensity over the course of treatment (60). The integration of intervention optimization with computational models of health behavior theories involves the addition of "controllers" to better regulate the system and "close the loop." As illustrated by Rivera and colleagues, an intervention essentially shifts the variability from the behavioral outcome to the controller. Modifying the type and intensity of the intervention over time to maintain a desirable level of the outcome is very consistent with the adaptive potential of automated, technology-based interventions (3). More importantly, these computational models can integrate theory testing and intervention testing, reducing the current disconnect between theory and practice.

CONCLUSIONS

Technology-based health behavior interventions hold considerable promise for delivering these interventions efficiently, with broad scalability, and with greater levels of personalization and adaptation than previously possible. The field, however, must not repeat the Public Health Service TB screening mistake of the 1950s and assume that greater convenience and access via a more "mobile" intervention is sufficient to change

health behaviors (6). Despite considerable limitations of current health behavior theories, application of these theories to intervention development result in better outcomes than interventions that are not theoretically based (13,14). Fortunately, there are exemplary examples of theory-driven, technology-based intervention development in both eHealth (28) and mHealth (36) that provide guidance for developers of technology-based interventions.

Technology-based interventions also provide new and exciting opportunities to test and advance health behavior theory. Technology-based interventions allow us to better isolate intervention components associated with specific theoretical mediators of change. Developing software modules for each theoretically derived intervention component allows for each intervention component to be removed or added, testing the effects of each component. Because computer software never gets tired or sick or thinks it knows better than the intervention developer, it can deliver the intervention components with true fidelity and isolate each component better than was possible with low-tech interventions.

Technology-based applications, especially mobile and wireless applications, also provide behavioral researchers with a stream of intensive longitudinal data to model and test theoretical concepts and their interrelationships over time. The availability of these intensive longitudinal data sets provides the opportunity for dynamic modeling approaches that can substantially improve the rigor of theory testing. Intensive longitudinal data also will change how health behavior theories are conceptualized, transforming them from predominately static, between-person explanations of behavior to dynamic, within-person explanatory and predictive models of behavior over time. Technology-based interventions not only can benefit from theory, but theory can benefit from the recent advances in technology to assess and change behavior.

REFERENCES

1. http://www.brainyquote.com/quotes/quotes/y/yogiberra141506.html
2. Abroms LC, Padmanabhan N, Thaweethai L, Phillips T. iPhone apps for smoking cessation: A content analysis. *American Journal of Preventive Medicine* 2011; 40(3):279–285.

3. Riley WT, Rivera DE, Atienza AA, Nilsen W, Allison SM, Mermelstein R. Health behavior models in the age of mobile interventions: Are our theories up to the task? *Translational Behavioral Medicine* 2011; 1(1):53–71.

4. Ritterband LM, Tate DF. The science of internet interventions. Introduction. *Annals of Behavioral Medicine* 2009; 38(1):1–3.

5. Kerlinger FM. *Foundations of Behavioral Research* (3rd ed.). New York: Holt, Rinehart, and Winston, 1986.

6. Rosenstock IM. Historical origins of the health belief model. *Health Education Monographs* 1974; 2:328–335.

7. Rosenstock IM. The health belief model and preventive health behavior. *Health Education Monographs* 1974; 2:354–386.

8. Ajzen I. The theory of planned behavior. *Organizational Behavior and Human Decision Processes* 1991; 50:179–211.

9. Ogden J. Some problems with social cognition models: A pragmatic and conceptual analysis. *Health Psychology* 2003; 22:424–428.

10. Bandura A, Walters RH. *Social Learning and Personality Development*. New York: Holt, Rinehart & Winston; 1963.

11. Bandura A. *Social Foundations of Thought and Action*. Englewood Cliffs, NJ: Prentice Hall; 1986.

12. Prochaska JO, Velicer WF. The transtheoretical model of health behavior change. *American Journal of Health Promotion* 1997; 12:38–48.

13. Webb TL, Joseph J, Yardley L, Michie S. Using the Internet to promote health behavior change: A systematic review and meta-analysis of the impact of theoretical basis, use of behavior change techniques, and mode of delivery on efficacy. *Journal of Medical Internet Research* 2010; 12:e4.

14. Glanz K, Bishop DB. The role of behavioral science theory in development and implementation of public health interventions. *Annual Review of Public Health* 2010; 31:399–418.

15. Stokols D. Translating social ecological theory into guidelines for community health promotion. *American Journal of Health Promotion* 1996; 10:282–296.

16. Noar SM, Benac CN, Harris MS. Does tailoring matter? Meta-analytic review of tailored print health behavior change interventions. *Psychological Bulletin* 2007;133:673–693.

17. Glanz K, Rimer BK, Lewis FM. Theory, research and practice in health behavior and health education. In K Glanz, BK Rimer, FM Lewis, *Health Behavior and Health Education*. San Francisco, CA, Jossey-Bass; 2002: 23–40.

18. O'Leary A. Self-efficacy and health. *Behavior Research Therapy* 1985; 4: 437–451.

19. Ashford S, Edmunds J, French DP. What is the best way to change self-efficacy to promote lifestyle and recreational physical activity? A systematic review with meta-analysis. *British Journal of Health Psychology* 2010; 15:265–288.

20. Hyde J, Hankins M, Deale A, Marteau TM. Interventions to increase self-efficacy in the context of addiction behaviours: A systematic literature review. *Journal of Health Psychology* 2008; 13:607–623.

21. Michie S, Richardson M, Johnston M, Abraham C, Francis J, Hardeman W, et al. The Behavior Change Technique Taxonomy (v1) of 93 hierarchically clustered techniques: Building an international consensus for the reporting of behavior change interventions. *Annals of Behavioral Medicine* 2013; 46:81–95.

22. Cassell MM, Jackson C, Cheuvront B. Health communication on the Internet: an effective channel for health behavior change? *Journal of Health Communication* 1998; 3:71–79.

23. Lustria ML, Cortese J, Noar SM, Glueckauf RL. Computer-tailored health interventions delivered over the Web: Review and analysis of key components. *Patient Education and Counseling* 2009; 74:156–173.

24. Strecher VK, Kreuter M, Den Boer J, Kobrin S, Hospers HJ, Skinner CS. The effects of computer-tailored smoking cessation messages in family practice settings. *Journal of Family Practice* 1994; 39:262–270.

25. Kreuter MW, Strecher VJ. Do tailored behavior change messages enhance the effectiveness of health risk appraisal? Results of a randomized trial. *Health Education Research* 1996; 11:97–105.

26. Strecher VJ. Computer-tailored smoking cessation materials: A review and discussion. *Patient Education Counseling* 1999; 36:107–117.

27. Kreuter MW, Strecher VJ, Glassman B. One size does not fit all: the case for tailoring print materials. *Annals of Behavioral Medicine* 1999; 21:276–283.

28. Strecher VJ, Shiffman S, West R. Moderators and mediators of a Web-based computer-tailored smoking cessation program among nicotine patch users. *Nicotine and Tobacco Research* 2006; 8(Suppl 1):S95–S101.

29. Pew Internet and American Life Project. Mobile Health 2012. Retrieved from http://pewinternet.org/reports/2012/mobile-health.aspx.

30. Heron KE, Smyth JM. Ecological momentary interventions: Incorporating mobile technology into psychosocial and behaviour treatments. *British Journal of Health Psychology* 2010; 15:1–39.

31. Patrick K, Intille SS, Zabinski MF. An ecological framework for cancer communication: Implications for research. *Journal of Medical Internet Research* 2005; 7:e2.

32. Dunton GF, Atienza AA. The need for time-intensive information in healthful eating and physical activity research: A timely topic. *Journal of the American Dietetic Association* 2009; 109:30–35.

33. Whittaker R, Borland R, Bullen C, Lin RB, McRobbie H, Rodgers A. Mobile phone-based interventions for smoking cessation (review). *Cochrane Database of Systematic Reviews* 2009; 4:CD006611.

34. Brendryen H, Kraft P. Happy ending: A randomized controlled trial of a digital multi-media smoking cessation intervention. *Addiction* 2008; 103:478–484.

35. Brendryen H, Drozd F, Kraft P. A digital smoking cessation program delivered via Internet and cell phone without nicotine replacement (happy ending): Randomized controlled trial. *Journal of Medical Internet Research* 2008; 10:e5.

36. Brendryen H, Kraft P, Schaalma H. Looking inside the black box: Using intervention mapping to describe the development of an automated smoking cessation intervention happy ending. *Journal of Smoking Cessation* 2010; 5:29–56.

37. Kelvin, WT. Presidential inaugural address to the General Meeting of the British Association, Edinburgh (August 2, 1871). In *Report of the Forty-First Meeting of the British Association for the Advancement of Science*, 1872. Retrieved from http://todayinsci.com/K/Kelvin_Lord/KelvinLord-Quotations.htm

38. Cella D, Riley W, Stone A, Rothrock N, Reeve B, Yount S, et al., on behalf of the PROMIS Cooperative Group. Initial item banks and first wave testing of the Patient–Reported Outcomes Measurement Information System (PROMIS) network: 2005–2008. *Journal of Clinical Epidemiology* 2010; 63:1179–1194.

39. Cook KF, O'Malley KJ. Roddey TS. Dynamic assessment of health outcomes: Time to let the CAT out of the bag? *Health Services Research* 2005; 40:1694–1711.

40. Stone AA, Turkkan JS, Bachrach CA, Jobe JB, Kurtzman HS, Cain VS. *The Science of Self-Report. Implications for Research and Practice.* Mahwah, NJ: Lawrence Erlbaum Associates; 2000.

41. Shiffman S, Stone AA, Hufford MR. Ecological momentary assessment. *Annual Review of Clinical Psychology* 2008; 4:1–32.

42. Rose M, Bjorner JB, Fischer F, Anatchkova M, Gandek B, Klapp BF, Ware JE. Computerized adaptive testing—ready for ambulatory monitoring? *Psychosomatic Medicine* 2012; 74:338–348.

43. Yang CC, Hsu YL. A review of accelerometry-based wearable motion detectors for physical activity monitoring. *Sensors (Basel)* 2010; 10:7772–7788.

44. Orr SP, Roth WT. Psychophysiological assessment: Clinical applications for PTSD. *Journal of Affective Disorders* 2000; 61:225–240.

45. Chan M, Esteve D, Fournois J-Y, Escriba C, Campo E. Smart wearable systems: Current status and future challenges. *Artificial Intelligence Medicine* 2012; 56:137–156.

46. Lillie EO, Patay B, Diamant J, Issell B, Topol EJ, Schork NJ. The n-of-1 clinical trial: The ultimate strategy for individualizing medicine? *Personalized Medicine* 2011; 8:161–173.

47. Hedeker D, Gibbons RD. *Longitudinal Data Analysis.* New York: Wiley, 2006.

48. Bollen KA, Curran PJ. *Latent Curve Models: A Structural Equation Perspective.* New York: Wiley; 2006.

49. Zeger SL, Irizarry R, Peng RD. On time series analysis of public health and biomedical data. *Annual Review of Public Health* 2006; 27:57–79.

50. Larrañaga P, Calvo B, Santana R, Bielza C, Galdiano J, Inza I, et al. Machine learning in bioinformatics. *Brief Bioinformation* 2006; 7:86–112.

51. Navarro-Barrientos JE, Rivera DE, Collins LM. A dynamical systems model for understanding behavioral interventions in weight loss. In SK Chai, JJ Salerno, & PL Mabry (Eds.). 2010 *International Conference on Social Computing, Behavioral Modeling, and Prediction* (SBP 2010) pp. 170–179. Heidelberg: Springer, 2010.

52. Orr MG, Thrush R, Plaut DC. The theory of reasoned action as parallel constraint satisfaction: Towards a dynamic computational model of health behavior. *PLOS One* 2013; 8:e62490.

53. Wiener N. *Cybernetics: On Communication and Control in Animals and Machines.* Cambridge, MA: MIT Press; 1948.

54. Hanneman RA. *Computer-Assisted Theory Building: Modeling Dynamic Social Systems.* Newbury Park, CA: Sage Publications; 1988.

55. Carver CS, Scheier MF. *On the Self-Regulation of Behavior.* Cambridge, MA: Cambridge University Press; 2001.

56. MacKinnon DP, Fairchild AJ, Fritz MS. Mediation analysis. *Annual Review of Psychology* 2007; 58:593–614.

57. Meyer B. *Object-Oriented Software Construction* (2nd ed.). Upper Saddle River, NJ: Prentice Hall; 1997.

58. Noar SM, Zimmerman RS. Health behavior theory and cumulative knowledge regarding health behaviors: Are we moving in the right direction? *Health Education Research* 2005; 20:275–290.

59. Collins LM, Murphy SA, Strecher V. The multiphase optimization strategy (MOST) and the sequential multiple assignment randomized trial (SMART): New methods for more potent eHealth interventions. *American Journal of Preventive Medicine* 2007; 32(5 Suppl):S112–S118.

60. Rivera DE, Pew MD, Collins LM. Using engineering control principles to inform the design of adaptive interventions: A conceptual introduction. *Drug and Alcohol Dependence* 2007; 88(Suppl 2):S31-S40.

SECTION II

Evidence-Based Approaches to Harnessing Technology to Promote Behavioral Health

3

Behavioral Monitoring and Assessment via Mobile Sensing Technologies

SANTOSH KUMAR, MUSTAFA AL'ABSI, J. GAYLE BECK, EMRE ERTIN, AND MARCIA S. SCOTT

INTRODUCTION

Recent advances in mobile sensing technologies are making it possible to collect physiological, behavioral, and social interaction data in the natural environment. These sensors can be worn in the mobile environment and can collect data anytime and anywhere. They can either be embedded in mobile phones that a person carries, or they can be worn on the body, in which case data are transmitted wirelessly to a mobile phone. Data from mobile sensors are usually processed at the mobile phone to infer the current state of health, behavior, and environment of the wearer and can be used to trigger prompts for self-report or to deliver an intervention, all in real time.

An attractive feature of wearable sensors is their ability for continuous monitoring in the natural environment, without active attention from the wearer. Data collected by these sensors are quite informative, as they can be used to infer a variety of human behaviors, context, and the environment. For example, continuous measurement of physical activity and posture can be obtained using triaxial accelerometers and gyroscopes placed on various parts of the body (1) or from those embedded in a smartphone (2). The location of an individual can be monitored continuously via global positioning systems (GPS) or Wi-Fi (3). In addition, exposure to environmental pollutants can be measured using tiny environmental sensors embedded in the mobile sensing equipment (4,5).

Mobile sensors have expanded the capability to detect physiological and mental responses to environmental stimuli beyond assessment in laboratory settings to day-to-day occurrences in natural settings. For instance, wearable and implantable sensors are being used to monitor disruption to homeostatic processes such as cardiovascular functioning (6), diabetes (7), and sleep apnea (8) in patients' homes, and physiological responses to occupational exposure to stress in work settings (9). Mobile non-contact impedance sensors are being developed for neuroimaging outside of laboratory settings (10). Measurement of physiological processes such as cardiac activity with electrocardiography (ECG), respiration, and electrodermal activity using wearable sensors can not only characterize the physiological dynamics but also provide information on a variety of behaviors, such as stress (11), conversation (12), smoking (13), and illicit drug use (14). In addition, intake of other addictive substances such as alcohol can be assessed using transdermal sensors, such as the SCRAM (Secure Continuous Remote Alcohol Monitoring) bracelet (15). Use of these devices can improve reliability and validity of measurement over participant self-reported substance use (16).

Given these qualities, mobile sensing technologies represent sophisticated tools to facilitate our understanding of the etiology of health and disease. Sensing data can be integrated with information from other sources including genomic data, biomarkers, and electronic medical records (from among many examples). This integration should provide a detailed picture of contextual and environmental influences on health and may help to answer difficult questions concerning the interplay between the individual and his or her environment in both health and disease (17).

In addition to advancing our understanding of the role of behavior and environment on health and disease outcome, mobile sensors can also enhance access to and delivery of healthcare. Care providers can be notified upon detection of vulnerable health states (e.g., falls among older adults) based on passive measurements from these sensors. To facilitate diagnosis and treatment, measurement of health states collected by these sensors can be shared with care providers (e.g., via integration into electronic health record system) without the patient having to visit the care facility. Such separation of care delivery from physical visits to a care facility can significantly reduce the burden on patients, providers, and the healthcare system and herald predictive, preventive, personalized, and participatory (P4) medicine (18).

Obtaining measures of health, behavior, and environment from wearable sensors, however, is a complex multistep process due to the nonspecific and noisy nature of sensor data. First, unobtrusively wearable sensors are needed that can be easily worn by participants for long periods of time in their natural environment for robust data collection. Second, methods are needed to convert the sensor data into measures of behavior and environment. To illustrate this entire process, we will use the example of our work on the AutoSense sensor system, which was developed to obtain continuous measures of stress and addictive behaviors in the natural field environment using wearable sensors (19).

This chapter first describes the AutoSense sensor system and the FieldStream mobile phone software that can be used to collect mobile health sensor data for assessment of behavioral health. It then describes the computational procedure for converting sensor data captured by AutoSense and FieldStream into measures of behaviors,

using the examples of stress, conversation, and smoking. Given the novelty of mobile sensor systems, there are still numerous challenges for making mobile health sensor data usable in health research and healthcare. The chapter concludes by discussing some of these research challenges that must be addressed to scale these technologies for broad use.

AUTOSENSE SENSOR SYSTEM

The AutoSense sensor suite was developed to obtain continuous measures of stress and addictive behaviors in the natural field environment under the NIH's Genes Environment and Health Initiative (GEI) (19). The AutoSense sensor suite consists of a chest band with six wireless sensors and an armband with four wireless sensors (see Figure 3.1). The Autosense chest band currently includes (a) a 2-lead ECG to measure heart rate, (b) a respiratory inductive plethysmograph (RIP) band for measurement of relative thorax volume and respiration frequency, (c) a three-axis accelerometer to assess motion and physical activity, (d) a galvanic skin response (GSR) sensor to tap arousal via skin conductance, (e) a thermometer to measure skin temperature, and (f) a thermometer to measure ambient temperature. All six sensors are hosted in a small plastic wearable enclosure, which is 0.5 inches thick and weighs approximately 1.5 oz. The chest band package is powered by a 500 mAh battery. The armband consists of (a) a transdermal WrisTAS alcohol sensor for measure alcohol consumption, (b) a three-axis accelerometer to capture wrist arm movements, (c) a skin temperature sensor, and (d) a GSR sensor to detect if the wrist sensor is on-body or off-body. The

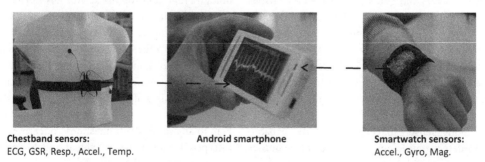

Chestband sensors:
ECG, GSR, Resp., Accel., Temp.

Android smartphone

Smartwatch sensors:
Accel., Gyro, Mag.

FIGURE 3.1: The AutoSense wearable sensor suite consists of wireless sensors for measurement of ECG, respiration, skin conductance at chest, temperature, and accelerometry in a chest suite, and wireless sensors to measure transdermal alcohol, temperature, skin conductance, and accelerometry in an arm suite.

armband package is 1×1 square inch in size and uses a small 210 mAh Li-Ion battery. Both sensing units wirelessly transmit measurements from all 10 sensors to an Android smartphone using a low-power ANT radio. The units last more than a week on a single battery charge even when sampling at 132 HZ and transmitting in the wireless channel at 32 packets per second. The entire platform can be easily extended to add new sensors such as environmental sensors or customized (mix-and-match sensors) for a particular research study. Commercially available mobile sensor suites such as BioHarness from Zephyr Technologies provide similar sensor measurements to those with AutoSense. Computational models developed to infer behaviors from AutoSense sensor data (described later in this chapter) are also applicable to sensor data collected by commercially available mobile sensors.

Sensors on the body are complemented by additional sensors on the phone (e.g., GPS, accelerometer). The GPS sensor data are collected to track the location and movement (e.g., transportation) episodes. The phone also acts as a local server for heavier computation and storage and for collecting self-reported information regarding thoughts, feelings, and other internal states. More details on the mobile phone software are described in the next section.

FIELDSTREAM MOBILE PHONE SOFTWARE SYSTEM

Mobile phone software is needed to interact with participants. The FieldStream mobile phone software was developed for this purpose, to complement the AutoSense sensor system. Several other such mobile phone software platforms, such as Ohmage (20) and Funf (21), provide similar functionality to that of FieldStream. In addition to collecting data from sensors, user activity such as call records, phone usage, and time spent with various apps on the phone can also be recorded with such software. The mobile phone frameworks are configurable so that they can be easily adapted to the specific requirements and protocol of a particular study.

The FieldStream mobile phone software serves multiple purposes. First, the data from the wearable sensors and those in the phone are stored in the mobile phone. Wearable sensor data

are streamed in real time over the wireless channel to the mobile phone, where they are time synchronized with the sensor data collected from the phone (for GPS and accelerometers).

Second, FieldStream software also integrates ecological momentary assessment (EMA) to collect self-reported data (e.g., mood states, urges to use licit or illicit substances). In response to an EMA prompt, the individual answers a series of questions to assess internal states. The prompts can be generated randomly, in response to initiation by subjects, or in response to an event of interest that is detected by the sensing device (e.g., a sudden increase in stress level). Collecting self-report, physiological, behavioral, and location data directly on the mobile phone makes it possible to synchronize these different data sources to generate a time series across multiple assessment domains. This fine-grained time series has the potential not only to be used to clarify associations among physiological, behavioral, and environmental events but also to provide interventions, such as proactively intervening prior to an unhealthy behavior (e.g., smoking lapse or impulsive eating).

A third purpose of the FieldStream software is that it allows real-time visualization of the sensor signals. This feature permits verification that the system is working properly before commencing data collection (see Figure 3.2). More importantly, it also holds promise for using mobile technology to deliver health-related interventions. For example, an individual could be provided with immediate feedback regarding changes in their physiology, as a means of providing input about changing their behavior or using relaxation skills. This type of intervention within the laboratory is referred to as biofeedback (22), and it has been shown to improve a number of health-related conditions (e.g., headache [23], hypertension [24]).

Fourth, the FieldStream software monitors the status of the wireless connection, attachment quality of specific sensors, and tightness of the respiration band, providing input regarding measurement quality. Prompts are delivered to the wearer to fix any issues that are detected, by providing a guided step-by-step procedure. The quality of data collected is checked automatically by the FieldStream software, which compares the morphology of the physiological signals (i.e., ECG and respiration) to their expected shapes. The FieldStream software

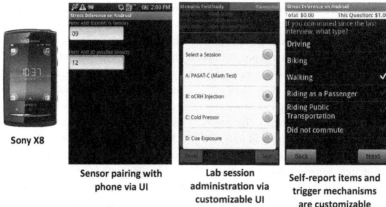

Sony X8

| Sensor pairing with phone via UI | Lab session administration via customizable UI | Self-report items and trigger mechanisms are customizable |

Sponsor: NetSE: Large grant from NSF

FIGURE 3.2: Screenshots of the FieldStream mobile phone framework used to conduct lab and field studies with wearable physiological sensors and ecological momentary assessment (EMA) self-report. The first screen shows a screenshot that allows the study staff to select which sensor they want to visualize and check its quality before sending participants out in the field. The second screen shows the signals from respiration sensors in real time. The third screen shows that incentives earned by participating in the study are displayed upon completing an EMA self-report to keep the participant motivated. The fourth screen shows the amount of good-quality sensor data and number of self-reports completed as a way to monitor compliance with a given study protocol.

also measures sensor wearing time, the number of hours of good-quality, usable sensor data, and the number of EMA reports provided by the subject. If desired, this information can be displayed on the mobile phone each day the subject participates in the study.

Finally, the use of mobile phones makes it possible to monitor and improve compliance with assessment. Compensation of participants in research studies can be broken down into micro-incentives and displayed periodically to subjects to keep them motivated (25). This type of incentive program can help to engage participants throughout longer intervals of data collection. The FieldStream software, for example, displays the total compensation accumulated upon completing each EMA report when participants are collecting data in the field. In studies conducted with the FieldStream software, incentives have been tied to the wearing of the sensors (for at least 60% of time since last self-report) and to completing the self-report when prompted. A bonus incentive can be provided if self-report is completed in a timely manner (within 5 minutes of the prompt).

These features help obtain high-quality data and good compliance from study participants. For example, in a study of daily smokers ($n = 30$, 15 female), each participant wore the AutoSense sensors during awake hours for 1 full week in

their natural environment (26). Each individual received up to 20 prompts for EMA reports and were also asked to report each smoking and drinking episode. This approach resulted in an average of 9.84 hours per day per subject of good-quality physiological data, using heart rate and respiration. The average response rate for EMAs was 94% (26).

INFERRING BEHAVIORAL STATES FROM MOBILE SENSORS

We now describe the computational procedure for converting the data collected from AutoSense sensors and FieldStream mobile phone software into behavioral states. Mobile sensors such as AutoSense collect data at a high sampling frequency, which enables analysis of fine-grained data patterns that may contain unique signatures of various health states, emotional and behavioral states, and contexts. But building computational models to identify such signatures is challenging. First, no sensor directly provides a measure of target health state, behavior, or environment. Second, measurement from a sensor is affected not only by the target phenomena but also by several other phenomena and activities. For example, measurement of ECG can capture the autonomic arousal due to stress, but the autonomic nervous system is also activated by physical activity, conversation, caffeine, and other activities. Similarly, capturing arm movements from a wristwatch can indicate a hand-to-mouth motion during smoking, but it needs to be distinguished from similar movements during eating. Hence, extracting a measure of interest requires identifying and extracting the unique fingerprints of the target health state or behavior in the measurements of a sensor or, even better, by fusing information obtained from multiple sensors. Machine learning models (27) such as support vector machines (SVM) that can identify complex subtle patterns in high-frequency measurements can be used to discover such signatures.

To illustrate the process of inferring behavioral states from mobile sensors, we present our experience in developing computational models for estimating stress from fine-grained patterns in the interval between successive beats of the heart (i.e., R-peaks in ECG, which refers to the top of the R-wave component of the heart beat) and respiration (11), detecting conversation episodes from respiration (12), and detecting smoking puffs from respiration (13). Each of these models is described in the next three subsections.

Continuous Measure of Stress from AutoSense

Continuous assessment of stress in the field could capture important information about the impact of psychosocial stressors on individuals and how they cope with these stressors. Existing technology and methods to assess the effects of stress in natural settings are limited to self-report or collection of biofluids such as saliva for hormonal assays. None of these methods provide a continuous and passive measure of stress. As such, these methods are limited in their scope, validity, and flexibility. To identify the fingerprint of a physiological stress response, a lab and field study was conducted (11) using AutoSense sensors and FieldStream mobile phone software. In this study, 21 participants completed a lab protocol of inducing stress that included public speaking (4 minutes of instruction, 4 minutes of preparation, and 4 minutes of delivery), two mental arithmetic challenge sessions (4 minutes each in seated and standing positions), and a cold pressor test (90 seconds). The lab assessment sessions were preceded by 30 minutes of resting baseline and followed by 30 minutes of resting recovery. The four stress sessions were separated by 5-minute rest periods, to prevent carryover effects.

Assessment of ECG (heart rate), respiration, and accelerometry occurred continuously via AutoSense, while EMA self-reports of stress were collected 14 times during the entire session on a mobile phone with FieldStream software. A computational model of stress was developed from these data based on the physiological responses. This model was validated with the EMA data capturing self-reported rating of stress.

To develop and evaluate the model for inferring physiological stress, several features were computed. Those aspects of signals that embed specific patterns of signals are called "features." Heart rate and heart rate variability are example of features, which have sometimes been used to indicate stress. It has been noted (11) that obtaining a measure of stress requires computing several other features from the fine-grained physiological data for it to be specific and sensitive to capturing autonomic activation due to stress. In this work, from each minute of ECG, intervals between successive R-peaks (called R-R intervals) and frequency components (for heart rate variability computation) were obtained. From each minute of respiration, the respiration cycles were identified, enabling the computation of inspiration duration, expiration duration, respiration duration, and stretch, as shown in Figure 3.3.

From these data, several features were computed. They include the ratio between (labeled "IE Ratio") and sum of (labeled "respiration duration") inspiration duration and expiration duration and minute ventilation, which is the volume of air inhaled or exhaled in a minute.

To mitigate between-person differences in physiological measures, each feature was normalized to the mean and standard deviation of the individual. Further, for robustness, statistics such as mean, median, quartile deviation, and 80th percentile were computed from normalized values of each feature. A machine learning model was then developed to identify unique patterns for each individual from these features in order to distinguish physiological signals obtained during a stress period from that of a non-stress period. Machine learning models (27) such as SVM project the measures onto an even higher dimensional space to find a linear classifier that can separate the two categories (i.e., stress vs. non-stress). In the

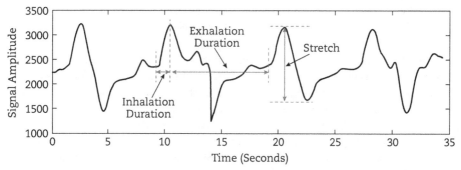

FIGURE 3.3: Features extracted from respiration signals to help identification of specific patterns.

case of physiological stress modeling, using such a machine learning model provides 90% accuracy in distinguishing stress intervals from non-stress intervals.

For developing the stress model, the lab stress protocol was used. More specifically, data collected during the minutes when participants were engaged in a stress task were labeled as a "stressed" class, and those collected outside of the period of the stress task were labeled as a "non-stressed" class. Accuracy is determined on the basis of ability of the model to identify whether a given minute of physiological measurement was collected during a stress session or a non-stress session in the laboratory. To assess the generalizability of this stress model in the field setting, we evaluated the correlation of the stress model with self-reported ratings of stress in both the lab setting and in the field setting.

To evaluate a correlation of the stress model with self-reported stress, a hidden Markov model (HMM) was used to estimate the subjective perception of stress (11). In this model, the perception of stress is modeled as a hidden state, which is estimated from the observed, physiological stress. An accumulation-decay model is assumed in this work that hypothesizes that repeated exposures to stressor(s), whose response may be exhibited by physiology, accumulate to form the subjective perception of stress, which decays over time, in the absence of a stressor. In this accumulation–decay model, the rate of accumulation and decay are assumed to be person-dependent and are estimated from self-reported ratings obtained from a subject. The model thus developed is called the perceived stress model, which can be used to impute self-reported stress for each minute in which a self-report was not obtained. Given

that self-report often can only be conveniently obtained several times a day, the perceived stress model is able to provide imputed data which are continuous.

In an effort to assess the utility of this modeling approach, the perceived stress model was evaluated in the lab session involving 21 participants as described earlier (11). For each subject, a correlation was computed between their 14 self-reported ratings of stress and data produced from the stress model. The median correlation between the subjective stress and physiological stress models was found to be $r = 0.72$.

The perceived stress model then was evaluated for its generalizability to the natural field environment. The same participants who completed the lab study wore the sensors for 2 days in their usual environment, where they were prompted 20 times a day to provide self-reported stress ratings. An average rating of self-reported stress and an average stress value from the model were computed for the 2 days of field study. One r value was computed for all the participants, each of whom contributed one average rating of self-reported stress and another average stress value from the model. The average stress rating from the perceived stress model was compared with that from these self-reports, with a resulting correlation of $r = 0.71$. These data suggest that the approach to modeling stress from AutoSense correlates reasonably well to self-reported stress in the natural environment.

The assessment of stress in the field environment can be made more robust by incorporating accelerometer signals, where over 30% of the signals are impacted by physical activity. Physical activity can activate physiological systems that are also activated by exposure to stress. Machine learning models using accelerometry can be trained to identify episodes of data that are impacted by physical activity. Incorporating accelerometry in modeling stress is an area of continuing research. Future research will also assess the reproducibility of this stress measure in other participants and will investigate the possible clinical utility of the stress measure in, for example, predicting lapse in newly abstinent smokers.

Automated Measure of Conversation Episodes from AutoSense

Another example of the process of inferring behavior from mobile sensors is reflected in the use of sensors measuring respiration to infer characteristics of conversations. Conversations change the way we breathe, hence physiological measurements (in particular, respiration pattern) may exhibit distinct patterns when one is speaking to conversational partners vs. expressing emotions as a result of a heated topic. In an initial study on conversational episodes, Rahman et al. (12) noted that respiration cycle measurements contain unique patterns that can be used to infer if the wearer of the sensor is speaking, listening to another person, or being quiet (12). Figure 3.4 shows examples of the respiration signal during speaking, listening, and quiet. As evidenced in this figure, the respiratory patterns are different in these three states. In particular, the signals during active listening in a two-party conversation are distinct from quiet intervals. Presumably, the listener's urge to speak or reciprocate influences respiratory pattern and interrupts the rhythm that characterizes quiet intervals.

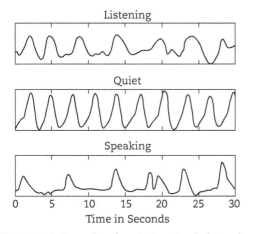

FIGURE 3.4: Examples of respiration signals during listening, quiet, and speaking.

To detect conversational states for a person wearing a respiration sensor, various features (seen in Figure 3.2) are extracted from respiration data captured by AutoSense. In addition to the features used in detecting stress, an additional feature proves useful in detecting conversation, called "B-Duration," which is defined as the time the signal spends within 2.5% of the valley amplitude when the signal hits a valley in a respiration cycle (12). During speaking, people tend to take a deep breath and continue to exhale while talking until they are out of air, and then take a deep breath again. This pattern can be observed in Figure 3.4, when the signal during speaking is compared with that from a quiet state.

Once features are extracted from the signal, they are parsed into 30-second segments and specific statistics such as mean, median, 80th percentile, etc. are computed. A 30-second segment usually consists of 10 respiration cycles and hence enables computation of robust statistics. Each 30-second segment can be classified as speaking, listening, or quiet, based on these values. Machine learning models then are trained over the feature statistics to identify each 30-second segment as quiet, listening, or speaking. A hidden Markov model is used to compose these composite features into conversational states. These procedures are described in greater detail in Rahman et al.'s study (12).

To test this approach of using sensors to measure and characterize conversational episodes, data from 46 hours of conversation were collected from 12 participants (12). In this study, an observer followed participants as they went about their daily life. The observer marked the conversational state by pressing buttons on a mobile phone that was wirelessly receiving respiration sensor data from participants, ensuring that these two data sources were synchronized in time. Results showed that this respiration sensor method achieved 83% accuracy in distinguishing the three conversation states (speaking, listening, and quiet). The application of a hidden Markov model improved the accuracy of detecting an entire conversation episode (that may consist of various speaking and listening states) to 87%. The conversation model was then applied to the respiration data collected from 21 college students who wore the AutoSense sensors for 2 full days in their natural environment. This is the same user study described above for developing a computational model for inferring stress. In this application, it was noted that the average duration of conversation was 3.83 minutes (±3.04) and the average time between successive conversations was 13.38 minutes (±23.86). On average, there were four conversations lasting 10 minutes or more during the entire day. These subjects spent 25% of their day in conversations.

Automated Measure of Smoking Episodes from AutoSense

The process of inferring behavior from mobile sensors is additionally illustrated in research focused on detecting smoking behavior via respiration pattern captured by the respiration sensor in AutoSense. Smoking usually involves deep inhalation and exhalation, a pattern that can be observed in respiration measurements. Respiratory cycles can be analyzed to detect the deep inhalation and exhalation patterns that are present while smoking a cigarette (13). The features extracted from respiration signals, as described earlier, are also useful in identifying smoking puffs. Because a smoking puff lasts only one respiration cycle, these features are computed for each individual respiration cycle. Figure 3.5 shows a sample of respiration signals during smoking and during other activities, such as running, stress, and conversation, when the respiratory signal may show a similar pattern. As noted in this figure, it is important to avoid coding smoking when other activities are responsible for the noted respiratory pattern. Typically, smoking puffs are associated with a deep and long inhalation followed by a long exhalation, relative to

neighboring respiration cycles. During running, the respiration cycles have deep inhalation and exhalation, but they are short in duration and the neighboring cycles are all similar. The respiration signals during conversation are similar to that during smoking, except that during conversation an individual spends more time near the expiration portion of the respiration cycle. The case of smoking and speaking presents a challenge for detection and continues to be an active topic of research.

These observations were used to develop a machine learning model that can identify respiration cycles corresponding to smoking puffs by comparing the features of a given respiration cycle with its neighboring respiration signals. This model was developed from examining 161 puffs from 13 smoking sessions of 10 participants (13) who wore AutoSense sensors and carried a mobile phone with FieldStream software during smoking. In this study, an observer labeled cigarette puffs by participants using a mobile phone with FieldStream that wirelessly collected respiration sensor data from AutoSense in real time. The model was able to distinguish smoking puffs from non-puff respiration cycles with 91% accuracy. To evaluate the robustness of this model, it was presented with respiration cycles from 46 hours of non-smoking data from 33 participants in which the participants were stressed, running, and engaged in conversation, which are all activities that produce respiration patterns most similar to smoking and hence act as confounding events. As evidenced by an 86.7% accuracy rate (91% precision, 81% true positive rate, and 8% false positive

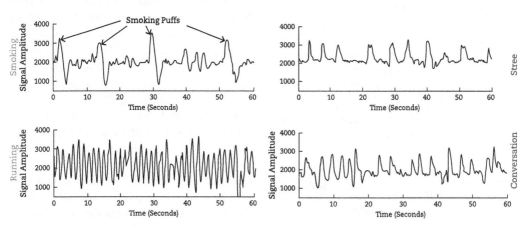

FIGURE 3.5: Respiration signals captured during smoking, running, stress, and conversation, to illustrate the different patterns observed during these activities. The respiration corresponding to smoking puffs is marked.

rate), the model was able to differentiate smoking respiration cycles from other activities. Additional research is needed to assemble individual smoking puffs into a larger smoking episode, which will be particularly useful in understanding environmental triggers to smoking (e.g., integrating this model with GPS data and assessing how location may influence subjective states such as craving). It is also critical to improve the specificity of the model in capturing smoking behaviors. Improvement in the sensitivity of the machine learning model can also assist in the detection of lapses among newly abstinent smokers, as this event may contain only a single smoking puff.

RESEARCH CHALLENGES FOR MOBILE MEASUREMENT OF HEALTH, BEHAVIOR, AND CONTEXT

Given the novelty and potential of mobile health, the development and evaluation of mobile sensing is a vibrant area of research within many disciplines, including the fields of computing, engineering, and behavioral science. We have discussed these issues in detail elsewhere (28,29). We next summarize some of the challenges that are most relevant for conducting behavioral assessment using mobile sensors.

Scaling Measurement by Reducing Burden on Study Personnel

Ongoing and future studies involve the use of mobile health sensing devices in the context of, for example, studying stress, smoking behaviors, alcohol use, physical activity, and related psychosocial, physical, and environmental factors (28,29). Devices such as AutoSense are able to last more than a week on a single charge of a small wearable battery, and therefore the user burden has largely been minimized. Study participants from risk populations such as daily smokers, heavy drinkers, and drug users have worn physiological sensors for 4 weeks in the field and provided thousands of hours of usable sensor data (26). Such preliminary studies provide evidence that mobile measurement of many different health states is feasible on a small scale for several weeks.

At present, the use of mobile measurement devices, however, requires close supervision by an investigative team to yield high-quality, valid data and is most suitable for laboratory or limited field studies. It is desirable to meet daily with participants to review the sensors and to check the data collected in the previous day. This high level of participant contact ensures a relative lack of missing or inaccurate data. During these daily meetings, research personnel change devices that may not be working properly, replace batteries, fix any loose connections, and motivate participants to continue or improve protocol adherence. However, the daily meetings pose a significant burden on participants and study staff and limit the size of user studies to four to five participants per week per staff member. To be able to conduct larger scale studies, these daily meetings need to be eliminated and replaced with automated monitoring of device malfunctions. Additional interventions targeting poor protocol adherence need to be developed for the mobile device itself; this step will eliminate face-to-face meetings with participants who are not adherent with the assessment protocol.

Data Quality

Data collected in the mobile environment are subject to various sources of noise, which can deteriorate quality. For wearable physiological sensors, these confounds include loose attachment, poor placement, physical movements, and sensor defects. Since measurements are collected in the natural environment, sensor attachment and placement may gradually worsen over the course of a day. While sensors on the phone such as GPS and accelerometers worn on the body are becoming more mature as they pose less stringent wearing constraints, physiological sensors requiring attachment at specific locations on the body such as with ECG are prone to more sources of data quality deterioration. Looking ahead, additional research is needed to develop methods to monitor data quality, to develop imputation methods to account for data that are missing because of movement, and ideally, to repair the source of the quality deterioration, without any manual intervention.

Validity and Reliability

Because mobile measurement provides a new class of assessment and incorporates the application of machine learning models to data collected in the natural environment, validation presents significant challenges. Traditional approaches to establishing the validity of a measure cannot easily be applied to mobile measurement. For example, benchmarking mobile measurement against laboratory physiological measurement is not possible in the natural environment. Moreover, the goals of mobile measurement are different from those of laboratory-based assessment, particularly given the emphasis on detection of specific behaviors (e.g., smoking), recognition of global states (e.g., stress), and discernment of interaction patterns among individuals. Additional conceptual work is needed to develop an approach and methodology to validate mobile measurement, in the absence of gold standards, and reconcile existing standards to demonstrate validity with these available in the field of biosensing methods.

Reliability of measurement also deserves additional attention, particularly as sensor placement may not be consistent across individuals or across days. Unlike laboratory settings, mobile measurement relies on the participant to place sensors and activate measurement devices, without close supervision. Strategies need to be developed to determine the stability of measurement (reliability), particularly in the face of an ever-changing environment. Underlying these concerns is the search for ways to adapt mobile measurement for the myriad uses that social and behavioral scientists desire, while retaining good measurement (psychometric) properties. These issues are further discussed elsewhere (29).

Reducing the Burden of Sensor Attachment

Miniaturization has made it possible to wear sensors unobtrusively for several weeks in the field environment. Currently, wearing of several physiological sensors requires skin contact, such as that for ECG or skin conductance. For mobile measurements to become truly population scalable, the sensing technology needs to advance further to eliminate the need for sensors. At present, accelerometers and GPS can be embedded within a mobile phone, permitting collection of data on movement and location. New sensing technologies such as radiofrequency micro-radar-based sensors such as EasySense (30) that are under development promise to eliminate the need for skin contact in measuring physiology. These new technologies are discussed in more detail elsewhere, together with other sensors that promise to

collect measures of health state that have not been possible until now (28).

Privacy, Security, and Confidentiality

Although mobile measurement offers exciting technology for assessment in the natural environment, it also includes new concerns about privacy, security, and confidentiality. The use of emerging machine learning models for assessing states such as stress, substance use, physical activity, social interactions, and location make it possible to obtain privacy-revealing states from individuals on the basis of their sensor measurements. Leakage of such data can lead to adverse physical, professional, social, and financial outcomes, particularly when such data are combined with publicly available information (31). Substantial research is needed to develop techniques for controlling access, interpretation, and transformation of such data. Greater consideration needs to be given to ways in which these data can truly be de-identified in scientific presentations and publications and when data are shared across studies. From a policy standpoint, greater understanding is needed concerning the impact of sharing of mobile measurement data. It is possible that public health policies such as HIPPA that currently do not assume such data as personally identifiable will need to be revised as well. We have discussed these issues in greater detail elsewhere (28,29). These issues are also addressed in more detail in Chapter 21 of this book.

Data Analytics

Mobile measurement offers a paradigm shift in the assessment of behavioral and physiological correlates of health and could advance efforts for the implementation of interventions. Ultimately, use of sensor technologies can lead to improved clinical utility through its potential for more efficient patient screening (6,32), by reducing the need for costly and time-consuming monitoring and follow-up by medical and technical experts (8,33). Prior studies have reported feasibility results from participants in field studies (34,35), but results in clinical settings warrant further examination (e.g., evaluation of coping with chronic stress [36]). Important considerations also must be given to informatics and statistical approaches for handling large datasets. Some statistical approaches and strategies for handling high dimensional data and methods for imputing and dealing with missing informative data have been developed (37,38), but significant work is needed to deal with data collected by mobile health sensors. This topic is addressed in more detail in Chapter 11 of this book.

JUST-IN-TIME INTERVENTIONS: THE FUTURE OF BEHAVIORAL HEALTHCARE

The emergence of smartphone applications that can process behavior- health–related measurements in real time can lead to a new class of interventions that can be delivered to individuals when and where needed. We can envision a future where this individualized delivery approach can vastly improve the effectiveness of interventions. Real-time measurement of health states and the environment also make it feasible to adapt interventions to the individual, the current health state of the individual, and the current state of the physical and social environment. Prospective use of sensor technologies in longitudinal studies can help to identify temporal signatures and inform potential causal attributions of stressors to long-term health outcomes (39). These methods, using frequent, repeated assessments, may be especially useful in future epigenetic studies that explore dynamic, complex, time-dependent (e.g., order of onset [35]) interactions between environmental exposures and physiological responding systems (40). Thus, beyond mere association of multiple data points of simultaneous measures of psychosocial and physiologic status, these methods have promise for use in understanding complex multidimensional phenomena, such as the integrated influence of biological, psychosocial, and physical effects on physiology (41). This theoretical concept encompasses the interactive contexts across social (e.g., developmentally relevant interpersonal interactions), material (e.g., available and accessible goods, services, and information relevant to social position), and ecological (e.g., social structures) domains within which environmental events and biological changes transpire across the life course. However, in order for the full potential of these technologies to be realized for these devices, more widespread adoption and adaptation will be needed to meet future study needs to inform empirical theory building, hypothesis generation and testing, and, ultimately, development and refinement of interventions for disease prevention and treatment.

REFERENCES

1. Wang Y, Chien C, Xu J, Pottie G, Kaiser W Gait analysis using 3D motion reconstruction with an activity-specific tracking protocol. IEEE International Conference on Acoustics, Speech and Signal Processing (ICASSP), May 26–31, 2013.
2. Bexelius C, Lof M, Sandin S, Trolle Lagerros Y, Forsum E, Litton JE. Measures of physical activity using cell phones: Validation using criterion methods. *Journal of Medical Internet Research* 2010; 12(1):e2.
3. Kim DH, Kim Y, Estrin D, Srivastava MB. SensLoc: Sensing everyday places and paths using less energy. *SenSys '10 Proceedings of the 8th ACM Conference on Embedded Networked Sensor Systems.* Zurich, Switzerland, 2010, pp. 43–56 [ACM Digial Library 1869989].
4. Chen C, Driggs Campbell K, Negi I, Iglesias RA, Owens P, Tao N, et al. A new sensor for the assessment of personal exposure to volatile organic compounds. *Atmospheric Environment* 2012; 54:679–687.
5. Vidal JC, Bonel L, Ezquerra A, Hernandez S, Bertolin JR, Cubel C, et al. Electrochemical affinity biosensors for detection of mycotoxins: A review. *Biosensors & Bioelectronics* 2013; 49:146–158.
6. Muller A, Goette A, Perings C, Nagele H, Konorza T, Spitzer W, et al. Potential role of telemedical service centers in managing remote monitoring data transmitted daily by cardiac implantable electronic devices: Results of the early detection of cardiovascular events in device patients with heart failure (detecT-Pilot) study. *Telemedicine Journal and E-Health* 2013; 19(6):460–466.
7. Renard E. Implantable continuous glucose sensors. *Current Diabetes Review* 2008; 4(3):169–174.
8. Tiihonen P, Hukkanen T, Tuomilehto H, Mervaala E, Toyras J. Evaluation of a novel ambulatory device for screening of sleep apnea. *Telemedicine Journal and E-Health* 2009; 15(3):283–289.
9. Jovanov E, Frith K, Anderson F, Milosevic M, Shrove MT. Real-time monitoring of occupational stress of nurses. Engineering in Medicine and Biology Society, EMBC, 2011 Annual International Conference of the IEEE, August 30–September 3, 2011.
10. Stopczynski A, Stahlhut C, Petersen MK, Larsen JE, Jensen CF, Ivanova MG, et al. Smartphones as pocketable labs: Visions for mobile brain imaging and neurofeedback. *International Journal of Psychophysiology* 2014; 91(1):54–66.
11. Plarre K, Raij A, Hossain SM, Ali AA, Nakajima M, Al'absi M, et al. Continuous inference of psychological stress from sensory measurements collected in the natural environment.

10th International Conference on Information Processing in Sensor Networks (IPSN), 2011 April 12–14, 2011.

12. Rahman MM, Ali AA, Plarre K, al'Absi M, Ertin E, Kumar S. mConverse: Inferring conversation episodes from respiratory measurements collected in the field. *Proceedings of the 2nd Conference on Wireless Health*, San Diego, CA 2011, p. 1–10 [ACM Digital Library 2077557].

13. Ali AA, Hossain SM, Hovsepian K, Rahman MM, Plarre K, Kumar S. mPuff: Automated detection of cigarette smoking puffs from respiration measurements. *Proceedings of the 11th ACM/IEEE International Conference on Information Processing in Sensor Networks*, Beijing, China, 2012, pp. 269–280 [ACM Digital Library 2185741].

14. Natarajan A, Parate A, Gaiser E, Angarita G, Malison R, Marlin B, et al. Detecting cocaine use with wearable electrocardiogram sensors. *Proceedings of the 2013 ACM International Joint Conference on Pervasive and Ubiquitous Computing*, Zurich, Switzerland, 2013, pp. 123–132 [ACM Digital Library 2493496].

15. Barnett NP, Tidey J, Murphy JG, Swift R, Colby SM. Contingency management for alcohol use reduction: A pilot study using a transdermal alcohol sensor. *Drug and Alcohol Dependence* 2011; 118(2-3):391–399.

16. Leffingwell TR, Cooney NJ, Murphy JG, Luczak S, Rosen G, Dougherty DM, et al. Continuous objective monitoring of alcohol use: Twenty-first century measurement using transdermal sensors. *Alcoholism, Clinical and Experimental Research* 2013; 37(1):16–22.

17. Green ED, Guyer MS. Charting a course for genomic medicine from base pairs to bedside. *Nature* 2011; 470(7333):204–213.

18. Hood L, Friend SH. Predictive, personalized, preventive, participatory (P4) cancer medicine. *Nature Reviews Clinical Oncology* 2011; 8(3):184–187.

19. Ertin E, Stohs N, Kumar S, Raij A, al'Absi M, Shah S. AutoSense: Unobtrusively wearable sensor suite for inferring the onset, causality, and consequences of stress in the field. *Proceedings of the 9th ACM Conference on Embedded Networked Sensor Systems*, Seattle, WA, 2011, pp. 274–287 [ACM Digital Library 2070970].

20. What is ohmage? Retrieved from http://ohmage.org/

21. Funf open sensing framework Retrieved from http://www.funf.org/

22. Field T. *Biofeedback. Complementary and Alternative Therapies Research*. Washington, DC: American Psychological Association; 2009, pp. 119–126.

23. Blanchard EB, Andrasik F. *Management of Chronic Headaches: A Psychological Approach*. New York: Pergamon Press; 1985.

24. McGrady A, Linden W. Biobehavioral treatment of essential hypertension. In: Schwartz MS, Andrasik F (eds.). *Biofeedback: A Practitioner's Guide* (3rd ed.). New York: Guilford Press; 2003, pp. 382–405.

25. Musthag M, Raij A, Ganesan D, Kumar S, Shiffman S. Exploring micro-incentive strategies for participant compensation in high-burden studies. *Proceedings of the 13th International Conference on Ubiquitous Computing*, Beijing, China, 2011, pp. 435–444 [ACM Digital Library 2030170].

26. Rahman M, Hossain SM, Ali A, Raij A, Hovsepian K, al'Absi M, et al. Bringing the lab to the field—a week-long wireless mHealth field study with an addictive population. Memphis, TN: University of Memphis, August 2012. Report No. CS-12-001.

27. Bishop CM. *Pattern Recognition and Machine Learning*. New York: Springer; 2006.

28. Kumar S, Nilsen W, Pavel M, Srivastava M. Mobile health: Revolutionizing healthcare through transdisciplinary research. *Computer* 2013; 46(1):28–35.

29. Kumar S, Nilsen WJ, Abernethy A, Atienza A, Patrick K, Pavel M, et al. Mobile health technology evaluation: The mHealth evidence workshop. *American Journal of Preventive Medicine* 2013; 45(2):228–236.

30. Al'absi M, Ertin E, Kumar S. EasySense. Retrieved from http://easysense.org/.

31. Raij A, Ghosh A, Kumar S, Srivastava M. Privacy risks emerging from the adoption of innocuous wearable sensors in the mobile environment. *Proceedings of the SIGCHI Conference on Human Factors in Computing Systems*, Vancouver, BC, Canada, 2011, pp. 11–20 [ACM Digital Library 1978945].

32. Darwish A, Hassanien AE. Wearable and implantable wireless sensor network solutions for healthcare monitoring. *Sensors* (Basel, Switzerland) 2011; 11(6):5561–5595.

33. Lutfi SL, Fernandez-Martinez F, Lorenzo-Trueba J, Barra-Chicote R, Montero JM. I feel you: The design and evaluation of a domotic affect-sensitive spoken conversational agent. *Sensors* (Basel, Switzerland) 2013; 13(8):10519–10538.

34. Johnson EI, Barrault M, Nadeau L, Swendsen J. Feasibility and validity of computerized ambulatory monitoring in drug-dependent women. *Drug and Alcohol Dependence* 2009; 99(1-3):322–326.

35. Swendsen J, Ben-Zeev D, Granholm E. Real-time electronic ambulatory monitoring of substance use and symptom expression in schizophrenia. *American Journal of Psychiatry* 2011; 168(2):202–209.

36. Peternel K, Pogacnik M, Tavcar R, Kos A. A presence-based context-aware chronic stress recognition system. *Sensors* (Basel, Switzerland). 2012; 12(11):15888–15906.

37. Houtveen JH, de Geus EJC. Noninvasive psychophysiological ambulatory recordings: Study design

and data analysis strategies. *European Psychology* 2009; 14(2):132–141.

38. Wilhelm FH, Grossman P. Emotions beyond the laboratory: Theoretical fundaments, study design, and analytic strategies for advanced ambulatory assessment. *Biological Psychology* 2010; 84(3):552–569.

39. Fossion P, Servais L, Rejas MC, Ledoux Y, Pelc I, Minner P. Psychosis, migration and social environment: An age—and—gender controlled study. *European Psychiatry* 2004;19(6):338–343.

40. Diez Roux AV. Integrating social and biologic factors in health research: A systems view. *Annals of Epidemiology* 2007;17(7):569–574.

41. Krieger N. Embodiment: A conceptual glossary for epidemiology. *Journal of Epidemiology and Community Health* 2005; 59(5):350–355.

4

Technology-Based Behavioral Interventions for Alcohol and Drug Use Problems

AIMEE N.C. CAMPBELL, FREDERICK MUENCH, AND EDWARD V. NUNES

INTRODUCTION

While substance abuse is widely recognized as a significant behavioral and mental health problem, it is unique in that its consequences can occur slowly over time (e.g., health problems, familial conflict) or result immediately from a single episode of use (e.g., driving under the influence, overdose), making it one of the most formidable personal and public health challenges facing scientists today. The substantial heterogeneity within substance-abusing samples, the cycling of relapse and recovery within individual cases, the range of severity in cases of individuals with substance use disorders, and the unfortunate reality that most individuals with substance use disorders never seek formal treatment collectively test the limits of face-to-face treatment as the sole substance abuse treatment option.

Technology-based behavioral interventions (TBI) have exponentially increased our ability to improve care across a range of physical and mental health disorders, including substance use disorders (1,2). Appetitive behaviors, such as substance abuse, are often driven by powerful environmental triggers that occur outside of treatment and can override change goals. With the boom in TBI, for the first time in history we can intervene with individuals in their natural environment when and where arousal and craving are most acute. Furthermore, we are no longer limited to narrow treatment models, but can build tailored just-in-time interventions personalized to the specific needs of individuals as they progress through the change process within this heterogeneous population.

Current TBI for substance use disorders typically fall within two broad technological domains,

each with various capabilities: computer-based interventions and mobile and wireless interventions. While most recent interventions integrate both modes of assessment and intervention delivery, the empirical literature has focused most extensively on computer-based interventions for problem drinking. Advances in mobile and wireless technology are relatively recent, and thus there has been a lag in outcome research, including possible concerns about how to treat illegal drug use through these media.

TBI for substance abuse typically fall into screening and one-time brief interventions in opportunistic settings (3), assessment and modular based interventions—both as stand-alone treatments and adjuncts to care (4)—mobile-based interventions that provide ongoing interventions for both low- and high-severity populations in need of continuing care and recovery support (5,6), and recovery and social support-based applications such as online support meetings, 12-step meeting finders, virtual sponsors, and recovery coaches (7,8).

This chapter will provide a brief overview of the existing TBI for substance use disorders; a review of the empirical literature across a range of populations and target behaviors; and design, methodology, and implementation considerations. In the first section of the chapter, we review the limitations of our current systems, models of assessment, and treatment, and how technology has met and can meet the needs of individuals with substance abuse problems. The second section reviews the empirical literature across a range of target behaviors, populations, and substances to summarize the current state of the art with regard to the effectiveness of computer-based and mobile digital interventions. The final section of the chapter presents considerations for design and research methods, specific implementation issues for clinicians providing specialty addiction care, and innovative, future directions for the application of digital technologies.

BARRIERS OF TRADITIONAL SUBSTANCE ABUSE PREVENTION AND TREATMENT SERVICES

While there is substantial variability in the intervention targets of many TBI for substance use disorders, in their simplest form they are designed to enhance factors associated with positive substance use outcomes and reduce the limitations of traditional substance abuse treatment (6). One of the most powerful opportunities that TBI offer is the ability to target specific barriers for specific populations to deliver highly personalized care. Following are some common barriers to successful outcomes identified in the substance abuse field and examples of how use of TBI is reducing or attempting to reduce those barriers.

Limited Accessibility of Care

Many individuals do not seek substance abuse treatment because they do not consider their use to be severe, they don't have insurance, treatment and transportation options in their area are limited, they lack motivation, or a combination of these factors (9,10). TBI combat each of these barriers to treatment access because they are available to anyone, anywhere, at any time (this is especially true of mobile and wireless technologies), and TBI tend to be free or low cost to the individual because they are housed in the cloud (11). TBI are uniquely capable of reaching the majority of substance users who may not be ready for formal specialty treatment or have the resources to attend but are using at hazardous levels, concerned about their use, attempting to cut back or reduce use, or at least interested in learning more about their substance use (3,12). For example, AlcoholScreening.org is one of the largest alcohol screening websites in the United States. The site has attracted over 1,000,000 visitors and continues to draw over 15,000 visitors per month (personal communication).

TBI can reach a wide range of help-seekers because individuals can access and utilize them with relative anonymity and privacy (13). They can also be located within opportunistic settings such as emergency rooms (14), primary care settings (15), and school-based settings (3), without burdening the resources of the system or requiring additional training or expertise for non–substance abuse treatment providers. The reach of TBI has widened exponentially with the mobile phone. Over 90% of adults now own a mobile phone, and while there is a large discrepancy between high- and low-income households, racial groups, and ethnicities in terms of home Internet access, there is no such discrepancy among cell phone users (16). Reaching populations that have traditionally been marginalized socioeconomically and maintaining continuous contact during the treatment and recovery change process can have tremendous personal and public health implications.

Stigma

There is evidence that individuals do not seek treatment because of stigma about substance use and general uneasiness or discomfort with face-to-face interactions. In particular, individuals tend to dislike group formats, which are the most prevalent intervention modality in traditional substance abuse treatment. Social penetration theory (17) describes the process of self-disclosure as a stage-based process in which individuals disclose more personal and unflattering information as the level of trust and intimacy increases. However, many individuals either fail to make it through the door or do not remain in treatment long enough to develop sufficient trust and intimacy for self-disclosure. Forty years of research indicates that individuals are more likely to disclose information about substance abuse and other high-risk behaviors (e.g., sexual risk) during computer interviews than during face-to-face interviews (18). While the mechanisms vary, there is evidence that the reduced risk of immediate negative feedback or judgment makes individuals feel that they are at a safe evaluative distance when disclosing to digital systems, even when they know the data are not anonymous. This distancing allows us to reach the most isolated individuals by slowly engaging them in the change process at their own pace. This is particularly important because, despite the motivational interviewing revolution and the ongoing shift to view addiction as a chronic medical condition paradigm, many traditional substance abuse treatments are predicated on an abstinence-only model and may be perceived as judgmental or shaming.

Lack of Standardization and Empirically Supported Treatment Dissemination

While the stigma of substance abuse is socially engrained, it can also be further cultivated by subpar treatment experiences and clinical staff faced with limited training opportunities and a lack of consistent supervision. Thus, although empirically supported treatments exist, they are infrequently provided as part of standard care (19–22). TBI are typically standardized using empirically supported intervention components. While face-to-face communication is significantly more nuanced—a phenomenon that cannot yet be replicated with virtual agents—TBI can deliver standardized information about substance use, self-regulatory skills training, rehearsal and refusal skills, and many more components of care that require specialized expertise (23,24). Standardization may be particularly useful for informational interventions to compliment in-person interventions for health topics such as HIV risk reduction within substance abuse settings (25). TBI do not simply regurgitate information to the individual. Rather, they apply methods of information retention and precision-based learning (26) and the expertise of user experience designers and other professionals to create an optimized user engagement and retention experience. The combination of these components allows for an enhanced delivery of services to supplement in-person care and support.

One Size Fits All

The treatment-matching literature indicates that certain individuals are more likely to respond to certain types of treatments and treatment components than others, yet even the most recent reports suggest that substance abuse treatment is still providing a one-size-fits-all approach to care (20). Given the range of severity, the variety of behavior change goals held by different individuals, and the research highlighting that individuals without abstinence goals rarely seek treatment, it is crucial

that individuals seeking care have access to multiple intervention strategies. Inherent in all digital technologies is the ability to personalize assessment and intervention to the needs of the end user by applying decision support rules based on static, real-time and dynamic self-report and passive assessment results. Interventions tailored to the individual, based on assessment results, have larger effect sizes, are perceived as more relevant, and produce better engagement in TBI than untailored interventions (27,28). Over the last 30 years, tailoring has been a trademark feature of TBI for substance abuse problems, primarily through normative personalized feedback for individuals not seeking specialty care (29,30). However, nearly every aspect of an intervention can be tailored, from medication suitability based on family history to individualized coping plans to just-in-time feedback based on current state to dynamic tailoring using machine learning based on ecological data trends over time. While the previous TBI literature is weighted toward static one-time tailoring, technology offers a framework on which to build dynamically context-driven assessments and tailored interventions that account for the temporal unfolding of the change process.

Difficulty Intervening When It Matters

TBI and, more specifically, mobile interventions can reach individuals continuously in their natural environment through automated contact and just-in-time assessment and intervention. The simple yet profound ability to send a message to an individual when and where they may need it most is changing how we deliver care. There is evidence that using prompting and reminders significantly improves outcomes across health behaviors (31–33) and that TBI that include a proactive messaging component have larger effect sizes than stand-alone interventions (31,34). Real-time active and passive ecological momentary assessment and intervention can be used to identify early warning signs of a developing problem or for crisis intervention (6). It is common in traditional substance abuse treatment to identify when clients may be isolating more than usual, experiencing negative affect, or having intense cravings. Based on a craving pattern, digital programs can compare previous responses to current responses and, if there is a discrepancy, text the individual to ask if they are having more cravings than in previous days. Gustafson and colleagues (6) developed an alert system based on global positioning to determine when someone is in a high-risk situation. Based on the individual's response, the system will connect them to crisis care if needed or generate provider or recovery coach or sponsor alerts. Thus, such systems can prove highly efficient when circumstances require direct intervention. This just-in-time component is another unique feature of mobile interventions that can be enhanced dramatically with additional passive sensing and ecological momentary assessment while using mathematical modeling and machine learning paradigms to develop truly adaptive real-time interventions (35,36).

Limited Social Support

Social support is one of the primary mediators of successful behavior change across all conditions, yet the ability to connect with individuals at the moment of need has been a core limitation of in-person interventions. This is true even of successful 12-step peer support models that require an individual to proactively reach out when they may be at risk for relapse. As noted earlier, a core component of just-in-time interventions is connecting individuals to social support when it is needed most. When developing a text messaging system for continuing care following treatment, Muench, Weiss, Kuerbis, and Morgenstern (37) found that 84% of individuals would send help messages to an automated system, 96% were interested in having a friend alerted during times of crisis, and 78% wanted a counselor alerted. While there have been few empirical data to date for TBI that connect individuals to providers, meetings, or recovery support systems, there are numerous apps that are specifically designed for this purpose. For example, there are simple GPS-enabled 12-step meeting finders that can connect individuals to peer support immediately. These apps have gained significant traction within the recovery community, in part because they constitute an extension of the features already engrained in self-help strategies. In addition to apps, there are numerous websites designed to deliver virtual 12-step meetings (e.g., virtual SMART recovery meetings) and virtual chat and discussion forums to assist individuals interested in moderation support.

CURRENT LIMITATIONS OF TECHNOLOGY-BASED INTERVENTIONS

TBI for substance use disorders are not without their limitations, which significantly overlap with the limitations described in other chapters. One of the primary concerns is that substance abuse records have special Health Insurance Portability and Accountability Act (HIPAA) guidelines, and mobile systems—connected systems in particular—are rarely secure enough to explicitly refer to disease states, highlighting the need for greater security. While secure systems have been developed, and systems delivered outside covered entities are not subject to regulations, this will continue to be a significant barrier to their integration into care. Privacy concerns are also salient to the end users. For example, 40% of individuals in substance abuse treatment did not want any mention of substance abuse in a substance abuse recovery-related text messaging system. Interestingly, 20% of individuals attempting to moderate their drinking felt similarly, suggesting that intervention developers must be sensitive to the end-user's feelings about stigma and confidentiality, even in the context of personal mobile devices.

Another important limitation is dropout, which has been termed the "law of attrition" in the world of technology-based interventions because it is so common to all mediums (38). This is true even when it is an extension of formal treatment. For example, Klein, Slaymaker, Dugosh, and McKay (39) examined the impact of a computerized continuing care intervention following inpatient treatment and found that engagement dropped to 50% after 1 month. By the end of the program, compliance was only 5%. The "law of attrition" underscores that it not realistic to rely solely on technology as a panacea. Cohen, Hunter-Reel, Hagman, and Mitchell (7) identified numerous self-tracking alcohol applications and blood alcohol count (BAC) calculators to aid in self-monitoring within the app store, but there is little evidence they are being used by individuals attempting to change their behavior. Future iterations of these tools can incorporate features that have been shown to increase engagement in systems, such as proactive prompts (e.g., text messages), incentives or vouchers, and TBI that include a human component for supportive accountability (40–43).

Unlike many behavioral health disorders such as asthma or diabetes for which behavioral health professionals are relatively absent from care, substance abuse providers deliver behavioral healthcare to clients directly. This may cause providers to be concerned about how TBI may replace some of their duties. Training and administrative support in how to integrate technologies into standard treatment, and education on how technology can enhance rather than compete with provider duties and can improve outcomes, will be important to create a culture shift in real-world settings.

EMPIRICAL SUPPORT FOR TECHNOLOGY-BASED BEHAVIORAL INTERVENTIONS

The purpose of this section is to provide a summary of the research evidence to date on TBI for substance use and abuse. This section is structured on the basis of target intervention behavior, from primary prevention to longer-term treatments and recovery management or continuing care. Specific settings are discussed separately within each target behavior, as relevant (e.g., colleges and universities, medical settings). The evidence base was assessed primarily through a review of meta-analyses and systematic reviews of adult substance abuse interventions, with specific examples of TBI with randomized controlled trial evidence. Because the outcome literature on mobile interventions is nascent, this section focuses primarily on controlled trials of computer-based substance abuse prevention and treatment interventions.

Prevention Interventions

Primary prevention occurs prior to the onset of problematic substance use. Individuals with risk factors or hazardous use (e.g., binge or heavy drinking episodes, drug use experimentation) who do not yet meet criteria for a substance use disorder may be targets of secondary prevention. Tertiary prevention addresses behavior that may meet the definition of a disorder but the individual may not have sought treatment, identified a problem, or experienced the most extreme consequences of the disorder.

Technology-based prevention interventions have primarily targeted alcohol use among at-risk college students. For the most part, these studies have been smaller, feasibility studies or comprised of convenience samples. The interventions are generally brief (usually one session) and assessment driven with a personalized, normative feedback component. The primary aim of these types of interventions is to target individuals who may be at risk of developing a substance use disorder (secondary prevention), to raise awareness and encourage behavior change (i.e., reduce negative consequences), or who may already be exhibiting signs of a substance use disorder, to encourage additional help-seeking (tertiary prevention). Technology-based prevention interventions can take a number of different forms, from online Websites (44) and computer-assisted programs (45) to mobile applications and messaging (5,46).

TBI can also be useful as a component of screening, brief intervention, and referral to treatment (SBIRT) models (47). SBIRT was developed as a secondary public-health prevention intervention to detect risky substance use before the onset of a disorder and to provide early intervention, or treatment, primarily in healthcare settings (47,48). Brief TBI can be delivered within emergency departments or as part of a primary care visit following a short screening. Overall, there is strong effectiveness evidence for SBIRT in addressing alcohol misuse and abuse but less for illicit drug use (47,48). However, there is tremendous potential for reaching the vast majority of problem drinkers who will not seek substance abuse specialty services but may be helped by a brief, less stigmatizing SBIRT-based TBI. Taken together, these simple, tailored interventions combat several of the barriers inherent to traditional care, by reducing stigma and cost, and increasing standardization and personalization of the content to match the severity of the problem.

College Populations

By far, the largest number of studies of brief, prevention-based interventions with a technology-based component have been completed with college-age, at-risk alcohol users. There are also efforts underway to test primary prevention interventions for illicit drug use, such as the adolescent prevention for cannabis/alcohol trial of schools in Australia (49), but the outcome literature on TBI in this domain is limited. College student samples are convenient to recruit for these types of studies because problem alcohol use is common within this population, and students are readily available for research participation through either general advertising, orientation events, or college courses.

Overall, the research demonstrates that brief TBI can reduce heavy drinking (e.g., number of drinking days, drinks per drinking days) and negative consequences associated with alcohol use, especially when compared to assessment-only controls. Two recent meta-analyses by Carey and colleagues provide a good summary of the evidence for brief alcohol interventions—primarily among college students. In a meta-analysis of 43 interventions of TBI to reduce alcohol use among college students (3), TBI reduced quantity of use and problems related to use compared to assessment-only controls with small effect sizes. However, TBI outcomes rarely differed significantly from those of the control conditions when the latter groups contained more than an assessment. In a more recent meta-analysis comparing face-to-face intervention and TBI (50), findings again demonstrated relative efficacy of TBI versus control ($N = 34$) on reducing alcohol use quantity, frequency, and peak intoxication at shorter-term follow-up (with outcomes not maintained longer term). There was a differential effect based on gender in that women were more likely to respond to the in-person brief intervention than to TBI, whereas men responded equally to both in the short term.

Other reviews generally support Carey and colleagues' findings (51). For example, Khadjesari, Murray, Hewitt, Hartley, and Godfrey (52) conducted a systematic review of 24 randomized control trials for alcohol reduction among adults, the majority of which examined brief interventions among college students. Again, brief interventions were effective versus assessment-only controls. However, the authors cautioned that lack of methodological rigor tempered these results. An additional meta-analysis (53) that included 42 computer-delivered interventions for alcohol and tobacco use ($n = 29$) found small weighted effect sizes overall ($d = 0.20$), with slightly higher effect sizes for alcohol studies ($d = .26$). Interestingly, effect sizes did not differ by inclusion of normative feedback, number of sessions, level of therapist involvement, or inclusion of entertainment elements. Not surprisingly, effect sizes were higher for studies in which the comparison condition was an attention or placebo control.

An example of a brief assessment and personalized normative feedback intervention that has been researched substantially is "eCHUG" (electronic Check-Up to Go)—a 20 minute Web-based intervention targeting alcohol use and consequences (45,54). The personalized feedback component offers information on quantity and frequency of use, normative comparisons, physical health information, negative consequences, advice, and local referrals and is designed to enhance motivation to change hazardous alcohol use (see http://www.echeckuptogo.com/usa/ for additional information and access to the intervention). Efficacy of eCHUG to reduce alcohol consumption compared to that of assessment-only controls has been demonstrated among college freshman completing the intervention at orientation (55), among higher-risk freshman recruited during a first-semester seminar (45), and among freshman who reported at least one heavy drinking episode in the past month (54). In this last study ($N = 106$), eCHUG produced greater reductions in alcohol use at 8 weeks compared to assessment-only controls, though at 16 weeks these outcomes diminished and no differences were detected for alcohol use consequences (54). Hustad, Barnett, Borsari, and Jackson (56) evaluated eCHUG versus a 3-hour Web-based educational program and an assessment-only control among incoming college freshman ($N = 82$). Individuals in both intervention conditions reported lower levels of alcohol use at 1-month follow-up compared to the control group. However, only the Web-based educational program demonstrated fewer consequences. In a separate but similar intervention, the College Drinker's Check-up ($N = 80$), Hester, Delaney, and Campbell (57) found that when compared to an assessment-only condition, the personalized feedback intervention reduced alcohol use more on three indicators (with effect sizes in the small to medium range at 1-month and 12-month follow-up).

Kypri and colleagues have conducted several large randomized, controlled trials of brief alcohol screening and intervention among college-aged students in Australia and New Zealand. In an Australian sample (58), 56% of 13,000 contacts responded to an online call for a brief alcohol screen. Of those screened, 34% met criteria for hazardous drinking and were offered a 10-minute motivational assessment and, in some cases, personalized feedback. At 1-month follow-up those receiving the intervention drank less often and had fewer drinks; effects persisted for drinking frequency and overall alcohol use at 6-month follow-up, although no significant differences were detected for alcohol-related harm. Kypri and colleagues (59) found similar outcomes among Maori college students in New Zealand. Of almost 6,700 students screened, 27% met hazardous drinking criteria. Those that received the intervention drank less often and consumed fewer drinks per occasion, and they reported fewer academic problems at 5-month follow-up compared to assessment-only controls.

Several small studies (one within a college setting) have also explored the use of text messaging to reduce hazardous drinking. Forty non–treatment-seeking college students used handheld computers to complete the assessment and then either received tailored texts on drinking amounts and consequences based on level of self-efficacy and expectancies or were placed in a non-text control condition (46). The texting condition was associated with fewer drinks per drinking day and lower expectancies of alcohol-related trouble.

In sum, it appears that brief, personal-feedback TBI are useful for problematic alcohol use among college-age students; additional research is required to determine if similar outcomes would be found for illicit drug use, such as cannabis or cocaine. Questions remain as to whether the addition of face-to-face provider time would improve effectiveness (60) and how best to develop interventions that help individuals sustain change over time, as there is evidence that all brief interventions, including TBI, are limited in their ability to produce long-term changes in behavior. Newer interventions that include readministration of feedback and ongoing mobile monitoring may improve these limitations. However, technology-based brief feedback interventions should be considered a useful tool for reaching large numbers of young, at-risk drinkers who would not typically seek specialty alcohol-related services, and at a significantly lower cost than that of face-to-face alternatives.

Nonclinical Adult Populations

Fewer studies have focused on use of TBI for alcohol use in general adult populations. Vernon and colleagues (61) completed a systematic review of general-public TBI for at-risk drinking that included seven online drinking assessments and eight computerized interventions and reported interesting use patterns. In general, they found that approximately 60,000 people visited an alcohol assessment site in a 6-month period, about half of whom completed the provided self-assessment. The average visitor age was 32 years (but this increased to 48 years on paid sites), with slightly more than half being men (60% on paid sites; 65% on free sites). Over 90% of people assessed as problem drinkers had not been diagnosed by a professional and 33% considered themselves to be alcoholic—a noteworthy finding in the context of trying to reach non–treatment-seeking populations. Seven of the eight computerized interventions showed improvements in at least one drinking outcome.

In an earlier study of an online website for screening and brief intervention for alcohol problems, Saitz et al. (44) found that almost half (44%) of visitors completed a screening. Of these, 66% were men and 90% reported hazardous levels of drinking. Visitors with hazardous levels of drinking were more likely to visit other parts of the website that offered information on additional help. This research suggests that large numbers of adults with problem drinking who might not normally seek face-to-face services may access and complete alcohol-use risk assessments.

An additional meta-analysis of nine randomized controlled trials (all with no contact controls) conducted in four high-income countries (U.S., Canada, the Netherlands, Germany) examined online e-self-help groups and brief feedback interventions to reduce hazardous drinking among individuals recruited via media outlets (60). They found a medium effect size overall for TBI and a small but significant difference favoring extended e-self-help groups over single-session feedback interventions, although there were smaller effects for the e-self-help groups among younger age groups.

Medical Settings

Similar types of interventions (i.e., assessment and brief feedback, text messaging) have been offered in SBIRT-type models within medical settings. Interventions for medical settings are brief and targeted, can offer addiction expertise beyond the purview of standard emergency or primary care staff, can build in follow-up procedures and appointments, and may have the potential to reduce return admissions.

At least two recent systematic reviews have examined brief TBI and assessments within primary care (15) and emergency departments (14). Within primary care, investigators found 22 randomized control trials of alcohol interventions with up to four sessions. Those receiving the brief interventions reported lower alcohol consumption than that in controls at 1-year follow-up or longer. Subgroup analyses revealed significant effectiveness of the interventions for men, but not for women. The emergency department review examined health interventions for substance abuse ($n = 8$), injury ($n = 7$) and mental health ($n = 4$). Four of the eight substance abuse–focused interventions were randomized controlled trials: two for adults and two for adolescents (62–65). Overall, there was high acceptability and feasibility for brief TBI, but only modest outcomes, although outcomes were diverse and varied in terms of clinical meaningfulness depending on the study. There is also evidence that very brief screening and single-session or automated TBI in medical settings may be useful in identifying at-risk individuals and be relatively easily integrated into care without significant burden on the system (66,67). For example, Suffoletto, Callaway, Kristan, Kraemer, and Clark (5) recruited young-adult hazardous drinkers ($N = 45$) from the emergency department via a brief alcohol screen and randomly assigned them to a) weekly text messaging–based feedback with goal setting, b) weekly text messaging assessment, or c) control. At 3-month follow-up participants in the feedback text group had 3.4 fewer heavy drinking days in the past 30 days compared to baseline. This single-group pilot, although small, demonstrates feasibility and potential for risk reduction using ongoing continuous mobile interventions—but larger trials are needed.

Pregnant Women and Women of Childbearing Age

Several studies conducted by Ondersma and colleagues have focused specifically on brief, computer-assisted interventions for substance-using postpartum women and women of childbearing age. A single 20-minute computer-delivered motivational interviewing session (with two additional mailings and vouchers for attendance) was compared to an assessment-only control group among 107 postpartum women (68). The computerized intervention reduced overall drug use with the exception of marijuana. This study was recently replicated (69) with 143 women, a longer follow-up period, and without the mailings and incentives. Findings support the original study; electronic screening and brief intervention resulted in significantly higher abstinence at 3-month follow-up compared to attention-matched controls (significant differences were not maintained at 6-month follow-up, although abstinence remained higher in the experimental arm). Days of illicit drug use also favored participants in the electronic screening and brief intervention group but did not reach significance. In another study, a brief, Web-based personalized feedback intervention was compared to general health information in a randomized trial among women of childbearing age to reduce risky alcohol use ($N = 150$). Follow-up 2 months post-intervention showed significant reductions in risky drinking for both treatment conditions (70). These studies, although small, are important given the target population and the fact that they focus on illicit drug use. TBI may be particularly appealing among pregnant and postpartum women in situations where the stigma and concern of punitive consequences may compel women not to seek assessment and treatment services for problem alcohol and drug use.

In sum, TBI in medical settings show promise in targeting individuals with problem alcohol use who might not otherwise be identified. Additional research is needed to identify gender-based differences in outcomes (15) and mechanisms responsible for successful change (15), and to provide consistency and meaning for selected outcomes (14) beyond feasibility and acceptability for computer-assisted intervention.

Prevention Summary

Recent reviews and studies of Web-based and computer-assisted interventions for problem drinking have revealed that, overall, brief TBI for alcohol prevention are superior to waitlist or no-treatment controls and roughly equivalent to alternative interventions for problem drinking (3,29,71–73). This finding has also been borne out for different types of treatments compared to assessment-only controls, educational interventions, and bibliotherapy (74–76). There is evidence of diminishing returns for brief interventions over time and positive shorter-term, but not longer-term, outcomes among TBI (52,76,77). Direct comparisons with face-to-face interventions were less frequent but tended to favor face-to-face interventions on quantity of use and reported problem outcomes, especially for individuals with higher problem severity. There are some individual studies that did find TBI to be as effective in most domains as brief therapies for problem drinking in college students (78,79). Face-to-face interventions may produce better outcomes, especially in the long term. However, TBI may have an advantage in being a lower-cost alternative, giving substantially better reach to non–treatment-seeking populations such as college students.

Drug and Alcohol Use Disorder Treatment Interventions

Overall, systematic and meta-analytic reviews of computer-assisted treatments for mental health and substance use disorders have reported promising findings, but methodological weaknesses temper enthusiasm at this point (29,80–83). Important questions also remain about the best methods of integrating computer-assisted treatments into standard substance abuse treatment care. Litvin, Abrantes, and Brown (84) reported on the successful adaptation of empirically supported face-to-face treatments (e.g., cognitive behavioral therapy and community reinforcement approach) in computer-assisted modalities, but they suggest that these types of interventions don't necessarily take full advantage of what technology has to offer (an exception to this may be newly emerging in technologies related to GPS and individualized, portable handheld applications). The current crop of alcohol and drug treatment TBI thus can provide valuable assistance for individuals with moderate levels of problem use (e.g., for those that do not require detox or addiction medications) and for those who, for various reasons, may not seek treatment (84). For other treatment seekers, TBI can be integrated in the following ways: as an adjunct to enhance or improve standard addiction treatment (that is, in addition to or as a supplement once a patient leaves treatment—continuing care), as a clinical extender (that is, as a substitution for a portion of standard treatment), or as a replacement for standard care (although most of these studies have included some brief face-to-face clinician time). Substitution and replacement models may be particularly beneficial because they could reduce the amount of time providers spend with clients, freeing them to see additional clients or spend more time with patients with more complicated needs. Adjunct models may enhance usual care and produce better outcomes.

Relatively few computer-assisted treatments have been tested among illicit substance users (29,81,85,86). Rigorous studies that address issues critical to community-based implementation are also needed. A recent systematic review of 12 studies included four studies of TBI for opioids (30). In addition to high levels of satisfaction, TBI for drug use demonstrated initial efficacy during treatment and some evidence for post-treatment continuation of effects. Bickel, Warren, Christensen, and Marsch summarized the computer-assisted treatment literature for drugs and found few controlled efficacy trials (1).

Replacement Model

In a review of a wide range of TBI for drugs ($N = 5$ studies) and alcohol ($N = 17$ studies) with varying degrees of professional provider contact, Newman, Szkodny, Llera, and Przeworski (87) concluded that general self-help and predominantly self-help computer-based cognitive and behavioral interventions are efficacious, but that some therapist contact is important for greater and more sustained reductions in substance use and addictive behaviors. Several studies have examined the "replacement model" of TBI, examining therapist-delivered interventions compared to the same intervention delivered online or via computer, and found similar drug use and satisfaction outcomes (a) among opioid-dependent samples, using the community reinforcement approach to behavior therapy and contingency management (23) and group counseling in person or by video (88); (b) for cognitive-behavioral therapy and motivational interviewing with patients with comorbid cannabis/alcohol abuse and depression (11); (c) for the community reinforcement approach, motivational enhancement therapy, and contingency management with cannabis treatment-seekers (89); and (d) with the community reinforcement approach among incarcerated individuals with substance use disorders (90). Across studies with available data, therapist time was vastly reduced (79–90%) when using primarily computer-delivered treatment, compared to that for therapist-delivered treatment (11,23,89). One limitation of these studies is the relatively small sample sizes (N = 37–135), with one exception (N = 494 across 10 prison sites) (90).

As an example of the replacement model, Bickel, Marsch, Buchhalter, and Badger (23) compared a computer-based community reinforcement approach (91,92) intervention plus contingency management (therapeutic education system, or TES) to a therapist-delivered mirrored intervention or treatment as usual. The TES consisted of 65 modules (or topics) and (optional) automated, intermittent, prize-based incentives (93). An initial training module taught patients how to use the Web-based program, followed by modules on basic cognitive-behavioral relapse prevention skills (e.g., drug refusal, managing thoughts about using). Subsequent modules taught skills aimed at improving psychosocial functioning (e.g., communication, mood management, and recreational activities) as well as prevention of HIV, hepatitis, and other sexually transmitted infections. The therapist- and computer-delivered interventions equally outperformed treatment as usual in terms of continuous weeks of abstinence from opioids, with computer-delivered TES using substantially less clinician time.

Partial Substitution Model

A recently completed effectiveness trial conducted within the National Institute on Drug Abuse's (NIDA's) Clinical Trials Network (94) demonstrated TBI within a partial substitution design—that is, substituting TBI for a portion of standard care. The study enrolled 507 participants from 10 outpatient treatment programs who were randomly assigned to 12 weeks of 1) usual care (consisting of at least two onsite sessions per week) or 2) modified usual care + Web-based community reinforcement approach and contingency management (TES) (23), whereby TES was substituted for approximately 2 hours of clinician time per week. Results showed significant positive findings favoring TES. Compared to treatment as usual, use of TES reduced dropout from treatment and increased abstinence in the last 4 weeks of treatment (OR = 1.62, p = .01), an effect that was more pronounced among patients with a positive urine drug and/or breath alcohol screen at baseline (n = 228; OR = 2.18, p = .003). A similar study

design using TES with opioid-dependent individuals in a single methadone maintenance treatment program (n = 160) was also recently completed and demonstrated significantly greater rates of opioid abstinence: 48% vs. 37% abstinence across all study weeks (4).

Adjunct to Care Model

Carroll and colleagues (24,95) demonstrated the efficacy of using a cognitive-behavioral therapy as an adjunct (or addition) to usual outpatient care. The team conducted a randomized, controlled trial of usual care with and without CBT4CBT (six 45-minute computer-assisted modules). Those in the CBT4CBT group had more negative drug urine test results (medium effect size). Cost analyses indicated that usual care + TBI could result in improved outcomes at a low cost (96).

In another example of TBI used as an adjunct to usual care, Moore et al. (97) examined the initial efficacy, feasibility, and acceptability of an interactive voice response (IVR; Recovery Line) intervention among methadone-maintained patients with secondary drug use (N = 36). Patients received 4 weeks of usual care or usual care + Recovery Line. The Recovery Line provided telephone-based learning and activity modules to support abstinence and coping skills, as well as daily assessments. There were overall high ratings of Recovery Line, but substantially less use than recommend daily calls (<10 of 28 days). Interestingly, patients were more likely to report abstinence on the days Recovery Line was used. No differences were detected on satisfaction, urine drug screen results, or coping strategies. Along with additional research on efficacy, reasons for lack of utilization as well as strategies to promote utilization are needed, given the initial positive results.

Adjunct models of TBI in drug treatment can also be used to focus on secondary issues such as engagement in treatment (e.g., used during waitlists, during down time in treatment, or during after-treatment hours) or HIV prevention. Further, adjunct models can be used for post-treatment or continuing care. Given the accessibility and availability limitations experienced by help seekers in the United States and the fact that 50–60% of individuals who enter treatment relapse within 6 months of completion (33,98), post-treatment alternatives for continuing care are desperately needed. Despite being generally beneficial, the most recent review of continuing care interventions suggests that there are specific techniques that promote effectiveness. McKay (33) has reported that effective continuing care interventions should be proactive (e.g., should not rely on the client to initiate care), long term (e.g., minimum of 12 months), and adaptive to client needs at various stages of change (e.g., more intense for those struggling to maintain change). Unfortunately, continuing care alternatives are hampered by limited staff time and nonbillable service provision. Thus, TBI hold promise in addressing the needs of patients following treatment.

Several studies have shown support for TBI as continuing care. Hester, Lenberg, Campbell, and Delaney (8) found that a Web application (Overcoming Addictions) was equally effective after 3 months for out-of-treatment problem drinkers in reducing alcohol use and related problems compared to SMART Recovery (which included a combination of face-to-face meetings, online meetings, forums, and resources). An acceptability study of interactive mobile text messaging was conducted with patients attending intensive outpatient treatment ($N = 50$) (37). Almost all of the patients (98%) expressed interest in using texts as a continuing care strategy. Patients tended to prefer benefit-driven to consequence-driven messages; this difference was based on patient perception of the benefit to be gained of behavior change (i.e., their expectancies). Thus, assessing and integrating personal attitudes and beliefs about behavior change may be an important element for messaging.

The novel smartphone-based system developed by Gustafson and colleagues (6), called A-CHESS, was designed to address the chronic-disease nature of alcoholism and the need for continuing support when patients exit treatment programs. This system includes features such as a needs assessment that identifies target areas for intervention (e.g., coping plans), tailored messaging, real-time in vivo assessments and feedback, mobile prompted check-ins, interactive discussion groups, and a panic button. It also utilizes a high-risk geolocation-based alert system that connects individuals with virtual and live counselors. These features are all accessible through the conduit of a mobile phone.

A-CHESS was tested as an intervention for the prevention of relapse to heavy drinking among individuals exiting treatment ($N = 349$). Almost all of the patients (94%) used A-CHESS within the first week after residential treatment, with 80% continuing to use the program at week 16. Patients with co-occurring mental health issues used the program slightly less (70% continued use at week 16) (99). Findings support the feasibility and acceptability of this intervention among this population, but further research is needed to determine whether these interventions improve post-treatment outcomes. Other interventions targeting post-treatment recovery management have had less success in maintaining engagement and retention. For example, Klein, Slaymaker, Dugosh, and McKay (39) examined a computerized continuing care intervention that included multimedia content and access to a recovery coach following inpatient treatment. Engagement with the intervention dropped 50% after 1 month and plummeted to 5% after 18 months. One of the primary differences between A-CHESS and this application was that A-CHESS used the mobile phone as the intervention medium instead of the computer. This highlights that more information is needed about the most effective methods to enhance engagement in these systems using various mediums for delivery.

Summary of Empirical Evidence

The evidence to date on TBI is extremely promising, especially with regard to brief interventions targeting problem substance use. There is substantial evidence that Web-based interventions can improve accessibility of interventions for individuals who are unlikely to seek in-person care but are engaging in hazardous use (12). There is further evidence that TBI are effective at disseminating empirically supported treatments in a standardized manner (30). Several studies have demonstrated that computer-based versions of interventions can be as effective as therapist-delivered versions, provided there is some clinician contact.

Future research should examine the efficacy and effectiveness of brief prevention interventions, as well as interventions to treat individuals who meet substance use disorder criteria, using stronger, methodologically rigorous procedures with larger sample sizes and active controls (52,80,86). Standardization of outcomes would also enhance the usefulness of review studies (51). Further, there is no empirical evidence through randomized, controlled designs that indicates a specific mediator of outcome for a just-in-time intervention tailored to someone's current state. While there are emerging trials that highlight acceptability and preference of certain TBI features like GPS, more research is needed to understand how these novel interventions impact outcomes and the mechanisms associated with their various components. Despite some limitations, the outcome research suggests that TBI can significantly reduce some of the barriers associated with our traditional models of treatment (e.g., one size fits all, stigma, cost). Newer intervention models could benefit from diverse delivery modalities (e.g., Web vs. mobile vs. telecare vs. in person) that integrate the most efficacious channels of care while accounting for the barriers to delivery for a particular individual.

FUTURE DIRECTIONS: METHODOLOGICAL CONSIDERATIONS AND EMERGING TECHNOLOGIES
Problems in Testing the Effectiveness of Technology-Based Behavioral Interventions

As the foregoing sections have outlined, a number of TBI have been developed in recent years for the prevention and treatment of alcohol and substance problems. These show considerable promise for surmounting barriers (e.g., stigma, accessibility, cost) and delivering behavioral therapy for this serious public health problem. However, a significant problem may be that the development of these technology-based interventions has outpaced our ability to conduct rigorous empirical evaluations of their effectiveness. A recent methodological review of randomized clinical trials of computer-assisted therapies for adult psychiatric disorders (80) was sobering in this regard. Seventy-five randomized clinical trials published between 1990 and 2010 were identified and rated for methodological quality. There was marked variability in study quality. No study was rated as satisfactory on all 14 quality items rated, and common weaknesses included lack of measurement of treatment exposure or adherence, poor rates of follow-up, violation of the intent to treat principle, and weak control conditions such as the "wait-list"

control. Further, studies with poor-quality scores and weaker control conditions were more likely to report positive findings—that is, to conclude that the TBI was effective. The field is done a disservice if the effectiveness of these interventions is overestimated and they become widely disseminated without good evidence of benefit (86).

One source of this problem may be the mismatch between the rapid pace of technology development and the rather ponderous pace of the classical approach of empirical testing of treatment interventions with randomized, controlled trials. For example, Bickel and colleagues developed the therapeutic education system (TES) over a decade ago. TES brings the community reinforcement approach, an elaborate, manual-guided cognitive-behavioral intervention for substance problems, into a computer-interactive learning environment, wedded with a contingency management intervention which the computer also manages, modeling a treatment package that has been particularly effective for treatment of cocaine dependence (100,101). The first controlled clinical trial testing its efficacy was published in 2008 (23), and other single-site trials (e.g., Marsch et al. [4]), as well as a multisite effectiveness trial (94,102), were only recently completed. This is not surprising, given the years typically required to secure funding and to plan, execute, analyze, and publish results from a rigorous clinical trial. However, during the same 10-year time frame technology has advanced tremendously, from faster computers, to the emergence of handheld devices, smartphones, and apps. Images of individuals sitting at desktop computers are now replaced with contemporary smartphone users accessing a vast menu of sophisticated apps at their fingertips (and, in fact, TES is now being made available as a mobile application).

Certainly, the randomized clinical trial remains the gold standard for testing of efficacy and effectiveness of any treatment intervention. However, the sophisticated and appealing smartphone applications of today are certainly not developed through an iterative process of randomized trials. Ideas are hatched, programs are written and launched, and the measure of success is utilization, which ultimately drives the potential for advertising dollars and profitability. Utilization is not the same as efficacy; however, it does indicate acceptability and exposure or adherence, which is a first step.

Perhaps the challenge to the field is to develop ways of testing efficacy within the model of rapid development and implementation of new technology-based applications. This may require moving beyond the classical randomized, controlled trial toward comparative effectiveness evaluations derived from nonrandomized observational data, and/or the principle of large sample trials, where simple outcome data are gathered automatically through the programs themselves or through the equivalent of standard electronic medical records (EMR). The question of whether observational data on comparative effectiveness is an adequate substitute for the randomized trial has been taken up in a number of branches of medicine over the years, with substantial evidence marshaled that observational studies are just as valid (103,104). There have also been cautionary tales, such as the data on postmenopausal hormone therapy: observational studies suggested it was a good thing, then a large randomized trial concluded the opposite, revealing substantial risks (105).

Nonetheless, it would seem that for TBI that develop and launch rapidly, we need to develop an equally nimble way of evaluating effectiveness. Applications that track users and gather outcome data from them on the target substance use and related behaviors should be able to deliver such rapid assessment. Issues of informed consent would need to be resolved. But conceivably, effectiveness could be evaluated through comparisons of interventions, or components within interventions, perhaps by delivering different interventions to different users who visit a given site or use a certain app. Thus, developing TBI with built-in data gathering and effectiveness evaluation would seem desirable as part of future intervention development efforts.

Emerging Technologies

To date, technology-based interventions for substance use disorders have largely fallen into the category of computer-interactive learning, or of some screening, motivational, or cognitive-behavioral therapy that has been automated. However, there is considerable potential in moving beyond this foundation to harness the full capabilities of technology (106–108). One example is wearable sensors able to detect motion, such as accelerometers that could track and recognize the hand and arm movements that indicate cigarette or alcohol use or drug taking. Similarly, sensors detecting physiological changes (e.g., vital signs) might be able to detect patterns signaling substance use, or stress levels that create risk for substance use. GPS could be integrated into interventions to track patients' movement into risky areas or track their general activity level. It might also be able to detect patterns of movement indicating episodes of drug and alcohol use. Web-based or handheld programs could be designed to give patients rapid feedback on their levels of drinking or on other symptoms (109,110). Detection of substance use or of high-risk situations could trigger immediate contact with patients through instant messaging, in an effort to prevent relapse. Ways of objectively and accurately monitoring medication adherence with such methods could also be extremely valuable in the treatment of addictions for which effective medications exist (e.g., disulfiram, naltrexone, buprenorphine) but depend on daily adherence.

Sustainability

A considerable future challenge regards the dissemination and sustainability of TBI in the substance abuse treatment system. One problem is funding and reimbursement. Community-based substance abuse treatment programs are presently funded largely by third-party payments, which generally recognize face-to-face clinical visits but not care delivered by a computer or other digital device. Thus, reimbursement for organization and delivery of TBI would be important to incentivize treatment programs to prescribe and recommend these interventions to their patients, not to mention to incentivize programmers and developers to supply and service these interventions on a large scale and to collaborate with investigators to innovate and create new and better interventions.

A related issue is the integration of TBI into the work of clinicians and treatment programs. As effective TBI for substance use problems accumulate, and as access to them increases (e.g., through Web-based or smartphone applications), clinicians will need to learn how to prescribe and monitor these interventions. Much as when a new class of medications for treating an addiction emerges, clinicians would need to learn about these new TBI tools, understand the benefits and limitations, and discern for whom to prescribe them. To date, interventions that have been tested within clinical programs have been tested as add-ons to or substitutes for usual care (see previous section), with only limited attention to how the clinicians in those programs would actually interface with the digital intervention (see, for example, reference 102) and how the intervention might be integrated into a long-term treatment plan. TBI for the addictions have been developed in part as a response to the challenges in training front-line clinicians to effectively deliver elaborate behavioral interventions. Yet, clinicians will ultimately need to be trained as effective prescribers. A clinician or treatment program armed with a menu (or tool box) of varied TBI is likely to be substantially better able to serve their patients and elevate the quality of care.

REFERENCES

1. Bickel WK, Warren K, Christensen, DR, Marsch LA. A review of computer-based interventions used in the assessment, treatment, and research of drug addiction. *Substance Use & Misuse* 2011; 46(1):4–9.

2. Heron KE, Smyth JM. Ecological momentary interventions: Incorporating mobile technology into psychosocial and health behaviour treatments. *British Journal of Health Psychology* 2010; 15(1):1–39.

3. Carey KB, Scott-Sheldon LAJ, Elliott JC, et al. Computer-delivered interventions to reduce college student drinking: A meta-analysis. *Addiction* 2009; 104(11):807–1819.

4. Marsch LA, Guarino H, Acosta M, Aponte-Melendez Y, Cleland C, Grabinski M, et al. Web-based behavioral treatment for substance use disorders as a partial replacement of standard methadone maintenance treatment. *Journal of Substance Abuse Treatment* 2014; 46(1):43–51.

5. Suffoletto B, Callaway C, Kristan J, Kraemer K, Clark DB. Text-message-based drinking assessments and brief interventions for young adults discharged from the emergency department. *Alcoholism, Clinical & Experimental Research* 2012; 36(3):552–560.

6. Gustafson DH, Shaw BR, Isham A, Baker T, Boyle MG, Levy M. Explicating an evidence-based, theoretically informed, mobile technology-based system to improve outcomes for people in recovery for alcohol dependence. *Substance Use & Misuse* 2011; 46:96–111.

7. Cohn AM, Hunter-Reel D, Hagman BT, Mitchell J. Promoting behavior change from alcohol use through mobile technology: The future of ecological momentary assessment. *Alcoholism, Clinical & Experimental Research*. 2011; 35(12):2209–2215.

8. Hester RK, Lenberg KL, Campbell W, Delaney HD. Overcoming Addictions, a Web-based appplication, and SMART Recovery, an online and in-person mutual help group for problem drinkers, part 1: Three-month outcomes of a randomized controlled trial. *Journal of Medical Internet Research* 2013; 15(7):e134.

9. Cunningham JA, Sobell LC, Chow VMC. What's in a label? The effects of substance types and labels on treatment considerations and stigma. *Journal of Studies on Alcohol* 1993; 54(6):693–699.

10. Rapp RC, Xu J, Carr CA, Lane DT, Wang J, Carlson R. Treatment barriers identified by substance abusers assessed at a centralized intake unit. *Journal of Substance Abuse Treatment* 2006; 30(3):227–235.

11. Kay-Lambkin FJ, Baker AL, Lewin TJ, Carr VJ. Computer-based psychological treatment for comorbid depression and problematic alcohol and/or cannabis use: A randomized controlled trial of clinical efficacy. *Addiction* 2009; 104(3):378–388.

12. Postel MG, de Jong CA, de Haan HA. Does e-therapy for problem drinking reach hidden populations? *American Journal of Psychiatry* 2005; 162(12):2393.

13. Rainie H, Packel D. More online, doing more: 16 million newcomers gain Internet access in the last half of 2000 as women, minorities, and families with modest incomes continue to surge online. Pew Internet & American Life Project, 2001. Retrieved from http://www.pewinternet. org/Reports/2001/More-Online-Doing-More/ Report.aspx

14. Choo EK, Ranney ML, Aggarwal N, Boudreaux ED. A systematic review of emergency department technology-based behavioral health interventions. *Academic Emergency Medicine* 2012; 19(3):318–328.

15. Kaner EF, Beyer F, Dickinson HO, Pienaar E, Campbell F, Schlesinger C, et al. Effectiveness of brief alcohol interventions in primary care populations. *Cochrane Database of Systemic Reviews* 2007; (2):CD004148.

16. Pew Research Center's Internet & American Life Project. Pew Research Center's Internet & American Life Project, Digital Divide, Broadband, Social Networking, Mobile. Washington, DC; 2013.

17. Altman I, Taylor D. *Social Penetration: The Development of Interpersonal Relationships.* New York: Holt, Rinehart, and Winston; 1973.

18. Des Jarlais DC, Paone D, Milliken J, et al. Audio-computer interviewing to measure HIV risk behaviour among injecting drug users: A quasi-randomised trial. *Lancet* 1999; 353:1657–1661.

19. Hall SM, Sorensen JL, Loeb PC. Development and diffusion of a skills-training intervention. In Baker TB, Cannon DS (Eds.), *Assessment and Treatment of Addictive Disorders*. New York: Praeger Publishers; 1988, pp. 180–204.

20. Center on Addiction and Substance Abuse (CASA). Addiction medicine: Closing the gap between science and practice. A report by the National Center on Addiction and Substance Abuse; 2012.

21. McLellan AT, Carise D, Kleber HD. Can the national addiction treatment infrastructure support the public's demand for quality care? *Journal of Substance Abuse Treatment* 2003; 25:117–21.

22. Lamb S, Greenlick MR, McCarty D (Eds.). *Bridging the Gap between Practice and Research: Forging Partnerships with Community-Based Drug and Alcohol Treatment*. Washington, DC: Institute of Medicine; 1998.

23. Bickel WK, Marsch LA, Buchhalter A, Badger G. Computerized behavior therapy for opioid dependent outpatients: A randomized, controlled trial. *Experimental & Clinical Psychopharmacology* 2008; 16:132–143.

24. Carroll KM, Ball SA, Martino S, Nich C, Babuscio T, Gordon MA, et al. Computer-assisted cognitive-behavioral therapy for addiction: A randomized clinical trial of 'CBT4CBT'. *American Journal of Psychiatry* 2008; 165(7):881–888.

25. Marsch LA, Bickel WK. The efficacy of computer-based HIV/AIDS education for injection drug users. *American Journal of Health Behavior* 2004; 28(4):316–327.

26. Aronson ID, Marsch LA, Acosta MC. Using findings in multimedia learning to inform technology-based behavioral health interventions. *Translational Behavioral Medicine* 2012; 3(3):234–243.

27. Noar SM, Benac CN, Harris MS. Does tailoring matter? Meta-analytic review of tailored print health behavior change interventions. *Psychological Bulletin* 2007; 133:673–693.

28. Strecher VJ, McClure J, Alexander G, Chakraborty B, Nair V, Konkel J, et al. The role of engagement in a tailored Web-based smoking cessation program: Randomized controlled trial. *Journal of Medical Internet Research* 2008; 10(5):e36.

29. Bewick BM, Trusler K, Barkham M, Hill AJ, Cahill J, Mulhern B. The effectiveness of Web-based interventions designed to decrease alcohol consumption—A systematic review. *Preventive Medicine* 2008; 47:17–26.

30. Moore BA, Fazzino T, Garnet B, Cutter CJ, Barry DT. Computer-based interventions for drug use disorders: A systematic review. *Journal of Substance Abuse Treatment* 2011; 40(3):215–223.

31. Fry JP, Neff RA. Periodic prompts and reminders in health promotion and health behavior interventions: Systematic review. *Journal of Medical Internet Research* 2009; 11(2): e16.

32. Walters ST, Ondersma SJ, Ingersoll KS, Rodriguez M, Lerch J, Rossheim ME, et al. MAPIT: Development of a Web-based intervention targeting substance abuse treatment in the criminal justice system. *Journal of Substance Abuse Treatment* 2014; 46:60–65.

33. McKay JR. Continuing care research: What we've learned and where we're going. *Journal of Substance Abuse Treatment* 2009; 36(2):131–145.

34. Krebs P, Prochaska JO, Rossi JS. A meta-analysis of computer-tailored interventions for health behavior change. *Preventive Medicine* 2010; 51(3):214–221.

35. Chakraborty B, Murphy SA. Dynamic treatment regimes. *Annual Review of Statistical Applications* 2014; 1:1.1–1.18.

36. Riley W, Rivera D, Atienza A, Nilsen W, Allison S, Mermelstein R. Health behavior models in the age of mobile interventions: Are our theories up to the task? *Translational Behavioral Medicine* 2011; 1(1):53–71.

37. Muench F, Weiss RA, Kuerbis A, Morgenstern J. Developing a theory driven text messaging intervention for addiction care with user driven content. *Psychology of Addictive Behaviors* 2013; 21(1):315–321.

38. Cunningham JA, Wild TC, Cordingley J, Van Mierlo T, Humphreys K. A randomized controlled trial of an Internet-based intervention for alcohol abusers. *Addiction* 2009; 104(12):2023–2032.

39. Klein AA, Slaymaker VJ, Dugosh KL, McKay JR. Computerized continuing care support for alcohol and drug dependence: A preliminary analysis of usage and outcomes. *Journal of Substance Abuse Treatment* 2012; 42(1):25–34.

40. Andersson G, Cuijpers P. Internet-based and other computerized psychological treatments for adult depression: A meta-analysis. *Cognitive Behaviour Therapy* 2009; 38(4):196–205.

41. Christensen H, Griffiths KM, Farrer L. Adherence in Internet interventions for anxiety and depression: Systematic review. *Journal of Medical Internet Research* 2009; 11(2):e13.

42. Mohr DC, Cuijpers P, Lehman K. Supportive accountability: A model for providing human support to enhance adherence to eHealth interventions. *Journal of Medical Internet Research* 2011; 13(1):e30.

43. Villano CL, Rosenblum A, Magura S, Fong C. Improving treatment engagement and outcomes for cocaine-using methadone patients. *American Journal of Drug and Alcohol Abuse* 2002; 28:213–230.

44. Saitz R, Helmuth ED, Aromaa SE, Guard A, Belanger M, Rosenbloom DL. Web-based screening and brief intervention for the spectrum of alcohol problems. *Preventive Medicine* 2004; 39(5):969–975.

45. Doumas DM, Anderson L. Reducing alcohol use in first-year university students: Evaluation of a Web-based personalized feedback program. *Journal of College Counseling* 2009; 12(1):18–32.

46. Weitzel JA, Bernhardt JM, Usdan S, Mays D, Glanz K. Using wireless handheld computers and tailored text messaging to reduce negative consequences of drinking alcohol. *Journal of Studies on Alcohol & Drugs* 2007; 68(4):534–537.

47. Substance Abuse and Mental Health Services Administration (SAMHSA). Screening, brief intervention and referral to treatment (SBIRT) in behavioral healthcare; 2011. Retrieved from http://www.samhsa.gov/prevention/sbirt/SBIRTwhitepaper.pdf.

48. Babor T, McRee B, Kassebaum P, Grimaldi P, Ahmed K, Bray J. Screening, brief intervention, and referral to treatment (SBIRT). *Substance Abuse* 2007; 28(3):7–30.

49. Newton NC, Andrews G, Teesson M, Vogl LE. Delivering prevention for alcohol and cannabis using the Internet: A cluster randomised controlled trial. *Preventive Medicine.* 2009; 48(6):579–584.

50. Carey KB, Scott-Sheldon LAJ, Elliott JC, Garey L, Carey MP. Face-to-face versus computer-delivered alcohol interventions for college drinkers: A meta-analytic review, 1998 to 2010. *Clinical Psychology Review* 2012; 32(8):690–703.

51. White A, Kavanagh D, Stallman H, Klein B, Kay-Lambkin F, Proudfoot J, et al. Online alcohol interventions: A systematic review. *Journal of Medical Internet Research* 2010; 12(5):e62.

52. Khadjesari Z, Murray E, Hewitt C, Hartley S, Godfrey C. Can stand-alone computer-based interventions reduce alcohol consumption? A systematic review. *Addiction* 2011; 106:267–282.

53. Rooke S, Thorsteinsson E, Karpin A, Copeland J, Allsop D. Computer-delivered interventions for alcohol and tobacco use: A meta-analysis. *Addiction* 2010; 105(8):1381–1390.

54. Walters ST, Vader AM, Harris TR. A controlled trial of Web-based feedback for heavy drinking college students. *Prevention Science* 2007; 8(1):83–88.

55. Doumas DM, Kane CM, Navarro T, Roman J. Decreasing heavy drinking in first year students: Evaluation of a Web-based personalized feedback program administered during orientation. *Journal of College Counseling* 2011; 14(1):5–20.

56. Hustad JT, Barnett NP, Borsari B, Jackson KM. Web-based alcohol prevention for incoming college students: A randomized controlled trial. *Addictive Behaviors* 2010; 35(3):183–189.

57. Hester RK, Delaney HD, Campbell W. The college drinker's check-up: Outcomes of two randomized clinical trials of a computer-delivered intervention. *Psychology of Addictive Behaviors* 2012; 26(1):1–12.

58. Kypri K, Hallett J, Howat P, McManus A, Maycock B, Bowe S, et al. Randomized controlled trial of proactive Web-based alcohol screening and brief intervention for university students. *Archives of Internal Medicine* 2009; 169(16):1508–1514.

59. Kypri K, McCambridge J, Vater T, Bowe SJ, Saunders JB, Cunningham JA, et al. Web-based alcohol intervention for Māori university students: Double-blind, multi-site randomized controlled trial. *Addiction* 2013; 108(2): 331–338.

60. Riper H, Spek V, Boon B, Conijn B, Kramer J, Martin-Abello K, et al. Effectiveness of E-self-help interventions for curbing adult problem drinking: A meta-analysis. *Journal of Medical Internet Research* 2011; 13(2):e42.

61. Vernon ML. A review of computer-based alcohol problem services designed for the general public. *Journal of Substance Abuse Treatment* 2010; 38(3):203–211.

62. Maio RF, Shope JT, Blow FC, et al. A randomized controlled trial of an emergency department-based interactive computer program to prevent alcohol misuse among injured adolescents. *Annals of Emergency Medicine* 2005; 45:420–429.

63. Neumann T, Neuner B, Weiss-Gerlach E, et al. The effect of computerized tailored brief advice on at-risk drinking in subcritically injured trauma patients. *Journal of Trauma* 2006; 61:805–1814.

64. Trinks A, Festin K, Bendtsen P, Nilsen P. Reach and effectiveness of a computer-based alcohol intervention in a Swedish emergency room. *International Emergency Nursing* 2010; 18:138–146.

65. Walton MA, Chermack ST, Shope JT, et al. Effects of a brief intervention for reducing violence and alcohol misuse among adolescents: A randomized controlled trial. *JAMA* 2010; 304:527–535.

66. Murphy MK, Bijur PE, Rosenbloom D, Bernstein SL, Gallagher EJ. Feasibility of a computer-assisted alcohol SBIRT program in an urban emergency department: Patient and research staff perspectives. *Addiction Science & Clinical Practice* 2013; 8(1):1–10.

67. Cucciare MA, Weingardt KR, Ghaus S, Boden MT, Frayne SM. A randomized controlled trial of a Web-delivered brief alcohol intervention in Veterans Affairs primary care. *Journal of Studies on Alcohol and Drugs* 2013; 74(3):428.

68. Ondersma SJ, Svikis DS, Schuster CR. Computer-based brief intervention: A randomized trial with post-partum women. *American Journal of Preventive Medicine* 2007; 32:231–238.

69. Ondersma SJ, Svikis DS, Thacker LR, Beatty JR, Lockhart N. Computer-delivered screening and brief intervention (e-SBI) for postpartum drug use: A randomized trial. *Journal of Substance Abuse Treatment* 2014; 46:52–59.

70. Delrahim-Howlett K, Chambers CD, Clapp JD, Xu R, Duke K, Moyer RJ, et al. Web-based assessment and brief intervention for alcohol use in women of childbearing potential: A report of the primary findings. *Alcoholism, Clinical & Experimental Research* 2011; 35(7):1331–1338.

71. Elliott JC, Carey KB, & Bolles JR. Computer-based interventions for college drinking: A qualitative review. *Additive Behavior* 2008; 33:994–1005.

72. White RE. Health information technology will shift the medical care paradigm. *Journal of General Internal Medicine* 2008; 23(4):495–499.

73. Lewis MA, Neighbors C. Optimizing personalized normative feedback: The use of gender-specific referents. *Journal of Studies on Alcohol and Drugs* 2007; 68(2):228.

74. Chiauzzi E, Green TC, Lord S, Thum C, Goldstein M. My student body: A high-risk drinking prevention Web site for college students. *Journal of American College Health* 2005; 53(6):263–274.

75. Kypri K, McAnally HM. Randomized controlled trial of a Web-based primary care intervention for multiple health risk behaviors. *Preventive Medicine* 2005; 41(3):761–766.

76. Kypri K, Saunders JB, Williams SM, McGee RO, Langley JD, Cashell-Smith ML, et al. Web-based screening and brief intervention for hazardous drinking: A double-blind randomized controlled trial. *Addiction* 2004; 99(11):1410–1417.

77. Kypri K, Langley JD, Saunders JB, Cashell-Smith ML, Herbison P. Randomized controlled trial of Web-based alcohol screening and brief intervention in primary care. Archives of Internal Medicine 2008; 168(5):530.

78. Barnett NP, Murphy JG, Colby SM, Monti PM. Efficacy of counselor vs. computer-delivered intervention with mandated college students. *Addictive Behaviors* 2007; 32(11):2529–2548.

79. Butler LH, Correia CJ. Brief alcohol intervention with college student drinkers: Face-to-face versus computerized feedback. *Psychology of Addictive Behaviors* 2009; 23(1):163.

80. Kiluk BD, Sugarman DE, Nich C, Gibbons CR, Martino S, Rounsaville BJ, et al. A methodological analysis of randomized clinical trials of computer-assisted therapies for psychiatric disorders: Towards improved standards for an emerging field. *American Journal of Psychiatry* 2011; 168(8):790–799.

81. Portnoy DB, Scott-Sheldon LAJ, Johnson BT, Carey MP. Computer-delivered interventions for health promotion and behavioral risk reduction: A meta-analysis of 75 randomized controlled trials, 1988-2007. *Preventive Medicine* 2008; 47:3–16.

82. Cuijpers P, Marks IM, Van Straten A, Cavanagh K, Gega L, Andersson G. Computer-aided psychotherapy for anxiety disorders: A meta-analytic review. *Cognitive Behavior Therapy* 2009; 38:66–82.

83. Spek V, Cuijpers P, Nyklicek I, Riper H, Keyzer J, Pop V. Internet-based cognitive-behaviour therapy for symptoms of depression and anxiety: A meta-analysis. *Psychological Medicine* 2007; 37:319–338.

84. Litvin EB, Abrantes AM, Brown RA. Computer and mobile technology-based interventions for substance use disorders: An organizing framework. *Addictive Behaviors* 2013; 38:1747–1756.

85. Copeland J, Martin G. Web-based interventions for substance use disorders: A qualitative review. *Journal of Substance Abuse Treatment* 2004; 26:109–116.

86. Carroll KM, Rounsaville BJ. Computer-assisted therapy in psychiatry: Be brave—it's a new world. *Current Psychiatry Reports* 2010; 12:426–432.

87. Newman MG, Szkodny LE, Llera SJ, Przeworski A. A review of technology-assisted self-help and minimal contact therapies for anxiety and depression: Is human contact necessary for therapeutic efficacy? *Clinical Psychology Review* 2011; 31(1):89–103.

88. King VL, Stoller KB, Kidorf M, Kindborn K, Hursh S, Brady T, Brooner RK. Assessing the effectiveness of an Internet-based video conferencing platform for delivering intensified substance abuse counseling. *Journal of Substance Abuse Treatment* 2009; 36:331–338.

89. Budney AJ, Fearer S, Walker DD, et al. An initial trial of a computerized behavioral intervention for cannabis use disorder. *Drug & Alcohol Dependence* 2011; 115(1):74–79.

90. Chaple M, Sacks S, McKendrick K, Marsch LA, Belenko S, Leukefeld C, et al. Feasibility of a computerized intervention for offenders with substance use disorders. *Journal of Experimental Criminology* 2014; 10:105–127.

91. Higgins ST, Sigmon SC, Wong CJ, Heil SH, Badger GJ, Donham R, et al. Community reinforcement therapy for cocaine-dependent outpatients. *Archives of General Psychiatry* 2003; 60:1043–1052.

92. Smith JE, Meyers RJ, Miller WR. The community reinforcement approach to the treatment of substance use disorders. *American Journal on Addictions* 2001; 10:S51–S59.

93. Petry NM, Peirce JM, Stitzer ML, Blaine J, Roll JM, Cohen A, et al. Effect of prize-based incentives on outcomes in stimulant abusers in outpatient psychosocial treatment programs: A National Drug Abuse Treatment Clinical Trials Network study. *Archives of General Psychiatry* 2005; 62:1148–1156.

94. Campbell ANC, Nunes EV, Matthews AG, Stitzer M, Miele GM, Polsky D, et al. Internet-delivered treatment for substance abuse: A multi-site randomized controlled clinical trial. *American Journal of Psychiatry* 2014; 171(6):683–690.

95. Carroll KM, Ball SA, Martino S, Nich C, Babuscio TA, Rounsaville BJ. Enduring effects of a computer-assisted training program for cognitive behavioral therapy: A 6-month follow-up of 'CBT4CBT'. *Drug & Alcohol Dependence* 2009; 100(1-2):178–181.

96. Olmstead TA, Ostrow CD, Carroll KM. Cost-effectiveness of computer-assisted training in cognitive-behavioral therapy as an adjunct to standard care for addiction. *Drug & Alcohol Dependence* 2010; 110(3):200–207.

97. Moore BA, Fazzino T, Barry DT, et al. The Recovery Line: A pilot trial of automated, telephone-based treatment for continued drug use in methadone maintenance. *Journal of Substance Abuse Treatment* 2013; 45(1):63–69

98. Simpson DD, Joe GW, Brown BS. Treatment retention and follow-up outcomes in the Drug Abuse Treatment Outcome Study (DATOS). *Psychology of Addictive Behaviors* 1997; 11(4):294–307.

99. McTavish FM, Chih MY, Shah D, Gustafson DH. How patients recovering from alcoholism use a smartphone intervention. *Journal of Dual Diagnosis* 2012; 8(4):294–304.

100. Budney AJ, Higgins ST: Therapy manuals for drug addiction, a community reinforcement plus vouchers approach: Treating cocaine addiction. Rockville, MD, National Institute on Drug Abuse, 1998.

101. Higgins ST, Sigmon SC, Wong CJ, Heil SH, Badger GJ, Donham R, et al. Community reinforcement therapy for cocaine-dependent outpatients. *Archives of General Psychiatry* 2003; 60:1043–1052.

102. Campbell ANC, Nunes EV, Miele GM, Matthews A, Polsky D, Ghitza U, et al. Design and methodological considerations of an effectiveness trial of a computer-assisted intervention: An example from the NIDA Clinical Trials Network. *Contemporary Clinical Trials* 2012; 33(2):386–395.

103. Berger ML, Dreyer N, Anderson F, Towse A, Sedrakyan A, Normand S. Prospective observational studies to assess comparative effectiveness: The ISPOR Good Research Practices Task Force Report. *Value in Health* 2012; 15:217–230.

104. Concato J, Shah N, Horwitz RI. Randomized, controlled trials, observational studies and the hierarchy of research designs. *New England Journal of Medicine* 2000; 342:1887–1892.

105. Santen RJ, Allred DC, Ardoin SP, Archer DF, Boyd N, Braunstein GD, et al. Postmenopausal hormone therapy: An endocrine society scientific statement. *Journal of Clinical Endocrinology and Metabolism* 2010; 95(7):S1-S66.

106. Boyer EW, Fletcher R, Fay RJ, Smelson D, Ziedonis D, Picard RW. Preliminary efforts directed toward the detection of craving of illicit substances: The iHeal project. *Journal of Medical Toxicology* 2012; 8(1):5–9.

107. Fletcher RR, Tam S, Omojola O, Redemske R, Kwan, J. Wearable sensor platform and mobile application for use in cognitive behavioral therapy for drug addiction and PTSD. Paper presented at the Engineering in Medicine and Biology Society, EMBC, 2011 Annual International Conference of the IEEE.

108. Raij B, Blitz P, Ali A, Fisk S, French B, Mitra S, et al. mStress: Supporting continuous collection of objective and subjective measures of psychosocial stress on mobile devices. Technical Report No. CS-10-004. Department of Computer Science, University of Memphis, 2010.

109. Aharonovich E, Greenstein E, O'Leary A, Johnston B, Seol SG, Hasin DS. HealthCall: Technology-based extension of motivational interviewing to reduce non-injection drug use in HIV primary care patients—a pilot study. *AIDS Care* 2012; 24(12):1461–1469.

110. Hasin DS, Aharonovich E, O'Leary A, Greenstein E, Pavlicova M, Arunajadai S, et al. Reducing heavy drinking in HIV primary care: A randomized trial of brief intervention, with and without technological enhancement. *Addiction* 2013; 108(7):1230–1240.

5

Using Behavioral Intervention Technologies to Reduce the Burden of Mood and Anxiety Disorders

STEPHEN M. SCHUELLER, MIRAJ CHOKSHI, AND DAVID C. MOHR

INTRODUCTION

Roughly half of all Americans will meet criteria for a mental disorder at some point in their life (1). The most common of these disorders are mood and anxiety disorders, with lifetime prevalence of 20.8% and 28.8%, respectively (1). Although effective, evidence-based interventions for these disorders exist, many people in need of services do not receive them (1). For example, in the United States, only two-thirds of those who experience a major depressive episode each year receive some form of treatment (2). Of those who do receive psychotherapy, only a small portion receive evidence-based practices or adequate care (3,4). National trends indicate that the use of psychotherapy has dropped within outpatient mental health facilities from 53.6% in 1998 to 43.1% in 2007 (5). Thus, it is critical to develop resources to promote the delivery of evidence-based practices.

Reducing the burden of mental illness, however, might not require creating entirely new interventions or principles per se, but focusing on new intervention paradigms that expand the modes of dissemination of evidence-based practices to ensure that more people benefit from the knowledge psychologists have developed (6–8). Current interventions rely almost entirely on *consumable interventions,* or interventions that once used can never benefit another person (9). Consumable interventions are interventions that are "used up" when they are provided to a patient. For example, a dose of medication or an hour of a therapist's time benefits only the patient receiving each and thus treatment costs increase with each additional patient served. Given the substantial burden of disease caused by mood and anxiety disorders, more work needs to focus on developing *non-consumable interventions,* or interventions whereby the cost per patient can actually decrease with each person served. For non-consumable interventions, the marginal cost, that is, the cost of providing the intervention to one more individual, eventually approaches zero (9). This is especially critical in light of recent changes in healthcare systems (e.g., the 2010 Affordable Care Act in the United States [10]) that expand coverage for mental health services and thus will place an additional burden on the system.

The provision of non-consumable interventions requires creating resources that can be delivered with minimal provider involvement; possibly even those that might be delivered with no human involvement whatsoever. Behavioral intervention technologies (BITs) could expand the availability of effective and scalable non-consumable interventions. BITs are applications of behavioral intervention theories and strategies implemented through the use of technology features (e.g., Internet sites, mobile applications, or apps, text messaging) that target behaviors in support of health and mental health (11). In this chapter, we focus on the empirical support for using BITs to address mood and anxiety disorders. A growing body of evidence suggests that BITs are effective at reducing the symptoms of depression and anxiety (12,13), useful across the spectrum of prevention (14), intervention (15), and recovery maintenance (16) and in a variety of settings (e.g., schools, communities, medical clinics). We explore this evidence base in more detail and illustrate features unique to BITs that are essential to consider when designing, implementing, and evaluating these technologies for use with mood and anxiety disorders.

First, we will provide a review and summary of existing BITs that have been used for the treatment and prevention of mood and anxiety disorders. Second, we will present existing technologies that have yet to undergo formal evaluation for use with clinical populations but could be applied to benefit treatment and prevention. Lastly, we will highlight a few key future directions that need to be considered in order to shape the development and implementation of BITs designed to address mood and anxiety disorders.

BITS FOR MOOD DISORDERS

A number of evidence-based interventions for mood disorders have been converted into BITs. They offer effective and inexpensive alternatives to non-technology-based treatments (17–19). These BITs present a therapeutic strategy or a combination of strategies relevant to the treatment or prevention of mood disorders. Early efforts often translated didactic content to computer or Web-based dissemination. More recent efforts, however, have used other technologies to find creative ways to provide and reinforce the behavior change principles underlying the treatment of mood disorders (e.g., text messaging [20,21] and smartphone applications [22]).

Psychoeducation as didactic content is an important component of many empirically supported interventions for mood disorders. Indeed, didactic content alone (e.g., BluePages) can improve patient's knowledge of treatment options for depression (23). One of the first randomized, controlled trials of an Internet site for the treatment of depression demonstrated a common strategy for adapting didactic content for Web dissemination (24). Existing content from cognitive-behavioral therapy group manuals (25,26) was modified to create self-guided tutorials that taught depression management skills. The website presented a book-like interaction that provided self-guided tutorials to help users acquire antidepressant skills. This structure allowed participants to navigate through the topics at their own pace. Participants who received the website, however, did not demonstrate significant

decreases in depressive symptoms compared to a control group that received a link to a healthcare website. This lack of significant results is not surprising, given that participants reported low usage of the intervention website (modal number of sessions = 1; mean = 2.6 [24]).

In an effort to overcome low usage rates, recent BITs that provide didactic content have been made more structured and interactive (e.g., MoodGYM [23,27]) or added coach support to otherwise self-guided websites (28). Methods of displaying and interacting with didactic content span passive multimedia experiences, from explanatory videos or animation (29–31) to interactive game elements (32,33).

Cognitive-behavioral therapy (CBT) is the most frequently used therapeutic approach in BITs for mood disorders (e.g., MoodGYM [23]; see references 12 and 13 for reviews). A key strategy used in CBT for mood disorders is cognitive restructuring, the process of identifying and modifying automatic negative thoughts. In face-to-face therapy, cognitive restructuring is typically supported through the use of paper-and-pencil thought records. Interactive features of BITs allow novel methods to perform this strategy. In one example, participants received a Thought Helper tool after they had been taught the basics of cognitive restructuring (24). Participants could enter a negative thought into a text box and then select from a predefined list of negative thoughts that best matched their own. After selecting this negative thought, the tool returned a list of possible positive counterthoughts and encouraged participants to create a personalized positive counterthought to correspond to their initial entry. Although a therapist can do this within a session, the technology-based approach transcends the therapist–client interaction by providing automated feedback that is streamlined and personalized yet delivered outside of the therapy room.

Gamification, the use of game elements in a ç context, has also been applied to cognitive restructuring (32). Games can be very engaging, and the popularity and ubiquity of games contained within various technological mediums (i.e., console-based video games, online games, mobile app games, social games) has made "gamifying" elements popular in BITs for mental health. An example is SPARX (Smart, Positive, Active, Realistic, X-factor thoughts), an interactive game for depressed youth. Players are immersed in a 3D fantasy world where they must battle GNATs (Gloomy Negative Automatic Thoughts) by shooting them down and classifying them as specific kinds of negative thoughts (31). SPARX provided in youth clinics, schools, and primary care was not inferior to treatment as usual and resulted in greater reductions in depressive symptoms. Rates of adherence to SPARX were good, with 86% of participants completing at least four of the seven modules and 60% completing all seven modules (31).

Another effective strategy to treat mood disorders is increasing pleasant activities (34). Increasing pleasant activities forms the basis of behavioral activation (35), and focusing on positive activities is a major component of positive psychotherapy (36). A preliminary study of computerized behavioral activation for the treatment of depression provided video content and interactive lessons to teach behavioral activation skills (37). Individuals with moderate to severe depression ($N = 15$) accessed the program by visiting a therapy clinic where rooms contained a workstation with the program preloaded onto it. Participants experienced a large ($d = 2.17$) and significant decrease in depressive symptoms, as measured by the Beck Depression Inventory, that was maintained at the 6-month follow-up assessment (37). Although sessions lasted an average of 45 minutes, only 7.84 minutes (on average) involved active interaction with study personnel. Thus, this program demonstrates that the workflow of a typical therapy session can be translated and delivered via a computer program for some types of therapy (i.e., behavioral activation).

Self-monitoring is another frequent strategy used in BITs for mood disorders. Self-monitoring is appealing to deploy via mobile phones or other devices that people carry throughout the day, because it allows people to conduct self-monitoring in the moment rather than retrospectively. Furthermore, people can use technologies in several ways (take pictures, send text messages, check in to mobile apps) that may be useful for self-monitoring. In a study of adolescents with mild or moderate depressive symptoms, a mobile app that promoted self-monitoring increased emotional self-awareness and decreased depressive symptoms (38). Participants monitored a variety of aspects, including activities, location, people,

mood, stressful events and reactions to those events, substance use, sleep, exercise, and diet. Promoting emotional self-awareness appeared to be an important mechanism of increased self-monitoring as greater increases in emotional self-awareness corresponded to greater decreases in depressive symptoms.

Similarly, other BITs can use passively collected data to illustrate links between one's behavior and mood. Combining data collected from ecological momentary assessment self-reports of mood and embedded sensors with machine learning techniques, researchers may be able to demonstrate the relationships between a patient's mood, emotions, states, activities, and environmental context (22). Mobilyze is a smartphone application that uses context-sensing and machine learning to predict a patient's mood and deliver just-in-time interventions responsive to low mood states (22). In a pilot trial, eight adults with major depressive disorder (MDD) received the mobile app and used it for an 8-week period. Participants who used this app reported significant decreases in depressive symptoms and were less likely to meet criteria for MDD at follow-up. Although, the application showed promise at predicting patient states (e.g., location, activity, social context), the prediction of mood was less promising. Further research is needed to determine the contextual features that best predict mood and indicate that some intervention might be warranted. Although it is likely that this is variable and individual-specific, given enough data, statistical modeling might be able to create individualized models that overcome this limitation. Thus, advances in technology and the use of novel analytic strategies might help solve this complicated problem.

Currently, most of the researched BITs for mood disorders use cognitive-behavioral principles as the basis for their programs (12). Cognitive-behavioral strategies lend themselves to the didactic and tool-based presentation encouraged by BITs. More recent BITs are starting to use principles from other therapeutic orientations (e.g., psychodynamic [39]), but more work is needed in areas outside of cognitive-behavioral treatments.

BITs for Anxiety Disorders

BITs for anxiety disorders are less developed and researched than BITs for mood disorders. Similar to BITs for mood disorders, many of the BITs for anxiety disorders, especially the early efforts, focused on using computers, the Internet, and other devices to deliver psychoeducational content or therapeutic messages to reduce symptoms of anxiety. Not surprisingly, these more passive interventions promote similar benefits to those seen in depressive symptoms, with small-to-moderate effects on symptoms of anxiety (12) and with similar limitations, including difficulties engaging and maintaining participants in large-scale implementation in community settings (27).

A critical element in the treatment of anxiety is exposure. Exposure therapy is one of the most well-supported evidence-based techniques for the treatment of anxiety disorders (40). Therapies that include exposure are considerably more effective for several anxiety disorders, including panic disorder (41), phobias (42), and obsessive-compulsive disorder (43). BITs that help support the creation and execution of successful exposure assignments can significantly enhance the treatment of anxiety disorders (44,45). Exposures for anxiety disorders include both in vivo and imaginal exposures that put people in real or imagined contexts to activate relevant fear structures and support learning to reduce anxiety. Imaginal exposure is often used when in vivo work cannot be conducted. BITs, however, can help create environments or situations that address specific aspects of a person's avoidance hierarchy that help bridge the gap between imaginal and in vivo exposure. This is often accomplished through virtual-reality treatment in which virtual environments are created in the service of exposure.

Research supports that virtual-reality exposure therapy is an effective treatment option for anxiety disorders. A meta-analysis of 13 studies found that virtual-reality exposure therapy produced large effect sizes when compared to control conditions ($d = 1.11$) and even outperformed in vivo treatments when directly compared ($d = 0.35$) (46). One proposed explanation was that virtual-reality treatments allow more personalized tailoring of the exposure situation to a patient's specific fear hierarchy. Indeed, virtual-reality exposure provides clinicians with a high degree of control over the material presented to a patient and can create experiences that are difficult or unpredictable to produce in the real world. For example, in virtual-reality exposure therapy for flying phobias

a patient can be subjected to a virtual plane flight that might tap their specific fears (i.e., flying during a storm with extreme turbulence), or a combat veteran with PTSD can be entered into a virtual warzone (47).

BITs can also help address psychological processes that contribute to anxiety disorders. A prime example is computer-guided attention retraining (48), which aims to reduce symptoms of anxiety through altering underlying cognitive biases believed to be a basic cognitive vulnerability for anxiety disorders (49). In the attention modification program (AMP), participants are trained through an attention task that pairs a probe with neutral faces to then direct their attention away from threatening faces. This paradigm effectively reduces symptoms of social phobia compared to placebo attention retraining when conducted in a controlled laboratory setting (49–51), but it has not produced significant differences relative to a control when disseminated via the Internet for home-based treatment (52). Although results of AMP are promising in short-term laboratory studies, more work needs to support its use for sustained benefits in real-world settings.

Lastly, an important aspect of treatment for anxiety disorder is increasing one's capacity to respond appropriately and adaptively to anxiety-provoking cues or situations in the environment. BITs facilitate this goal through repeated prompting and assessment and can monitor and provide feedback on aspects that a person might not be aware of (e.g., heart rate [53]). A palmtop computer program for the treatment of anxiety included a module that prompted a patient to record physiological, cognitive, or situational anxiety cues and to respond with appropriate coping strategies in response to initial signs of worry (54). This program was integrated into group treatment for social phobia to facilitate additional practice of skills. Outcome data were only presented for a single case; however, this patient benefited greatly, showing decreases in percentage of the day spent worrying and in social phobia symptoms, and a reduction in anxiety on the State-Trait Anxiety Inventory such that it was within a standard deviation of the mean for normative samples (54). In another illustration of a BIT to supplement treatment in the hopes of improving its efficacy, a portable heart-rate variability biofeedback device led to improved response for patients currently receiving medication or psychotherapy for anxiety (55).

Prevention

While the majority of research has focused on the treatment of depression and anxiety, BITs also hold considerable potential as tools for primary prevention of depression and anxiety, as well as prevention of recurrence, or maintenance of treatment gains. The Institute of Medicine's (IOM) report on preventing mental disorders presented a continuum of care options that spans promotion to recovery maintenance (56). BITs at each of these levels can expand their ability to improve the mental health of the population. Additionally, BITs can be integrated into existing systems using stepped-care models in which patients are initially provided unsupported, automated resources; those who do not respond receive programs supported by more highly trained individuals (first paraprofessionals, then professionals).

The promotion of positive mental health is a major focus of many BITs. Within psychology, this is the goal of the subfield of positive psychology (57). A majority of mobile apps that provide psychological guidance are based on a wellness perspective or positive psychology principles (58). One major reason for this is that, especially in the United States, many mental health apps are marketed directly to consumers and a wellness perspective may be more appealing (and profitable) than focus on mental illness and dysfunction. Fortunately, as emphasized by the IOM's continuum, promotion is relevant across the whole spectrum of interventions, and research indicates that methods that address positive thoughts, emotions, and behaviors also lead to significant reductions in depressive symptoms (59).

Increasing one's well-being might confer preventive benefits as well, as building psychological resources may ensure that individuals never experience a mood disorder in the first place (60). Indeed, an Internet site advertised to promote mental well-being to self-recruited users of a national health services website was able to boost scores on psychological well-being compared to scores for control group participants (19). BITs can be useful tools for preventing depression, as they are scalable and low-cost options, attractive for widespread dissemination (61), and depression prevention trials require large samples to find

significant reductions in incidence (62). Although cost-effectiveness data for Internet sites designed for mental health are still relatively lacking (63), the few studies addressing costs for the treatment of mood and anxiety disorders suggest favorable cost-benefit ratios compared to treatment as usual in primary care (64) and waiting lists in the general population (65). In terms of the scalability of these resources, once a site is developed it can be adapted and translated for a fraction of initial development costs. A study evaluating the cost-effectiveness of translating BluePages, a psychoeducational website designed to reduce and prevent anxiety and depression, into Norwegian found that it could be accomplished for 27% of the original development costs and that this was less than the cost assigned to one gained quality-adjusted life year (18). Based on the efficacy of this program and the cost, it would only be necessary to treat 46 subjects with depression to reach a break-even point (18).

Indeed, several examples of effective prevention programs exist. Mood Memos was a fully automated depression prevention program for participants with subthreshold depressive symptoms (14). Participants received weekly e-mails related to depression, with intervention participants receiving self-help strategies and control participants receiving general information. Intervention group participants reported significantly lower symptoms of depression after 6 weeks than those of control participants. This difference, however, was small ($d = 0.17$), and no significant differences were found in reductions of incidence. Nevertheless, given the low cost and ease of dissemination of such programs, they remain promising avenues for prevention efforts.

Screening

In the IOM framework, treatment is divided into case identification and treatment. BITs can be used as a screening tool to engage people in psychological services that might not otherwise seek treatment. In an Internet site for smoking cessation, only one out of three of the visitors to the site had previously used any healthcare resources prior to the Web intervention (66). Internet-based screening tools for depression can reach large portions of the population and provide tailored feedback that might encourage subsequent treatment seeking. One such screening tool recruited participants worldwide using ads delivered on the

Google search engine (67). During a 1-year period 24,965 participants provided enough data to evaluate the presence of a major depressive episode. Of these participants, 66.6% screened positive for a current major depressive episode and 7.8% indicated a suicide attempt in the past 2 weeks. Just over half of the participants (53.1%) reported seeking help for depression at some point in their lives and only a quarter of the participants with a current major depressive episode were receiving treatment. Unfortunately, participants in this study only received screening for depression and were offered no intervention resources. Such cases, where high response rates and data indicate a high need, represent ideal venues for deploying Internet interventions to provide a basic level of care. This study provides an example for how BITs may not replace traditional modes of intervention delivery, but instead open up a new market to serve individuals who are being untreated, thus reducing health disparities worldwide (9).

BITs can also significantly improve upon screening processes. For example, computerized adaptive testing has been developed that significantly reduces patient and clinician burden while boosting diagnostic accuracy (68). This research team showed that with computerized adaptive testing 12 items (that took 2 minutes 17 seconds per patient to administer) could produce sufficient information to diagnose depression while drawing from a bank of 389 depression items (68). Quick, efficient, diagnostic methods such as computerized adaptive testing can be integrated into Internet resources, primary care clinics, or other non-mental healthcare settings where populations can access BITs when indicated to drastically expand those reached by mental health services.

Recovery Support

BITs can also be used to follow up successful treatment and ensure that patients have access to resources to reduce the likelihood of subsequent episodes of mood or anxiety disorders. In one example, brief Internet chat groups were organized for patients following discharge from inpatient psychiatric care. Participants in the intervention group, who participated in the online chat groups, were significantly less likely than control participants to experience relapse (69). Interestingly, however, chat participants were less likely to use outpatient psychotherapy services following their

discharge, and the lowest rates of relapse were found in chat participants who did not engage in outpatient treatment (69). Given the relative cost of online chat groups vs. outpatient therapy, it is worth investigating and replicating this finding in diverse groups.

Another trial found that an Internet-based transdiagnostic treatment consisting of self-management lessons, online symptom monitoring, asynchronous coach communication, and an online support group helped reduce symptom deterioration and improve remission compared to treatment as usual following discharge from an inpatient hospitalization (16). BITs can be designed to be consistent with techniques and content from treatment and used to maintain gains and support transition to independent self-management of one's condition. Elucidating an evidence base for BITs for the maintenance phase remains an important area for future work.

Deployment Settings for BITs

Just as BITs are applied across the continuum of need for the promotion of well-being, prevention, treatment, and recovery maintenance of mood disorders and anxiety they can also be implemented in a variety of settings. BITs can serve as contained intervention or treatment tools that can be used as stand-alone resources by consumers or as an augment to existing clinical care. This self-contained nature of BIT resources allow them to be deployed directly to the general population (e.g., 19,27) or to be provided by practitioners—even those with little or no training in the delivery of evidence-based psychological practices (70,71).

As mood disorders lead to a disruption of functioning that impacts students' academic achievement and interpersonal interactions (72), schools are motivated to provide tools that improve the emotional health of their students. In the YouthMood Project, students accessed a previously validated Internet-based CBT program for depression during a class period once a week for 5 weeks (73). The purpose of this study was to examine adherence to the program, as it was investigating the ability of an Internet intervention to provide easy-access services to the student body. Teachers acted as supports for the program by offering information, support, and referral advice when warranted but provided no other psychosocial intervention. Completion of the program in the school setting was significantly higher than in a comparison condition that consisted of a community sample accessing the website on their own with no support; participants from the school-based sample completed three times as many exercises (9.38 vs. 3.10 [73]). Although the impact on depressive symptoms was not reported, this initiative used the effective and well-validated MoodGYM website (18,23,27).

BITs integrated into existing healthcare systems can greatly expand the scope of services provided. The U.K. National Health Service (NHS) and the National Institute of Clinical Excellence have adopted an online website as an evidence-based treatment for depression and anxiety (74) that has demonstrated efficacy in primary and specialized care settings (75–77). Beating the Blues is subsidized by the NHS and made available for free with a referral from one's general practitioner or for a fee for anyone else interested in the program. The Internet site includes 8 hour-long, interactive lessons and homework assignments based on cognitive-behavioral practices. Primary health professionals provide emergency aid, but mental health treatment is provided completely through the fully automated site (76,77).

In another example of services within primary care, adolescents (14–21 years of age) with subthreshold symptoms of depression as identified by their primary care provider were randomly assigned to receive an Internet intervention in combination with either brief advice or motivational interviewing (78). Both groups experienced decreases in depressive symptoms during the 12-week trial period, and the motivational interviewing group was significantly less likely to experience a subsequent major depressive episode. In both interventions, the physician's time delivering the intervention was brief (1.25 hours training via a video, 1–2 minutes to provide brief advice, 5–10 minutes to provide motivational interviewing).

Additionally, services can be provided to those seeking care in other, less formal, settings. One study examined the effect of providing people who called a national helpline service with a 6-week automated Internet-based CBT program (BluePages and MoodGYM) (71). Helpline workers received minimal training in the delivery of mental health resources; many people who call helplines do not expect to receive any services directly from the helpline. Callers who received the Internet intervention experienced a significant reduction in depressive symptoms relative to those who did not (71).

Lastly, BITs can also be deployed in traditional behavioral health treatment settings to improve individual quality of care. For the treatment of mood and anxiety disorders, these BITs are often aimed at increasing engagement in the therapy process and practice of therapy skills. BIT approaches can provide a different therapeutic experience than one can provide in standard face-to-face therapy. gNats Island is a computer game developed to support face-to-face CBT therapy by providing an opportunity for clinicians and interventions to sit side by side as patient's explore an interactive world that reinforces CBT lessons (79). The vast majority of clinicians who used this game reported believing it would be very to extremely useful in their work.

HARNESSING NEW TECHNOLOGIES TO ADVANCE THE TREATMENT OF MOOD AND ANXIETY DISORDERS

The aim of BITs is to translate clinical interventions into digital formats in order to achieve treatment aims of altering affect, behaviors, and cognitions to reduce symptoms of anxiety and depression. As we reviewed, most early BITs did so by delivering didactic content or simple tools through computers or Internet sites. This was effective at creating interventions that could help transcend space and time and deliver resources to people where no others existed and could be available 24 hours a day, at a time and place that is convenient. The next generation of BITs, however, should integrate behavior change principles to represent a synthesis of psychological theory and technological sophistication (80). In this section, we move beyond evidence-based practices to focus on novel lines of research that further expand treatment options.

Rapidly developing technologies are opening new avenues for addressing mood and anxiety disorders. We review here recent technologies that have potential for use in treatment for mood and anxiety disorders, but that currently lack empirical evidence supporting their use. We believe the most efficacious BITs for mood and anxiety disorders will continue to push the boundaries of behavioral theory with creative applications of relevant technologies. Thus, highlighting potential lines of research with applications for treatment is critical to guide the development of the next generation of interventions.

A characteristic of mood and anxiety disorders is that mood or anxiety tends to be a predominant state within the individual. Mood states fluctuate over time such that problematic levels of depression or anxiety are not always present. As such, an open empirical question is whether knowledge of one's current affective state can improve the efficacy of interventions. Recent emerging technologies have focused on diverse strategies to detect individuals' mood states. Researchers are increasingly investigating ways to use embedded sensors (e.g., accelerometers, Bluetooth sensors, video cameras, microphones, light sensors) and passive recording of behavioral data such as call logs, messages sent, or application usage to improve mental health and provide "just-in-time" ecological momentary interventions (e.g., 2,81,82). Our research team is currently updating early work on context-sensing applications for the treatment of depression (22). *Context-sensing* refers to the use of embedded sensors within smartphones to infer information (e.g., location, time, weather, activity) that might be useful in the prediction of mood and personalization of treatment recommendations. The next generation of BITs for mood and anxiety disorders might not only make use of self-reports of mood and anxiety symptoms but also provide feedback to a patient as to the prediction of what symptoms they might be experiencing based on other contextual information. Furthermore, sensors might become commonplace in more places than just smartphones, as several research teams are investigating the user of home and body sensor networks to gather more information about people and their behavior in naturalistic settings (e.g., 53,83–85).

Advances in natural language processing and machine learning have led to the development of virtual communication partners to aid in the treatment of mood and anxiety disorders. These "partners" have been deployed as training tools for new therapists (86) and explored as alternatives to face-to-face therapy when barriers prevent access (87). In the treatment of PTSD, these virtual partners can guide patients through exposure therapy and mimic the typically therapist-led process

of processing trauma narratives within sessions (87). Our research team is currently developing and evaluating virtual communication partners to teach assertiveness skills that can be practiced in virtual role-play within challenging situations, with the hope of reducing symptoms of depression and anxiety. Although, the current state of natural language processing limits the scope of interactions that can be programmed, virtual agents remain a promising avenue for future BITs for mood and anxiety disorders (see also Chapter 10, this volume).

FUTURE DIRECTIONS AND CONCLUSIONS

BITs show great promise for the treatment of mood and anxiety disorders. A key obstacle facing mental healthcare is how to provide effective and scalable interventions to support individuals' health behaviors across multiple settings. Each year in the United States approximately 40 million adults will experience an anxiety disorder and 20.9 million will experience a mood disorder (1). In the Affordable Care Act (10), essential health benefits for all Americans include mental health disorder services, including behavioral health services, preventive health and wellness services, and chronic disease management. Unfortunately, given the limited number of trained health professionals in the United States, it is unlikely that this burden will be addressed by face-to-face services provided by trained professionals alone. Behavioral intervention technologies address this problem by offering low-cost, scalable and innovative platforms for delivery of novel interventions to address aspects of mood and anxiety disorders.

Development of effective and scalable BITs is a collaborative process. Professionals with expertise in behavior change principles must team up with those having expertise in the design, evaluation, and implementation of technology to create the next generation of BITs. Elicitation of feedback from target end-users in all phases of design, development, and evaluation helps ensure that BITs are engaging and will be used by the intended audience. As technology develops and user expectations change, BITs must continue to evolve, to put the latest technology in the hands of consumers. More work needs to be done to leverage the unique expertise of psychologists, engineers, computer scientists, and others working in this area to create BITs that are usable and perceived as useful, and that produce positive change for those suffering from mood and anxiety disorders. Concerted effort toward this goal can help actualize the potential of BITs to be an important resource in the portfolio of reducing the burden of mood and anxiety disorders worldwide.

REFERENCES

1. Kessler RC, Chiu WT, Demler O, Merikangas KR, Walters EE. Prevalence, severity, and comorbidity of 12-month DSM-IV disorders in the National Comobidity Survey replication. *Archives of General Psychiatry* 2005; 62:617–627.
2. Office of Applied Studies. *Results from the 2007 National Survey on Drug Use and Health: National findings* (DHHS Publication No. SMA 08-4343, NSDUH Series H-34). Rockville, MD: Substance Abuse and Mental Health Services Administration (SAMHSA); 2008. Retrieved from http://oas.samhsa.gov.
3. Fullerton CA, Busch AB, Normand SLT, McGuire TG, Epstein AM. Ten-year trends in quality of care and spending for depression: 1996 through 2005. *Archives of General Psychiatry* 2011; 68:1218–1226.
4. Marcus SC, Olfson M. National trends in the treatment for depression from 1998 to 2007. *Archives of General Psychiatry* 2010; 67:1265–1273.
5. Olfson M, Marcus SC. National trends in outpatient psychotherapy. *American Journal of Psychiatry* 2010; 167:1456–1463.
6. Christensen A, Miller WR, Muñoz RF. Paraprofessionals, partners, peers, paraphernalia, and print: Expanding mental health service delivery. *Professional Psychology* 1978; 9:249–270.
7. Kazdin AE, Blase SL. Rebooting psychotherapy research and practice to reduce the burden of mental illness. *Perspectives on Psychological Science* 2011; 6:21–37.
8. Simon GE, Ludman EJ. It's time for disruptive innovation in psychotherapy. *Lancet* 2009; 374:594–595.
9. Muñoz RF. Using evidence-based Internet interventions to reduce health disparities worldwide. *Journal of Medical Internet Research* 2010; 12:e60.
10. Patient Protection and Affordable Care Act. 2010. Retrieved from http://www.gpo.gov/fdsys/pkg/PLAW-111publ148/html/PLAW-111publ148.htm.
11. Mohr DC, Burns MN, Schueller SM, Clarke G, Klinkman M. Behavioral intervention technologies: Evidence review and recommendations for future research. *General Hospital Psychiatry* 2013; 35:332–338.
12. Andersson G, Cuijpers P. Internet-based and other computerize psychological treatments for adult depression: a meta-analysis. *Cognitive Behaviour Therapy* 2009; 38:196–205.
13. Cuijpers P, Marks IM, van Straten A, Cavanagh K, Gega L, Andersson G. Computer-aided psychotherapy for anxiety disorders: A meta-analytic review. *Cognitive Behaviour Therapy* 2009; 38:66–82.
14. Morgan AJ, Jorm AF, Mackinnon AJ. Email-based promotion of self-help for subthreshold depression: Mood Memos randomised controlled trial.*British Journal of Psychiatry* 2012; 200:412–418.
15. Donker T, Bennett K, Bennett A, Mackinnon A, can Straten A, et al. Internet-delivered interpersonal psychotherapy versus Internet-delivered cognitive behavioral therapy for adults with depressive symptoms. Randomized controlled noninferiority trial. *Journal of Medical Internet Research* 2013; 15:e82.
16. Ebert D, Tarnowski T, Gollwitzer M, Sieland B, Berking M. A transdiagnostic Internet-based maintenance treatment enhances the stability of outcome after inpatient cognitive behavioral therapy: A randomized controlled trial. *Psychotherapy and Psychosomatics* 2013; 82:246–256.
17. Andersson G, Cuijpers P, Carlbring P, Lindefors N. Effects of Internet-delivered cognitive behaviour therapy for anxiety and mood disorders. *Review Series Psychiatry* 2007; 9:9–14.
18. Lintvedt OK, Griffiths KM, Eisemann M, Waterloo K. Evaluating the translation process of an Internet-based self-help intervention for prevention of depression: A cost-effectiveness analysis. *Journal of Medical Internet Research* 2013; 15:e18.
19. Powell J, Hamborg T, Stallard N, Burls A, McSorley J, Bennett K, et al. Effectiveness of a Web-based cognitive-behavioral tool to improve mental well-being in the general population: Randomized controlled trial. *Journal of Medical Internet Research* 2013; 15:e2.
20. Aguilera A, Muñoz RF. Text messaging as an adjunct to CBT in low-income populations: A usability and feasibility pilot study. *Professional Psychology: Research and Practice* 2011; 42:472–479.
21. Agyapong VI, Ahern S, McLoughlin DM, Farren CK. Supportive text messaging for depression and comorbid alcohol use disorder: Single-blind randomised trial. *Journal of Affective Disorders* 2012; 141:168–176.
22. Burns MN, Begale M, Duffecy J, Gergle D, Karr CJ, Giangrande E, Mohr DC. Harnessing context sensing to develop a mobile intervention for depression. *Journal of Medical Internet Research* 2011; 13:e55.
23. Christensen H, Griffiths KM, Jorm AF. Delivering interventions for depression by using the Internet: Randomised controlled trial. *British Medical Journal* 2004; 328:265–268.

24. Clarke G, Reid E, Eubanks D, O'Connor E, DeBar LL, Kelleher C, et al. Overcoming Depression on the Internet (ODIN): A randomized controlled trial of an Internet depression skills intervention program. *Journal of Medical Internet Research* 2002; 4:e14.

25. Clarke GN, Lewinsohn PM. The Adolescent Coping with Stress Class: Leader Manual. Portland, OR: Kaiser Permanente Center for Health Research; 1995.

26. Clarke GN, Lewinsohn PM, Hops H. Instructor's Manual for the Adolescent Coping with Depression Course. Eugene, OR: Castalia; 1990.

27. Christensen H, Griffiths K, Groves C, Korten A. Free range users and one hit wonders: Community users of an Internet-based cognitive behaviour therapy program. *Australian and New Zealand Journal of Psychiatry* 2006; 40:59–62.

28. Mohr DC, Duffecy J, Jin L, Ludman EJ, Lewis A, Begale M, McCarthy, Jr M. Multimodal e-mental health treatment for depression: A feasibility trial. *Journal of Medical Internet Research* 2010; 12:e48.

29. Duffecy J, Sanford S, Wagner L, Begale M, Nawacki E, Mohr DC. Project onward: An innovative e-health intervention for cancer survivors. *Psychooncology* 2013; 22(4):947–951.

30. Meyer B, Berger T, Caspar F, Beevers CG, Andersson G, et al. Effectiveness of a novel integrative online treatment for depression (Deprexis): Randomized controlled trial. *Journal of Medical Internet Research* 2009; 11:e15.

31. Merry SN, Stasiak K, Shepherd M, Frampton C, Fleming T, Lucassen MF. The effectiveness of SPARX, a computerised self help intervention for adolescents seeking help for depression: Randomised controlled non-inferiority trial. *British Medical Journal* 2012; 344:e2598.

32. Deterding S, Sicart M, Nacke L, O'Hara K, Dixon D. Gamification: Using game-design elements in non-gaming contexts. In *CHI '11 Extended Abstracts on Human Factors in Computing Systems*. New York: ACM; 2011. Retrieved from http://dl.acm.org/citation.cfm?id=1979742&picked=prox

33. Doherty G, Coyle D, Sharry J. Engagement with online mental health interventions: An exploratory clinical study of a treatment for depression. In *Proceedings of the 2012 ACM Annual Conference on Human Factors in Computing Systems* (pp. 1421–1430). New York, NY; 2012.

34. Zeiss AM, Lewinsohn PM, Muñoz RF. Nonspecific improvement effects in depression using interpersonal, cognitive, and pleasant events focused treatments. *Journal of Consulting and Clinical Psychology* 1979; 47:427–439.

35. Dimidjian S, Barrera Jr, M, Martell C, Muñoz RF, Lewinsohn PM. The origins and current status of behavioral activation treatments for depression. *Annual Review of Clinical Psychology* 2011; 7, 1–38.

36. Seligman ME, Rashid T, Parks AC. Positive psychotherapy. *American Psychologist* 2006; 61:774–788.

37. Spates CR, Kalata AH, Ozeki S, Stanton CE, Peters S. Initial open trial of a computerized behavioral activation treatment for depression. *Behavior Modification* 2013; 37:259–297.

38. Kauer SF, Reid SF, Crooke AHW, Khor A, Hearps SJC, Jorm AF, et al. Self-monitoring using mobile phones in the early stages of adolescent depression: Randomized controlled trial. *Journal of Medical Internet Research* 2012; 14:e67.

39. Johansson R, Ekbladh S, Hebert A, Lindström M, Möller S, Petitt E, et al. Psychodynamic guided self-help for adult depression through the Internet: A randomised controlled trial. *PLoS ONE* 2012; 7:e38021.

40. Zalta AK, Foa EB. Exposure therapy: Promoting emotional processing of pathological anxiety. In W. O'Donohue, JE. Fisher (Eds.). *Cognitive Behavior Therapy: Core Principles for Practice.* New York: John Wiley & Sons; 2012:75–104.

41. Gould RA, Otto MW, Pollack MH. A meta-analysis of treatment outcome for panic disorder. *Clinical Psychology Review* 1995; 15:819–844.

42. Schulte D, Künzel R, Pepping G, Schulte-Bahrenberg T. Tailor-made versus standardized therapy of phobic patients. *Advances in Behaviour Research & Therapy* 1992; 14:67–92.

43. Abramowitz JS. Effectiveness of psychological and pharmacological treatments for obsessive-compulsive disorder: A quantitative review. *Journal of Consulting and Clinical Psychology* 1997; 65:44–52.

44. Marks IM, Kenwright M, McDonough M, Whittaker M, Mataix Cols D. Saving clinician's time by delegating routine aspects of therapy to a computer: A randomised controlled trial in phobia/panic disorder. *Psychological Medicine* 2004; 34:9–18.

45. Nakagawa A, Marks IM, Park J, Bachofen M, Baer L, Dottl SL, Greist JH. Self-treatment of obsessive-compulsive disorder guided by manual and computer-conducted telephone interview. *Journal of Telemedicine and Telecare* 2000; 6:22–26.

46. Powers MB, Emmelkamp PMG. Virtual reality exposure therapy for anxiety disorders: A meta-analysis. *Journal of Anxiety Disorders* 2008; 22:561–569.

47. Rizzo A, Difede J, Rothbaum BO, Reger G, Spitalnick J, Cukor J, Mclay R. Virtual Iraq/Afghanistan: Development and early evaluation of a virtual reality exposure therapy system

for combat-related PTSD. *Annals of the New York Academy of Sciences* 2010; 1208:114–125.

48. Amir N, Weber G, Beard C, Bomyea J, Taylor CT. The effect of a single-session attention modification program on response to a public-speaking challenge in socially anxious individuals. *Journal of Abnormal Psychology* 2008; 117:860–868.

49. Hakamata Y, Lissek S, Bar-Haim Y, Britton JC, Fox NA, Leibenluft E, et al. Attention bias modification treatment: A meta-analysis toward the establishment of novel treatment for anxiety. *Biological Psychiatry* 2010; 68:982–990.

50. Amir N, Beard C, Taylor CT, Klumpp H, Elias J, Burns M, et al. Attention training in individuals with generalized social phobia: A randomized controlled trial. *Journal of Consulting and Clinical Psychology* 2009; 77:961–973.

51. Schmidt NB, Richey JA, Buckner JD, Timpano KR. Attention training for generalized social anxiety disorder. *Journal of Abnormal Psychology* 2009; 118:5–14.

52. Carlbring P, Apelstrand M, Sehlin H, Amir N, Rousseau A, Hofmann SG, Andersson G. Internet-delivered attention bias modification training in individuals with social anxiety disorder—A double blind randomized trial. *BMC Psychiatry* 2012; 12:66.

53. Rennert K, Karapanos E. Faceit: Supporting reflection upon social anxiety events with life-logging. In *CHI'13 Extended Abstracts on Human Factors in Computing Systems* (pp. 457–462). New York: ACM; 2013, April. Retrieved from http://dl.acm.org/citation.cfm?id=2468356

54. Przeworski A, Newman MG. Palmtop computer-assisted group therapy for social phobia. *Journal of Clinical Psychology* 2004; 60:179–188.

55. Reiner R. Integrating a portable biofeedback device into clinical practice for patients with anxiety disorders: Results of a pilot study. *Applied Psychophysiology and Biofeedback* 2008; 33:55–61.

56. O'Connell ME, Boat T, Warner KE. (Eds.). *Preventing Mental, Emotional, and Behavioral Disorders among Young People: Progress and Possibilities*. Washington, DC, National Academies Press; 2009.

57. Seligman MEP, Csikszentmihalyi M. Positive psychology: An introduction. *American Psychologist* 2000; 55:5–14.

58. Morris ME, Aguilera A. Mobile, social, and wearable computing and the evolution of psychological practice. *Professional Psychology: Research and Practice* 2012; 43:622–626.

59. Sin NL, Lyubomirsky S. Enhancing well-being and alleviating depressive symptoms with positive psychology interventions: A practice-friendly meta analysis. *Journal of Clinical Psychology* 2009; 65:467–487.

60. Fredrickson BL. Cultivating positive emotions to optimize health and well-being. *Prevention & Treatment* 2000; 3: Article 1.

61. Cuijpers P, Beekman ATF, Reynolds CF. Preventing depression: A global priority. *JAMA* 2012; 307:1033–1034.

62. Muñoz RF, Cuijpers P, Smit F, Barrera AZ, Leykin Y. Prevention of major depression. *Annual Review of Clinical Psychology* 2010; 6:181–212.

63. Tate DF, Finkelstein EA, Khavjou O, Gustafson A. Cost effectiveness of Internet interventions: Review and recommendations. *Annals of Behavioral Medicine* 2009; 38,:40–45.

64. McCrone P, Knapp M, Proudfoot J, Ryden C, Cavanagh K, Shapiro DA, et al. Cost-effectiveness of computerized cognitive-behavioural therapy for anxiety and depression in primary care: Randomised controlled trial. *British Journal of Psychiatry* 2004; 18:55–62.

65. Warmerdam L, Smit F, van Straten A, Riper H, Cuijpers P. Cost-utility and cost-effectiveness of Internet-based treatment for adults with depressive symptoms: Randomized trial. *Journal of Medical Internet Research* 2010; 12:e53.

66. Muñoz RF, Aguilera A, Schueller SM, Leykin Y, Pérez-Stable EJ. From online randomized controlled trials to participant preference studies: Morphing the San Francisco Stop Smoking site into a worldwide smoking cessation resource. *Journal of Medical Internet Research* 2012; 14:e64.

67. Leykin Y, Muñoz RF, Contreras O. Are consumers of Internet health information "cyberchondriacs"? Characteristics of 24,965 users of a depression screening site. *Depression and Anxiety* 2012; 29:71–77.

68. Gibbons RD, Weiss DJ, Pilkonis PA, Frank E, Moore T, Kim JB, Kupfer DJ. Development of a computerized adaptive test for depression. *Archives of General Psychiatry* 2012; 69:1104–1112.

69. Bauer S, Wolf M, Haug S, Kordy H. The effectiveness of Internet chat groups in relapse prevention after inpatient psychotherapy. *Psychotherapy Research* 2011; 21:219–226.

70. Craske MG, Rose RD, Lang A, Welch SS, Campbell-Sills L, Sullivan G, et al. Computer-assisted delivery of cognitive behavioral therapy for anxiety disorders in primary care settings. *Depression and Anxiety* 2009; 26:235–242.

71. Farrer L, Christensen H, Griffiths KM, Mackinnon A. Internet-based CBT for depression with and without telephone tracking in a national helpline: Randomised controlled trial. *PLoS ONE* 2011; 6:e28099.

72. Andrews B, Wilding JM. The relation of depression and anxiety to life-stress and achievement in students. *British Journal of Psychology* 2004; 95:509–521.

73. Neil AL, Batterham P, Christensen H, Bennett K, Griffiths KM. Predictors of adherence by adolescents to a cognitive behavior therapy website in school and community-based settings. *Journal of Medical Internet Research* 2009; 11:e6.

74. National Institute for Clinical Excellence. Computerised cognitive behaviour therapy for depression and anxiety. Review of Technology Appraisal 51. London: National Institute for Clinical Excellence; 2006.

75. Learmonth D, Rai S. Taking computerized CBT beyond primary care. *British Journal of Clinical Psychology* 2008; 47:111–118.

76. Proudfoot J, Goldberg D, Mann A, Everitt B, Marks I, Gray JA. Computerized, interactive, multimedia cognitive-behavioural program for anxiety and depression in general practice. *Psychological Medicine* 2003; 33:217–227.

77. Proudfoot J, Ryden C, Everitt B, Shapiro D, Goldberg D, Mann A, et al. Clinical effectiveness of computerized cognitive behavioural therapy for anxiety and depression in primary care. *British Journal of Psychiatry* 2004; 185:46–54.

78. Van Voorhees BW, Fogel J, Reinecke MA, Gladstone T, Stuart S, Gollan J, et al. Randomized clinical trial of an Internet-based depression prevention program for adolescents (Project CATCH-IT) in primary care: 12 week outcomes. *Journal of Developmental Behavioral Pediatrics* 2009; 30:23–37.

79. Coyle D, McGlade N, Doherty G, O'Reilly G. Exploratory evaluations of a computer game supporting cognitive behavioural therapy for adolescents. In *Proceedings of the 2011 Annual Conference on Human Factors in Computing Systems* (pp. 2937–2946). New York: ACM; 2011, May.

80. Schueller, SM, Muñoz RF, Mohr DC. Realizing the potential of behavioral intervention technologies. *Current Directions in Psychological Science* 2013;22:478–483.

81. Heron KE, Smyth JM. Ecological momentary interventions: Incorporating mobile technology into psychosocial and health behaviour treatments. *British Journal of Health Psychology* 2010; 15:1–39.

82. Rachuri KK, Musolesi M, Mascolo C, Rentfrow PJ, Longworth C, Aucinas A. EmotionSense: A mobile phones based adaptive platform for experimental social psychology research. In *Proceedings of the 12th ACM International Conference on Ubiquitous Computing* (pp. 281–290). New York: ACM; 2010, September.

83. Goodwin MS, Velicer WF,,Intille SS. Telemetric monitoring in the behavior sciences. *Behavior Research Methods* 2008; 40:328–341.

84. Intille SS, Lester J, Sallis JF, Duncan G. (2012). New horizons in sensor development. *Medicine and Science in Sports and Exercise* 2012; 44:S24–31.

85. Massey T, Marfia G, Potkonjak M, Sarrafzadeh M. Experimental analysis of a mobile health system for mood disorders. *IEEE Transactions on Information Technology in Biomedicine* 2010; 14:241–247.

86. Rizzo A, Kenny PG, Parsons TD. Intelligent virtual patients for training clinical skills.. *Journal of Virtual Reality and Broadcasting* 2011; 8: 3.

87. Rizzo A, Sagae K, Forbell E, Kim J, Lange B, Buckwalter JG, et al. SimCoach: An intelligent virtual human system for providing healthcare information and support. In *The Interservice/Industry Training, Simulation & Education Conference (I/ITSEC)* (Vol. 2011, No. 1: 1–11). Arlington, VA: National Training Systems Association; 2011, January.

6

Technologies for People with Serious Mental Illness

DROR BEN-ZEEV, ROBERT E. DRAKE, AND RACHEL M. BRIAN

INTRODUCTION

In the United States, a minority of people with serious mental illnesses (SMI), such as psychotic disorders and major mood disorders, receive evidence-based treatments (1). Only 60% of people with the most severe psychiatric disorder, schizophrenia, report receiving any services in the previous 6–12 months (2). Rates of receiving any services are even lower for psychosocial interventions, as opposed to pharmacological care. Many people drop out of the mental health system after their initial contact and avoid the system over time because of stigma, dissatisfaction with previous services, and unawareness of the potential benefits that may be achievable with appropriate treatment (3).

For those who remain in the mental health system, services research has shown that people with SMI are unlikely to receive effective interventions, known as evidence-based practices (4). Those receiving evidence-based psychosocial interventions may fall below 5% (1). Efforts to implement evidence-based practices in the United States are moving toward improving larger systems of care, including developing and improving electronic records, decision supports, and the chronic-care model (5). Nevertheless, these efforts are often stalled because of financing problems (e.g., Medicaid regulations are not aligned with evidence-based practices), health system reform (e.g., attempts to integrate physical and behavioral healthcare), workforce problems (e.g., rapid turnover), and regulatory problems (e.g., fears of Medicaid audits).

Mental health leaders have widely advocated the use of new technologies to improve the quality of services in the United States (6,7). Several chapters in this volume present technological tools that can be deployed among people with psychiatric disabilities (see, e.g., Chapters 4, 5, and 10), and an emerging literature is focusing on technology-based resources specifically designed for people with severe psychiatric disorders, their family members, and supports (8,9). These include Web-based cognitive behavioral interventions for coping with auditory hallucinations (10), online peer support and social therapy for first-episode psychosis (11), Internet-based family intervention programs (12,13), computerized "relational agents" designed to enhance medication adherence and physical activity (14), clinic-based computerized patient kiosks for self-assessment (15), virtual-reality paradigms for vocational rehabilitation (16,17), and smartphone applications (apps) for self-management of schizophrenia (18). In the following section, we describe how these approaches may help people with SMI overcome some of the traditional barriers to receiving high-quality care.

EXISTING BARRIERS AND POSSIBLE TECHNOLOGY-BASED SOLUTIONS
Understanding and Accessing Treatment Systems

People with SMI and their family members experience great difficulties in understanding and effectively utilizing complex treatment systems (6). Technologies may help them to access information in ways that are more intuitive and easier to understand, and to find appropriate treatment system resources that fit their needs. For example, electronic system-guides or automated kiosks (19) can be made accessible as a website on the Internet or via self-help touchscreen stations available in a variety of settings, such as public libraries, pharmacies, and primary care centers. Automated service system guides could support users in identifying the areas in which they are having difficulties, using familiar understandable language and minimal professional jargon. Once the individual identifies perceived needs, the electronic guide could present information on relevant interventions, explain how they could be helpful, identify local programs, provide contact information or immediate links to the appropriate provider or website, and convey information for effective advocacy. For example, a person experiencing mental health problems could use the guide to locate a counselor, doctor, housing provider, or supported employment program.

Obtaining Accurate and Understandable Information

Even when people access services through a traditionally offered clinical program, they may receive insufficient information about their mental health problems and the potential treatment options. Providers often have difficulty staying abreast of new interventions, and many believe that people with SMI are not able to understand options and make informed choices (20). Consequently, clinicians may present options in a biased way, or recommend the interventions that they are most familiar with, rather than those that are most effective. For every behavioral health problem, several interventions exist—many with potential positive effects and possible negative side effects as well. When no clear best treatment is apparent, the person's goals, preferences, and personal choices should be prominent in the decision-making process (21). The optimal way to present these options and their related effects accurately and fairly may be through information technology. Electronic decision support systems can be administered on computers at user-stations in a clinic waiting area before consumers meet with a provider. Incorporating multimodal (e.g., audio, video, text) and multilingual information delivery strategies may help clients to feel informed and empowered to exercise their sense of agency. Electronic systems could also help clients prepare for meetings with clinicians ahead of time via home computers or cell phones, and to express their treatment choices and concerns in a concise and informed fashion (22).

Supporting Treatment Engagement

After people with SMI enter treatment, participation in and adherence to interventions often fluctuate or erode all together (23–25). For example, use of medications waxes and wanes for most people. Ongoing treatment adherence may be explained by symptoms, interpersonal and social interactions, or unconscious or implicit motivations (26). Technological platforms could facilitate outreach to enhance participation and adherence; for example, text messaging could be used to deploy basic motivational interviewing strategies to encourage people who are inconsistent in their service use to examine the costs and benefits and increase internal drivers to continue care. Electronic health records can also be used to automatically send text or automated voice reminders of upcoming scheduled appointments.

Learning and Maintaining Coping Behaviors

Behavior change interventions, particularly skills training interventions targeting illness management for people with SMI (e.g., medication adherence, functional and social skills), aim to transfer skills learned in the clinic to the home environment (27). Homework between sessions clearly enhances the impact of psychosocial interventions (28). But cognitive impairments and motivational problems related to SMI may limit one's ability to recall, initiate, and maintain behaviors that are trained in clinic settings. Remote technologies can provide supports for transfer of skills to real-world settings through e-mails, illness management software, smartphone applications, or text message reminders. In addition, many of the skill training interventions specify actions to be taken in the presence of an event, feeling state, or warning sign of illness exacerbations; technological interventions may be delivered at the moment these experiences occur and thus facilitate use during particularly vulnerable, high-risk times (29).

Improving Treatment Effectiveness and Availability

Treatments that incorporate relevant technologies may enhance outcomes in several ways. People with SMI could use the technologies to quickly and easily access information, involve family members and other supporters, and engage in an intervention at their own pace (e.g., cognitive remediation exercises, practice coping strategies to manage symptoms, social skills training, family psychoeducation). Technologically based assessments provide rapid feedback to users (i.e., average symptom severity during the week, change in symptom severity, appearance of warning signs, daily substance use) on a computer or smartphone screen (18). When people receive regular information about their progress, they can evaluate and customize their own treatment, likely increasing engagement or, conversely, choose to seek out alternatives better suited for them when the status quo is not satisfactory. Individuals may choose to repeat or spend more time on areas within an electronically administered intervention they find challenging, revisit ones in order to access content that helps them cope with a current concern (e.g., hearing voices, racing thoughts), or become more engaged in an intervention that meets their needs and helps them better manage their illness.

Telecommunications can also open lines for direct support. Clinicians, for example, can adjust their response methods when an individual is in crisis or in need of acute care (30). Electronic systems can serve as health navigators, facilitating communication with providers, perhaps improving therapeutic alliance and treatment outcomes. Providers can gain a better sense of times of vulnerability for their patients and respond in more ways, through the use of technology (i.e., phone calls, video conferencing, or text messages). Technologies may also be used to engage family members and other supports, even those at a great geographical distance. For example, websites designed specifically for people with SMI could host forums for family members with a therapist moderating discussions. Online resources could include common questions and answers, educational reading materials, and lists of community activities and events (12).

Because evidence-based psychosocial treatments for people with SMI (e.g., cognitive-behavioral therapy, family therapy, illness-management training) are rarely available, technologies may play a key role in increasing access to these services (e.g., telehealth to rural areas). For those already receiving evidence-based psychosocial treatments, use of technologies can help extend the duration of interventions (e.g., providing self-guided sessions) or increase the intensity of treatment (e.g., providing online interactive content between sessions) (10).

Overcoming Barriers of Stigma

Technologies can enable consumers to access information and engage in interventions according to their preferred schedule and in their natural environments (12), thus decreasing the stigma associated with seeking mental health services and increasing the likelihood of service utilization (23). Currently, people with SMI are often unwilling to access care through specialty mental health providers and treatment centers because exposure can exacerbate self-stigma (31). Use of technologies significantly alters the experience of mental healthcare. Instead of traveling to a clinic, technology-facilitated telemedicine can be provided in the person's own environment and culture, permitting a clearer exchange of information, and greater control over disclosure. Instead of a jargon-filled, rapid, and often unclear exchange, communication can involve strategies with which the person is intimately familiar, through ongoing practice at home. Interventions can be delivered via technological platforms (e.g., smartphones) widely used by the general population for other purposes. Thus, users can choose to engage in interventions and guided illness-management in public without attracting unwanted attention, using an instrument that does not have the appearance and associated stigma of a medical device (18).

Affordability

Technological advancements may reduce treatment costs. On the individual level, use of technologies may prompt and assist consumers to engage in health-promoting behaviors outside of psychotherapy sessions or other clinic-based activities in the convenience of one's own environment, thus overcoming barriers of differing work and family schedules, as well as that of transportation. Technologies can also be deployed to enhance traditional therapeutic and supportive services, for example, by allowing supporters (e.g., family members) to be more engaged in their loved ones' ongoing treatment, reinforcing therapeutic principles such as identifying and solving problems, overcoming barriers to behavior change, or facilitating practice and use of learned skills through activities or games. Improving interactivity and access to self-management and independent coping strategies via technology may reduce the need for direct face-to-face contact with mental healthcare providers, which in turn, can affect treatment costs and service demand.

On the mental healthcare systems level, early investment in distribution and utilization of basic technologies and infrastructure (e.g., Medicare recently started providing consumers with mobile phones and call minutes) may help to reduce utilization of costly services, such as emergency room visits for psychiatric care or acute psychiatric hospitalization. Development and maintenance cost considerations should be taken into account, however, when deciding whether to adopt or build technology-based programming. Some smaller institutions, or non-profits, may not have the financial or technical resources to develop (i.e., software developers, content developers) and support (i.e., servers, databases) programming. One possible solution would be to develop a federally supported intervention suite of programs that could be leveraged by smaller entities (32).

Taken together, technological solutions can address numerous challenges that emerge at different stages of mental healthcare for individuals with SMI. We summarize these in Table 6.1.

MOBILE HEALTH (MHEALTH) APPROACHES
Mobile Technologies Are Ubiquitous

The UN's International Telecommunications Union reported that the number of mobile phone subscriptions worldwide has already reached at least six billion (33); it likely reached 6.8 billion by the end of 2013 (34). Developing countries use close to three-quarters of all mobile phones, and developed countries use more mobile phones than the population, with many people using more than one mobile device. A recent survey of 1,592 individuals with SMI receiving community-based services in the United States found that 72% owned a mobile device (i.e., cellular phone, smartphone, or text messaging device for people with hearing impairments), a rate only 12% lower than that of the general adult population. Moreover, many respondents expressed interest in receiving additional services (e.g., clinical check-ins with providers, psychoeducation, and medication and appointment reminders) via their mobile device (35). Remarkably, there is evidence suggesting that approximately 70% of people who are homeless have mobile phones (36). The penetration of mobile technologies among vulnerable

---

TABLE 6.1. PROPOSED TECHNOLOGY-BASED APPROACHES FOR DIFFERENT STAGES OF MENTAL HEALTH SERVICE USE*

| | Stages of Mental Health Service Use | | | |
	Seeking Care	Choosing Treatment	Engaging in Treatment	Sustaining Care
Objectives	Accessing services Understanding systems of care	Understanding mental health conditions Obtaining unrestricted and unbiased treatment options	Overcoming barriers linked with stigma Utilizing remote services Learning coping skills	Ongoing feedback Engaging family members and other supports Practicing coping skills Cost reduction
Technologies	Electronic treatment systems guides Clinic work stations and online information kiosks	Consumer-friendly informational websites Electronic decision support systems	Phone and video telehealth services Mobile devices for real-time/real-place interventions Computer-based treatment for use as needed	Automated text message or email reports and reminders Online forums, secure social networks Instant messaging, video conferencing Smartphone self-management programs, automated electronic "booster" sessions

* Adapted from an earlier version that appeared in the *American Journal of Psychiatric Rehabilitation*, published by Taylor & Francis. Reproduced with permission of Taylor & Francis in the format republished in a book/textbook via Copyright Clearance Center.

populations creates new opportunities for assessment and treatment, extending well beyond the clinic or treatment center.

Mobile technologies such as cellular phones and smartphones are particularly well suited for psychiatric monitoring, assessment, and illness management, because they are typically carried on the person and turned on, and often have impressive computational capacities and connection to the Internet (37). Thus, in addition to their originally intended commercial uses, mobile devices can also facilitate access to self-monitoring resources, time-sensitive health information, prompts, reminders, and personalized illness-management tools in real time and in real-world environments (38,39).

Mobile devices such as microcomputers, smartphones, and wearable sensors (e.g., for measurement of movement, location, galvanic skin response, heart rate) may elucidate the day-to-day factors that affect ongoing clinical status. Traditionally, in order to understand how psychiatric patients think, feel, and function, clinicians and researchers would ask individuals to provide retrospective reports of symptoms, functioning, and personal life events. Despite their broad use, retrospective reports are problematic; they are typically collected in laboratory or clinic settings, not in the real-world environments in which symptoms or life events actually take place. Consequently, their ecological validity (i.e., the extent that findings in artificial settings reflect experiences in the real world) is questionable. In addition, they require patients to recollect (e.g., "How many times did you leave the house last month?") or aggregate ("On average, how often do you hear voices during the day?") their experiences—tasks that are susceptible to social desirability influences, memory biases, and other inaccuracies (40). Finally, retrospective reports are static; they provide a single estimate of dynamic functions—illness expression and mental health over time (41). Mobile health (mHealth) approaches like ecological momentary assessment (EMA) utilize microcomputers or smartphones to gather information about one's self-reported thoughts, feelings, activities, and settings, as they occur in real-world environments. With these data, researchers can map the temporal sequence or co-occurrence of events over a given period of data collection, identifying immediate and/or short-term relationships between variables. Recent studies using mobile approaches have already produced important insights into the causes and correlates of various health-related behaviors, such as triggers for cigarette smoking in individuals attempting to quit (42), predictors of suicidal ideation (43) and self-injurious behavior (44), and associations between substance use and symptom exacerbation in schizophrenia (45). Studies also show that certain phenomena widely considered chronic or constant in SMI actually ebb and flow both in frequency and severity, suggesting more malleability than previously believed (46–50).

The data collected with mobile technologies can facilitate more effective, person-tailored treatments (9,51). Mobile interventions vary according to the degree to which interaction with a clinician is involved—that is, they can be completely automated (algorithm-driven text messaging or smartphone applications) (18,52), can involve asynchronous communication with a clinician, such as the periodic delivery of reports about symptoms (e.g., 53), or can collect data for live interactions with a clinician (e.g., 51). Mobile devices could support skills practice between meetings with a clinician, providing individual guidance, allowing access to peer or family assistance regardless of location, and ultimately increasing the effectiveness of interventions and providing some assistance when face-to-face support is unavailable.

The impressive computational capacities of contemporary smartphones allow for the integration of several approaches and modalities into a comprehensive mHealth package on a single device. For example, Ben-Zeev and colleagues (18) developed FOCUS, a smartphone system for self-management of schizophrenia, that has both system-initiated and on-demand resources for self-management of a range of problems including psychotic symptoms, medication non-adherence, social dysfunction, sleep irregularities, and mood disturbances (Figure 6.1).

The system uses audio prompts, visual aids (e.g., photos, cartoons, colors), and written text to deliver evidence-based self-management coping strategies in the form of interactive questions and suggestions. FOCUS can be used as needed in an automated manner, but it can also be used to collect, process, and transmit individuals' self-assessment and system use data so that these

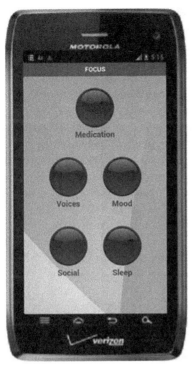

FIGURE 6.1: The FOCUS smartphone system intervention selection screen.

can be viewed as an update report by a clinician using a secure website, shortly after collection. If a clinician believes that an individual is in crisis, he or she can call directly on the smartphone and provide real-time consultation. Thus, the system integrates automated, asynchronous communication and real-time live support, all in one platform (18).

PTSD Coach is another example of an mHealth application designed to help trauma survivors recognize symptoms and utilize personalized self-management tools for posttraumatic stress disorder (PTSD) (54). Developed by the Department of Veterans Affairs, this mobile application includes PTSD information, self-management tools, coping strategies, assessments, trackers, and social support to manage symptoms from trauma. PTSD Coach allows users to choose relaxing images and songs already stored on personal phones to be used within the application intervention to provide salient forms of relaxation. Social support is provided in a number of ways, through choosing a social support person via personal contact list, or through the application directing users to nationally provided resources.

Researchers are at the early stages of harnessing wearable and smartphone sensors (e.g., accelerometer, GPS, microphone) for passive behavioral data collection (e.g., movement, location, speech); all the user would need to do to facilitate continuous data capture would be to carry the device. These exciting methodologies could potentially decrease patient response burden and increase data accuracy. Emerging evidence suggests that mobile device sensor streams can be used to make inferences about one's social functioning, physical activity level, sleep, and mental well-being (55,56). Sensor-derived models may one day be used to detect shifts from one's typical behavioral pattern or rhythm (e.g. changes in sleep, drop in social interaction) and perhaps serve as early warning systems for impending mood episodes in bipolar disorder or psychotic relapse in schizophrenia, triggering just-in-time intensive services and preventive care.

DEVELOPMENT AND TESTING
Usability

People with SMI often have cognitive impairments, salient symptoms, limited literacy, and other difficulties that affect engagement in electronic-based interventions and resources (57,58). Systems with inadequate consideration of these needs may be difficult to learn, or misused or underused, and likely to fail to achieve their objectives (59). To ensure usability, interventions need to be developed in accordance with design principles for e-resources for people with SMI—for example, minimal steps to access content; memory aids to facilitate navigation; screens that avoid distracting and superfluous elements; simple screen arrangements and sentences; concrete wording to minimize the need for abstract thinking; and minimal but adequate amount of total text used to convey meaning (60).

Ethics, Privacy, and Safety

With the growing capacity for delivering services and rapid transfer of clinical data from offsite locations, the maintaining of confidentiality and privacy poses new challenges, such as a need for sophisticated data transfer and encryption methods (61). In response to the steadily growing use of mobile technologies in various clinical and research settings, the U.S. Food and Drug Administration has released a draft on how it intends to monitor and regulate the use of mobile medical devices and applications in the near future (62). One issue, for example, is that technology-based interventions may collect time-sensitive data during times when clinicians are not at work. Individuals with SMI may use social network websites that are in the public domain and broadly accessible as a medium to communicate distress or crisis (63). In these circumstances, the ethical obligation to respond is unclear (43,63).

Interdisciplinary Research and Training Models

Designing innovative interventions that integrate services and technologies requires expertise in multiple fields. Academic institutions will need to offer training for students that couples complementary areas (e.g., computational neuroscience, engineering psychology, and information technology courses offered in medical schools and clinical psychology programs), and interdisciplinary teams will need to include researchers familiar with both clinical aspects (e.g., physicians, psychiatric rehabilitation specialists, and clinical psychologists) and technological domains (hardware and software engineers, computer scientists, design experts, and human–computer interaction experts) (64). Integrating disciplines may prove quite challenging. For example, new NIH mHealth training institutes bring together behavioral and social scientists, clinical researchers, engineers, and computer scientists, using a team approach. The grouping of multidisciplinary teams stimulates discussion and integration in the development of novel mobile technologies. While the process is challenging, past research shows that interdisciplinary teams generate better research solutions than do single-discipline teams (65).

Long-Term Engagement

Because SMI is by definition a long-term condition, an advantage of technology-based interventions, particularly automated ones, is their use for an ongoing rather than fixed duration. However, data from many Internet-based interventions suggest attrition rates as high as 40–50%, partly due to static content and participant loss of interest (32). A review of anxiety and depression-focused Internet intervention adherence indicated several reasons for attrition: Low motivation, technical problems, symptom severity, physical illness, lack of face-to-face contact, preference for taking medication, perceived lack of treatment effectiveness, improvement of condition, and program burden were all mentioned as reasons for individuals discontinuing their use of programs (66).

A central challenge of mental health research on technology-based interventions is to develop strategies that maximize user engagement, through adapting and personalizing content based on accumulating data and changing physical and emotional conditions. Tailoring of program content is one way in which programs have increased relevance, acceptance, receptivity, and processing of information (67). By providing individualized and customized feedback specific to targeted behaviors and cultural factors, individuals are more receptive when processing information than when information is static (67,68).

Incentive strategies and continued communication to increase participation are other possible ways of reducing attrition. Methods from marketing and computer science may help to identify system-user rewards for engagement, such as games or caring for virtual pets (69). In addition, a variety of automated or manual push messages (e.g., e-mails, postcards, text messages, phone calls) that remind participants to continue using the intervention are methods that have also proven to be helpful with program adherence among people with mental health conditions (70).

Cost, Access, and Use

Although technological interventions promise to reduce healthcare costs, most research groups typically produce systems that are closed, rigid, and proprietary. Consequently, few standard platforms exist, time and resources are devoted to devising and testing basic technological infrastructure instead of reusing existing components, and new developments emerge as a patchwork of incompatible applications. Shifts toward developing open-sourced software can already be seen in private industry, such as Android, a mobile operating system platform supported by Google (71). Android's open source code allows individuals to freely modify, reuse, or repurpose the software, including writing unique applications using its platform, through a provided software development kit (SDK). Several other private companies, including Oracle (http://www.oracle.com), a leader in hardware and software development, and MySQL (http://www.mysql.com), one of the largest open source database companies in the world, are also driving open source initiatives.

Several other software applications, architectures, and systems are currently being developed with the intention of creating open-sourced platforms for wide distribution and utility. Open-sourced software not only provides lower cost access to software programs but its natural transparency could also possibly provide greater reliability and accuracy because the coding is available to everyone. Any errors would likely be picked up by increased numbers of external users, as opposed to quality testing of a smaller team's closed software codes.

CONCLUSIONS

Emerging technologies can help individuals with SMI better understand and utilize complex treatment systems, obtain information on mental health conditions and interventions, improve their treatment engagement, learn and maintain effective coping strategies, and overcome some of the barriers associated with the stigma of seeking services. The current evidence base in this area is still quite limited; the barriers and possible solutions to broad implementation in real-world settings have not been addressed. New technologically driven approaches entail inherent challenges in terms of usability, safety and confidentiality, research design, and affordability. Interdisciplinary training for providers and researchers, as well as multidisciplinary teamwork to bridge gaps across technical, methodological, and clinical areas of expertise, will be essential for effective research and use of technologies in the assessment and treatment of SMI in years to come.

REFERENCES

1. Drake R, Essock S. The science-to-service gap in real-world schizophrenia treatment: The 95% problem. *Schizophrenia Bulletin* 2009; 35(4):677–678.
2. Mojtabai R, Fochtmann L, Chang S, Kotov R, Craig T, Bromet E. Unmet need for mental healthcare in schizophrenia: An overview of literature and new data from a first-admission study. *Schizophrenia Bulletin* 2009; 35(4):679–695.
3. Kreyenbuhl J, Nossel I, Dixon L. Disengagement from mental health treatment among individuals with schizophrenia and strategies for facilitating connections to care: A review of the literature. *Schizophrenia Bulletin* 2009; 35(4):696–703.
4. Wang P, Demler O, Kessler R. Adequacy of treatment for serious mental illness in the United States. *American Journal of Public Health* 2002; 92(1):92–98.
5. Wagner EH, Austin BT, Davis C, Hindmarsh M, Schaefer J, Bonomi A. Improving chronic illness care: Translating evidence into action. *Health Affairs* 2001; 20(6):64–78.
6. Institute of Medicine. *Improving the Quality of Health Care for Mental and Substance-Use Conditions.* Washington DC: National Academies Press; 2006.
7. New Freedom Commission on Mental Health Achieving the Promise. Transforming mental health care in America. Final Report. DHHS Publ. No. SMA-03-3832. Rockville, MD: Substance Abuse and Mental Health Services Administration; 2003.
8. Alvarez-Jimenez M, Gleeson J, Bendall S, Lederman R, Wadley G, Killackey E, McGorry P. Internet-based interventions for psychosis: A sneak-peek into the future. *Psychiatric Clinics of North America* 2012; 35(3):735–747.
9. Depp C, Mausbach B, Granholm E, Cardenas V, Ben-Zeev D, Patterson T, et al. Mobile interventions for severe mental illness: Design and preliminary data from three approaches. *Journal of Nervous and Mental Disease* 2011; 198(10):715–721.
10. Gottlieb J, Romeo K, Penn D, Mueser K, Chiko B. Web-based cognitive-behavioral therapy for auditory hallucinations in persons with psychosis: A pilot study. *Schizophrenia Research* 2013; 145(1-3):82–87.
11. Alvarez-Jimenez M, Bendall S, Lederman R, Wadley G, Chinnery G, Vargas S, Gleeson J. On the HORIZON: Moderated online social therapy for long-term recovery in first episode psychosis. *Schizophrenia Research* 2013; 143(1):143–149.
12. Rotondi A, Anderson C, Haas G, Eack S, Spring M, Ganguli R, et al. Web-based psychoeducational intervention for persons with schizophrenia and their supporters: One-year outcomes. *Psychiatric Services* 2010; 61(11):1099–1105.
13. Glynn S, Randolph E, Garrick T, Lui A. A proof of concept trial of an online psychoeducational program for relatives of both veterans and civilians living with schizophrenia. *Psychiatric Rehabilitation Journal* 2010; 33(4):278–287.
14. Bickmore T, Puskar K, Schlenk E, Pfeifer L, Sereika S. Maintaining reality: Relational agents for antipsychotic medication adherence. *Interacting with Computers* 2010; 22(4):276–288.
15. Cohen A, Chinman M, Hamilton A, Whelan F, Young A. Using patient-facing kiosks to support quality improvement at mental health clinics. *Medical Care* 2013; 51(3):S13–S20.

16. Bell M, Weinstein A. Simulated job interview skill training for people with psychiatric disability: Feasibility and tolerability of virtual reality training. *Schizophrenia Bulletin* 2011; 37(S2):S91–S97.

17. Tsang M, Man D. A virtual reality-based vocational training system (VRVTS) for people with schizophrenia in vocational rehabilitation. *Schizophrenia Research* 2013; 144(1-3):51–62.

18. Ben-Zeev D, Kaiser S, Brenner C, Begale M, Duffecy J, Mohr D. Development and usability testing of FOCUS: A smartphone system for self-management of schizophrenia. *Psychiatric Rehabilitation Journal* 2013; 36(4):289–296.

19. Stein J, Navab B, Frazee B, Tebb K, Hendey G, Maselli J, Gonzales R. A randomized trial of computer kiosk-expedited management of cystitis in the emergency department. *Acadamic Emergency Medicine* 2011; 18(10):1053–1059.

20. Drake R, Cimpean D, Torrey W. Shared decision making in mental health: Prospects for personalized medicine. *Dialogues in Clinical Neuroscience* 2009; 11(4):455–463.

21. Drake R, Deegan P, Rapp C. The promise of shared decision making in mental health. *Psychiatric Rehabilitation Journal* 2010; 34(1):7–13.

22. Drake R, Deegan P. Shared decision making is an ethical imperative. *Psychiatric Services* 2009; 60(8):1007.

23. Corrigan P. How stigma interferes with mental health care. *American Psychologist* 2004; 59(7):614–625.

24. Gilmer T, Dolder C, Lacro J, Folsom D, Lindamer L, Garcia P, Jeste D. Adherence to treatment with antipsychotic medication and health care costs among Medicaid beneficiaries with schizophrenia. *American Journal of Psychiatry* 2004; 161(4):692–699.

25. Goldman G, Gregory R. Preliminary relationships between adherence and outcome in dynamic deconstructive psychotherapy. *Psychotherapy: Theory, Research, Practice, Training* 2009; 46:480–485.

26. Corrigan P, Rusch N, Ben-Zeev D, Sher T. Rational patient and beyond: Implications for treatment adherence in people with psychiatric disabilities. *Rehabilitation Psychology* 2014; 59(1):85–98.

27. Mueser K, Deavers F, Penn D, Cassisi J. Psychosocial treatments for schizophrenia. *Annual Review of Clinical Psychology* 2013; 9:465–497.

28. Mausbach B, Moore R, Roesch S, Cardenas V, Patterson T. The relationship between homework compliance and therapy outcomes: An updated meta-analysis. *Cognitive Therapy and Research* 2010; 34(5):429–438.

29. Rizvi S, Dimeff L, Skutch J, Carroll D, Linhean M. A pilot study of the DBT coach: An interactive mobile phone application for individuals with borderline personality disorder and substance use disorder. *Behavior Therapy* 2011; 42:589–600.

30. Corrigan P, Roe D, Tsang H. *Challenging the Stigma of Mental Illness: Lessons for Advocates and Therapists*. London: Wiley; 2011.

31. Lawrence S, Willig J, Crane H, et al. Routine, self-administered, touch-screen computer based suicidal ideation assessment linked to automated response team notification in an HIV primary care setting. *Clinical Infectious Disease* 2010; 50(4):1165–1173.

32. Bennett G, Glasgow R. The delivery of public health interventions via the Internet: Actualizing their potential. *Annual Review of Public Health* 2009; 30:273–292.

33. International Telecommunications Union. *The World in 2011: ICT Facts and Figures*. Geneva, Switzerland; 2011.

34. International Telecommunications Union. *The World in 2013: ICT Facts and Figures*. Geneva, Switzerland; 2013.

35. Ben-Zeev D, Davis K, Kaiser S, Krzos I, Drake R. Mobile technologies among people with serious mental illness: Current use and opportunities for future services. *Administration and Policy in Mental Health and Mental Health Services Research* 2012; 40(4):340–343.

36. Post L, Vaca F, Doran K, et al. New media use by patients who are homeless: The potential of mHealth to build connectivity. *Journal of Medical Internet Research* 2013; 15(9):e195.

37. Proudfoot J. The future is in our hands: The role of mobile phones in the prevention and management of mental disorders. *Australian and New Zealand Journal of Psychiatry* 2013; 47(2):111–113.

38. Harrison V, Proudfoot J, Wee P, Parker G, Pavlovic D, Manicavasagar V. Mobile mental health: Review of the emerging field and proof of concept study. *Journal of Mental Health* 2011; 20(6):509–524.

39. Luxton D, McCann R, Bush N, Mishkind M, Reger G. mHealth for mental health: Integrating smartphone technology in behavioral healthcare. *Professional Psychology: Research and Practice* 2011; 42(6):505–512.

40. Kimhy D, Myin-Germeys I, Palmier-Claus J, Swendsen J. Mobile assessment guide for research in schizophrenia and severe mental disorders. *Schizophrenia Bulletin* 2012; 38(3):386–395.

41. Ben-Zeev D, McHugo G, Xie H, Dobbins K, Young M. Comparing retrospective reports to real-time/real-place mobile assessments in individuals with schizophrenia and a nonclinical comparison group. *Schizophrenia Bulletin* 2012; 38(3):396–404.

42. Shiffman S, Kirchner T. Cigarette-by-cigarette satisfaction during ad libitum smoking. *Journal of Abnormal Psychology* 2009; 118(2):348–359.

43. Ben-Zeev D, Young M, Depp C. Real-time predictors of suicidal ideation: Mobile assessment of hospitalized depressed patients. *Psychiatry Research* 2012; 197(1-2):55–59.

44. Nock M, Prinstein M, Sterba S. Revealing the form and function of self-injurious thoughts and behaviors: A real-time ecological assessment study among adolescents and young adults. *Journal of Abnormal Psychology* 2009; 118(4):816–827.

45. Swendsen J, Ben-Zeev D, Granholm E. Real-time electronic ambulatory monitoring of substance use and symptom expression in schizophrenia. *American Journal of Psychiatry* 2011; 168(2):202–209.

46. Ben-Zeev D, Ellington K, Swendsen J, Granholm E. Examining a cognitive model of persecutory ideation in the daily life of people with schizophrenia: A computerized experience sampling study. *Schizophrenia Bulletin* 2011; 37(6):1248–1256.

47. Ben-Zeev D, Morris S, Swendsen J, Granholm E. Predicting the occurrence, conviction, distress, and disruption of different delusional experiences in the daily life of people with schizophrenia. *Schizophrenia Bulletin* 2012; 38(4):826–837.

48. Depp C, Kim D, de Dios L, Wang V, Ceglowski, J. A pilot study of mood ratings captured by mobile phone versus paper-and-pencil mood charts in bipolar disorder. *Journal of Dual Diagnosis* 2012; 8(4):326–332.

49. Oorschot M, Lataster T, Thewissen V, Wichers M, Myin-Germeys I. Mobile assessment in schizophrenia: A data-driven momentary approach. *Schizophrenia Bulletin* 2012; 38(3):405–413.

50. Thewissen V, Bentall R, Lecomte T, van Os J, Myin-Germeys I. Fluctuations in self-esteem and paranoia in the context of daily life. *Journal of Abnormal Psychology* 2008; 117(1):143–153.

51. Myin-Germeys I, Birchwood M, Kwapil T. From environment to therapy in psychosis: A real-world momentary assessment approach. *Schizophrenia Bulletin* 2011; 37(2):244–247.

52. Granholm E, Ben-Zeev D, Link P, Bradshaw K, Holden J. Mobile assessment and treatment for schizophrenia (MATS): A pilot trial of an interactive text-messaging intervention for medication adherence, socialization, and auditory hallucinations. *Schizophrenia Bulletin* 2012; 38(3):414–425.

53. Spaniel F, Hrdlička J, Novák T, Kožený J, Höschl C, Mohr P, Motlová LB. Effectiveness of the information technology-aided program of relapse prevention in schizophrenia (ITAREPS): A randomized, controlled, double-blind study. *Journal of Psychiatric Practice* 2012; 18(4):269–280.

54. U.S. Department of Veterans Affairs. Mobile App: PTSD Coach. 2011, March 25. Retrieved from http://www.ptsd.va.gov/public/pages/PTSDCOach.asp

55. Zhenyu C, Lane N, Cardone G, Lin M, Choudhury T, Campbell A. Unobtrusive sleep monitoring using smartphones. In *Proceedings of Pervasive Health*, 2013, Venice, Italy.

56. Rabbi M, Ali S, Choudhury T, Berke E. Passive and in-situ assessment of mental and physical well-being using mobile sensors. In *Proceedings of Ubicomp*, 2011, Beijing, China.

57. Black A, Serowik K, Schensul J, Bowen A, Rosen M. Build a better mouse: Directly observed issues in computer use for adults with SMI. *Psychiatric Quarterly* 2013; 84(1):81–92.

58. Brunette M, Ferron J, Devitt T, Geiger P, Martin W, Pratt S, Santos M, McHugo G. Do smoking cessation websites meet the needs of smokers with severe mental illnesses? *Health Education Research* 2012; 27(2):183–190.

59. Maguire M. Methods to support human-centered design. *International Journal of Human-Computer Studies* 2001; 55(4):587–634.

60. Rotondi A, Sinkule J, Haas G, Spring M, Litschge C, Newhill C, Ganguli R, Anderson C. Designing websites for persons with cognitive deficits: Design and usability of a psychoeducational intervention for persons with severe mental illness. *Psychological Services* 2007; 4(3):202–224.

61. Silva B, Rodrigues J, Canelo F, Lopes I, Zhou L. A data encryption solution for mobile health apps in cooperation environments. *Journal of Medical Internet Research* 2013; 15(4):e66.

62. U.S. Department of Health and Human Services Food and Drug Administration. Mobile medical applications guidance for industry and food and drug administration staff. 2013. Retrieved from http://www.fda.gov/downloads/MedicalDevices/DeviceRegulationandGuidance/GuidanceDocuments/UCM263366.pdf

63. Lehavot K, Ben-Zeev D, Neville R. Ethical considerations and social media: A case of suicidal postings on Facebook. *Journal of Dual Diagnosis* 2012; 8(4):341–346.

64. Kumar S, Nilsen W, Pavel M, Srivastava M. Mobile health: Revolutionizing healthcare through transdisciplinary research. *Computer* 2013;28–35.

65. Stokols D, Hall K, Taylor B, Moser R. The science of team science: Overview of the field and introduction to the supplement. *American Journal of Preventive Medicine* 2008; 35:S77–S89.

66. Christensen H, Griffiths K, Farrer L. Adherence in Internet interventions for anxiety and depression: Systematic review. *Journal of Medical Internet Research* 2009; 11(2):e13.

67. Hawkins R, Kreuter M, Resnicow K, Fishbein M, Dijkstra A. Understanding tailoring in communicating about health. *Health Education Research* 2008; 23(3):454–466.

68. Whaley A, Davis K. Cultural competence and evidence-based practice in mental health services: A complementary perspective. *American Psychology* 2007; 62:563–574.

69. Byrne S, Gay G, Pollack J, et al. Caring for mobile phone-based virtual pets can influence youth eating behaviors. *Journal of Children and Media* 2012; 6(1):83–99.

70. Clarke G, Eubanks D, et al. Overcoming depression on the internet (ODIN) (2): A randomized trial of a self-help depression skills program with reminders. *Journal of Medical Internet Research* 2005; 7:e16.

71. Google, Inc. Get the Android SDK. 2013. Retrieved from http://developer.android.com/sdk/index.html

7

Applying Technology to Medication Management and Adherence

LEAH L. ZULLIG, RYAN J. SHAW, AND HAYDEN B. BOSWORTH

THE PROBLEM OF MEDICATION NON-ADHERENCE

Medication non-adherence is one of the most significant challenges to public health today (1). In order for medication to work properly, it must be taken consistently as prescribed. However, poor medication adherence is rampant, negatively impacting both individual and community-level health. In fact, it has been consistently demonstrated that approximately 20–30% of prescription medications are never filled (2,3); 40% of patients do not fill an original prescription (4–6); over 50% prematurely discontinue medications within 1 year (4,7,8); and an average of 50% of chronic disease medications are not taken as prescribed (2,3). Furthermore, adverse events, including hospitalizations and death, are associated with inadequate pill refill rates for many common chronic conditions such as hypertension and hyperlipidemia (4,9–11). The effects of medication non-adherence are far-reaching and include increased cost related to increased utilization of healthcare services, reduced care quality, and poor patient outcomes (4,12–14). Proper medication adherence can potentially improve patients' health and quality of life, save patients from unnecessary expenses, and reduce unnecessary healthcare utilization and cost to the healthcare system.

Medication non-adherence is costly, both to individual patients and the healthcare system. It has been estimated that medication non-adherence costs the U.S. healthcare system between $100 billion and $298 billion annually (14,15). As the U.S. population continues to age (16), the burden of chronic disease has dramatically increased (17), and reliance on medication

management for control of chronic diseases has also escalated (18). Aggravating the problem, overall healthcare costs have soared (19), and the ability to pay for medications is one factor that is responsible for non-adherence (20). Therefore, proper medication adherence should lead to subsequent reductions in healthcare costs. For example, one study determined that for many chronic diseases, including diabetes and hypercholesterolemia, a high level of medication adherence was associated with lower disease-related medical costs. Moreover, cost offsets (where higher medication costs were more than offset by reductions in medical costs) were observed for all-cause medical costs, and adherent patients had lower hospitalization rates (21).

IMPORTANT ROLE OF TECHNOLOGY AS A SOLUTION TO MEDICATION ADHERENCE

Existing interventions that have proven effective at promoting proper medication management tend to be costly (22,23), labor intensive (24), and ineffective in promoting long-term change (25,26). Emerging technology-driven interventions provide an important strategy to increase medication adherence, while simultaneously overcoming many of these previous deficits. Technological solutions can be used to intervene across the continuum of non-adherence, ranging from simplifying prescription refills, to providing daily reminders, facilitating patient–provider communication, and creating a social environment supportive of medication adherence. For example, technology can provide precise data about when and how medications are refilled and administered, which may be more reliable than self-reported information.

Technology-driven interventions may reduce reliance on human resources, be accessible to a broader group of patients, and save cost.

By harnessing technology to aid in adherence, non-adherent patients (and those at risk for non-adherence) can be easily identified and, with the aid of technological solutions, adherence can be improved. Engaging appropriate technological solutions has many advantages. They can be inexpensive, span geographic distances, and be delivered directly to patients in a manner that is most convenient for them (2). Technology can facilitate communication between patients and their providers (27) and can be used to provide tailored feedback and/or triggers based on patient preferences or when intervention is needed (28).

TYPES OF TECHNOLOGY

There are a number of technologies to improve medication adherence. The types of technology and how they are applied are in a constant state of evolution. We highlight here three primary categories of technology: (a) pill-monitoring technology—electronic pill caps, smart blister packaging, and digital pills; (b) mobile health technology—including text messaging, smartphone applications, or apps, interactive voice response, electronic health records (EHRs), and multimodal approaches; and (c) online resources and social media. Although these are merely a sample of available strategies, they illustrate the diversity of technological tools available today. These interventions can be employed to improve medication adherence for many chronic conditions, including hypertension, diabetes, obesity, tuberculosis, and human immunodeficiency virus (HIV), among others.

Pill-Monitoring Technologies

Electronic pill sensors can be used to facilitate medication monitoring and prompt patients to take medication at appropriate times. There are many forms of pill monitoring, including electronic pill caps, smart blister packs, and digital pills. Electronic pill caps are probably the most widely utilized technology in this category. These caps record the date and time that a pill bottle was opened, providing an objective measure of medication adherence. This information can be used to report on pill-taking patterns and inform patient counseling. Electronic pill caps, often called medication event monitoring systems, or MEMs, have been applied to measure medication adherence for many chronic conditions, including HIV (29), cancer (30), depression (31), schizophrenia (32), and hypertension (33).

Smart blister packs are another method to monitor medication adherence. These are either disposable cards that contain multiple pills (e.g., a 30-day supply) with a sensor on the back of the packaging or an adhesive label of sensor "stickers" that can be applied to an existing, standard blister pack. Regardless of its form, the sensor tracks the time and location when each pill is removed from its package.

Variations of both the electronic pill caps and smart blister packs incorporate reminder systems; they may illuminate or emit an auditory tone if a patient fails to take medication at a predetermined time. Both technologies use short-range wireless technology to generate reports about medication adherence and associated behavioral patterns, such as timing of taking medications and consistency with daily medication-taking routines. This information can be useful in differentiating between non-adherent patients (those who truly do not take their medication) and non-respondent patients (those that do not communicate with their clinicians about taking their medications). Making this distinction is important, because different intervention strategies and intervention intensity may be required depending on a patient's specific behaviors related to medication non-adherence.

One industry example of an electronic pill cap harnessing multiple strategies to promote adherence is the GlowCap™, manufactured by Vitality (34). The GlowCap™ has a computer chip in the lid that communicates with a cellular-connected plug-in nightlight. The cap itself and/or the plug-in nightlight serve as a reminder system. Depending on their preference, patients can be notified that it is time to take their medication via a glowing light, a tune, automated calls, text messages, or e-mails. The reminders can be repeated for up to four doses a day and the messages can intensify depending on the persistence of non-adherence (e.g., escalate from subtle to insistent: devices glow, then produce audible noise, then send a text notification). Patients can also order a refill of their medication by pressing a button on the base of the GlowCap™ lid. The lid sends a request to the patient's pharmacy over the cellular network, which sets up an automatic call-back for the patient to confirm the request (34).

Preliminary evidence suggests that GlowCap™ can be effective in increasing medication adherence. Although the results have not been published in a peer-reviewed journal, Partners Healthcare's Center for Connected Health conducted a 6-month, three-arm randomized controlled trial. Patients with hypertension were randomized to one of three groups: 1) a control group that did not receive any communication or GlowCap™ services; 2) an intervention group that received visual and audio GlowCap™ reminders, plus phone call reminders for missed doses, and medication refill reminders and progress reports e-mailed to the patient, designated family member, and/or their primary care provider; or 3) an intervention-plus group which received the services noted in the intervention group, as well as a financial incentive if they met or exceeded a target of 80% adherence (35,36). At 6 months, the control group had an adherence rate of 71%, and the intervention and intervention-plus groups had adherence rates of 98% and 99%, respectively (35,36). This equates to approximately 27% increase, on average, in medication adherence rates among hypertensive patients. The cost-effectiveness of this intervention has not been studied.

As another example of electronic pill-monitoring technology, Rosen, Rigsby, Salahi, Ryan, and Cramer assessed electronic pill-monitoring technology (37) among 79 patients that were prescribed metformin for the management of hyperglycemia. Patients' adherence levels were first assessed during a 4-week baseline period using an electronic pill cap. Non-adherent patients, those who did not take doses as prescribed within a 4-hour time frame, were randomized to either 4 months of cue-dose training or to a control group. Cue-dose training entails reviewing pill cap data with patients and advising them to link medication-taking with an element of their daily routine such as brushing their teeth or mealtimes. Cue-dose training was associated with a statistically significant mean increase of 15% more metformin doses taken as prescribed compared to the control group. Nine patients and five providers involved in the cue-dosing training group provided feedback on their experiences. Participants reported that medication adherence was discussed

for approximately 6 minutes on average and that the pill cap data were moderately helpful (as assessed by a 5-point Likert scale) in informing this discussion (37). Use of this technology can facilitate improvements in medication adherence and may foster counseling and education that can further enhance adherence.

The Phillips Medication Dispensing Service provides a different approach to pill monitoring (38). The medication dispenser may be particular useful among adults with cognitive difficulties, people with limited mobility, and/or take complex medication regimens that require consistent reminders. To use the device, the patient or their caregiver loads the medication into individual cups with a lid. These cups are loaded into the medication dispensing service. The machine dispenses up to 60 cups and is capable of storing up to 40 days of medication and 6 daily doses. At programmed time intervals, the dispensing machine emits a sound and lights up to alert the patient that it is time to take his or her pills. The patient presses a button and the medication cup is delivered. If desired, the dispensing service can also be programmed to present instructions on how to take the medication. The machine is connected to the patient's telephone line. If the patient misses a dose, the medication dispensing service can contact a caregiver, family member, or another contact (38).

Digital Pills

"Digital pills" are essentially ingestible sensors, which are currently about the size of a grain of sand (39). A silicon chip is attached on top of a pill. These digitized pills consist of materials found in common foods; they contain small amounts of copper and magnesium that interact with stomach fluids inside the body to produce a voltage that can be read through the skin (40). Patients wear a disposable patch, similar in appearance to a Band-Aid. Because of its battery life, the patch is replaced every 7 days. This patch detects a signal from the pill and transmits date- and time-stamped information to any Bluetooth-enabled device. The device could be the patient's or a caregiver's mobile phone, or it could reside in a physician's office. The sensor can communicate when a pill has been taken (or not taken). The pill and sensor can also detect vital signs such as a patient's heart rate, body temperature, rest, and physical activity level. It can safely be used alongside other medical devices, such as a pacemaker.

The scalability of digital pills will depend on their cost. There is little information about the cost of digital pills, either in terms of total cost or return on investment. Leading manufacturers are vague about cost, only indicating that the cost is dependent on "the context" in which the pill is used (39). The quality of the data supporting digital pills is another unknown. Although the digital pill may have a positive impact on medication adherence, the data regarding digital pills exclusively originate from the pill manufacturers (40).

There are additional challenges associated with digital pills. They require a significant level of coordination between patients, clinicians, and pharmaceutical manufacturers. The U.S. Food and Drug Administration only recently approved placebo digital pills (e.g., manufactured by Proteus Digital Health) (40). In addition, digital pills must be non-toxic, safe and effective in clinical testing, and they must pass electrical safety requirements. Digital pills also require labeling for maximum number of daily ingestions (41). Once these initial challenges have been overcome, research studies are needed to determine acceptability, efficiency, and cost-effectiveness of digital pills in promoting medication adherence.

Conductive Inks

Conductive inks have been used for a variety of purposes, including radiofrequency identification tags used for many modern transportation tickets. These inks generally consist of metallic nanoparticles, such as silver, to form an antenna that wirelessly transmits information about its location. Industrial conductive ink products may not be appropriate for patient monitoring because conductivity is poor and most ink contains toxic components. However, researchers at the University of Florida have pioneered conductive ink that is non-toxic and that will degrade after use (42). This "safer" conductive ink could be used to monitor medication adherence. For example, the conductive ink could be applied to the exterior of a pill. Because the ink is safe to ingest, it can transmit information about the pill's location both inside and outside of the human body. This invention may be revolutionary in inpatient and outpatient settings, as well as promote optimal adherence during

clinical trial participation. Rather than relying on memory recall, this conductive ink technology ensures that patients and clinicians have accurate information about medication-taking (42).

Mobile Health (mHealth) Technologies

Mobile health (mHealth) technologies provide a promising way to inexpensively reach a broad spectrum of patients. mHealth encompasses an array of tools including (a) text messaging, (b) interactive voice response, (c) smartphone applications, and (d) multimodal mHealth approaches. These tools may integrate some of the aforementioned systems, like reminders, in addition to providing educational or motivational information. A key advantage of mHealth is that it can overcome many common barriers to in-person care. These include patient-initiated barriers such as lack of transportation, geographic distance, employment and/or childcare obligations, and absenteeism or missed appointments, as well as health system–initiated barriers such as long appointment wait times, lack of availability of physicians, and high cost. Messages can easily be tailored in terms of delivery format (e.g., text messaging vs. interactive voice response), timing of delivery, and content of the message, to appeal to patients with differing medication adherence needs and personal preferences.

mHealth approaches have the additional advantage of accessibility to many different patient populations. For example, mobile phone penetration worldwide averages 58%, and this is expected to increase (43,44). In many developing geographic areas, such as Latin America and the Caribbean, nearly 80% of adults have mobile phones (44). Virtually all homes in the United States (97%) have telephones (45), making telephone-based care an attractive modality for medication adherence interventions. For many patients, the telephone is an acceptable medium for delivery of a self-management support program (43,46,47). In Honduras, Piette, Mendoza-Avelares, Milton, Lange, and Fajardo identified that approximately 88% of respondents with chonic disease were willing to receive automated telephone remidners about upcoming appointments, more than 83% were willing to receive information about medication adherence, and nearly 80% were willing to receive automated health status monitoring for their symptoms and self-care needs. Moreover,

over 81% were willing to participate in automated self-management education (43). In addition to acceptability, telephone-based interventions have been proven effective in changing patient behaviors (2,43,48,49). For example, a randomized trial of a telephone-based behavioral intervention found that among hypertensive patients in the telephone-based intervention group, self-reported medication adherence increased by 9%, vs. 1% in the group receiving usual care (50).

Text Messaging

Short message service (SMS), or text messaging, has been used to motivate medication adherence for patients with HIV, asthma, tuberculosis, mental health conditions, diabetes, and hypertension, among others. Text messaging can be used to communicate urgent health needs between patients and clinicians (51), which may result in improved adherence and outcomes. Text messaging can also be employed to monitor adherence in real time and prompt patients with reminders to take their medications.

A randomized, controlled trial conducted in the Netherlands evaluated the effect of SMS reminders of adherence to oral antidiabetics in patients using a real-time medication monitoring system (52). One hundred and four patients with type II diabetes with suboptimal medication adherence to oral antidiabetics were enrolled. Approximately half of the patients received SMS reminders if they failed to take their medication and approximately half received no reminders. The days without dosing were not significantly different between the two groups. However, over the 6-month study period, patients who received the reminders took more doses than those who did not receive SMS reminders. The difference was moderate: 50% vs. 39% within a 1-hour window and up to 81% vs. 70% within a 4-hour window (52). Although this is not a dramatic difference, it suggests that the timeliness with which patients take medications can be improved through the use of SMS reminders. Such timeliness may be critical to manage conditions where the timing and consistency of medication administration is imperative, such as with antiretrovirals.

Although the study on antidiabetic adminstration suggests some promise, the overall success of SMS is unclear. Trials using SMS to improve adherence to antihypertensive medication have met with mixed results (53). Similarly, results are mixed regarding the effectiveness of SMS to incite changes in healthcare utilization for people with chronic diseases (54). The effectiveness of SMS may be affected by both their timinig and length, as well as by the specific condition being addressed. For example, trials using SMS to promote medication adherence to antiretrovirals seem to be be more successful than for some other conditions (55). While more evidence is needed regarding the impact of text messaging on medication adherence, it seems most effective when certain conditions are met: (a) when there is follow-up, (b) when the message is personally tailored, and (c) when the frequency, wording, and content are highly relevant (56). In the example regarding SMS reminders for antidiabetic medications, one reason for the success of the intervention could be the frequency and content of the messages.

Interactive Voice Response (IVR)

IVR is a technology that allows people to interact with an automated computer system through speech or by entering information on a phone keypad. IVR can be used to triage those whose needs can be met exclusively by the computer from those who require communication with a professional (in the context of healthcare, possibly a nurse or pharmacist). IVR has broad non-health-related uses. Common applications include checking bank balances, flight schedules, or theater show times through the use of an automated IVR system. Because of its widespread use, the U.S. population is generally familiar with IVR technology, making it an attractive technology to aid medication adherence.

Although medication adherence work has focused on precursors to cardiovascular disease (CVD; e.g., hypertension, hyperlipidemia, and diabetes), IVR can also be leveraged to improve medication adherence for clinical conditions beyond precursors to CVD. IVR may be particularly useful for complex medication regimens such as oral chemotherapy. The instructions on how to take cancer-related medications can be confusing (e.g., take 5 to 12 pills 2 to 3 times daily with 2 weeks on and 1 week off followed by 2 weeks on). Further complicating the matter, symptom severity may inhibit adherence. One study using an IVR system plus a nursing intervention found a 23.3% non-adherence rate to oral chemotherapy medications due either to symptoms or forgetting to take medication (57). Interestingly, the majority of adherent and non-adherent patients reported that the IVR was helpful in monitoring their oral chemotherapy regimen (58% adherent; 60% non-adherent), while 40% of non-adherent patients reported that IVR was burdensome (compared to 0% of adherent patients). When asked if they would recommend IVR to their oncologist to remind patients to take pills, adherent and non-adherent patients were divided (58% of adherent patients would recommend vs. 40% of non-adherent patients). For future interventions developers should seek to understand the role of purely automated IVR vs. IVR coupled with interaction with an interventionist and for which types of patients and/or disease states IVR is most effective. Although work may be needed to fine-tune IVR as a singular intervention strategy, these findings suggest that IVR may be an acceptable and effective tool for improving medication adherence.

Smartphone Applications

In the United States, more than 87% of the population uses a mobile phone (58). As mobile phones offer more advances in computing ability, mobile phones have transitioned beyond solely providing basic voice and text messaging features. Many mobile phones now incorporate a sophisticated operating system allowing users to download and add programs. These phones, commonly called "smartphones," are capable of running applications and connecting to the Internet, and they contain a plethora of features, including digital and video cameras, media players, global positioning system (GPS) navigation, touchscreens, and speech recognition. With the advent of smartphones and mobile devices such as iPads and tablets, an app can be used to deliver healthcare and promote self-management.

Many apps can be leveraged to promote health. Smartphones can be used to list patients' medication, schedule pill reminders, and help order refills. A review by Gayar et al. (2013) examined the use of cell phone apps to help patients with type 1 or type 2 diabetes self-manage their condition (59). They found that the apps supported self-management tasks such as exercise, insulin and oral medication dosage, blood glucose testing, and diet. Other tasks included decision support, alerts, tagging of input data such as blood glucose levels, and integration with social media. Figure 7.1 demonstrates the use of an app to remind a patient to take their oral diabetes medication (metformin).

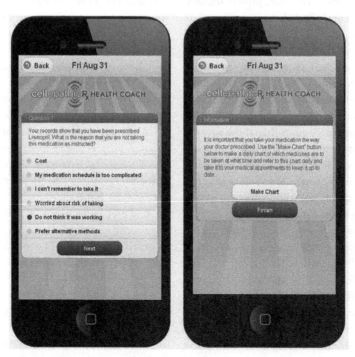

FIGURE 7.1: A smartphone application address medication adherence.

Multimodal mHealth Approaches

mHealth strategies, such as reminder systems and IVR, can be combined to improve patient care in a manner considered most appropriate by the patient. As an example, McGillicuddy and colleagues (60) monitored patient-reported generalized perceived stress and medication adherence among kidney transplant patients. Participants were also asked about their personal mobile phone use. As part of the study, patients were furnished with a multimodal prototype system, which included a smartphone. In addition to a smartphone, the project's prototype system also involved a wireless medication tray and a wireless blood pressure monitor. The medication tray could remind the patient to take his or her medication in several forms—via lights, tones, text message, or a phone call. To assess medication adherence without relying on patient self-report, the medication tray also tracked when patients were taking the medication. Adherence information could be transmitted directly to the patient, their provider, or both. Patients were given a choice about how they wanted to receive medication-related instructions from their healthcare provider. Patients preferred phone call, voicemail, and text messages, in that order. Only 7% ($n = 7/98$) of patients reported prior knowledge of mobile phone–based remote monitoring. The majority of patients (79%, total $n = 78/99$) had a positive attitude toward use of the system, provided that they incurred no costs. Participants were comfortable being monitored by mHealth technology, and they felt their privacy could be adequately protected.

The work of McGillicuddy et al. is innovative and provides an excellent example of a multimodal, technology-driven intervention to improve medication adherence among a vulnerable population of kidney transplant patients (60). Given limited financial resources, it may not be possible to furnish smartphones to all patients experiencing medication adherence issues. Understanding whether patients currently use and personally own a smartphone is an important consideration for rolling out this or similar interventions. In the kidney transplant patient cohort, 90% of patients owned a mobile phone, and non-white patients were more likely than white patients to own a smartphone.

Furthermore, there was no report on the clinical or cost-effectiveness of this intervention. Although judging feasibility and acceptability of mHealth to patients is a key first step, even more critical is determining the effectiveness of mHealth to improve medication adherence.

Online Resources and Social Media

Online resources and social media provide a unique forum for patients to obtain information and connect with others. Although there are many websites focused on providing specific information about conditions, products, and medications, technology has shifted to allow for more peer-to-peer information exchanges. Nearly half (46%) of all adults and 62% of Internet-using adults report using social media sites, such as Facebook or MySpace (61). One study reported that a minority of adults (13%) go online to connect with others who have similar health problems. This was significantly more common among adults living with a chronic health condition than generally healthy adults (23% vs. 15%) (61).

In the context of medication adherence, online communities and social media can be critical resources, as they may provide a community supportive of staying adherent. One example is Patients Like Me (www.patientslikeme.com), which provides educational material on a multitude of chronic conditions, an online community to connect with other patients, and a tracking system for self-monitoring. Researchers conducted a survey on the use of social media and mobile technologies to enhance adherence to antiretroviral therapy among people living with HIV (62). Survey respondents favored Facebook because it helped people feel like they were not alone and presented "real" photographs, offering a more lifelike perspective (62). Additionally, survey participants reported that social networking websites enabled them to socialize with others (45% of participants) and provided information relevant to their condition (e.g., HIV; 22% of participants). However, privacy was a noteworthy barrier for 26% of participants (62).

Websites like YouTube (www.youtube.com) that feature videos, Twitter (www.twitter.com), and blogs may provide a growing forum for patients to learn strategies for improved medication adherence from health professionals, pharmaceutical and device manufacturers, as well as their peers. Online resources, particularly social media, are rapidly evolving and increasing in popularity. Thus social media has the potential for reaching a broad patient audience.

ELECTRONIC HEALTH RECORDS

Electronic health records (EHRs) are reshaping the landscape of clinical care delivery, including medication management. In 2011, approximately 54% of office-based physicians used EHRs in the United States (63). Also in 2011, nearly half of physicians who were not using EHRs indicated that they planned to do so in the coming year. Perhaps because of evolving health policy and reimbursement changes, implementation of EHRs has rapidly increased. Another study conducted in 2012 indicated that 72% of office-based physicians had adopted EHR technology (64). The use of EHRs is expected to increase.

EHRs serve as the backbone of technological approaches to improve medication adherence. EHRs enable electronic prescription ordering, provide a conduit for communication between provider and pharmacy, offer clinical reminders, facilitate communication across providers to avoid medication duplication and reduce the likelihood of medication error, and may provide a portal for patients to access and/or add to their health data. We highlight here examples of EHRs from an integrated health system, the Veterans Affairs (VA) healthcare system, which effectively uses EHRs to facilitate medication adherence.

The VA healthcare system was a pioneer in adopting EHRs. The VA's EHR system, known as the Computerized Patient Record System (CPRS), has a successful history spanning from 1997 to today. CPRS serves as a platform for an array of clinical functions, including laboratory and medication ordering. It also interfaces with electronic pharmacy benefits management systems. In 2003, the VA initiated two programs with potential to positively impact medication adherence. The first was an online patient portal and electronic personal health record system called MyHealtheVet (https://www.myhealth.va.gov/index.html). MyHealtheVet enables patients to become active participants in their healthcare,

promoting medication adherence. Users of the system are able to enter their medications (including herbs and over-the-counter medications such as aspirin), request VA prescription refills, view a complete history of their VA medications, and view and/or print a list of all medications, including both VA-administered medications and any that the patient manually entered. Users are also able to send secure text messages to their healthcare team for non-urgent questions such as changes in medication, renewing a medication prescription, or changing symptoms (65).

Another tool based on the VA's EHR is the Home Telehealth Program. This program targets patients with chronic conditions, many of whom rely on medications for disease management, and provides them with home monitoring equipment that transmits health data (e.g., blood pressure values) bidirectionally between the VA and patients' homes via telephone and the Internet (66). Although this intervention does not directly address medication adherence, assessing patients' clinical values (such as blood pressure) remotely may provide an early warning sign of non-adherence and a cue to intervene. For example, patterns in a patient's blood pressure readings over time can be monitored. If a patient's blood pressure changes, perhaps gradually increases, this may be a sign of medication non-adherence or a need to modify the medication regime. Home monitoring can provide an early indicator of non-adherence, presenting clinical data in between office visits, which may improve patient care.

The push to use EHRs for medication adherence is moving beyond hospitals and health systems and into the neighborhood pharmacy. Drug makers such as Merck are teaming up with pharmacies such as CVS Caremark to monitor and motivate their customers. Through the use of the EHRs, pharmacies are able to determine if patients are refilling their medications, and refilling prescriptions is a factor in determining medication adherence (67).

The abilities to view medications and to electronically order prescription refills at any time of day from the convenience of one's home are expected to have a positive impact on medication adherence. To prevent non-adherence due to refill problems, pharmacies and EHR systems can partner to make obtaining refills easier. This could prompt refill alerts, triggered to patients, their pharmacy, or both. The partnership between pharmacies and EHRs may make obtaining refills easier, thus minimizing potential non-adherence. Such strategies include providing longer prescriptions (e.g., 90-day supply instead of a 30-day supply), automatic refills, and alerting patients when a new prescription from their provider is needed.

While existing EHRs are invaluable, EHRs are evolving. As part of the American Recovery and Reinvestment Act of 2009, the Health Information Technology for Economic and Clinical Health (HITECH) Act to promote the adoption and meaningful use of health information technology (IT) was enacted. This significant investment in health IT has pushed the adoption and meaningful use of health IT, particularly EHRs, by U.S. providers and hospitals through incentive payments and penalties. These incentive payments are based on meaningful use. Meaningful use is the set of standards defined by the Centers for Medicare and Medicaid Services Incentive Programs that governs the use of EHRs and allows incentive payments by meeting specific criteria. HITECH has not only pushed the adoption of EHRs, but by 2016, the third stage of meaningful use will tie incentive payments under the Medicare and Medicaid programs on the use of Health IT for improved patient outcomes. This third stage specifies that patients must have access to self-management tools and that technology should be used to improve health outcomes and population health. The technological tools for medication adherence described in this chapter allow for the collection of data on medication adherence and can serve as technological tools for patient self-management.

IMPORTANCE OF APPROPRIATENESS AND ACCEPTABILITY

No single technology will be the holy grail of medication adherence. What may work for one group may not work for another. Because of patient preferences, for instance, technologies to improve medication adherence among teenagers may not be appropriate for elderly patients. For example, teenagers may use text messaging often in their daily routine whereas the elderly may be

less apt to do so; this may impact which technological approach is best suited for a specific patient population. Harris, Hood, and Mulvaney note that technologies used by teens include mobile phone text messaging, applications, and video conferencing through software such as Skype™ (68). Reaching elderly populations may require a different set of technologies because of physical limitations. According to the Pew Research Center (61), many seniors find mobile phones complex, have difficulty managing small mobile phone buttons, or cannot read text on mobile phone screens. This may require tools such as big-button mobile phones, extra-loud speakers for reminder systems, and one-touch commands. The technological tool chosen should align with the needs and preference of the target population.

Furthermore, many studies focus on one specific product, which may not have broad appeal. For example, we previously described the GlowCap™, a pill-monitoring technology that uses multiple strategies to improve adherence (34). While the GlowCap™ is a cutting-edge product, it relies exclusively on a single cellular network. Although it is not necessary that patients use that particular network, patients have to pay a separate monthly fee for the service. Consequently, while patients may be generally amenable to the idea of pill monitoring, they may prefer a different product style. When designing technology-driven interventions, one must be mindful of the appropriateness and acceptability of the particular technology to the target population. Moreover, the social validity of a technological intervention—whether it is socially acceptable, relevant, and useful from the patients' perspective—must be assessed in the context of development efforts.

LIMITATIONS OF CURRENT KNOWLEDGE

There are several gaps in our current understanding of how technology, particularly mHealth, can be leveraged most effectively as an instrument to increase medication adherence. More information is needed regarding the clinical effectiveness, cost-effectiveness, and broad dissemination potential of these interventions. Developers of most mHealth interventions aim to establish feasibility or acceptability of the intervention. The evidence for clinical effectiveness of technology-driven interventions is mixed and may be impacted by lack of clarity regarding how they should be administered. Interventions vary in length of the study, frequency of contact, direction of communication (e.g., uni- or bidirectional), and general context. Further examination is required to examine the long-term benefits of these programs.

Additionally, many mHealth technologies, including text messaging, interactive voice response, and applications, rely on cellular phones. This leads to four potential limitations: accessibility, unknown cost-effectiveness, privacy, and interoperability. Regarding accessibility, while cellular phones are a common part of daily life in many cultures worldwide, they are dependent on network availability. The cost of supporting devices may be a barrier to elderly, minority, rural, and low-income populations (69). Those who do not have cellular coverage in their homes may be unable to use this technology. Many interventions hinge on patients having the desired technological devices (e.g., smartphone vs. standard mobile phone; specific product or brand) and require some degree of technology literacy. This may be a particular problem for the elderly or those not technologically savvy and may limit broad dissemination of interventions that have been pilot tested in a specific population. Making this especially problematic, it is possible that those at increased risk for medication adherence are also the least likely to understand the target technology. For example, medication adherence is a common issue among seniors with multiple chronic conditions, a population who may find smartphones to be difficult to understand and use properly. They may have more basic phone models and limited coverage plans and may fail to carry their phones with them regularly. These behaviors would make a text messaging or app-based intervention difficult to deliver.

Although there is much promise with the use of apps for medication management, there is limited testing, and rigorous research is still in its early stages. Limitations of apps include lack of personalized feedback, usability issues, and limited integration with patients' EHRs. Most apps simply provide reminders to help stimulate adherence and fail to integrate lifestyle factors that affect conditions like diabetes. Additional research and development is needed to take full advantage of the capabilities of apps. This includes making data collection passive and information delivered to patients proactive so that, for example, an app can recognize when medication is not taken or needs to be taken based on vital signs (e.g., blood pressure, heart rate, respiratory rate).

Variability in reporting makes it difficult to systematically evaluate the cost-effectiveness of technology-driven studies or to synthesize the elements that make an intervention effective for wider dissemination. However, interventions capitalizing on technology are purportedly cost-effective for two primary reasons. First, most are relatively inexpensive. This is especially true of telephone-based modalities such as text messaging and IVR. Second, mHealth has potential for broad reach and reduced need for expensive human resources. Although these assertions are plausible, there is a dearth of scientific evidence for their support. This may partially be a function of inconsistent information regarding their clinical effectiveness.

Similarly, there are mixed messages regarding cost-effectiveness. An assessment of text-messaged reminders to improve attendance at a health promotion clinic showed that text messages were more cost-effective than telephone calls (70). A well-conducted analysis studied the cost-effectiveness of a computer-delivered intervention designed to increase patients' health literacy as a strategy to improve their HIV medication adherence. Data were obtained from an electronic pill bottle, which recorded each time it was opened. This information was used to estimate adherence, and the intervention was determined to be clinically effective. After considering sizeable development costs, including computer programming and other development costs, as well as lost patient-wages for time spent participating in the study, the intervention was also found to be cost-effective. However, the intervention was most cost-effective when delivered to a relatively large group of participants (71). The ideal number of participants to maximize cost-effectiveness is not known. Some interventions have coupled technology-driven interventions with financial incentives. For example, Volpp and colleagues used an electronic reminder system in tandem with a daily lottery-based financial incentive system to improve warfarin adherence (72). Similarly, Sorensen et al. provided voucher-based incentives to patients who opened electronic pill caps on their antiretroviral medications (73). While these incentivized technology-driven interventions proved successful in the short term, whether the medication adherence improvement is sustained once incentives are removed is not well documented. The limited existing analyses examining cost-effectiveness have not begun to describe the numerous technology-intensive delivery modalities available nor the synergistic effect of combined, multimodal interventions.

Privacy is also a concern with these technologies. There are no clear guidelines about privacy. Yet patient privacy must be a major consideration in the design and development of these new technologies. This is particularly true for text messaging, as user authentication is not available for an individual message at this time, beyond having a password to access some phones. Mobile health interventions may often use a third party to transmit text messages (SMS), video messages, voice messages, or other data into an app. It is imperative that personal health information that is transmitted be limited.

Other challenges exist as well. Interoperability of mobile phone apps, electronic pill caps, and electronic health records is not always possible. These systems often do not link with each other. While a patient may use a mobile phone app as a reminder system, the information on whether or not the patient took the medication through the electronic pill cap is not necessarily transmitted to the mobile phone app. Even less likely is that either of these technologies will communicate with the EHR. Many data sources, such as a phone app, may store information exclusively on the user's phone or on a private network. This creates a problem: not only are the data stored in a single place, but clinicians may not have access to this adherence information. The responsibility of sharing information with providers may lie with the patients. Patients who are already non-adherent may be less likely to share information with their providers, thus preventing clinicians from intervening in their patients' medication management when they are on the verge of becoming non-compliant or need help most. The ability to integrate these technologies and allow clinicians access to their adherence data in real time is needed.

CONCLUSIONS

Advances in information technology are providing a variety of tools for patients and clinicians to use for medication adherence. As mobile technology and access to the Internet have become increasingly ubiquitous, we are able to leverage more interactive capabilities that facilitate communication between patients and their providers across geographic locations. The potential benefits of technology to improve medication adherence while minimizing additional cost are numerous. As technology advances and patients become increasingly comfortable with the role of technology in promoting health, we anticipate that the evidence supporting technology-driven interventions will advance and that technological solutions will be further integrated into patient-centered clinical care.

REFERENCES

1. Hill MN, Miller NH, Degeest S, Materson BJ, Black HR, Izzo JL Jr, et al. Adherence and persistence with taking medication to control high blood pressure. *Journal of the American Society of Hypertension* 2011; 5(1):56–63.
2. Bosworth HB. How can innovative uses of technology be harnessed to improve medication adherence? *Expert Review of Pharmacoeconomics & Outcomes Research* 2012; 12(2):133–135.
3. Bosworth HB, Oddone EZ, Weinberger M (Eds.). *Patient Treatment Adherence: Concepts, Interventions, and Measurement.* New York: Psychology Press; 2012.
4. Granger BB, Bosworth HB. Medication adherence: Emerging use of technology. *Current Opinion in Cardiology* 2011; 26(4):279–287.
5. Murray MD, Tu W, Wu J, Morrow D, Smith F, Brater DC. Factors associated with exacerbation of heart failure include treatment adherence and health literacy skills. *Clinical Pharmacology and Therapeutics* 2009; 85(6):651–658.
6. Steiner JF, Ho PM, Beaty BL, Dickinson LM, Hanratty R, Zeng C, et al. Sociodemographic and clinical characteristics are not clinically useful predictors of refill adherence in patients with hypertension. *Circulation Cardiovascular Quality and Outcomes* 2009; 2(5):451–457.
7. Shah ND, Dunlay SM, Ting HH, Montori VM, Thomas RJ, Wagie AE, et al. Long-term medication adherence after myocardial infarction: Experience of a community. *American Journal of Medicine* 2009; 122(10):961 e7–13.

8. Vanelli M, Pedan A, Liu N, Hoar J, Messier D, Kiarsis K. The role of patient inexperience in medication discontinuation: A retrospective analysis of medication nonpersistence in seven chronic illnesses. *Clinical Therapeutics* 2009; 31(11):2628–2652.

9. Bailey JE, Wan JY, Tang J, Ghani MA, Cushman WC. Antihypertensive medication adherence, ambulatory visits, and risk of stroke and death. *Journal of General Internal Medicine* 2010; 25(6):495–503.

10. Burzotta F, Trani C, Todaro D, Mazzari MA, Porto I, De Vita M, et al. Outcome of patients treated by a novel thin-strut cobalt-chromium stent in the drug-eluting stent era: Results of the SKICE (Skylor in real world practice) registry. *Catheterization and Cardiovascular Interventions* 2009; 73(4):457–465.

11. Eussen SR, van der Elst ME, Klungel OH, Rompelberg CJ, Garssen J, Oosterveld MH, et al. A pharmaceutical care program to improve adherence to statin therapy: A randomized controlled trial. *Annals of Pharmacotherapy* 2010; 44(12):1905–1913.

12. Benner JS, Glynn RJ, Mogun H, Neumann PJ, Weinstein MC, Avorn J. Long-term persistence in use of statin therapy in elderly patients. *JAMA* 2002; 288(4):455–461.

13. Feldman R, Bacher M, Campbell N, Drover A, Chockalingam A. Adherence to pharmacologic management of hypertension. *Canadian Journal of Public Health* 1998; 89(5):116–118.

14. Lewis A. Non-compliance: A $100 billion problem. *Remington Report* 1997; 5(4):14–15.

15. Viswanathan M, Golin CE, Jones CD, Ashok M, Blalock SJ, Wines RC, et al. Interventions to improve adherence to self-administered medications for chronic diseases in the United States: a systematic review. *Annals of Internal Medicine,* 2012; 157(11):785–795.

16. Administration on Aging. Aging statistics 2013. Retrieved from http://www.aoa.gov/Aging_Statistics/.

17. Centers for Disease Control and Prevention. Chronic diseases: The power to prevent, the call to control. 2009. Retrieved from http://www.cdc.gov/chronicdisease/resources/publications/aag/pdf/chronic.pdf.

18. Howard DH, Thorpe KE, Busch SH. Understanding recent increases in chronic disease treatment rates: More disease or more detection? *Health Economics, Policy, and Law* 2010; 5(4):411–435.

19. Kaiser Family Foundation. Health care costs: A primer. Publ. No. 7670-03. Menlo Park, CA: Kaiser Family Foundation; 2012. Retrieved from http://kaiserfamilyfoundation.files.wordpress.com/2013/01/7670-03.pdf.

20. Schoen C, Osborn R, Doty MM, Squires D, Peugh J, Applebaum S. A survey of primary care physicians in eleven countries, 2009: Perspectives on care, costs, and experiences. *Health Affairs (Project Hope)* 2009; 28(6):w1171–w1183.

21. Sokol MC, McGuigan KA, Verbrugge RR, Epstein RS. Impact of medication adherence on hospitalization risk and healthcare cost. *Medical Care* 2005; 43(6):521–530.

22. Chapman RH, Kowal SL, Cherry SB, Ferrufino CP, Roberts CS, Chen L. The modeled lifetime cost-effectiveness of published adherence-improving interventions for antihypertensive and lipid-lowering medications. *Value in Health* 2010; 13(6):685–694.

23. Esposito D, Bagchi AD, Verdier JM, Bencio DS, Kim MS. Medicaid beneficiaries with congestive heart failure: Association of medication adherence with healthcare use and costs. *American Journal of Managed Care* 2009; 15(7):437–445.

24. Haynes RB, Yao X, Degani A, Kripalani S, Garg A, McDonald HP. Interventions to enhance medication adherence. *Cochrane Database of Systematic Reviews* 2005; 4:CD000011.

25. Melloni C, Alexander KP, Ou FS, LaPointe NM, Roe MT, Newby LK, et al. Predictors of early discontinuation of evidence-based medicine after acute coronary syndrome. *American Journal of Cardiology* 2009; 104(2):175–181.

26. Newby LK, LaPointe NM, Chen AY, Kramer JM, Hammill BG, DeLong ER, et al. Long-term adherence to evidence-based secondary prevention therapies in coronary artery disease. *Circulation* 2006; 113(2):203–212.

27. Mandl KD, Kohane IS, Brandt AM. Electronic patient–physician communication: Problems and promise. *Annals of Internal Medicine* 1998; 129(6):495–500.

28. Cutler DM, Everett W. Thinking outside the pillbox—medication adherence as a priority for health care reform. *New England Journal of Medicine* 2010; 362(17):1553–1555.

29. Krummenacher I, Cavassini M, Bugnon O, Schneider MP. An interdisciplinary HIV-adherence program combining motivational interviewing and electronic antiretroviral drug monitoring. *AIDS Care* 2011; 23(5):550–561.

30. Oldenmenger WH, Echteld MA, de Wit R, Sillevis Smitt PA, Stronks DL, Stoter G, et al. Analgesic adherence measurement in cancer patients: Comparison between electronic monitoring and diary. *Journal of Pain and Symptom Management* 2007; 34(6):639–647.

31. Lee MS, Lee HY, Kang SG, Yang J, Ahn H, Rhee M, et al. Variables influencing antidepressant medication adherence for treating outpatients with depressive disorders. *Journal of Affective Disorders* 2010; 123(1-3):216–221.

32. Acosta FJ, Bosch E, Sarmiento G, Juanes N, Caballero-Hidalgo A, Mayans T. Evaluation of noncompliance in schizophrenia patients using electronic monitoring (MEMS) and its relationship to sociodemographic, clinical and psychopathological variables. *Schizophrenia Research* 2009; 107(2-3):213–217.

33. Zeller A, Schroeder K, Peters TJ. Electronic pillboxes (MEMS) to assess the relationship between medication adherence and blood pressure control in primary care. Scandinavian Journal of Primary Health Care 2007; 25(4):202–207.

34. Vitality Inc. GlowCap. 2013. Retrieved from http://www.glowcaps.com/product/

35. Dolan B. Study: GlowCaps up adherence to 98 percent. *Mobile Health News*; 2010. Retrieved from http://mobihealthnews.com/8069/study-glowcaps-up-adherence-to-98-percent/.

36. Cornstock J. GlowCaps now sold through CVS, new randomized control trial launches. *Mobile Health News*; 2013. Retrieved from http://mobihealthnews.com/20750/glowcaps-now-sold-through-cvs-new-randomized-control-trial-launches/.

37. Rosen MI, Rigsby MO, Salahi JT, Ryan CE, Cramer JA. Electronic monitoring and counseling to improve medication adherence. *Behaviour Research and Therapy* 2004; 42(4):409–422.

38. Philips Medication Dispensing Service; May 30, 2013. Retrieved from http://www.managemypills.com/content/.

39. Murray P. No more skipping your medicine—FDA approves first digital pill. *Forbes*, August 9, 2012.

40. Proteus Digital Health; 2013. Retrieved from http://proteusdigitalhealth.com

41. Overley J. FDA eases up on 'smart pills' for wireless monitoring. *Law 360*; 2013. Retrieved from http://www.law360.com/articles/441977/fda-eases-up-on-smart-pills-for-wireless-monitoring

42. University of Florida, Office of Technology Licensing. Conductive ink for marking pills to electronically track patient adherence. UF #13134; 2013. Retrieved from http://technologylicensing.research.ufl.edu/technologies/13134/conductive-ink-for-marking-pills-to-electronically-track-patient-adherence

43. Piette JD, Mendoza-Avelares MO, Milton EC, Lange I, Fajardo R. Access to mobile communication technology and willingness to participate in automated telemedicine calls among chronically ill patients in Honduras. *Telemedicine Journal and e-Health* 2010; 16(10):1030–1041.

44. World Information Society. World Information Society 2007 report: Beyond WSIS 2007. Retrieved from http://www.itu.int/osg/spu/publications/worldinformationsociety/2007/report.html

45. U.S. Census Bureau. Selected housing characteristics: 2010 American Community survey 1-year estimates. Retrieved from http://factfinder2.census.gov/faces/tableservices/jsf/pages/productview.xhtml?src=bkmk.

46. Bosworth HB, Olsen MK, Neary A, Orr M, Grubber J, Svetkey L, et al. Take Control of Your Blood Pressure (TCYB) study: A multifactorial tailored behavioral and educational intervention for achieving blood pressure control. *Patient Education and Counseling* 2008; 70(3):338–347.

47. Friedman RH. Automated telephone conversations to assess health behavior and deliver behavioral interventions. *Journal of Medical Systems* 1998; 22(2):95–102.

48. Friedman RH, Kazis LE, Jette A, Smith MB, Stollerman J, Torgerson J, et al. A telecommunications system for monitoring and counseling patients with hypertension. Impact on medication adherence and blood pressure control. *American Journal of Hypertension* 1996; 9(4 Pt 1):285–292.

49. Pinto BM, Friedman R, Marcus BH, Kelley H, Tennstedt S, Gillman MW. Effects of a computer-based, telephone-counseling system on physical activity. *American Journal of Preventive Medicine* 2002; 23(2):113–120.

50. Bosworth HB, Olsen MK, Neary A, Orr M, Grubber J, Svetkey L, et al. Take Control of Your Blood Pressure (TCYB) study: A multifactorial tailored behavioral and educational intervention for achieving blood pressure control. Patient Education and Counseling 2008; 70(3):338–347.

51. Mbuagbaw L, Thabane L, Ongolo-Zogo P. Opening communication channels with people living with HIV using mobile phone text messaging: Insights from the CAMPS trial. *BMC Research Notes* 2013; 6(1):131.

52. Vervloet M, van Dijk L, Santen-Reestman J, van Vlijmen B, van Wingerden P, Bouvy ML, et al. SMS reminders improve adherence to oral medication in type 2 diabetes patients who are real time electronically monitored. *International Journal of Medical Informatics* 2012; 81(9):594–604.

53. Wei J, Hollin I, Kachnowski S. A review of the use of mobile phone text messaging in clinical and healthy behaviour interventions. *Journal of Telemedicine and Telecare* 2011; 17(1):41–48.

54. de Jongh T, Gurol-Urganci I, Vodopivec-Jamsek V, Car J, Atun R. Mobile phone messaging for facilitating self-management of long-term illnesses. *Cochrane Database of Systematic Reviews* 2012; 12:CD007459.

55. Horvath T, Azman H, Kennedy GE, Rutherford GW. Mobile phone text messaging for promoting adherence to antiretroviral therapy in patients with HIV infection. Cochrane Database of Systematic Reviews 2012; 3:CD009756.

56. Tomlinson M, Rotheram-Borus MJ, Swartz L, Tsai AC. Scaling up mHealth: Where is the evidence? *PLoS Medicine* 2013; 10(2):e1001382.

57. Decker V, Spoelstra S, Miezo E, Bremer R, You M, Given C, et al. A pilot study of an automated voice response system and nursing intervention to monitor adherence to oral chemotherapy agents. Cancer Nursing 2009; 32(6):E20–E29.

58. dotMobi. Global mobile statistics 2014 Home: All the latest stats on mobile Web, apps, marketing, advertising, subscribers, and trends . . . 2014. Retrieved from http://mobithinking.com/mobile-marketing-tools/latest-mobile-stats—mobilemessaging

59. El-Gayar O, Timsina P, Nawar N, Eid W. Mobile applications for diabetes self-management: Status and potential. *Journal of Diabetes Science and Technology* 2013; 7(1):247–262.

60. McGillicuddy JW, Weiland AK, Frenzel RM, Mueller M, Brunner-Jackson BM, Taber DJ, et al. Patient attitudes toward mobile phone-based health monitoring: Questionnaire study among kidney transplant recipients. *Journal of Medical Internet Research* 2013; 15(1):e6.

61. Fox S, Jones S. The social life of health information. Pew Research Internet Project, June 11, 2009. Retrieved from http://www.pewinternet.org/2009/06/11/the-social-life-of-health-information/

62. Horvath KJ, Danilenko GP, Williams ML, Simoni J, Amico KR, Oakes JM, et al. Technology use and reasons to participate in social networking health websites among people living with HIV in the US. AIDS and Behavior 2012; 16(4):900–910.

63. Jamoom E, Beatty P, Bercovitz A, Woodwell D, Palso K, Rechtsteiner E. Physician adoption of electronic health record systems: United States, 2011. *NCHS Data Brief* 2012; 98:1–8.

64. Hsiao CJ, Hing E. Use and characteristics of electronic health record systems among office-based physician practices: United States, 2001-2012. *NCHS Data Brief* 2012; 111:1–8.

65. Nazi KM, Hogan TP, Wagner TH, McInnes DK, Smith BM, Haggstrom D, et al. Embracing a health services research perspective on personal health records: Lessons learned from the VA My HealtheVet system. *Journal of General Internal Medicine* 2010; 25(Suppl 1):62–67.

66. Darkins A, Ryan P, Kobb R, Foster L, Edmonson E, Wakefield B, et al. Care coordination/home telehealth: The systematic implementation of health informatics, home telehealth, and disease management to support the care of veteran patients with chronic conditions. *Telemedicine Journal and e-Health* 2008; 14(10):1118–1126.

67. Moukheiber Z. Merck, CVS Caremark, PhRMA and others band together to promote medication adherence. *Forbes*, April 22, 2013.

68. Harris MA, Hood KK, Mulvaney SA. Pumpers, skypers, surfers and texters: Technology to improve the management of diabetes in teenagers. *Diabetes, Obesity & Metabolism* 2012; 14(11):967–972.

69. Rice RE, Katz JE. Comparing Internet and mobile phone usage: Digital divides of usage, adoption, and dropouts. *Telecommunications Policy* 2003; 27(8):597–623.

70. Chen ZW, Fang LZ, Chen LY, Dai HL. Comparison of an SMS text messaging and phone reminder to improve attendance at a health promotion center: A randomized controlled trial. *Journal of Zhejiang University Science B* 2008; 9(1):34–38.

71. Ownby RL, Waldrop-Valverde D, Jacobs RJ, Acevedo A, Caballero J. Cost effectiveness of a computer-delivered intervention to improve HIV medication adherence. *BMC Medical Informatics and Decision Making* 2013; 13:29.

72. Volpp KG, Loewenstein G, Troxel AB, Doshi J, Price M, Laskin M, et al. A test of financial incentives to improve warfarin adherence. *BMC Health Services Research* 2008; 8:272.

73. Sorensen JL, Haug NA, Delucchi KL, Gruber V, Kletter E, Batki SL, et al. Voucher reinforcement improves medication adherence in HIV-positive methadone patients: A randomized trial. *Drug and Alcohol Dependence* 2007; 88(1):54–63.

8

Technological Approaches to Assess and Treat Cigarette Smoking

JESSE DALLERY, ALLISON KURTI, AND SARAH MARTNER

INTRODUCTION

Cigarette smoking continues to take an enormous toll on society. During the 50 years since the first Surgeon General's report on the health consequences of smoking, more than 20 million Americans have died prematurely from tobacco-related diseases (1). Currently, over 42 million continue to smoke in the United States, but over 70% express some desire to quit (1). The 2014 Surgeon General's report recommends several "end-game" tobacco control strategies such as reducing the levels of nicotine in cigarettes, increasing the use of smoke-free areas, restricting advertising, increasing the price of cigarettes, and increasing the prevalence of "barrier-free cessation support." These strategies also apply to global efforts to stem the smoking epidemic (2).

Technology can play a key role in an end-game tobacco-control strategy, particularly in the realm of barrier-free cessation support. First, the results from technology-based assessment can help inform and improve the nature of cessation support (3,4). Advances in wearable sensors and mobile technology are permitting a fine-grained picture of the dynamic determinants of smoking, relapse, and cessation (5). These advances may lead to more personalized and effective cessation interventions (6). Second, technology-based treatment can reduce or eliminate geographic barriers to treatment (7). The Internet, social network websites, and mobile telephones are providing new avenues to deliver evidence-based psychosocial treatments to people who have been historically hard to reach. Third, technology may enable treatment delivery to a wider number of smokers than through traditional in-person methods, which

could also improve the cost-effectiveness of these treatments.

In this chapter, we review several major advances in the technology-based assessment and treatment of cigarette smoking. Because the use of technology-based tools should be guided by scientific theory—as well as inform theory (8)—we begin with a brief review of extant biobehavioral theoretical frameworks as they relate to cigarette smoking. Next, we discuss methods to assess smoking behavior, in addition to methods to assess the socioenvironmental correlates of smoking. We then review Internet- and mobile phone–based interventions to promote cessation. Because there are already several excellent reviews of these interventions (9–13), we discuss primarily these reviews. We also highlight several noteworthy and more recent technology-based interventions to provide some specific illustrations. We then discuss technology-based interventions for special populations, such as smokers with severe mental illness or HIV/AIDs, and adolescent and rural smokers.

THEORETICAL FRAMEWORKS AND CIGARETTE SMOKING

Several theoretical frameworks have been used to guide the development of technology-based interventions. A complete review of extant theories is beyond the scope of this chapter. Rather, we wish to provide a broad view of the nature and scope of some of the more common frameworks. These theories include social cognitive theory, cognitive-behavioral theories, learning theories, and the transtheoretical model. These complementary and cohesive theories encompass a wide range of variables and constructs related to smoking.

Social cognitive theory has been used to describe the acquisition, maintenance, and remediation of smoking (14–16). The model acknowledges both environmental and personal factors affecting smoking. Environmental factors include the social situation, social support, and the presence of role models. Personal factors include biological and cognitive dimensions. The cognitive dimensions include outcome expectations (pros and cons of smoking), self-efficacy (ability to resist smoking in tempting situations), and intentions (motivation or readiness to quit) (14).

Cognitive-behavioral treatments (CBT) emphasize the role of stressful life circumstances, cognitive distortions, and environmental triggers that influence cigarette smoking (17,18). For example, work-related stress or other interpersonal conflicts will be more likely to motivate an individual to smoke if he or she lacks relevant cognitive and behavioral coping skills. For such an individual, smoking may be a form of self-medication that temporarily alleviates negative affect produced by stressors. CBT for smoking cessation might include coping skills training (e.g., strategies to manage urges to smoke), problem-focused coping (e.g., cognitive reframing), behavioral contracting (e.g., a contract with a significant other specifying consequences for quitting smoking), and other relapse prevention strategies (19–21).

Learning theories view smoking as being determined by biobehavioral processes (i.e., operant and respondent processes) (18,22). Respondent processes may account for situations in which cigarette "craving" is elicited, such as seeing a familiar bar or tasting coffee (23). Operant processes may account for the maintenance of smoking via positive (e.g., euphoria) and negative reinforcement (e.g., alleviation of withdrawal symptoms). In addition, situations that have been associated with reinforcement-derived smoking in the past may occasion stimulus control over smoking (in which certain situations, people, or other stimuli occasion smoking), and thus treatment may focus on mitigating or altering stimulus control. Treatment strategies based on operant approaches also seek to provide alternative reinforcers (e.g., positive consequences contingent on abstinence) that compete with the immediate, reinforcing value of smoking (10). Modern learning theory also emphasizes the roles of thoughts and feelings in influencing smoking and, in particular, on weakening the influence of maladaptive thoughts and feelings in maintaining smoking or a relapse to smoking (24,25).

The transtheoretical model of smoking is a stage-based theory of behavior change (26–28). The stages are precontemplation (not intending to quit smoking), contemplation (cessation is being considered but not definitely planned), preparation (cessation attempt is imminent), action (actively amidst a quit attempt), and maintenance (cessation has been achieved). Movement through the stages is related to changes in decisional balance, self-efficacy, and several processes of change. The notions of the decisional balance (e.g., pros and cons of smoking or quitting) and self-efficacy are similar to the relevant constructs in social cognitive theory. While a full discussion of the processes of change is beyond the scope of this chapter, we would note that they include activities such as consciousness raising about the problem behavior, self-reevaluation related to smoking, changing stimulus control, managing reinforcement for behavior change, and bolstering helping relationships (27).

In a recent review of theory-based interventions for health behavior, including smoking, Riley et al. (29) questioned whether existing theories were "up to the task" of generating effective cessation interventions in the era of digital, information, and mobile technology. The problem is that most theories emphasize the roles of largely static dispositional constructs in behavior change, rather than how these constructs, and behavior, change dynamically over time. A more dynamic view would permit interventions to be tailored in real time based on ongoing technology-based assessment. The authors argued for revised and new conceptual frameworks "that have dynamic, regulatory system components to guide rapid intervention adaptation based on the individual's current and past behavior and situational context" (29, p. 54). Indeed, we envision that theory will change to accommodate the nature of technology, and technology will inevitably change theory by providing new insights into the causes of smoking and its remission (see Chapter 2, this volume).

TECHNOLOGY-BASED ASSESSMENT
Ecological Momentary Assessment

Currently, ecological momentary assessment (EMA) is the most common method to conduct technology-based assessment of antecedents of smoking and smoking behavior itself (4). EMA assessments (a) occur in naturalistic settings, (b) focus on the participant's internal experiences and external situations, (c) sample behavior over long durations (e.g., weeks), and (d) occur repeatedly on a daily basis. EMA can therefore reveal variation in smoking and correlated events over time and across contexts (30).

Most applications of EMA use handheld computers or smartphones (4). For example, Shiffman and colleagues used handheld computers to assess the relation between negative mood and ad libitum cigarette smoking (5). Smokers were asked to record their mood and other variables immediately prior to smoking. As a control, they were also prompted to record their mood at other, random times during the day, irrespective of whether they were about to smoke. There were no meaningful differences in levels of negative mood before smoking compared to other, randomly chosen times of day. EMA has been used to examine a range of other predictors of ad libitum smoking, including alcohol, coffee, smoking cues, certain situations (e.g., working vs. doing nothing), and the urge to smoke (31,32). Smokers used palmtop computers to record context and affect prior to smoking, and also at random times when not smoking. Smoking was moderately associated with particular activities (e.g., drinking coffee) and locations (e.g., in a car or bar or restaurant), and urge to smoke was the strongest predictor of smoking.

Recent EMA efforts exemplify not only fine-grained assessment of antecedents of smoking but also sophisticated analytic strategies. Although EMA has not revealed a relationship between negative affect and ad libitum smoking among current smokers, it has revealed a relationship between negative affect and lapse and relapse to cigarette smoking among those undergoing a quit attempt. The temporal resolution of these relationships is striking: Several studies have shown predictive relations between elevated negative affect, smoking urges, and a relapse of 3 hours (33), 2 hours (34), and 15 minutes (33) prior to

smoking. Shikyo, Naab, Shiffman, and Li (35) used a time-varying effect model to assess lagged relations between negative affect and smoking urges in adult smokers. Smokers were categorized as low nicotine dependent and high nicotine dependent. The effect of negative affect depended on the time lag, with stronger immediate effects (e.g., within 1 hour) of affect on urge for low dependent smokers, but the relation persisted for longer durations for high dependent smokers (e.g., the relation persisted for up to 3 hours).

Combining technology that detects smoking with other sensing technology (e.g., global positioning systems [GPS], accelerometers) may facilitate the detection of environmental events that precipitate smoking (e.g., the smoker is at a bar), therein permitting the delivery of "just-in-time" interventions to prevent smoking (6). Functionality present in most mobile phones can be used to assess environmental antecedents to smoking. Mobile phones can track a user's location via GPS (36), which can generate automated signals when a user is entering a risky area (e.g., a bar). For example, the user may indicate previous drinking locations, and coping messages or other support could be delivered automatically when the individual enters these areas. Microphones in mobile phones have also been used to infer whether an individual is alone or surrounded by others (37). McClernon, Roy, and Choudhury (3) have discussed how mobile phones could be used to detect a number of antecedents to smoking, including driving in a car (assessed via accelerometer input), the presence of other people (assessed via microphone or Bluetooth detection of other mobile devices in the area), or standing outside (assessed via camera). The authors also noted that multiple inputs could be integrated to identify an antecedent. For example, leaving a bar could be assessed on the basis of a mobile phone's clock (e.g., 10:00 PM), GPS, and/or accelerometer.

Overall, EMA methods reveal a more fine-grained picture of the relations between environmental events and cigarette smoking for individual smokers. These findings are critical in testing existing theories of smoking. For example, more frequent EMA assessments of self-efficacy and smoking may clarify their relation. Indeed, several recent reports suggest a more complicated relationship between self-efficacy and smoking than the simple, unidirectional relationship that was previously assumed (38,39). Specifically, one EMA study suggested that self-efficacy predicted abstinence, and abstinence predicted changes in self-efficacy (38). EMA findings are also critical in generating more effective, tailored interventions. In particular, EMA methods are being linked with ecological momentary interventions, such that assessment results can trigger intervention delivery (e.g., access to therapeutic support) in real time in the smoker's naturalistic environment.

Detecting Smoking with Technology

Given the numerous inexpensive, noninvasive techniques to verify smoking now available, the Society for Research on Nicotine and Tobacco (40) Subcommittee on Biochemical Verification recommends verifying smoking status in most or all cases (with one exception being large studies with limited face-to-face contact with participants). Thus, knowledge about various verification methods—as well as their associated advantages and disadvantages—will facilitate researchers' ability to choose optimal methods given their purposes.

One common way to verify smoking status is by measuring cotinine. Cotinine is a metabolite of nicotine that is present in plasma, saliva, and urine (40). Cotinine can be assayed semiquantitatively using immunoassay test strips (e.g., urine, NicAlert®) and quantitatively using liquid chromatography–tandem mass spectrometry or gas chromatography–mass spectrometry (41). The latter two methods are relatively expensive, are time and labor intensive, and require highly trained staff; thus, the former two methods are more common. NicAlert® is advantageous in that it is inexpensive, and results are available to researchers within minutes of collecting the (urine or saliva) sample. In addition, cotinine's long half-life (10–30 hours) permits detection for several days after cessation (40). Although NicAlert® reliably yields an estimation of tobacco use, disadvantages of this method are that various drugs and dietary substances (e.g., isoniazid, niacin) can cause false positives (42).

A second way to verify smoking status is by measuring carbon monoxide (CO) in expired air. Commercially available devices (e.g., Pico Smokerlyzer; Bedfont Scientific Ltd.) do this by measuring the rate of conversion of CO to carbon dioxide when the smoker exhales air over a catalytically active electrode (40). CO provides a reliable index of recent smoking, particularly heavy smoking (43), but its short half-life (2–3 hours) requires frequent sampling, and controversy remains with respect to the cutoff that best distinguishes smokers from nonsmokers (44). Specifically, smokers whose expired breath CO samples are <8 or 10 ppm (along with self-reported abstinence for at least 24 hours) are typically considered abstinent in clinical research (45). However, Perkins, Karelitz, and Jao (45) demonstrated that sensitivity and specificity measures were optimal at a CO criterion of <4 ppm. As discussed by Meredith and colleagues (46), the cutpoint may depend on the make and model of the CO meter.

In terms of which method most accurately indexes smoking status, cotinine versus breath CO, Jarvis et al. (47) suggest that sensitivity and specificity are highest for cotinine, but relying on breath CO in most clinical studies is acceptable. More recent research suggests that the combination of breath CO and NicAlert® may be the optimal biochemical verification method (41,48,49). The nature of the study must also be taken into account when selecting a biochemical verification method. For example, Dallery, Glenn, and Raiff (50) conducted an Internet-based contingency management intervention to reduce cigarette smoking, in which smoking was verified remotely. For practical reasons (e.g., ease of use, interpretability of smoking data submitted over the Internet via web camera), breath CO was selected for use in this study (see later discussion for further details about this method).

Finally, researchers may also consider using new technology to verify smoking status. For example, Meredith et al. (46) recently developed a mobile phone–based breath CO meter prototype that attaches to and communicates with a smartphone through an audio port. Breath CO measures calculated by the mobile meter were correlated with measures calculated by a commercially available breath CO meter, and the mobile meter accurately distinguished smokers from nonsmokers. Another technology-based smoking verification method is the Zephyr BioHarness, a wearable sensor that infers smoking from ECG, respiration, and skin temperature (51). These data can then be automatically uploaded to a smartphone in a smoking cessation intervention. Similarly, mPuff (52) detects smoking from respiration measurements and can distinguish smoking from stress, speaking, and walking. Finally, Sazonov, Lopez-Meyer, and Tiffany (53) recently described the prototype for the Personal Automatic Cigarette Tracker (PACT), a sensor system that includes a respiratory inductance plethysmograph to monitor breathing and a hand-to-mouth gesture sensor to detect cigarettes at the mouth. When tested in the laboratory study, PACT reliably distinguished smoking from other 12 other common daily activities.

Unlike traditional verification methods (which detect smoking *after* it has occurred), the development of technology that identifies *when* smoking is occurring (51,52) may permit the delivery of interventions to prevent continued smoking. Moreover, technology-based verification of smoking lessens the effort required on the smoker's part to reliably monitor his or her own smoking behavior.

TECHNOLOGY-BASED TREATMENT
Reviews of Internet-Based Methods

Internet-based treatments can transcend geographic barriers to treatment. Some broad characteristics of most extant interventions include progress-monitoring tools, goal setting, online quizzes with feedback, and providing links to various resources and peer support (e.g., discussion boards [54]). Most interventions that have been tested in randomized controlled trials (RCTs) and reviewed in this chapter were developed based on evidence-based practice guidelines (55). The theories from which these interventions have been derived include social cognitive theory, cognitive-behavioral theories, learning theories, and the transtheoretical model.

Several systematic reviews suggest that Internet-based interventions have the potential to promote abstinence in adult populations (56,57). For example, Shahab and McEwen (12) reviewed 11 RCTs. Most of the RCTs reviewed compared an interactive, Internet-based intervention with either self-help booklets, no intervention, face-to-face interventions, or less interactive websites (12). Other studies in the review examined the use of an Internet intervention as a supplement to other treatment, using the other treatment alone as a control. RCTs in this review were widely variable in respect to both their methods and outcomes. This variability limited the reviewers from evaluating specific therapeutic components across

interventions. Therefore, the review focused on outcomes (e.g., abstinence and attrition rates) of each intervention relative to the comparison group or control, and potential moderators and mediators (e.g., motivation to quit, the use of NRT, and length of treatment). Results of the review suggest interactive and tailored Internet-based interventions resulted in higher rates of abstinence when compared to self-help materials and e-mails. There were no significant increases in cessation rates for the Internet interventions compared with face-to-face interventions. Similarly, trials in which an Internet intervention was included in addition to face-to-face interventions showed no gains in abstinence rates compared to face-to-face interventions alone. Pooled results suggested that fully automated interventions tended to have better outcomes than non-automated interventions (e.g., interacting with peers, coaches, experts). Overall, users' ability to access the sites and users' reported satisfaction and acceptability of the Internet-based interventions were high.

A second major review was a Cochrane review of 20 randomized trials of Internet-based interventions (9). Of these, 10 compared an Internet intervention to either a non-Internet intervention (e.g., self-help materials) or no intervention, and 10 compared an Internet intervention with a different Internet intervention (e.g., Smokefree.gov vs. a bulletin board; tailored vs. non-tailored interventions). Few trials demonstrated long-term effects of the Internet intervention when compared to non-Internet interventions or no intervention controls. The trials that compared different Internet-based interventions focused mostly on level of interactivity, complexity, or tailoring. Similar to results from Shahab and McEwen (12), Civljak, Sheikh, Stead, and Car (9) suggest that Internet-based interventions that provide support and tailored information might be more effective at promoting cessation than static websites, and utilizing such sites in addition to other methods (e.g., face-to-face interventions and/or NRT) might further enhance their cessation-promoting capability.

One example of a popular Internet-based approach to cessation is QuitNet®. QuitNet® is one of the most popular websites for smokers and is frequently a top result in search engines. It is designed in accordance with recommendations from the U.S. Public Health Service's *Treating Tobacco Use* and *Dependence: Clinical Practice Guideline* (55). The website provides users with diagnostic tools and tailored materials, problem solving and skills training, information about pharmacotherapy, and a social network with expert counseling (58). One uncontrolled evaluation of QuitNet® reported that only 7% of enrollees were abstinent at 3-month follow-up. Additionally, results revealed a high attrition rate (58). Rabius, Pike, Wiatrek, and McAlister (59) compared cessation rates of participants randomly assigned to QuitNet®, four other tailored websites, or a minimally interactive site. Follow-up surveys revealed no significant differences in abstinence rates between the websites.

Examples of Internet-Based Interventions Derived from Specific Theoretical Frameworks

Smoking cessation interventions derived from CBT typically include content that addresses issues such as self-efficacy, coping strategies, and adherence to nicotine replacement therapy (NRT). One website that is inspired by CBT is BecomeAnEx.org. The website focuses on teaching strategies to identify and cope with smoking cues, along with providing social support and pharmacotherapy resources. The website contains an online forum for smokers to communicate with one another, videos, interactive content, and a personalized quit plan. McCausland et al. (60) identified nine key components of the website: registering, creating a profile, setting a quit date, tracking cigarettes, trigger separation practice (i.e., increasing the time between triggers and smoking), playing educational videos, visiting the support page, and completing at least one support exercise. The authors reported that 20.7% of registered users utilized five of nine key components of the website, and only 2% of registered users utilized all nine components. Although participants may have accessed other components that were not identified as "key" components, these results indicated low retention rates and underutilization of the intervention. A recent cohort study of BecomeAnEX.org reported 7- and 30-day abstinence rates of 11.13% and 9.87%, respectively, at 6-month follow-up (61).

In another study of Internet-based CBT, Swan (62) randomized participants to one of three conditions: Web-based counseling, telephone-based counseling, or combined telephone and Web-based counseling. Participants in all conditions received varenicline (Chantix©). The Web-based intervention was designed to mirror the telephone-based intervention and included an interactive quit plan, information about quitting, several progress monitoring tools, and a discussion board. Short-term abstinence rates were higher in the phone-based counseling condition than in the Web-based condition, yet all three groups had similar 30-day abstinence rates at 6-month follow-up (27–30%). The high abstinence rates from this study support, albeit with limitations, the notion that CBT for smoking can be administered effectively via the Internet.

Although many Internet-based interventions are based on CBT, only a few interventions are based on learning theories. One example of an intervention derived from learning theory is acceptance and commitment therapy, which was recently adapted to the Internet (24). ACT for smoking focuses on acknowledging and accepting emotions, thoughts, and other triggers for smoking without allowing them to control subsequent behavior. ACT uses six core processes to develop such "psychological flexibility": acceptance, cognitive diffusion, being present, self as context, values, and committed action. Without going into detail, these processes focus on two main activities: mindfulness and acceptance of thoughts and feelings, and identifying values and behavior change procedures to commit to these values (e.g., smoking cessation). WebQuit.org is the first Internet-based ACT intervention for smokers (24). Core processes of ACT were embedded in the website by using personalized quit plans along with videos of former smokers sharing success stories and modeling acceptance. In a between-subjects comparison of WebQuit.org and the Department of Health and Human Services website, Smokefree.gov, results indicated greater satisfaction and utilization (measured by duration of website visits) of the ACT intervention than the control website. More important, cessation rates were higher for the Web-based ACT intervention than the Smokefree.gov website (23% vs. 10%) at 3-month follow-ups. Also, acceptance of cues for smoking (i.e., urges precipitated by stimuli associated with smoking with smoking itself not engaged in) at 3-month follow-up was greater for WebQuit.org relative to Smokefree.gov website. In fact, changes in acceptance from baseline to 3-month follow-up explained much of the effect of the web-based ACT intervention. Thus, the core process of acceptance appears to be an effective ingredient in a successful quit attempt: short-term abstinence is influenced by smokers' ability to acknowledge cravings without acting on them. These results are promising, yet they must be interpreted with caution considering the infancy of this intervention and the lack of a long-term follow-up.

Another intervention based on learning theories is contingency management (CM). CM has been evaluated as a tool to initiate smoking cessation (10,50,63,64). In CM interventions, smokers earn positive consequences for objectively verified reductions in smoking. As described in the section above on detecting smoking, breath CO samples are used to verify smoking in Internet-based CM. The sampling procedure requires users to submit two breath CO samples per day via web camera over a secure website, called Mōtiv8. On this website, participants can view a cumulative progress graph and a record of all monetary earnings and transactions. When earnings were provided contingent on smoking abstinence (i.e., a negative CO sample) in the Dallery et al. (50) study, a majority of the participants in the intervention reduced their smoking and submitted negative CO samples.

Monetary consequences may limit the sustainability of CM interventions. Hence, additional methods have been investigated to lessen the costs associated with CM. For example, Dallery, Meredith, and Glenn (64) used a deposit contract method. The procedure required an up-front deposit by the participant, which could be earned back based on evidence of abstinence. In a small pilot study, the deposit contract procedure produced equivalent rates of abstinence relative to a no-deposit group, and it resulted in cost savings. Similarly, Raiff, Jarvis, and Rapoza (65) proposed a novel, low-cost method to deliver reinforcers in the context of a video game. Game-based consequences such as points, badges, and progressing through levels would be accessible based on evidence of smoking abstinence. Such a program would represent an innovative integration of CM with game-based procedures (66,67).

Tailored Internet-Based Interventions

Treatment that is effective for one individual will not necessarily be effective for another. Consequently, methods have been developed to generate more personalized interventions based on assessment of a number of variables; this method is referred to as tailoring. The most basic level of tailoring (also termed "targeting" [68]) is to use demographic information such as a user's race, ethnicity, sex, or age to design an intervention. For example, an intervention targeted to a participant's gender might display success stories with pictures of ex-smokers of the same gender.

More sophisticated approaches use information derived from initial and/or iterative assessments to inform feedback based on a theoretical framework. For example, a participant in the precontemplation stage might receive motivational messages, whereas a participant in the action stage may receive feedback related to their progress. As another example, feedback in the form of messages can be tailored to be evaluative (feedback based on expert evaluations), motivational (feedback regarding progress), or normative (providing peer performances as a benchmark for progress (54).

Existing tailored interventions typically include a combination of simple and more complex approaches (i.e., targeting and tailoring). Lustria, Cortese, Noar, and Glueckauf (54) reviewed 30 tailored interventions, 7 of which were RCTs for smoking cessation. The most common variables used for tailoring were demographic characteristics, smoking behaviors (e.g., number of cigarettes smoked per day), use of change and coping strategies, self-efficacy, and attitudes and intentions about quitting. The theoretical frameworks underlying assessments and feedback in five of the seven RCTs were the transtheoretical model and social cognitive theory. Two studies had no clear theoretical framework. Although outcome measures varied across studies, in general, tailoring resulted in greater abstinence rates and satisfaction ratings than non-tailored interventions. For example, Strecher, Shiffman, and West (68) assigned smokers to a generic or tailored website. The generic website contained content based on CBT and information about smoking cessation products. The tailored website was similar, but also included follow-up newsletters and a supportive person who received e-mails with tailored advice to give to the participant. Tailored materials—which were based on demographics, smoking history, motives for quitting, and perceived difficulties of quitting—were also provided. There was greater satisfaction with the tailored website than with the generic website. In addition, participants using the tailored website had higher rates of abstinence than did those using a generic website at 6-week follow-up (29.0% vs. 23.9%) and at a 3-month follow-ups (22.8% vs. 18.1%).

In a later study, Strecher et al. (69) examined the impact of the degree of tailoring by manipulating three components: tailored success stories, efficacy expectations, and outcome expectations. Each component could be either highly tailored or minimally tailored. Low-tailored success stories included the participant's name in the greeting and matched the gender of the storyteller and participant. High-tailored success stories included those variables, along with several more variables (e.g., age, marital status, social support, perceived barriers, and stage of change). Low-tailored efficacy messages addressed two broad barriers to quitting that were indicated by the participant. High-tailored efficacy messages addressed two more individualized barriers to quitting, and also tailored the messages sent to that participant using several variables (e.g., stress and coping skills, home environment). The depth of outcome expectations was manipulated by providing feedback related to participants' motives for quitting (low-tailored) or their intrinsic and extrinsic motives, health histories, perceived and actual health status, and additional outcomes (high-tailored). Participants were randomly assigned to receive 0–3 high-depth components. For example, a participant assigned to receive two high-depth components might receive high-tailored success stories, high-tailored efficacy expectations, and low-tailored outcome expectations. The personalization of the introductory message source was also manipulated. That is, participants read an impersonal introductory message with a photograph of a building representing the organization (low-personalization) or a friendly introductory message with a photograph of the support team (highly personalized). Overall, increasing the level of tailoring appeared to have a positive effect on cessation rates. Participants receiving no high-depth components had 6-month cessation rates of 28%, whereas 38.6% of participants receiving all (three) high-depth components were abstinent at 6-month follow-up. Cessation rates were most influenced by high-tailored success stories and a more personalized message source.

Initial findings suggest that tailoring might improve the efficacy of interventions, but simply making an Internet intervention more personalized does not guarantee its success. Wangberg, Nilsen, Antypas, and Gram (70) randomized participants to either a multicomponent Internet-based intervention, or the Internet intervention plus 150 tailored messages. Several variables (e.g., self-efficacy, quit date, and social support) were used to tailor messages. The tailored intervention induced abstinence in the short term relative to controls (15.2% vs. 9.4%), but at 12-month follow-up these effects disappeared (11.2% vs. 11.7%). Mason, Gilbert, and Sutton (15) reported similar results. In this study, comparisons were made between participants who received either tailored cessation advice and progress reports or non-tailored information, delivered via the intervention website. Tailoring was based on smoking-related beliefs, personal characteristics and smoking patterns, self-efficacy, and outcome expectations. Tailored information (9.1% abstinent) was not more effective than non-tailored information (9.3% abstinent) as measured by self-reported prolonged abstinence at 3 months.

There is some evidence to suggest that the seemingly promising effects of tailoring are due not to tailoring itself, but rather to the fact that tailored interventions increase participants' engagement and utilization of the cessation program. For example, Hutton et al. (11) concluded there was moderate evidence in support of tailored websites when compared to static websites. However, they noted that participants had greater interaction with the tailored programs than with the static programs. It is unclear whether tailoring increased interaction and effectiveness, or whether greater interaction resulted in increased efficacy. It is worth mentioning here that recent studies have found a relationship between engagement in an Internet-based intervention and abstinence rates (61,71). Thus, more work needs to be done to tease apart the effects of tailoring and other factors such as program interaction and exposure.

MOBILE PHONE–BASED TREATMENT
Consumer-Based Applications

With increasing numbers of people using smartphones, the opportunity for people to use applications (apps) as health promotion tools continues to grow. Indeed, of the 10,000+ iApps at Apple iTunes devoted to some aspect of health promotion, recent research identified 252 iOS apps and 148 Android apps designed specifically to promote smoking cessation. In addition, the volume of these downloads is high—over 700,000 downloads per month on Google Play alone (72). These apps utilize diverse approaches to facilitate cessation: My Last Cigarette emphasizes the long-term, cessation-related improvements pertaining to smokers' health and lifespans, whereas Quit it Lite informs smokers about the money they save each day that they abstain. Cessation Nation emphasizes both the short- and long-term rewards associated with quitting smoking, along with offering smokers a distracting game to play when cravings strike. A different approach entirely is taken with tweetsmoking, an app that facilitates sharing of messages about smokers' successes (e.g., consecutive days abstinent), failures (e.g., lapses), and concerns associated with quitting (e.g., weight gain, coping with craving).

As the technological sophistication of iPhones themselves continues to increase, the interactive features offered by quit smoking apps are expected to increase as well (73). For example, the forward-facing cameras and FaceTime videoconferencing software included on newer iPhones allow users to communicate with healthcare providers and potentially other smokers from remote locations. Importantly, research suggests that leveraging technology in conjunction with person-to-person cessation programs is the most effective tobacco cessation method (74). Thus, future, mobile phone–based apps that capitalize on these technologies to provide smokers with social support opportunities may be a promising means of reducing smoking.

The extent to which existing cessation apps adhere to the U.S. Public Health Service's 2008 *Clinical Practice Guidelines for Treating Tobacco Use and Dependence* (55) was evaluated by Abroms and colleagues (72). In this work, 47 of the most popular cessation apps were reviewed, and they were grouped into various categories (e.g., "calculators" that tracked dollars saved and health benefits accumulated since quitting, "hypnosis" apps that used hypnosis techniques, and "calendars" that tracked days before and after a quit date). All apps were coded for adherence to the 20 Clinical Practice Guidelines (e.g., recommended the use of approved medications, counseling, and connecting to a Quitline) using a 0 to 3 scale (0 = feature was not present, 3 = feature is fully present). Results indicated a mean adherence score of 7.8 (range = 0–30). Some of the unaddressed guidelines included referring the user to a recommended treatment, recommending medications and/or counseling, and providing opportunities to recruit social support. Interestingly, those apps for which adherence scores were lowest (e.g., calendars, hypnosis) were among the most frequently downloaded. As iPhone purchases continue to rise among low-socioeconomic status populations, where smoking prevalence is disproportionately high, the development of apps that adhere to evidence-based standards will be important. It will also be important for design considerations to be taken into account, such that the apps that adhere to current guidelines are attractive to smokers.

Science-Based Mobile Interventions

Whereas Internet-based interventions are delivered to devices that individuals do not typically carry throughout the day (e.g., desktops, laptops), mobile interventions interact with individuals frequently and in the context of ongoing behavior. As such, mobile phone–based smoking cessation interventions can be delivered in a dynamic fashion, tailored to an individual's frequently changing behaviors and environmental contexts. Riley and colleagues (75) reviewed the current literature on mobile technology health behavior interventions, where "mobile technology" was defined as computer devices that an individual carries on him- or herself throughout the day. With respect to smoking cessation, seven studies were identified, all of which were computer tailored at treatment initiation (e.g., users indicated times at which high-risk situations typically occurred, using an associated Internet site) and consisted primarily of text message output. In five of the seven studies, various theories (e.g., social cognitive theory, transtheoretical model) guided the development of the text message's content. Quit rates in these studies ranged from 8% to 53%, thus effectiveness varied considerably across studies.

Like Riley et al.'s review (75) review, a recent Cochrane review of randomized studies also reported varying effectiveness across different mobile phone–based interventions. Specifically, Whittaker et al. (13) discussed five interventions consisting purely of text messaging (three studies), text messaging plus an Internet QuitCoach (one study), and video messaging delivered via mobile phone (one study). Results were aggregated across the five studies and revealed that mobile interventions increased long-term quit rates relative to control programs. However, three of the mobile phone–based interventions had little or no effect. Collectively, Riley et al.'s and Whittaker et al.'s reviews suggest that mobile phone–based interventions may promote abstinence in the short term, but further research is needed to establish the long-term success of these interventions.

Although Riley et al. (29) and Whittaker et al. (76) characterized the interventions in their reviews as mobile interventions, the individual studies in both reviews are dissociable in terms of whether they involved text messaging alone (77,78) or multiple components (e.g., e-mail, text messages, phone-based counseling (79). For example, Free et al. (77) developed "txt2stop," a purely SMS-based smoking cessation program in which smokers received text messages comprising motivational messages and behavioral-change support. Messages were delivered before and after the quit date, in response to specific issues (e.g., "think you'll put on weight when you quit? We're here to help—We'll TXT weight control and exercise tips, recipes, and motivation tips"), and when smokers requested a message in response to cravings or lapses (e.g., "cravings last less than 5 minutes on average. To help distract yourself, try sipping a drink slowly until the craving is over"). Biochemically verified continuous abstinence at 6 months was significantly increased in the intervention group (10.7%) relative to a control group that received text messages unrelated to quitting smoking (4.9%, RR 2.20, 95% CI 1.80–2.68).

In contrast to purely text message–based programs, Brendryen and Kraft's (79) 54-week Happy Ending program is delivered through both cell phones and the Internet, therefore reflecting a hybrid (mobile phone plus Internet) approach to cessation. Each day in the Happy Ending program, participants accessed a Web page unique to that program day, along with receiving one audio message and up to three text messages. Automated relapse prevention therapy was delivered to participants who reported smoking, and an interactive voice response (IVR)-based craving helpline was available 24 hours a day. Compared to a self-help booklet control group in which 24% of participants were abstinent at 12-month follow-up, 38% of participants in the Happy Ending group were abstinent. Other positive features of the intervention include its adherence to Clinical Practice Guidelines (e.g., setting a quit date, motivational messages, recommendations to utilize craving helplines and NRT), being 100% automated, and increasing self-efficacy among current smokers and ex-smokers.

Riley, Obermayer, and Jean-Mary's (80) technology-based smoking cessation intervention targeting college students also reflects a hybrid approach. The intervention was developed on the basis of self-regulation and transtheoretical theories, and included both an Internet and text-messaging component. The Internet component included educational modules, progress-monitoring tools, and e-mail alerts sent to preselected individuals who provided social support and encouragement to the participant. However, the main function of the Internet component was to generate personalized text messages based on a user-specified quit date and likely times for smoking cues. Messages were then delivered one to three times per day at times that the individual indicated smoking being likely (e.g., "after eating, try gum or mints instead of a cigarette"). Six weeks after initiating the program, 45% of participants were abstinent based on self-report (42% based on cotinine verification).

In their review of interventions involving text-messaging alone, as well as hybrid phone and Internet interventions, Whittaker et al. (13) concede that the therapeutically effective components in hybrid interventions (e.g., text messages vs. phone-based counseling) are unclear. However, because these interventions seem to offer some clear benefits, future research on their effectiveness is warranted. These benefits include the anonymity and confidentiality that mobile interventions afford, and the ability to access them anywhere and at any time (76,81,82). In addition, mobile phone–based interventions can be disseminated to large groups of people at a lower cost than face-to-face interventions, leading some to deem them "high-reach, cost-effective" smoking cessation treatments (57,79,83). More important, mobile phone–based interventions may be the optimal delivery method for individuals who have been historically hard to reach in face-to-face interventions (e.g., adolescents, socioeconomically disadvantaged smokers, smokers with inconsistent housing [84–86]). Of course, these considerations remain empirical questions.

SPECIAL POPULATIONS AND TECHNOLOGY-BASED TREATMENT
Adolescent Smokers

Advances in technology have made smoking interventions available to certain populations who are difficult to treat. Perhaps the best example of such a population is adolescents. Adolescents are not likely to utilize cessation services such as NRT or advice from health professionals (78). By comparison, 95% of teens aged 12–17 use the Internet and 78% use mobile phones (87). In fact, most adolescents use the Internet *on* their mobile phones (74%) (87,88). These data suggest that technology-delivered cessation interventions may be an appropriate approach for this population.

Because of adolescents' use of Internet and mobile technology, one would expect them to be receptive to such interventions. There is some research to support this notion: Websites used as supplements to in-person treatments have increased cessation rates over those with treatments that rely on in-person meetings alone (89,90). Conversely, other evidence suggests that existing treatments delivered via websites alone may be insufficient for maintaining cessation among adolescents (91–95). In a systematic review of 21 RCTs for Internet-based interventions, Hutton and colleagues (11) identified five trials in which adolescents were the target population. Interventions in these five trials were based on social cognitive theory, social learning theory, and motivational interviewing. Upon assessing the results, the authors reported there was

insufficient evidence supporting these interventions for adolescents.

Suls, Luger, Curry, Mermelstein, and Sporer (96) suggest that the discrepancy in results for adolescent smokers is not a result of lack of effectiveness of the treatment per se, but rather a result of underutilization of treatment. Therefore, more attention should be focused on motivating adolescents to initiate and sustain their use of Internet-based treatments. Crutzen et al. (97) recommend using incentives, reminders to participate in treatment components (e.g., completing exercises, watching videos), and tailoring to increase the likelihood that an adolescent will engage more fully in an Internet-based smoking cessation treatment.

Indeed, there is evidence that supports the use of incentives for initiating abstinence in adolescents. For example, a small pilot study found that Internet-based CM promoted abstinence in four adolescent smokers (98). Participants earned cash reinforcers contingent on 3 CO submissions per day that were ≤5 ppm. Considering the lack of adolescents' utilization of in-person and other Internet-based treatments, the high rate of submission compliance (97.2% of required samples) observed in this study is noteworthy.

Smokers with Serious Mental Illness

Another population requiring special attention is smokers with serious mental illness (SMI). For example, Hartz et al. (99) found that the risk of smoking was much greater for individuals with severe psychotic disorders (74–80%) than for controls (33%, OR 4.61, 95% CI 4.31–4.94). Even though this population is recognized to be at risk, they are underrepresented in smoking cessation research. As a result, no clinical guidelines have been developed to treat smoking in this population (for a review, see reference 100).

Another important consideration with respect to smokers with serious mental illness if possible at this point is that technology-based smoking cessation tools that most people consider user-friendly may not be so for smokers with SMI. In an effort to understand how effectively people with SMI are able to use websites for smoking cessation, Brunette et al. (101) asked 16 patients (primarily diagnosed with schizophrenia) to use four different websites. These websites met the U.S. Department of Health and Human Services (102) guidelines for Web design and usability and included BecomeAnEx. org, PMUSA.com, smokefree.gov, and whyquit. com. Researchers assessed expert ratings of content and usability (based on guidelines and previous research) and patients' ability to navigate the website (i.e., complete two tasks related to finding information on the website). Expert evaluations rated smokefree.gov as the highest scoring website in terms of content; however, a majority of participants did not satisfy the requirements for the website to be considered usable. Participants were better able to navigate PMUSA.com than other websites, and yet this website received low marks from experts on quality of content. All four websites in the Brunette et al. study were difficult to navigate for the sample of individuals with SMI, even for websites that experts deemed to be usable and composed of quality content. Therefore, Brunette and colleagues recommend website design that is simple and easy to read (e.g., large buttons, text at fifth-grade reading level) and reduces the need for clicking (e.g., using a shallow hierarchy, displaying menus by hovering the cursor over relevant content) (101).

Because of their increased risk of dependence, developing effective cessation interventions for smokers with SMI is an area that warrants more attention. A greater evidence base is needed to develop specific guidelines for interventions that target SMI smokers. Such guidelines should consider the usability of technology-based interventions, as this has been identified as one of the most prominent limitations of existing interventions.

Smokers Living with HIV/AIDS

People living with HIV/AIDS are up to three times more likely to be smokers than the general population (103). They also are more likely to suffer from negative consequences (e.g., heart and lung disease) of smoking than smokers without HIV (104). Traditional interventions that are typically effective for smokers without HIV are ineffective for HIV-positive smokers, perhaps because of "the complex array of medical and psychosocial factors that complicate their lives" (105). Advances in technology-based interventions narrow this gap. Humfleet, Hall, Delucchi, and Dilley (106) found that a computer-based CBT treatment plus NRT was at least equally as effective as self-help plus NRT and counseling plus NRT among HIV-positive participants. Moreover,

the cessation rates in this study were also similar to cessation rates for treatments in the general population.

There is evidence to suggest that mobile phone–based interventions might reach more users than Internet-based interventions. Chander and colleagues (107) surveyed HIV-positive smokers receiving care at Johns Hopkins HIV Clinic about their use of information technology. The survey revealed that 48% of HIV-positive smokers used the Internet; a larger percentage (73%) owned a cell phone. Vidrine, Marks, Arduino, and Gritz (108) conducted an RCT among people receiving cessation treatment at a large HIV care center and compared usual care with a cell phone intervention. The cell phone intervention consisted of 11 proactive counseling sessions plus usual care over a period of 3 months. At 3-month follow-up, those receiving the cell phone intervention were over four times more likely to be abstinent than those receiving a standard care approach. These differences were essentially eliminated at a 6- and 12-month follow-up (109). In short, modest results have been found across the few studies that assessed tech-based interventions for smoking among people living with HIV/AIDS.

Rural Smokers

Another population of importance is rural smokers. Increased rates of smoking coupled with limited access to healthcare and public transportation among this population present challenges which traditional interventions are unable to overcome. The ability to reach smokers in any location is undoubtedly the best-selling feature of technology-based smoking interventions. For example, Stoops et al. (110) treated 68 rural Appalachian smokers using Internet-based CM. Participants who received vouchers contingent on abstinence were three times more likely to submit negative CO samples than control participants. Retention in this study was 85%, which is a high rate relative to other Internet-based interventions, in which retention rates were as low as 6.1% (111). Despite the prevalence of smoking among this population, focus groups and key informant interviews indicate that Appalachian residents welcome smoking cessation treatments (112). This population differs from the populations mentioned previously in that availability of smoking cessation resources appears to be the greatest barrier to treatment.

CONCLUSIONS

Cigarette smoking remains a vexing public health issue. The promise of technology to stem the smoking epidemic comes from two sources: enhanced assessment and treatment of smoking. Technology-enabled assessment promises to uncover the dynamic determinants of smoking, relapse, and cessation. Increasingly, such assessment will become more personalized and idiographic. The results will also help guide decisions about treatment, perhaps in real time, completing the link to personalized, just-in-time treatment. Several researchers have called for a new health model that enables "automated hovering" of patients' behavior while they engage in everyday activities (113), and technology is already in place to perform some forms of automated hovering of smoking behavior. Because most choices about health, including smoking, are made during everyday activities, assessing and influencing such choices constitutes the "single greatest opportunity to improve health and reduce premature deaths" in the United States (114, p. 1222). As this chapter has illustrated, automated hovering of smoking has been enabled by technology-based tools such as sensors and mobile devices. In addition to hovering, technological tools afford "automated nudging" about decisions to smoke.

The ubiquity of technology, however, is just one part of the equation to promote behavior change. The second part is a science of behavior to inform developers and researchers about how technology can nudge behavior. In a major review of mobile-health interventions, also known as mHealth, Kaplan and Stone (115) noted that "many application developers seem unaware that there is a basic science of behavior change" (p. 491). Fortunately, there are several evidence-based developments that adhere to what is known about influencing decisions to smoke. And, increasingly, these developments emphasize real-time assessment, and thus personalized, therapeutic content to influence behavior. Topol (116) outlined a similar outcome in "The Creative Destruction of Medicine: How the Digital Revolution Will Create Better Healthcare." He described how the emergence of mobile phones, Internet connectivity, digital sensors, social networks, and other advances in medicine such as genomics have created a "super-convergence" of technology and medical science. He predicted that this super-convergence will lead to a new medical science focused on personalized diagnostics and treatment in real time, and with minimal geographical restrictions. A similar possibility exists for the field of technology-based interventions for smoking cessation.

REFERENCES

1. U.S. Department of Health and Human Services. The Health Consequences of Smoking—50 Years of Progress: A Report of the Surgeon General, 2014. U S Department of Health and Human Services, Centers for Disease Control and Prevention, National Center for Chronic Disease Prevention and Health Promotion, Office on Smoking and Health, 2014.
2. World Health Organization. WHO Report on the Global Tobacco Epidemic, 2013: Enforcing bans on tobacco advertising, promotion and sponsorship. World Health Organization.
3. McClernon FJ, Roy Choudhury R. I am your smartphone and I know you are about to smoke: The application of mobile sensing and computing approaches to smoking research and treatment. *Nicotine & Tobacco Research* 2013; 15(10):1651–1654.
4. Shiffman S, Stone AA, Hufford MR. Ecological momentary assessment. *Annual Review of Clinical Psychology* 2008; 4:1–32.
5. Shiffman S. Ecological momentary assessment (EMA) in studies of substance use. *Psychological Assessment* 2009; 21(4):486.
6. Heron KE, Smyth JM. Ecological momentary interventions: Incorporating mobile technology into psychosocial and health behaviour treatments. *British Journal of Health Psychology* 2010; 15(1):1–39.
7. Marsch LA, Dallery J. Advances in the psychosocial treatment of addiction: The role of technology in the delivery of evidence-based psychosocial treatment. *Psychiatric Clinics of North America* 2012; 35(2):481–493.
8. Webb TL, Sniehotta FF, Michie S. Using theories of behaviour change to inform interventions for addictive behaviours. *Addiction* 2010; 105(11):1879–1892.
9. Civljak M, Sheikh A, Stead LF, Car J. Internet-based interventions for smoking cessation. *Cochrane Database System Review* 2010; 9:CD007078.
10. Dallery J, Raiff BR. Contingency management in the 21st century: Technological innovations to promote smoking cessation. *Substance Use & Misuse* 2011; 46(1):10–22.

11. Hutton HE, Wilson LM, Apelberg BJ, Tang EA, Odelola O, Bass EB, et al. A systematic review of randomized controlled trials: Web-based interventions for smoking cessation among adolescents, college students, and adults. *Nicotine & Tobacco Research* 2011; 13(4):227–238.

12. Shahab L, McEwen A. Online support for smoking cessation: A systematic review of the literature. *Addiction* 2009; 104(11):1792–1804.

13. Whittaker R, Borland R, Bullen C, Lin RB, McRobbie H, Rodgers A. Mobile phone-based interventions for smoking cessation. *Cochrane Database System Review* 2009; 4:CD006611.

14. Bandura A. *Social Foundations of Thought and Action: A Social Cognitive Theory.* Upper Saddle River, NJ: Prentice-Hall; 1986.

15. Mason D, Gilbert H, Sutton S. Effectiveness of Web-based tailored smoking cessation advice reports (iQuit): A randomized trial. *Addiction* 2012; 107(12):2183–2190.

16. Van Zundert, Rinka M. P., Nijhof LM, Engels RCME. Testing social cognitive theory as a theoretical framework to predict smoking relapse among daily smoking adolescents. *Addictive Behaviors* 2009; 34(3):281–286.

17. Hendricks PS, Delucchi KL, Hall SM. Mechanisms of change in extended cognitive behavioral treatment for tobacco dependence. *Drug & Alcohol Dependence* 2010; 109(1-3):114.

18. Moos RH. Theory-based active ingredients of effective treatments for substance use disorders. *Drug & Alcohol Dependence* 2007; 88(2-3):109–121.

19. Brandon TH, Copeland AL, Saper ZL. Programmed therapeutic messages as a smoking treatment adjunct: Reducing the impact of negative affect. *Health Psychology* 1995 01;14(1):41–47.

20. Hall SM, Humfleet GL, Munoz RF, Reus VI, Prochaska JJ, Robbins JA. Using extended cognitive behavioral treatment and medication to treat dependent smokers. *American Journal of Public Health* 2011; 101(12):2349–2356.

21. Sugarman DE, Nich C, Carroll KM. Coping strategy use following computerized cognitive-behavioral therapy for substance use disorders. *Psychology of Addictive Behaviors* 2010; 24(4):689–695.

22. Cooper JO. *Applied Behavior Analysis.* Upper Saddle River, NJ: Pearson/Merrill-Prentice Hall; 2007.

23. Rose JE. Nicotine and nonnicotine factors in cigarette addiction. *Psychopharmacology (Berlin)* 2006; 184(3-4):274–285.

24. Bricker J, Wyszynski C, Comstock B, Heffner JL. Pilot randomized controlled trial of Web-based acceptance and commitment therapy for smoking cessation. *Nicotine & Tobacco Research* 2013; 15(10):1756–1764.

25. Dougher MJ, Hackbert L. Establishing operations, cognition, and emotion. *Behavior Analyst* 2000; 23(1):11–24.

26. Prochaska JO, DiClemente CC. Stages and processes of self-change of smoking: Toward an integrative model of change. *Journal of Consulting and Clinical Psychology* 1983; 51(3):390–395.

27. Prochaska JO, Velicer WF, DiClemente CC, Fava J. Measuring processes of change: Applications to the cessation of smoking. *Journal of Consulting and Clinical Psychology* 1988; 56(4):520–528.

28. Prochaska JO, Wright JA, Velicer WF. Evaluating theories of health behavior change: A hierarchy of criteria applied to the transtheoretical model. *Applied Psychology: An International Review* 2008; 57(4):561–588.

29. Riley WT, Rivera DE, Atienza AA, Nilsen W, Allison SM, Mermelstein R. Health behavior models in the age of mobile interventions: Are our theories up to the task? *Translational Behavioral Medicine* 2011; 1(1):53–71.

30. Shiffman S, Stone AA, Hufford MR. Ecological momentary assessment. *Annual Review of Clinical Psychology* 2008; 4:1–32.

31. Shiffman S, Gwaltney CJ, Balabanis MH, Liu KS, Paty JA, Kassel JD, et al. Immediate antecedents of cigarette smoking: An analysis from ecological momentary assessment. *Journal of Abnormal Psychology* 2002; 111(4):531–545.

32. Shiffman S, Paty JA, Gwaltney CJ, Dang Q. Immediate antecedents of cigarette smoking: An analysis of unrestricted smoking patterns. *Journal of Abnormal Psychology* 2004; 113(1):166–171.

33. Cooney NL, Litt MD, Cooney JL, Pilkey DT, Steinburg HR, Oncken CA. Alcohol and tobacco cessation in alcohol-dependent smokers: Analysis of real-time reports. *Psychology of Addictive Behaviors* 2007; 21(3):277–286.

34. Berkman ET, Dickenson J, Falk EB, Lieberman MD. Using SMS text messaging to assess moderators of smoking reduction: Validating a new tool for ecological measurement of health behaviors. *Health Psychology* 2011; 30(2):186–194.

35. Shiyko M, Naab P, Shiffman S, Li R. Modeling complexity of EMA data: Time-varying lagged effects of negative affect on smoking urges for subgroups of nicotine addiction. *Nicotine & Tobacco Research* 2014; 16(Suppl 2):S144–S150.

36. Kerr J, Duncan S, Schipperijn J. Using global positioning systems in health research: A practical approach to data collection and processing. *American Journal of Preventive Medicine* 2011; 41(5):532–540.

37. Lane ND, Mohammod M, Lin, M. Yang X, Lu H, Ali S, et al. BeWell: A smartphone application to monitor, model and promote wellbeing. Presented

at the 5th International Conference on Pervasive Computing Technologies for Healthcare (Pervasive Health 2011); 2011.

38. Perkins KA, Parzynski C, Mercincavage M, Conklin CA, Fonte CA. Is self-efficacy for smoking abstinence a cause of, or a reflection on, smoking behavior change? *Experimental & Clinical Psychopharmacology* 2012; 20(1):56.

39. Romanowich P, Mintz J, Lamb RJ. The relationship between self-efficacy and reductions in smoking in a contingency management procedure. *Experimental & Clinical Psychopharmacology* 2009; 17(3):139–145.

40. Benowitz NL, Jacob P, Ahijevych K, Jarvis MJ, Hall S, LeHouezec J, et al. Biochemical verification of tobacco use and cessation. *Nicotine & Tobacco Research* 2002; 4(2):149–159.

41. Marrone GF, Shakleya DM, Scheidweiler KB, Singleton EG, Huestis MA, Heishman SJ. Relative performance of common biochemical indicators in detecting cigarette smoking. *Addiction* 2011; 106(7):1325–1334.

42. Ubbink JB, Lagendijk J, Hayward Vermaak W. Simple high-performance liquid chromatographic method to verify the direct barbituric acid assay for urinary cotinine. *Journal of Chromatography B: Biomedical Sciences and Applications* 1993; 620(2):254–259.

43. Heatherton TF, Kozlowski LT, Frecker RC, Rickert W, Robinson J. Measuring the heaviness of smoking: Using self-reported time to the first cigarette of the day and number of cigarettes smoked per day. *British Journal of Addiction* 1989; 84(7):791–800.

44. Jarvis M, Tunstall-Pedoe H, Feyerabend C, Vesey C, Saloojee Y. Biochemical markers of smoke absorption and self reported exposure to passive smoking. *Journal of Epidemiology and Community Health* 1984; 38(4):335–339.

45. Perkins KA, Karelitz JL, Jao NC. Optimal carbon monoxide criteria to confirm 24-hr smoking abstinence. *Nicotine & Tobacco Research* 2013; 15(5):978–982.

46. Meredith SE, Robinson A, Erb P, Spieler CA, Klugman N, Dutta P, et al. A mobile-phone-based breath carbon monoxide meter to detect cigarette smoking. *Nicotine & Tobacco Research* 2014; 16(6):766–773.

47. Jarvis M, Tunstall-Pedoe H, Feyerabend C, Vesey C, Saloojee Y. Biochemical markers of smoke absorption and self reported exposure to passive smoking. *Journal of Epidemiology and Community Health* 1984; 38(4):335–339.

48. Schepis TS, Duhig AM, Liss T, McFetridge A, Wu R, Cavallo DA, et al. Contingency management for smoking cessation: Enhancing feasibility through use of immunoassay test strips measuring cotinine. *Nicotine & Tobacco Research* 2008; 10(9):1495–1501.

49. Acosta MC, Buchhalter AR, Breland AB, Hamilton DC, Eissenberg T. Urine cotinine as an index of smoking status in smokers during 96-hr abstinence: comparison between gas chromatography/ mass spectrometry and immunoassay test strips. *Nicotine & Tobacco Research* 2004; 6(4):615–620.

50. Dallery J, Glenn IM, Raiff BR. An Internet-based abstinence reinforcement treatment for cigarette smoking. *Drug & Alcohol Dependence* 2007; 86(2-3):230–238.

51. Choi H, Chakraborty S, Charbiwala ZM, Srivastava MB. Sensorsafe: A framework for privacy-preserving management of personal sensory information. In *Secure Data Management*. New York: Springer; 2011, pp. 85–100.

52. mPuff: automated detection of cigarette smoking puffs from respiration measurements. In *Proceedings of the 11th International Conference on Information Processing in Sensor Networks*. New York: ACM; 2012.

53. Sazonov E, Lopez-Meyer P, Tiffany S. A wearable sensor system for monitoring cigarette smoking. *Journal of Studies on Alcohol and Drugs* 2013; 74(6):956.

54. Lustria MLA, Cortese J, Noar SM, Glueckauf RL. Computer-tailored health interventions delivered over the Web: Review and analysis of key components. *Patient Education and Counseling* 2009; 74(2):156–173.

55. Fiore M. *Treating Tobacco Use and Dependence: 2008 Update: Clinical Practice Guideline*. Darby, PA: DIANE Publishing; 2008.

56. Myung S, McDonnell DD, Kazinets G, Seo HG, Moskowitz JM. Effects of Web-and computer-based smoking cessation programs: Meta-analysis of randomized controlled trials. *Archives of Internal Medicine* 2009; 169(10):929.

57. Walters ST, Wright JA, Shegog R. A review of computer and Internet-based interventions for smoking behavior. *Addictive Behaviors* 2006; 31(2):264–277.

58. Cobb NK, Graham AL, Bock BC, Papandonatos G, Abrams DB. Initial evaluation of a real-world Internet smoking cessation system. *Nicotine & Tobacco Research* 2005; 7(2):207–216.

59. Rabius V, Pike KJ, Wiatrek D, McAlister AL. Comparing Internet assistance for smoking cessation: 13-month follow-up of a six-arm randomized controlled trial. *Journal of Medical Internet Research* 2008; 10(5):e45.

60. McCausland KL, Curry LE, Mushro A, Carothers S, Xiao H, Vallone DM. Promoting a Web-based smoking cessation intervention: Implications for practice. *Cases in Public Health Communication & Marketing* 2011; 5:3–26.

61. Richardson A, Graham AL, Cobb N, Xiao H, Mushro A, Abrams D, et al. Engagement promotes abstinence in a Web-based cessation intervention: Cohort study. *Journal of Medical Internet Research* 2013; 15(1):e14.

62. Swan GE, McClure JB, Jack LM, Zbikowski SM, Javitz HS, Catz SL, et al. Behavioral counseling and varenicline treatment for smoking cessation. *American Journal of Preventive Medicine* 2010; 38(5):482–490.

63. Dallery J, Glenn IM. Effects of an Internet-based voucher reinforcement program for smoking abstinence: A feasibility study. *Journal of Applied Behavioral Analysis* 2005; 38(3):349–357.

64. Dallery J, Meredith S, Glenn IM. A deposit contract method to deliver abstinence reinforcement for cigarette smoking. *Journal of Applied Behavioral Analysis* 2008; 41(4):609–615.

65. Raiff BR, Jarvis BP, Rapoza D. Prevalence of video game use, cigarette smoking, and acceptability of a video game–based smoking cessation intervention among online adults. *Nicotine & Tobacco Research* 2012; 14(12):1453–1457.

66. King D, Greaves F, Exeter C, Darzi A. 'Gamification': Influencing health behaviours with games. *Journal of the Royal Society of Medicine* 2013; 106(3):76–78.

67. McCallum S. Gamification and serious games for personalized health. *Studies in Health Technology Information* 2012; 177:85–96.

68. Strecher VJ, Shiffman S, West R. Randomized controlled trial of a Web-based computer-tailored smoking cessation program as a supplement to nicotine patch therapy. *Addiction* 2005; 100(5):682–688.

69. Strecher VJ, McClure JB, Alexander GL, Chakraborty B, Nair VN, Konkel JM, et al. Web-based smoking-cessation programs: Results of a randomized trial. *American Journal of Preventive Medicine* 2008; 34(5):373–381.

70. Wangberg SC, Nilsen O, Antypas K, Gram IT. Effect of tailoring in an Internet-based intervention for smoking cessation: Randomized controlled trial. *Journal of Medical Internet Research* 2011; 13(4):e121.

71. Schwarzer R, Satow L. Online intervention engagement predicts smoking cessation. *Preventive Medicine* 2012; 55(3):233–236.

72. Abroms LC, Westmaas JL, Bontemps-Jones J, Ramani R, Mellerson J. A content analysis of popular smartphone apps for smoking cessation. *American Journal of Preventive Medicine* 2013; 45(6):732–736.

73. Pulverman R, Yellowlees PM. Smart devices and a future of hybrid tobacco cessation programs. *Telemedicine Journal and e-Health* 2014; 20(3):241–245.

74. Zbikowski SM, Hapgood J, Barnwell SS, McAfee T. Phone and Web-based tobacco cessation treatment: Real-world utilization patterns and outcomes for 11,000 tobacco users. *Journal of Medical Internet Research* 2008; 10(5):e41.

75. Riley W, Rivera D, Atienza A, Nilsen W, Allison S, Mermelstein R. Health behavior models in the age of mobile interventions: Are our theories up to the task? *Translational Behavioral Medicine* 2011; 1(1):53–71.

76. Whittaker R, McRobbie H, Bullen C, Borland R, Rodgers A, Gu Y. Mobile phone–based interventions for smoking cessation. *Cochrane Database System Review* 2012; 11:CD006611.

77. Free C, Knight R, Robertson S, Whittaker R, Edwards P, Zhou W, et al. Smoking cessation support delivered via mobile phone text messaging (txt2stop): A single-blind, randomised trial. *Lancet* 2011; 378(9785):49–55.

78. Rodgers A, Corbett T, Bramley D, Riddell T, Wills M, Lin R, et al. Do u smoke after txt? Results of a randomised trial of smoking cessation using mobile phone text messaging. *Tobacco Control* 2005; 14(4):255–261.

79. Brendryen H, Kraft P. Happy Ending: A randomized controlled trial of a digital multi-media smoking cessation intervention. *Addiction* 2008; 103(3):478–484.

80. Riley W, Obermayer J, Jean-Mary J. Internet and mobile phone text messaging intervention for college smokers. *Journal of American College Health* 2008; 57(2):245–248.

81. Balch GI, Tworek C, Barker DC, Sasso B, Mermelstein RJ, Giovino GA. Opportunities for youth smoking cessation: Findings from a national focus group study. *Nicotine & Tobacco Research* 2004;6(1):9–17.

82. Fjeldsoe BS, Marshall AL, Miller YD. Behavior change interventions delivered by mobile telephone short-message service. *American Journal of Preventive Medicine* 2009; 36(2):165–173.

83. Strecher VJ. Computer-tailored smoking cessation materials: A review and discussion. *Patient Education and Counseling* 1999; 36(2):107–117.

84. Franklin V, Waller A, Pagliari C, Greene S. " Sweet Talk": Text messaging support for intensive insulin therapy for young people with diabetes. *Diabetes Technology & Therapeutics* 2003; 5(6):991–996.

85. Faulkner X, Culwin F. When fingers do the talking: A study of text messaging. *Interacting with Computers* 2005; 17(2):167–185.

86. Leena K, Tomi L, Arja R. Intensity of mobile phone use and health compromising behaviours—how is information and communication technology connected to health-related lifestyle in adolescence? *Journal of Adolescence* 2005; 28(1):35–47.

87. Madden M, Lenhart A, Cortesi S, Gasser U. 2012 Teens and Privacy Management Survey. 2013 Retrieved from http://pewinternet.org/Reports/2013/Teens-and-Mobile-Apps-Privacy/Methods/2012-Teens-and-Privacy-Management-Survey.aspx

88. Madden M, Lenhart A, Cortesi S, Gasser U. Teens and Mobile Apps Privacy. 2013 Retrieved from http://pewinternet.org/Reports/2013/Teens-and-Mobile-Apps-Privacy.aspx

89. Chen H, Yeh M. Developing and evaluating a smoking cessation program combined with an Internet-assisted instruction program for adolescents with smoking. *Patient Education and Counseling* 2006; 61(3):411–418.

90. Mermelstein R, Turner L. Web-based support as an adjunct to group-based smoking cessation for adolescents. *Nicotine & Tobacco Research* 2006; 8(Suppl 1):S69-S76.

91. Buller DB, Borland R, Woodall WG, Hall JR, Hines JM, Burris-Woodall P, et al. Randomized trials on consider this, a tailored, internet-delivered smoking prevention program for adolescents. *Health Education & Behavior* 2008; 35(2):260–281.

92. Norman CD, Maley O, Li X, Skinner HA. Using the Internet to assist smoking prevention and cessation in schools: A randomized, controlled trial. *Health Psychology* 2008; 27(6):799.

93. Patten CA, Croghan IT, Meis TM, Decker PA, Pingree S, Colligan RC, et al. Randomized clinical trial of an Internet-based versus brief office intervention for adolescent smoking cessation. *Patient Education and Counseling* 2006; 64(1):249–258.

94. Stoddard AM, Fagan P, Sorensen G, Hunt MK, Frazier L, Girod K. Reducing cigarette smoking among working adolescents: Results from the SMART study. *Cancer Causes & Control* 2005; 16(10):1159–1164.

95. Woodruff SI, Conway TL, Edwards CC, Elliott SP, Crittenden J. Evaluation of an Internet virtual world chat room for adolescent smoking cessation. *Addictive Behaviors* 2007; 32(9):1769–1786.

96. Suls JM, Luger TM, Curry SJ, Mermelstein RJ, Sporer AK, An LC. Efficacy of smoking-cessation interventions for young adults: A meta-analysis. *American Journal of Preventive Medicine* 2012; 42(6):655–662.

97. Crutzen R, de Nooijer J, Brouwer W, Oenema A, Brug J, de Vries NK. Strategies to facilitate exposure to internet-delivered health behavior change interventions aimed at adolescents or young adults: A systematic review. *Health Education & Behavior* 2011; 38(1):49–62.

98. Reynolds B, Dallery J, Shroff P, Patak M, Leraas K. A Web-based contingency management

program with adolescent smokers. *Journal of Applied Behavioral Analysis* 2008; 41(4):597–601.

99. Hartz SM, Pato CN, Medeiros H, Cavazos-Rehg P, Sobell JL, Knowles JA, et al. Comorbidity of severe psychotic disorders with measures of substance use. *JAMA Psychiatry* 2014; 71(3):248–254.

100. Banham L, Gilbody S. Smoking cessation in severe mental illness: What works? *Addiction* 2010; 105(7):1176–1189.

101. Brunette MF, Ferron JC, Devitt T, Geiger P, Martin WM, Pratt S, et al. Do smoking cessation websites meet the needs of smokers with severe mental illnesses? *Health Education & Research* 2012; 27(2):183–190.

102. U.S. Department of Health and Human Services. The Research-Based Web Design & Usability Guidelines. 2006.

103. Tesoriero JM, Gieryic SM, Carrascal A, Lavigne HE. Smoking among HIV positive New Yorkers: Prevalence, frequency, and opportunities for cessation. *AIDS and Behavior* 2010; 14(4):824–835.

104. Rahmanian S, Wewers ME, Koletar S, Reynolds N, Ferketich A, Diaz P. Cigarette smoking in the HIV-infected population. *Proceedings of the American Thoracic Society* 2011; 8(3):313.

105. Niaura R, Chander G, Hutton H, Stanton C. Interventions to address chronic disease and HIV: Strategies to promote smoking cessation among HIV-infected individuals. *Current HIV/AIDS Reports* 2012; 9(4):375–384.

106. Humfleet GL, Hall SM, Delucchi KL, Dilley JW. A randomized clinical trial of smoking cessation treatments provided in HIV clinical care settings. *Nicotine & Tobacco Research* 2013; 15(8):1436–1445.

107. Chander G, Stanton C, Hutton HE, Abrams DB, Pearson J, Knowlton A, et al. Are smokers with HIV using information and communication technology? Implications for behavioral interventions. *AIDS and Behavior* 2012; 16(2):383–388.

108. Vidrine DJ, Marks RM, Arduino RC, Gritz ER. Efficacy of cell phone–delivered smoking cessation counseling for persons living with HIV/AIDS: 3-month outcomes. *Nicotine & Tobacco Research* 2012; 14(1):106–110.

109. Gritz ER, Danysh HE, Fletcher FE, Tami-Maury I, Fingeret MC, King RM, et al. Long-term outcomes of a cell phone-delivered intervention for smokers living with HIV/AIDS. *Clinical Infectious Diseases* 2013; 57(4):608–615.

110. Stoops WW, Dallery J, Fields NM, Nuzzo PA, Schoenberg NE, Martin CA, et al. An Internet-based abstinence reinforcement smoking

cessation intervention in rural smokers. *Drug & Alcohol Dependence* 2009; 105(1-2):56–62.

111. Swartz L, Noell J, Schroeder S, Ary D. A randomised control study of a fully automated Internet-based smoking cessation programme. *Tobacco Control* 2006; 15(1):7–12.

112. Kruger TM, Howell BM, Haney A, Davis RE, Fields N, Schoenberg NE. Perceptions of smoking cessation programs in rural Appalachia. *American Journal of Health Behavior* 2012; 36(3):373.

113. Asch DA, Muller RW, Volpp KG. Automated hovering in health care—watching over the 5000 hours. *New England Journal of Medicine* 2012; 367(1):1–3.

114. Schroeder SA. Shattuck Lecture. We can do better—improving the health of the American people. *New England Journal of Medicine* 2007;357(12):1221–1228.

115. Kaplan RM, Stone AA. Bringing the laboratory and clinic to the community: Mobile technologies for health promotion and disease prevention. *Annual Review of Psychology* 2013;64:471–498.

116. Topol, EJ. *The creative destruction of medicine how the digital revolution will create better health care.* New York: Basic Books;2012.

9

Technology-Based Interventions to Promote Diet, Exercise, and Weight Control

CARMINA G. VALLE AND DEBORAH F. TATE

INTRODUCTION

Over the past 15 years, there has been an accumulation of evidence for the feasibility and efficacy of behavioral treatment programs and, more specifically, health promotion programs delivered via the Internet. However, computer-assisted therapies for obesity began well before the Internet age, by harnessing the power of lightweight portable computers in the mid-1980s. Many early computer programs were simply means of self-monitoring, but more comprehensive computerized treatment packages designed to mimic traditional therapy for obesity were also developed. Such programs offered a new means for patients to record self-monitoring information, set goals, receive prompts or cues to action, and receive proximal feedback and reinforcement for incremental steps toward weight loss (1,2). Compared with bibliotherapy, which was the self-help treatment format popular at the time, the computer offered advantages, namely the ability to provide interactions between the patient and computer that mimicked those that might occur with a behavior therapist, and the potential to deliver obesity treatment with less direct therapist contact. Burnett (1) reported one of the initial studies using a computer for behavioral treatment of obesity in which 12 subjects (6 matched pairs) were randomly assigned to use either an interactive microcomputer program to enter self-monitoring data, receive feedback, and praise or further instructions to modify eating contingent on performance, or pencil-and-paper self-monitoring techniques. After 8 weeks, mean weight losses were significantly greater in the computer-based treatment, averaging 3.7 kg vs. 1.5 kg for the paper monitoring condition. In a follow-up study (2), the computer program was

described as encouraging daily goal setting, prompting and delivering motivational messages on a random schedule. It also included a meal-planning tool and calorie-tracking diary, a feature to train users to slow their rate of eating, and displayed several different graphs of progress. Though early technology-delivered treatment packages were devoid of the images, videos, and dynamic content that are commonplace in Internet- and mobile-delivered interventions of 2013, the functionality built into these early systems included interactive elements that remain fundamental to achieving outcomes today.

In the ensuing years, many terms have proliferated to describe interventions involving use of devices connected to the Internet for intervention delivery, including Web-based, e-Health, interactive health communication approaches; online treatment; Internet counseling and Internet interventions; and technology-based and, increasingly, mHealth or mobile interventions. In 2006, Ritterband and Thorndike (3) proposed a useful definition of Internet interventions to distinguish them from patient education websites that contain online information. Key characteristics of Internet interventions include being based on effective behavioral or cognitive behavioral therapies, being highly structured, as well as interactive and personalized to the user, and often including tailored assessments with feedback and recommendations for change over time. Similarly, the *Cochrane Review of Interactive Health Communication Applications* (IHCAs; [4]) defined IHCAs as computer programs that include at least one component beyond information—such as behavior change support, decision support, or peer support—and acknowledged the trend toward delivery via the Internet rather than through stand-alone computers. While no consensus exists, the underlying tenants of these definitions suggest that Internet behavior change programs are more than information delivered via Internet-connected devices; these programs contain many of the behavioral strategies that underlie effective interventions delivered in more traditional face-to-face settings.

Most systematic reviews and meta-analyses suggest that Internet-delivered interventions are more effective than controls or minimal treatments for a broad range of behaviors (5,6) and specifically for weight loss (7,8) and physical activity behavior (9). It is generally recognized that this first generation of studies was focused on demonstrating efficacy, and comparison groups were often minimal or no-treatment control groups, appropriate for early-stage research in the field. It is less well known what aspects of technology interventions make them relatively more or less effective. This chapter aims to synthesize the technology functions that have been identified in the empirical literature as "active ingredients" in changing diet and physical activity behavior or changing weight outcomes, and will provide a basis from which this field can expand.

Rather than conducting a comprehensive review of technology-based interventions, we provide illustrative examples of behavioral interventions that aimed to change both diet and physical activity behaviors, including trials that focused on weight loss, weight gain prevention, and weight maintenance after weight loss. Following from Ritterband and Thorndike (3), we define Internet behavioral interventions as a program or specific set of activities (including learning, skill-building, behaving) designed to encourage people to achieve an objective related to weight loss, weight gain prevention, or dietary and physical activity changes. We selected a sample of studies representative of the current literature that was identified from comprehensive searches of PubMed and EMBASE databases for articles published through September 2013. Search strategies and terms employed in previous systematic reviews of mobile and Internet technology-based interventions (10,11) were used to identify potential articles for inclusion. We also searched references lists of recent systematic review articles (12–14) for

relevant articles. Studies were included if they met the following criteria: applied interactive technologies used by study participants for monitoring health status or improving health outcomes; randomized controlled trial; follow-up outcome data reported at least 12 weeks after randomization; healthy adult participants; primary outcomes of weight and/or diet or physical activity behaviors; technology-based behavioral interventions that aimed at changing both diet and physical activity behaviors compared to a group that also received a technology-based program; study groups that differed in one or more functions used to support behavior change with technology (as opposed differing only in behavior targeted). We excluded studies that focused on using technology for assessment or technology interventions and applications utilized by healthcare professionals and/or providers.

TECHNOLOGY-BASED INTERVENTIONS COMPARED WITH INTERVENTIONS OR CONTROLS NOT USING TECHNOLOGY

The body of evidence regarding technology-based interventions demonstrates that, compared with usual care, minimal contact, waitlist control groups, in-person, or non-technology interventions (e.g., print, face-to-face), technology-based interventions have been effective in producing changes in diet and physical activity behaviors. Recent systematic reviews of eHealth and mHealth interventions have addressed specific delivery modes or devices applied (e.g., websites), technology capabilities (e.g., text messages), and specific disease populations (see 4,10,11,15). As these reviews cover studies with research designs and comparison groups that tested *whether* technology can be used to change diet and physical activity behaviors, we provide a brief summary of the evidence and have excluded these studies from our analyses. With the goal of understanding *how* we can best use technology to facilitate behavior change techniques that promote healthy diet, physical activity, and weight control and maximize public health impact, we focus our review and analyses here on studies in which a technology-based intervention was compared with another group that also received technology-based components.

Technology-Based Interventions vs. Usual Care, Minimal Contact

Several studies have evaluated technology-based interventions vs. comparison groups that used little or no technology, including usual care, minimal contact, or waitlist control groups. These interventions have aimed to produce weight loss (16–24), to promote weight gain prevention or weight maintenance (25–28), and to enhance dietary and physical activity behaviors (29–33). Modes of communication have included the Internet, telephone, and mobile phones to deliver intervention content and strategies through websites, e-mails, counseling, interactive voice response, text messages, short message service (SMS), multimedia message service (MMS), and videos. In comparing technology-based interventions with usual care, some studies have tested the effectiveness of using technology to promote weight loss or maintenance in primary care (16,17,26,34), military (19), and workplace settings (20,27), and specifically among men (22,35). When compared with usual care or no treatment conditions, these technology-based interventions have consistently resulted in short-term weight losses and lower levels of weight regain (8).

Technology-Based Interventions vs. In-person Interventions

When compared with in-person interventions, technology-based interventions have been less effective in producing weight loss (8,36,37). Similarly, weight maintenance interventions that are delivered in person, both with minimal or more frequent in-person contact, have achieved better prevention of weight regain than technology-based interventions (8,38–40).

Technology-Based Interventions as an Adjunct to In-person Interventions

Several studies have used technology-based strategies in conjunction with in-person standard behavioral weight loss interventions (41–47) or in conjunction with, and in comparison to, usual care or minimal care (47–51). These studies have shed light on the added effects to in-person programs of PDA- or computer-based self-monitoring with or without tailored feedback (41–43,46,51), an intervention website (50), text messaging programs (48,49), and intermittent or continuous physical activity monitoring with an armband (44,45,47). By isolating the effects of technology or mode for self-monitoring behaviors, several studies have demonstrated that the use of PDAs, accelerometers, or objective physical activity monitors can improve upon weight losses achieved through in-person treatment alone (42,45,47,51), potentially through enhancing adherence to self-monitoring behaviors (41). The magnitude of technology use for self-monitoring (e.g., intermittent, continuous physical activity monitoring, self-weighing frequency) needed to improve adherence and optimize diet and physical activity behavior changes requires further elucidation.

Although traditionally effective self-monitoring for weight loss required monitoring diet and activity behaviors, new research suggests that objective daily weight monitoring might be another effective metric to monitor. A study by Steinberg et al. (23) demonstrated that a 6-month weight loss intervention that involved daily self-weighing with digital scales, weekly e-mails with behavioral weight loss lessons and tailored feedback, and online weight graphs led to clinically significant weight loss (M = −6.55%, 95% CI: −7.7, −5.4) over 6 months. Although this randomized trial, among 91 overweight or obese healthy adults, evaluated the intervention compared with a delayed control group, participants in the control group also received digital scales to weigh themselves as they normally would. Findings that the intervention group self-weighed on average 6.1 +1.1 days per week and had positive perceptions of daily self-weighing offer insights regarding the frequency of self-weighing using digital scale technology that may be sufficient, in conjunction with behavioral weight loss lessons, online weight graphs, and tailored feedback, for supporting the achievement of clinically significant weight loss. Future studies that isolate the added effects of technology use to in-person interventions could be beneficial for improving our understanding of the optimal levels of technology use necessary to promote positive behavior change. Future studies should also evaluate simpler forms of monitoring that are aided by wearable and other technologies to determine if they are as effective as the well-studied, though tedious, task of monitoring all food intake and activity behaviors for weight loss.

TECHNOLOGY-BASED INTERVENTION COMPARED WITH TECHNOLOGY-BASED CONTROL

In reviewing studies that compared technology-based interventions with a study arm or arms that also utilized technology, we recognize that many modes of technology can be used to affect behavior change via theory- and evidence-based mechanisms and techniques. Given the rapid development of technology and the many challenges to conducting research that is responsive to these advances, identifying and understanding the technological capabilities or functions that support behavior change, rather than studying the technology mode in and of itself, will better address research gaps and facilitate research on technology-based behavioral interventions moving forward. We used elements of a taxonomy of behavior change techniques specific to healthy eating and physical activity interventions (52) to guide our characterization of functions used to support behavior change applied through the use of technology. Thus, the following sections are organized by the various functions or behavior change strategies utilized in diet and physical activity interventions for weight control, emphasizing the need for research that evaluates the functions of technology that successfully promote behavior change rather than testing delivery through the technology itself.

To enhance our understanding of how technology can best be used to promote behavior change, perhaps the most informative study designs are additive, dismantling, or comparative effectiveness trials. Studies that have employed these designs to compare technology-based interventions with another technology-based intervention augmented with additional technology functions or strategies contribute to our understanding of specific intervention components applied through technology that may be most effective for producing behavior change. Table 9.1 outlines weight control studies that have evaluated the effects of a technology-based function as an adjunct to a technology-based intervention, highlighting the differences between intervention groups and the

additional technology-based intervention component or function that was evaluated. In the following sections, we provide some exemplars that, by study design, have isolated the additive effects of singular or several functions or strategies used to support behavior change with technology.

Self-Monitoring

Of the 19 studies reviewed, the most frequent function of technology for behavior change was self-monitoring of dietary intake, physical activity, and/or weight, with 84% ($n = 16$) of the studies utilizing technology to support this behavioral strategy (53–68). Given that evidence to date demonstrates that frequency of self-monitoring behaviors is significantly and consistently associated with weight loss (69), this is not surprising. Technology enables researchers to provide intervention participants with tools for self-monitoring and to objectively measure participants' adherence to self-monitoring. A wide variety of tools to self-monitor dietary intake, physical activity, and weight exist, continue to emerge, and are commercially available through computer- or phone-based applications that allow for more efficient entry of information. Rather than recording energy consumption and expenditure by hand, computer software and applications can automatically calculate energy balance based on food and exercise entries recorded by participants. In addition, emerging digital devices allow for frequent or continuous monitoring of activity and weight (e.g., armbands, accelerometers, wireless or cellular phone–enabled scales). These tools enable the rapid collection of objective participant data, which in turn enables the participant to gain knowledge of his or her own behavior. It also enables researchers to use the data in several ways: (a) to provide individualized feedback on self-monitoring and progress toward a behavior or outcome (e.g., computer-generated graphs); (b) to evaluate participant adherence; and (c) to elucidate underlying mechanisms or mediators of intervention efficacy. The large amounts of data that can be generated in the process of implementing and evaluating a technology-based intervention raise questions on how, when, and what data should be analyzed. Other research gaps in the current literature on the use of self-monitoring strategies for diet, physical activity, and weight control interventions include the generalizability of previous findings to more diverse populations (e.g., racial and ethnic minorities, disease populations), the level or frequency of self-monitoring sufficient to support behavior change (69), and the optimal timing or interval within which to provide feedback on monitoring data.

Although self-monitoring is frequently used and has served as the foundation for some behavioral interventions in weight control (40,69), few studies have focused on examining the effect of self-monitoring as an adjunct or in comparison to a technology-based intervention on weight-related outcomes. Shapiro et al. (60) conducted a randomized trial, among 170 overweight and obese adults, of a text-messaging intervention for weight loss over 12 months. The study compared a theory- and evidence-based intervention, Text4Diet™, which used daily interactive SMS and MMS text messages, with a control group that received monthly e-newsletters. Self-monitoring of diet and physical activity was supported through the provision and use of pedometers and digital scales, and further encouraged through text messages requesting daily step count data and weekly weight data and the ability to submit self-monitoring data via website. Additional intervention text messages provided educational content, personalized feedback on progress, and weekly encouragement, and participants also received monthly e-newsletters and access to a website with diet and physical activity tips, logs, resources, and personal weight trends. Study results did not support the efficacy of the intervention for weight loss, as groups did not differ on weight loss outcomes at 6 and 12 months. However, findings did demonstrate that greater adherence to self-monitoring, as measured by proportion of SMS responses to queries about educational content, daily step count, and weekly weight, was associated with greater weight loss over time; the authors suggest that text messages may be a helpful technology tool for improving self-monitoring.

Wing, Crane, Thomas, Kumar, and Weinberg (68) demonstrated in a series of two randomized controlled trials that the addition of daily self-monitoring of diet, exercise, and weight with automated feedback to an Internet-based weight loss program can improve weight loss outcomes in a community setting. In Study 1, 170 adult participants were randomized to receive the standard Shape Up Rhode Island (SURI) Internet-based community program or the SURI program with video lessons related to weight loss. In Study 2, 128 participants were randomized to either the standard SURI program or the SURI program supplemented with video lessons, access to a website to record self-monitoring data, and computerized feedback (SURI Enhanced). While there were no significant group differences in weight loss in Study 1, Study 2 demonstrated that the SURI Enhanced program led to significant mean weight losses that were over two times greater than among those receiving the standard SURI program alone (3.5 + 3.8 kg vs. 1.4 + 2.7 kg; p <.01) and to high rates of adherence to submitting online weight and calorie intake records (78% and 74% of days, respectively), which were associated with weight loss outcomes ($r = 0.43, 0.42$, respectively). Although the effect of the self-monitoring behaviors alone could not be isolated in Study 2, the authors note that the effectiveness of the enhanced program may partly be attributable to the automated feedback leading to increases in the number of lessons viewed and the likelihood of self-monitoring. The findings also provide insight on the potential for using technology to support behavioral strategies in larger scale public health campaigns without significant costs.

Tailoring and Feedback

Tailoring of intervention content was also a frequently used function applied through technology in over 80% ($n = 16$) of the intervention studies. In almost all of these studies, feedback on progress or behavioral goals was provided in conjunction with and tailored on the basis of self-monitoring data reported for weight, dietary intake, and physical activities (24,55–63,65,68,70,71). Feedback is one of several tailoring strategies that may be provided in the context of multicomponent computer-tailored interventions that offer several individualized components and facilitate widespread delivery of an individualized program (see Lustria, Cortese J, Noar, and Glueckauf [72] for conceptual framework describing a variety of tailoring approaches). Along with feedback, other message-tailoring strategies utilized in technology-delivered behavioral interventions are personalization (i.e., using an individual's personal information to enhance message relevance) and adaptation (i.e., message content is matched to an individual's levels or perceptions of

TABLE 9.1. WEIGHT LOSS, WEIGHT GAIN PREVENTION, WEIGHT MAINTENANCE TECHNOLOGY-BASED INTERVENTION STUDIES

Study	Study Characteristics Setting, Target Group, Modes of Technology Delivery	Intervention and Comparison Description	Functions Used to Support Behavior Change with Technology	Components Evaluated by RCT Design	Outcomes, Implications, Retention, Adherence
Brindal et al., 2012 (53)	$N = 8,112$ overweight or obese adults; population based; website, e-mail	**Information (I):** Web-based WL program with diet information; not interactive **Supportive (S):** I, plus interactive supportive features: weight tracker, real-time feedback on weight progress and dietary compliance, interactive meal planner, social networking platform **Personalized-supportive (PS):** I + S, plus personalized automated meal planner based on recipe and earlier preferences	Self-monitoring Feedback (based on user input, tailored initially and iteratively, automated) Social support (personalized plans)	S vs. I: weight tracker, real-time feedback on weight progress and dietary compliance, interactive meal planner, social networking platform **Enhanced monitoring, FB, SS** PS vs. S: Plus personalized meal planner based on user preferences **Personalized plans**	No significant differences in WL between groups ($p = .42$). **Enhanced monitoring, FB, SS, meal planner did not improve WL.**
Collins et al., 2012 (70) Collins et al., 2013 (54)	$N = 309$ overweight or obese adults; community based; website, e-mail, SMS, telephone	**Control:** wait-list, re-randomized to basic or enhanced after 12 weeks **Basic:** standard commercial Web-based WL program, including diet and PA diary; menu plans; grocery list; weekly PA plan; tips; challenges; community forum; weekly e-mail newsletters; dietary intake goals; feedback graphs; weekly weight reporting; automated reminders to record weight **Enhanced:** Basic, plus personalized automated weight loss goals and advice on behavior change; weekly automated tailored feedback, reminders to use website and diary, and report weight (e-mail, SMS, phone)	Self-monitoring Tailoring Social support Modeling Goal setting Planning Feedback (based on user input, tailored initially and iteratively, automated) Tailored goals Reminders (automated, human)	Enhanced: personalized WL goals; tailored e-feedback; reminders **Feedback** **Tailored goals** **Reminders**	Significant WL in both basic and Enhanced vs. Control ($p < .001$) at 12 weeks. No differences between Basic and Enhanced groups at 12 weeks. Significant WL in Basic and Enhanced groups at 24 weeks, with no differences between groups. **Adding personalized WL goals, tailored e-feedback, and automated reminders to commercial Web-based WL program did not improve WL at 24 weeks.**

Gabriele et al., 2011 (55)	104 overweight adults; university employees; website, e-mail	**Minimal support (MS):** calorie book, exercise expenditure chart, 12 self-monitoring booklets; Internet-based weight loss program, including weekly e-mail with behavioral weight loss lesson, quiz, and link to online survey to report self-monitoring data; weekly e-mail with tailored feedback (graphs of weight, calorie and exercise trends, quiz answers) and support **Nondirective support (NS):** MS, plus participant chooses goals weight loss, calorie, and PA goals; lesson order; discussion topics; and strategies to use; prompt to communicate with e-coach **Directive support (DS):** MS, plus structured e-coach support; standard lesson order; e-coach provides caloric intake and PA prescription, short-term goals, specific plan for overcoming barriers; prompt to communicate with e-coach, complete weekly self-monitoring survey, and review previous goals	Self-monitoring Tailored feedback (based on user input, tailored initially and iteratively, human) Social support Reminders Goal setting	NS vs. MS: nondirective human e-mail counseling **Type of tailored feedback** DS vs. MS: directive human e-mail counseling **Type of tailored feedback**	Significantly greater WL in DS vs. ND and MS in females over 12 weeks. Significantly more self-monitoring reports by DS vs. MS and NS. **Among females, adding directive e-coach support to an Internet-based program produced more WL than adding nondirective e-coach support or Internet-based program alone.**
Gold et al., 2007 (56)	124 overweight and obese adults; community setting; website	**eDiets:** 12-month access to commercially available online WL website, including basic WL information, calorie prescription, weekly weight report, automated feedback on weight progress, meal plan tailored on user preferences, recipes, grocery lists, exercise diary, social support features (therapist-moderated online meetings, chat rooms, discussion boards, FAQs, peer mentoring) **Vtrim:** website with therapist-led, structured behavioral WL program for 6 months, weight maintenance program for 6 months, including structured behavioral lessons/activities; weekly meeting to reinforce lessons; individualized calorie goal; PA recommendation; weekly weight reporting; food journal; online food database; e-mailed therapist feedback on homework; weekly therapist feedback on journal; discussion board. Same components in maintenance, but biweekly meetings and therapist feedback	Self-monitoring Feedback (based on user input, tailored initially and iteratively, automated vs. human) Social support	Vtrim: structured behavioral lessons/activities, online meeting, therapist feedback, PA recommendation eDiets: automated feedback, tailored meal plan **Intervention package:** **Human feedback, Online meetings,** **Structured behavioral lessons**	Significantly greater WL in VTrim vs. eDiets.com ($p < .005$) at 6 months and better maintenance ($p < .034$) at 12 months. **Multicomponent Internet program, including structured behavioral lessons, online meetings, and therapist feedback, produced greater WL than Internet program without these features.**

(Continued)

TABLE 9.1. CONTINUED

Study	Study Characteristics Setting, Target Group, Modes of Technology Delivery	Intervention and Comparison Description	Functions Used to Support Behavior Change with Technology	Components Evaluated by RCT Design	Outcomes, Implications, Retention, Adherence
Hersey et al., 2012 (57)	1,755 overweight adults; non–active-duty military; TRICARE healthcare system; website, telephone, e-mail	RCT1: written manual (bookHEALTH) focused on skills for lifestyle change (problem solving, goal setting, self-monitoring, enlisting social support); tip sheets; website to support skill development (eHEALTH); weekly Internet or telephone submission of weight, dietary intake and PA RCT2: RCT1, plus an interactive version of eHEALTH with tailored automated feedback when submitted self-monitoring data RCT3: RCT1 & RCT2, plus brief coaching support using motivational interviewing techniques to facilitate problem solving and reinforcement (via alternating telephone call and personalized e-mail every 2 weeks)	Self-monitoring Social support (coaching) Feedback (based on user input, tailored initially and iteratively, computerized vs. coach) Problem solving Reinforcement Goal setting	RCT2 vs. RCT1: Tailored automated feedback on progress **Feedback** RCT3 vs. RCT2: Brief telephone/e-mail coaching support **Feedback** **Problem solving** **Reinforcement**	Significant WL in all 3 groups after 12 months, and after 15–18 months, with no differences between groups. **Adding automated tailored feedback, with or without e-mail and telephone coaching support, to a manual and Web program did not improve WL.** Cost-effectiveness ratios were $900 to $1,100/ quality-adjusted life year (QALY) for RCT1 and RCT2 and $1,900/QALY for RCT3.
Micco et al., 2007 (58)	123 overweight and obese adults; community based; Internet, in person	**Internet (I):** 12-month behavioral WL program: 2 in-person orientation sessions; diet and PA prescription; study website (VTrim) with behavior therapy via lessons and homework; online chat group discussions about lessons (weekly in months 1–6, biweekly in months 7–12); online journal submission (diet, PA); tailored feedback e-mail from facilitator on journal and homework; automated reinforcement for lesson completion/ journal entry)	Social support Self-monitoring Feedback (based on user input, tailored initially and iteratively, human) Reinforcement (automated)	Monthly in-person group feedback and support **Feedback/social support mode**	No significant group differences in WL at 6 months ($p = .15$) or 12 months ($p = .17$). **Adding minimal in-person support to an Internet program did not improve WL.**

Reference	Population; setting	Intervention	Components	Results
Rothert et al. 2006 (59)	2,862 eligible overweight and obese adults; large healthcare delivery system; website	**Internet + In-person treatment (I + IPS):** I, plus, monthly in-person group meeting instead of online group meeting, in-person facilitator different from online facilitator) **Information only:** website with information and sections on weight (definitions, management, weight loss programs, strategies) and other health topics (e.g., diabetes, asthma) **Tailored Expert System (TES):** 6-week computer-automated, tailored weight management program, including weight management plan; advice on barriers and stress management; ability to enlist supportive buddy; tailored action plan; e-mail prompt when follow-up content available (action plan, reinforcements, overcoming barriers, support, self-monitoring resources)	Feedback (tailored on user input, initially and iteratively, automated) Social support Action plan Self-monitoring Prompt to follow-up	Tailored intervention package: weight management plan, stress management advice, action plans, supportive buddy, prompts **Feedback** **Social support** **Action plan** **Prompts**	Significantly greater self-reported WL in TES group vs. IO group at 3 months and 6 months. Significantly more TES participants reported reading website information vs IO. **Adding tailored automated feedback, social support, tailored action plan, and prompts improved WL over self-help information.**
Shapiro et al., 2012 (60)	Overweight and obese adults (n = 170); community; text messages; website	**Control:** monthly e-newsletters (publicly available diet and PA information) **Text4Diet:** daily interactive and personally weight-relevant text-messages, 4×/day for 12 months, included tips, facts, motivation, prompts for self-monitoring data (weekly weight, daily steps) and knowledge questions, portion control pictures, feedback graphs, personalized step goal, weekly encouragement; pedometer; digital scale; monthly e-newsletters (publicly available diet and PA information); access to website (health tips, recipes, food and PA logs, weight chart)	Self-monitoring Feedback (based on user input, tailored initially and iteratively, automated) Prompts	Intervention package: **Self-monitoring** **Feedback** **Prompts**	No significant group differences in WL over 6 months or 12 months. Higher adherence (% responses to text messages) was associated with more WL over time. **Intervention package delivered via text messaging did not improve WL.**

(Continued)

TABLE 9.1. CONTINUED

Study	Study Characteristics Setting, Target Group, Modes of Technology Delivery	Intervention and Comparison Description	Functions Used to Support Behavior Change with Technology	Components Evaluated by RCT Design	Outcomes, Implications, Retention, Adherence
Tate et al., 2006 (62)	192 overweight adults, community setting; website, e-mail	**No counseling (NC):** one group session with standard behavioral weight control lesson, diet and PA recommendation, 1 week of meal replacements, coupons for meal replacements, and encouragement to self-monitor; access to publicly available interactive website with weight graphs, prompts to report weight and tips via e-mail, recipes, e-buddy peer support network) **Computer-automated feedback (AF):** NC, plus separate website with electronic diary (weight, caloric intake, meal replacements, and exercise), message board; weekly e-mail with behavioral lesson and reminder to complete diary; weekly, automated tailored feedback on Web page (based on predefined algorithms and weight loss diary) **Human e-mail counseling (HC):** NC, plus separate website with: electronic diary (weight, caloric intake, meal replacements, and exercise), message board; weekly e-mail with behavioral lesson and reminder to complete diary; weekly individualized feedback from counselor via e-mail (no predefined content); personal e-mail follow-up to non-reporters.	Self-monitoring Feedback (based on user input, tailored initially and iteratively, human vs. automated) Prompts Social support	AF vs. NC: **Computer-automated feedback** HC vs. NC: **Human feedback** AF vs. HC: **Feedback on diary (AF only)** **E-mail inquiry if no diary submission (HC only)**	Significantly greater WL in both AF and HC vs. NC group ($p = .005$, $p = .001$), with no difference between AF and HC ($p = .95$) at 3 months. Significantly greater WL in HC vs. NC group ($p < .001$) at 6 months. AF not significantly different vs. NC or HC at 6 months. Total logins and online diary submissions correlated with WL. **Adding automated feedback or human e-counseling to basic Internet program produced comparable WL at 3 months. Adding human e-counseling to basic Internet program improved WL at 6 months.**

Study	Sample/setting	Intervention	Techniques		Results
Tate et al., 2003 (61)	92 overweight adults at risk of type 2 diabetes; clinical center; website	**Basic Internet program:** one face-to-face introductory group session with standard behavioral weight control lesson, diet and PA recommendation, and encouragement to self-monitor; calorie book; PA and exercise diaries; website, including weight loss tutorial, weekly tip and link, directory of links to Internet weight loss resources; message board; weekly e-mail with weight loss information and reminder to submit weight **Internet behavioral e-counseling:** above, plus e-mail counseling with feedback on self-monitoring, reinforcement, recommendations, and general support (5×/week in month 1, weekly in months 2–12); online self-monitoring diaries to report weekly weight, caloric intake, and exercise (daily in month 1, then weekly); personal e-mail follow-up to non-reporters	Self-monitoring Social support Feedback (based on user input, tailored initially and iteratively, human) Prompt to follow-up Reinforcement	**Feedback** **Reinforcement** **Prompts**	Significantly greater WL in behavioral e-counseling group vs. basic Internet group at 12 months ($p = .04$). **Adding e-mail counseling to Internet program with other content improved WL.**
Tate et al. 2001 (63)	$N = 91$ healthy, overweight adult hospital employees; website, e-mail	**Internet education (IE):** one face-to-face introductory group session with standard behavioral lesson on weight control, diet and PA recommendations, basic weight loss information; website with directory of links to Web resources on diet, PA, self-monitoring and behavioral topics **Internet behavior therapy (IBT):** IE, plus 24 weekly e-mails with behavioral lessons, individualized therapist feedback, reinforcement and general support; online self-monitoring diaries to report weekly weight, caloric intake and exercise; e-mail prompts to self-monitor; bulletin board	Self-monitoring Social support Feedback (based on user input, tailored initially and iteratively, human) Reinforcement Prompt to self-monitor	Intervention package: **Self-monitoring** Feedback **Social support** **Reinforcement** Prompts	Significantly greater WL in behavior therapy group vs. education group over time ($p <.001$). Login frequency significantly correlated with WL outcomes in both groups. **Adding behavioral intervention package to Internet education improved WL.**

(*Continued*)

TABLE 9.1. CONTINUED

Study	Study Characteristics Setting, Target Group, Modes of Technology Delivery	Intervention and Comparison Description	Functions Used to Support Behavior Change with Technology	Components Evaluated by RCT Design	Outcomes, Implications, Retention, Adherence
Turner-McGrievy et al., 2009 (80)	N = 78 overweight adults; community setting; podcast, website, e-mail (reminders) telephone (reminders)	**Control Podcast:** 2 podcasts per week for 12 weeks, currently available, popular podcast: weight loss discussions, emphasized cognitive restructuring to achieve healthy weight **Enhanced Podcast:** two behavioral, theory-based podcasts per week for 12 weeks provided nutrition and PA information, information on consequences of trying to lose weight (audio blog of man/woman trying to lose weight), goal-setting activity, behavioral lessons through information and soap opera, encouragement to monitor weight, calories and PA; e-mail and phone reminders to access study website, new podcast and report podcast uses	Modeling Goal setting Prompt to follow-up	Theory-based intervention package: **Modeling** **Goal setting** **Prompt**	Enhanced group had significantly greater WL at 12 weeks (p <.001 between groups). No difference in reported number of podcasts listened to by group. **Enhanced, theory-based podcast intervention package produced greater WL than general podcast.**
Turner-McGrievy et al., 2011 (64)	N = 96 overweight adults; community setting; podcast, mobile application, social networking site	**Enhanced Podcast:** one face-to-face group overview, 2 podcasts per week for 3 months (same as above), 2 shorter podcasts per week for months 4–6 provided nutrition and exercise information on overcoming barriers and problem solving; calorie book; access to podcast site. **Enhanced Podcast + Mobile:** above (except calorie book), plus mobile application to self-monitor diet and PA; Twitter application: moderator prompts twice per day, encouraged to post themselves and follow peers in cohorts of 11–12 (months 1–3) and then all peers (months 4–6)	Modeling Goal setting Prompts Self-monitoring Social support	**Self-monitoring** **Social support** **Prompts**	No significant group difference in WL at 6 months (p = .98). **No additional benefits of mobile monitoring app and social networking site interaction above enhanced, theory-based podcast intervention package on WL.**

Author, year	Sample/setting	Intervention	Behavioral targets	Support/components	Results
Webber et al., 2008 (67)	66 adult overweight/obese women; community setting; website	**Minimal:** initial face-to-face weight loss session, calorie book, self-monitoring diaries, diet and exercise goals, 16-week Internet behavioral WL program (weight loss tips, lessons, message board, links to websites, online self-monitoring diaries for weekly weight and daily diet and PA levels **Enhanced:** Same as Minimal, 16 weekly online chat group sessions moderated using motivational techniques	Self-monitoring Social support Counseling support (human)	Motivationally enhanced online group chat **Counseling support** **Social support**	Over 16 weeks, significant WL in both groups ($p < .001$), no significant differences between groups ($p = .19$). Numbers of website visits, self-monitoring diaries completed, posts to message boards associated with greater WL in both groups. **Addition of weekly motivationally enhanced online chats to Internet behavioral program did not improve WL.**
Wing et al., 2010 (68)	179 adults, 128 adults enrolled in statewide weight loss competition; community-based; website	**Study 1:** **Standard Shape Up RI (SURI):** online team-based health improvement program, pedometer, wristband, paper logbook, SURI website access (submit self-monitoring data), e-mail with directory of publicly available websites **SURI + lessons:** SURI, 12 weekly multimedia lessons on nutrition, PA, behavior change strategies, interactive activities (e.g., quizzes), links to related documents and websites **Study 2:** **SURI:** Same as above **SURI Enhanced:** SURI, 12 weekly multimedia lessons with additional interactive activities, 1 group session, printed food diary, calorie reference book, submission of weight, diet, PA data on SURI website, weekly automated computer feedback based on user data	Self-monitoring Tailored feedback (based on user input, automated initially and iteratively)	SURI + lessons vs. Standard: Multimedia behavioral weight loss lessons SURI enhanced vs. Standard: Multimedia behavioral weight loss lessons **Self-monitoring** **Tailored feedback**	In study 1, no group difference in WL (SURI + lessons: $1.9 + 2.8$ kg vs. $1.3 + 2.9$ kg; $p = .20$) (ITT). In study 2, SURI enhanced group had significantly greater WL ($3.1 + 3.7$ kg vs. $1.2 + 2.5$ kg; $p < .01$) compared to standard program (ITT). **Addition of video behavioral weight loss lessons, self-monitoring, and tailored feedback to online community-based program improved WL.**

(Continued)

TABLE 9.1. CONTINUED

Study	Study Characteristics Setting, Target Group, Modes of Technology Delivery	Intervention and Comparison Description	Functions Used to Support Behavior Change with Technology	Components Evaluated by RCT Design	Outcomes, Implications, Retention, Adherence
Wylie-Rosett, 2001 (24)	588 adults in health maintenance organization; computer software, telephone, face to face	**Workbook:** self-help weight loss materials with self-help pages directing to relevant sections **Computer-tailored program (CT):** Workbook, computer software system to guide workbook use, tailored behavioral goals, barrier identification, end-of-session prompt to continue/modify self-monitoring goals and select behavioral goals, weekly logins in months 1–3, monthly logins in months 4–12. **Counseling:** Workbook, computerized tailoring, 6 group workshop sessions and up to 18 telephone or face-to-face counseling sessions to reinforce workbook and computer system	Goal setting Prompts Tailored behavioral goals (based on user input, automated initially) Barrier identification	CT vs. Workbook: **Tailored behavioral goals** **Goal setting** **Barrier identification** **Prompts** Counseling vs. Workbook: **Tailored behavioral goals** **Goal-setting** **Barrier identification** **Prompts** **Group counseling** **Individual counseling** Counseling vs. CT: **Group counseling** **Individual counseling**	Significant WL in all groups at 12 months. Significantly greater WL in Counseling group vs. Workbook group. No significant difference between CT and Workbook. **Computer-delivered intervention package with counseling produces greater WL than self-help workbook.**

Weight Gain Prevention / Weight Maintenance

van Genugten et al., 2012 (65)	539 overweight adults; general population and employees from large companies; website	**Generic website:** 3 modules with general information on WGP; 1) increasing motivation for WGP; 2) information about and choosing behavior change; 3) general information on healthy diet and safe PA; e-mail reminders to visit website every 2 weeks **Computer-tailored website:** 4 modules, 1 per week based on self-regulation steps; 1) pros/cons of WGP, individualized feedback, guided goal setting to set 1 diet/PA goal, make implementation plan; 2–3) evaluated progress toward change, feedback on performance, modified action plans if necessary;	Feedback (based on user input, automated tailoring initially and iteratively) Goal setting Action planning Self-monitoring Reinforcement Behavioral contract Social support Reminders to logon	Tailored treatment package: **Feedback** **Goal-setting** **Action planning** **Self-monitoring** **Reinforcement** **Behavioral contract** **Social support**	Over 6 months in all available observed data, no significant changes in BMI, and no differences between groups on BMI. **Tailored treatment package no more effective for WGP than generic information website over 6 months.** 65.2% retention at 6 months

van Wier et al., 2009 (66) van Wier et al., 2011 (71)	1,386 employees, recruited from seven companies; website, e-mail, telephone 6-month program	4) promoted maintenance of self-regulation, self-monitoring tools, reinforcement; End) personalized contract with behavior goals, action plans; peer-to-peer forum; recipes; links to websites. E-mail reminders to visit website every 2 weeks **Usual care:** 3 publicly available lifestyle brochures (overweight, healthy diet, PA), calorie chart **Phone group:** 10 print educational modules with assignments (information, behavioral modification techniques), pedometer, phone counseling after completed module (every 2 weeks) **Internet group:** interactive website with 10 educational modules with assignments, pedometer, personalized Web pages, e-mail counseling after completed module, e-mail or SMS reminder to log on	Counseling (human) Tailored feedback (Internet: based on user input, automated just-in-time, human) Prompt Self-monitoring	Phone vs. Usual care: Print behavioral lessons Phone counseling Pedometer Internet vs. Usual care: Online behavioral lessons Tailored Web pages E-mail counseling Pedometer Internet vs. Phone: Counseling mode Tailored Web content Prompts **Counseling mode** **Tailored content** **Prompts**	No significant differences between Phone and Internet groups on weight loss at 6 months. Significant weight loss in all groups at 2 years. No significant differences between groups at 2 years. **Among all participants at 2 years, no difference between Phone and Internet groups on WL.** 57% retention at 2 years

Diet and Physical Activity

Dickinson et al., 2013 (76)	N = 169 patients from primary care practices; website	**Basic website:** health risk assessment, feedback with health behavior recommendations, education materials (diet, PA, smoking, alcohol), tips on behavior change, education on communicating with physician **Enhanced website:** plus action planning section with prompts to make personalized plan for changing targeted behaviors, discussion forum, "Ask the Expert," e-mail and automated phone prompts to revisit action plan	Social support Prompts Feedback (based on user input, automated initially) Action planning	**Action planning Social support** **Prompts**	No significant differences between groups on healthful eating scores and PA levels. **Adding action planning, social support and prompts did not improve healthful diet or PA level.**

BMI, body mass index; FB, feedback; PA, physical activity; SS, social support; WGP, weight gain prevention; WL, weight loss.

psychosocial/theoretical determinants of targeted behavior) (72,73). Systematic reviews indicate the effectiveness of computer-tailored interventions delivered over the Web for improving healthy dietary, physical activity, and weight behaviors compared with non-tailored conditions (74,75). In the studies reviewed here, feedback messages were often tailored at baseline, using data from baseline assessments, and iteratively, using self-monitoring data reported throughout the study to provide users with ipsative feedback on progress (i.e., compares current performance with previous). In addition to feedback, computer-delivered tailoring has been used to provide individually tailored weight management plans (59), tailored behavioral goals (24,65), personalized action plans (59,65), and personalized behavioral contracts (65). Descriptors such as personalized, individualized, and tailored were often used interchangeably without sufficient description of the technique. As such, we used an organizing framework from a systematic review of Web-delivered computer-tailored behavioral interventions to help characterize tailoring functions used in the studies reviewed (72). A few studies exemplify approaches that allow for evaluation of a multicomponent tailored health program or intervention package (e.g., tailored intervention package vs. generic), examination of the added benefit of tailored message components (e.g., feedback), comparison of delivery mode of tailored feedback or type of counseling contact (e.g., computer-automated Web vs. expert e-mail counseling), or evaluation of the nature of coaching or counseling contact (e.g., directive or nondirective support) in implementing a technology-based intervention.

van Genugten et al. (65) examined a Web-delivered computer-tailored intervention for preventing weight gain among overweight adults. The authors compared an Internet-delivered computer-tailored intervention for weight management with a generic website among 539 overweight adults from the general population. The intervention included four modules providing tailored content, including feedback on behavior, feedback on previous performance, personal behavior goals and action plans, and a personalized contract, and a peer-to-peer forum. At 6 months, there were no significant differences between groups on anthropometric measurements and dietary and physical activity behaviors, which

may partly be attributable to low intervention adherence, with 15% of intervention participants completing four intervention modules vs. 46% of comparison participants completing three modules from the generic website. Overall, findings highlight the need for more research to enhance adherence to technology-based interventions.

Tailored feedback may be presented in a manner that is descriptive (i.e., reports individual's data or behaviors), comparative (i.e., contrasts individual's data with others') or evaluative (makes judgments about individuals' data) (73), or it can use a combination of these approaches. Indeed, participants most often are encouraged to self-monitor in the context of and as a predecessor to receiving tailored feedback on progress and behavioral strategies to employ in response to information gained through self-monitoring. In the Healthy Eating and Active Living in TRICARE Households (HEALTH) demonstration project, Hersey et al. (57) tested the added benefit and cost-effectiveness of computerized feedback with or without e-mail or telephone coaching compared with written materials and a basic website for weight loss in non-active-duty military participants. Over 1,700 overweight adult beneficiaries of the TRICARE healthcare program for uniformed service members were randomized to receive RCT1) a basic Internet program (eHEALTH) with written materials on improving diet and physical activity; RCT2) plus an interactive version of eHEALTH with tailored computerized feedback on weekly self-reported logs; or RCT3) plus brief telephone or e-mail coaching every 2 weeks. Among study completers, there were significant mean weight losses among all three groups after 12 months (−4.0% to −5.3%) and after 15 to 18 months (−3.5% to −5.1%), with no difference between groups, and multiple imputation analyses showed a comparable pattern of statistical significance. Low retention rates, ranging from 58% to 29% from 6 to 18 months, and low adherence, ranging from 44% to 49% completing weekly logs, limit generalizability of the findings. However, cost-effectiveness estimates suggest that the program was relatively inexpensive, with the two more minimal approaches costing $30–$40 per 1% weight loss ($900 to $1,100 per quality-adjusted life year) and RCT3 costing $70 per 1% weight loss ($1,900 per quality-adjusted life year). The addition of brief personalized coaching support may have helped to improve adherence, which was significantly higher among RCT3 participants than for the other groups, but still suboptimal (53% or less), and to improve weight loss, although not significantly.

Comparing the source of tailored feedback was the focus a three-group randomized trial by Tate, Jackvony, and Wing (62), which tested the added efficacy of human e-mail counseling or computer-tailored automated feedback to an Internet weight loss program compared with a minimal Internet control group. One hundred ninety-two overweight or obese adults were randomized to receive 1) one weight loss group session, access to a publicly available interactive website, coupons for meal replacements; 2) plus human e-mail counseling, an additional website (with electronic self-monitoring diaries and message boards), and weekly e-mail with a behavioral lesson and reminder to complete the electronic diary; or 3) plus computer-automated feedback, the same additional website, and same weekly e-mail lesson and reminder. After 3 months among completers, weight losses in the e-mail counseling and computer-automated feedback groups were comparable and significantly greater than in the no counseling group (−6.1 + 3.9 kg, −5.3 + 4.2 kg, −2.8 + 3.5 kg). The human e-counseling group was more effective than no counseling for weight loss after 6 months (−7.3 + 6.2 kg vs. −2.6 + 5.7 kg; $p < .001$), while the computer-automated feedback group did not differ from either group (−4.9 + 5.9 kg). Given that weight losses in the automated feedback group averaged 5 kg, which is approximately 5% and enough to confer health benefits, and the potential for computer-automated feedback as a lower cost alternative to providing population-level weight control treatments, additional research is needed to enhance computer-tailored feedback.

With the earliest studies of Internet behavioral weight loss programs demonstrating the added benefit of human e-counseling or coaching support (61,62), more recent studies have focused on examining the nature of e-counseling contact or coaching support (55–58). Gabriele, Carpenter, Tate, and Fisher (55) examined the effects of type of e-coaching support on weight loss outcomes in a 12-week trial of 104 overweight adults randomly assigned to receive an Internet intervention with directive, nondirective, or minimal support. The

Internet-based weight loss intervention was delivered to all participants over 12 weeks and included 2 e-mails per week (behavioral weight loss lesson, feedback graphs on progress) and a weekly Web-based survey for reporting self-monitoring data. The minimal support group received no additional support, while the directive support participants received lessons in a standard order, as well as structured goals and discussion topics selected by the e-coach, and were actively reminded by the e-coach about previous goals and to complete the weekly survey. Nondirective support participants had the flexibility to change the standard order of their e-mail lessons, to select their own behavioral and weight loss goals, and to discuss topics of their choice. Results showed that in comparison with the nondirective and minimal support conditions, the directive condition was more effective for weight loss and reducing waist circumference in females.

Social Support and Social Networking

Social support is another commonly targeted theoretical construct and strategy used to encourage weight control and changes in dietary and PA behaviors. Fourteen of the 19 studies identified (74%) used technology-based components to enable supportive communication. In addition to support offered by individual therapists or counselors via e-mail (55,57,61–63) or on a website (62), studies utilized technology to encourage social support through discussion forums, message boards, or online chats (53,56,58,61–63,65,67,70,76), by providing a social networking platform on intervention websites (53), or by utilizing an existing social networking site (64). Other studies facilitated social support through strategies that enlisted supportive buddies or peers (59,62). Some studies used randomized, additive designs that tested the effects of social support components alone (67), or as part of a multicomponent intervention (64).

The increasing adoption and growing popularity of social media and social networking sites, such as Twitter and Facebook, offer opportunities to supplement and deliver technology-based interventions for behavior change using existing technology platforms. Research is newly emerging in this area, with the earliest studies taking innovative approaches to testing the feasibility and preliminary efficacy of behavioral interventions using Twitter to facilitate social support (64) and Facebook as a delivery channel (77–79). There have been mixed results on the effects of online social networks or group discussions for encouraging social support for weight loss, weight maintenance or diet, and physical activity behavior changes in adding to the effects of a basic program.

Turner-McGrievy and Tate (64) compared two 6-month, minimal-contact weight loss interventions with no tailored feedback among 96 overweight adults: podcast-only or podcast plus enhanced mobile media. All participants received theory-based podcast-only components, including two podcasts per week over 3 months, which previously had been shown to be effective for producing short-term modest weight loss compared with a popularly available weight-loss podcast at 3 months (−2.9 + 3.5 kg vs. −0.3 + 2.1 kg; $p <.001$) (80), followed by two minipodcasts (shorter) per week for months 3–6. Additionally, the podcast + mobile group was asked to use a downloadable application on their mobile device to self-monitor their diet and physical activity and to use Twitter to "follow" other weight loss group peers, post comments, and read and respond to moderator prompts. At 6 months, mean weight loss outcomes were not different between groups (both −2.7%; $p = .98$), though social support sources were different, with more podcast-only participants endorsing friends (28% vs. 10%; $p = .045$) and more podcast + mobile participants endorsing online sources of support (25% vs. 0%; $p = .001$). The authors concluded that a self-monitoring app without feedback and mobile communication and discussion prompts via Twitter did not improve weight loss achieved through a minimally intensive podcast intervention. Secondary analyses of Twitter engagement among the enhanced intervention group revealed that frequency of Twitter posts predicted % weight loss at 6 months (i.e., every 10 Twitter posts was associated with approximately −0.5 % weight loss; $p <.001$), and self-reported weight loss in the first month of the study predicted frequency of Twitter posts over the 6 months (81). Secondary analyses also revealed that intervention participants had used Twitter mostly to provide informational social support to weight loss peers (81).

Other studies have found no additional benefit of facilitated social discussions. Webber, Tate, and Michael Bowling (67) examined the added benefit of weekly online group discussions moderated by a trained facilitator using motivational interviewing to an Internet-based behavioral weight loss program. Among 66 adult women randomized to one of two motivationally enhanced Internet weight loss interventions, mean weight loss was significant over time, with no difference between the group with minimal motivational enhancement and the group receiving more motivation (5.2 +4.7 kg vs. 3.7 + 4.5kg; $p = .19$). Both groups had received an initial face-to-face weight loss session, a 16-week Internet program including a study website, weekly lessons, online self-monitoring, Web links, and message boards. Additionally, the enhanced group received weekly online moderator-led group discussions, led in a style designed to enhance autonomous motivation using motivational interviewing principles in an Internet chat. Results indicated that the chat groups did not enhance weight loss. Interestingly, while none of the enhanced-motivation participants met with each other outside of the study, 15% of minimal-motivation participants reported meeting face to face with other participants for support and exercise activities, and frequency of these contacts was significantly correlated with weight loss. This occurrence of eliciting support from peers, in the absence of therapist- or moderator-prompted interaction among participants randomized to receive a more minimal technology-based intervention, was also observed in a recent randomized trial of a Facebook-based physical activity intervention for young adult cancer survivors (79).

Although Valle, Tate, Mayer, Allicock, and Cai (79) focused on promoting physical activity in this 12-week study among 86 young adult cancer survivors, the use of Facebook groups in both the intervention and active comparison groups offer insights into the potential for using existing social networking sites to engage participants and enlist peer support for behavior change. Participants in the self-help comparison Facebook group received weekly Facebook messages with links to publicly available websites, a pedometer, and peer group interaction without discussion prompts, while participants in the intervention Facebook group received weekly Facebook lessons with more detailed behavioral lessons, access to a self-monitoring website, a pedometer, and moderated-led group interaction with discussion prompts posted by a trained study facilitator.

Despite differences in the nature of moderator contact, both moderated and peer-only groups posted a comparable number of Facebook comments, and a significantly greater proportion of peer-only participants reported that members of their group were supportive compared with moderator-led participants. Overall, these studies highlight the need for research to elucidate how individuals use online social networks, which strategies can improve engagement in these networks, and how to facilitate various types of online social support that promote behavior change.

Reminders and Prompts

Sixty-eight percent of the 19 studies (*n* = 13) reviewed used technology to provide reminders or prompts to engage with intervention content (24,55,59–64,70,76,80). Reminders have been delivered through various technology modalities, such as e-mail (55,59,61–65,70,71,76,80), SMS (60,70), telephone calls (70,71,76,80), or social networking site posts (64), and were initiated by a human counselor (55,61–63) or computer automated (24,62,70). The purpose of reminders and prompts varied across studies and included reminders or prompts to use an online diary or report self-monitoring data (60–63,70); encourage use of an intervention website or new content (59,65,70,71,76,80); review progress (76); update action plans (76); prompt review of goals (55); or complete short, weekly online questionnaires (55,64).

Collins et al. (70) evaluated the effects of enhancing a commercially available Web-based weight loss program with escalating reminders, personalized e-feedback, and personalized weight loss goals by comparing this enhanced program with the Web program alone (basic) and a wait-list control group among 309 adults. The basic group participants had access to a completely Web-based program that included several features, such as goal setting, tailored daily caloric goals, food and exercise diaries, weight and body measurement self-monitoring, graphs of body measurement trends, meal and exercise plans, community forums, e-mail newsletters, and weekly automated reminders to record weight. In addition to this program, enhanced group participants received escalating reminders prompting them to record their weekly weight, visit the website, and use the online diaries. These reminders were sent initially through e-mail, then SMS, and participants ultimately received a phone call if they had not recorded their weekly weight. At 12 weeks, both enhanced and basic groups had significant weight losses and reduced body mass index (BMI) compared with the waitlist control group. However, there were no significant differences between the two intervention groups, indicating that the escalating reminders and tailored feedback produced no additional effects on weight outcomes beyond those achieved through the basic program at 12 or 24 weeks. Follow-up findings demonstrated that retention at 24 weeks and website logins at 12 and 24 weeks were significantly higher in the enhanced group than in the basic group, which suggests that the reminders may have enhanced engagement with the intervention, but utilization did not lead to greater weight loss. This is in contrast to findings from Tate et al. (62), where automated tailored feedback on weight loss progress and behavioral adherence did produce better weight loss than a basic program at 12 weeks. Consistent with other studies, these findings suggest that the use of personalized feedback and reminders may facilitate better engagement and intervention adherence, but questions about technology features and type and dose of reminders remain.

van Wier et al. (66) offered participants the option to receive reminders to log in to a Web-based weight management intervention by text messages, in addition to receiving e-mail reminders twice a week. In one of the few studies of worksite weight control programs for overweight adults assessing long-term outcomes and technology-based modes of delivery (*n* = 1386), van Wier et al. (66,71) compared the effectiveness of a 6-month intervention delivered via phone or Internet with usual care (self-help brochures) at 6 months and 2 years. Participants were randomized to one of three groups, which received 1) publicly available self-help brochures on healthy diet, physical activity, and weight control; 2) self-help brochures, pedometer, intervention workbook with 10 modules, 10 counseling phone calls; or 3) self-help brochures, pedometer, intervention website with 10 modules, 10 counseling e-mails, e-mail or text message reminders two times per week to access the website. Results at 2 years showed that the Internet intervention produced modest weight losses among study completers compared with the control group, but there were no group differences in weight outcomes among all study participants (71). Consistent with other population-based Internet-based behavioral interventions, high attrition and intervention adherence were limitations, with 43% attrition at 2 years, half of Internet group participants completing 1 to 2 sessions (out of 10), and only 18% completing all 10 counseling sessions. Although the phone group completed more counseling calls (34% completed 10 calls), the Internet group gained significantly less weight than the phone group from 6 to 24 months. The authors propose that an Internet-based program is potentially more effective for maintaining initial weight loss than a phone-based program. Whether this sustained intervention effect could be partially attributed to mode of counseling or additional reminders was not speculated on, and data on Internet program participants' preferences for and receipt of reminders via e-mail or text messages were not provided. Given the potential for widespread dissemination of worksite interventions using technology-based strategies, further research that considers participant preferences for communication, enhances adherence and website usage, and promotes healthy weight, diet, and physical activity in the workplace setting is warranted.

Goal Setting and Action Planning

Goal setting and/or action planning were common behavioral strategies used in 53% of the studies ($n = 7$, $n = 3$, respectively) (55,57,59,64,65,70,76,80). Some interventions used technology to automate the tailoring and delivery of personalized weight loss and/or behavior change goals (that were either computer automated and tailored on the basis of participant reports) (24,65,70) or utilized technology to convey specific goals through e-mails or podcasts (55,80). Other studies educated participants on the importance of goal setting, encouraged them to set goals, and provided tools to guide goal setting, but specific goal selection was at the discretion of participants (55,57,64,65,70).

In the previously described study by van Genugten et al. (65), the computer-tailored intervention for weight maintenance, which was compared to a generic website, was developed primarily on the basis of self-regulation theory, and comprised strategies and a technology platform for goal setting, planning, self-monitoring, and automated feedback. The Web-based program included features to support guided goal setting and personal selection of behaviors change goals. Study findings demonstrated that the computer-tailored intervention was not different from the generic website with respect to preventing weight gain over 6 months, perhaps due to low adherence and use of the intervention website. As with most other studies, the goal-setting function was part of a multicomponent intervention, and the isolated effects of using this feature on weight and behavioral outcomes were not reported. Given existing technology platforms and the advent of applications and devices that enable real-time and continuous collection of objective data on intervention usage and adherence, the identification of active ingredients or technology functions that are most effective for promoting behavior can and should be pursued.

Dickinson et al. (76) specifically examined the potential benefit of an action-planning component added to a basic website for promoting improved eating and physical activity and reduced smoking and alcohol use, in a primary care setting. Participants ($n = 169$) were randomized to receive a Web-based health risk assessment with personalized feedback and online resources promoting behavior change (basic website), or the basic website with additional action-planning modules to support planning and implementation of changes in diet, physical activity, smoking, and alcohol use behaviors (enhanced website). From baseline to 3 and 6 months, healthful eating scores and physical activity improved in both groups, but there were no significant differences between groups. Potential explanations for the lack of an added effect of action planning were that the basic website alone was adequate for promoting behavior change, the methods used for the action-planning component were insufficient to produce change, and supplementing the Web-delivered action planning component with in-person support might have improved outcomes (76). While the study was limited by a low recruitment rate and high attrition, the additive design was conducive to isolating the effect of the action planning component and helped call attention to the need for research on the type and level of human interaction and reinforcement necessary to support adherence to action planning.

Reinforcement, Modeling, Behavioral Contracts, Problem Solving

Technology was used to provide reinforcements over one-quarter of the studies ($n = 5$) (57,58,61,62,65), and other specific behavior change strategies that were supported by technology and used less often were modeling (64,70,80,82) ($n = 3$), problem solving or barrier identification (24,57) ($n = 2$), and behavioral contracts (65) ($n = 1$). One of the proven techniques for behavioral weight control is problem-solving therapy, particularly during the maintenance phase (82). In our review, few studies have translated this technique for automated delivery, although one of the strategies that human e-mail counselors have employed is identifying barriers and problem-solving solutions with participants (61,62). Considering that modeling behavior is a well-established strategy to enhance self-efficacy related to diet and physical activity behaviors, one of the most commonly targeted theoretical constructs, video, audio, and gaming technology represent opportunities to address modeling as a strategy for promoting effective behavior change. Although we excluded intervention studies using video games because of their predominant focus on either dietary or fitness and exercise behaviors, there is an emerging body of research on gaming for health (83–85). Additionally, games and stealth interventions have taken innovative approaches to promoting healthy diet and physical activity behaviors as secondary benefits of activities that otherwise might focus on entertainment, enjoyment, or a social movement (86,87).

FUTURE DIRECTIONS

As the field of behavioral interventions for healthy diet, physical activity, and weight moves forward in conjunction with evolving technology, there are several unanswered questions that require attention. Research that examines technology functions that are most effective for promoting adherence and engagement with intervention content is needed to understand optimal dose, types, frequency, timing, and nature of functions for supporting dietary and physical activity behavior change. Study designs that permit isolated testing of specific theoretical constructs or key determinants of behavior change that are applied using technology are important for identifying active ingredients of interventions that can be efficiently and cost-effectively delivered and disseminated to improve public health behavior change. Among some of the studies we reviewed, it is possible that finding no added benefit of a particular technology function for supporting behavior change was related to insufficient statistical power to detect differences in outcomes. Newer research designs such as MOST—multiphase optimization strategy (88)—are particularly suited to building technology interventions and including those components that are "active ingredients" in order to optimize them on outcomes such as efficacy, cost, or even adherence (also see Chapter 8, this volume). Few studies designed and evaluated technology-based interventions with the intent of future widespread dissemination, and larger population-based studies delivered in workplace or health organization settings commonly suffered from high attrition and low adherence. Additional research examining completely automated real-time interventions that do not require human interaction or identify minimal and sufficient levels of interaction with counselors or coaches is also warranted.

CHALLENGES AND OPPORTUNITIES

The dynamic growth of technologies presents unlimited potential for developing, testing, and disseminating behavioral interventions that employ technology functions to support weight control, dietary, and physical activity behavior change. Newer technologies allow for greater ease of data collection, study assessments, and delivery of software or application updates. Novel intervention approaches and multiple modes of delivery have the potential to improve compliance with intervention recommendations and technology- or distance-based engagement with interventionists and peers, and offer flexibility and tailoring to user preferences at unprecedented levels. These opportunities introduce considerable challenges with respect to the enormous amount of data that can now be assessed throughout the course of behavioral intervention studies; advances in managing, monitoring, analyzing, and ensuring privacy of data collected continuously and in real time are necessary.

While examining the use of the latest technology innovation is critical and will make novel contributions to the field, we emphasize that in many cases newer technologies have similar capabilities used in the past (i.e., the functions that support behavior change are common to emerging technologies). Concerted efforts should be made to better understand the functions of technology interventions that afford the essential elements of effective programs for behavior change. In other words, it may not be necessary to repeat study designs that examined self-monitoring with PDAs compared to paper methods using mobile apps, since the underlying functions—mobile Internet-connected device for monitoring diet and physical activity with feedback—are essentially the same. Thus, greater advances to the field will be realized if research questions are posed around what the technology is being used to facilitate in terms of behavior change, rather than what the latest technology happens to be.

More rigorous research is needed that tests technology-based interventions in comparison with another group receiving a technology-based program, moves beyond a single delivery channel to using multiple modes of delivery to achieve a common function, and establishes the efficacy of technology interventions in real-world settings. Whereas Internet and technology adoption was historically disparate across population subgroups (e.g., age, race or ethnicity), current estimates indicate widespread adoption and use of several technologies such as smartphones, social networking sites, and text messaging. Consequently, it may be more important to test behavioral interventions delivered via various technology channels, given the existing potential for technology to help address health inequities. With the rapid evolution of technology, being flexible, adaptable, and creative in designing and implementing behavioral interventions is essential for success.

With an array of technologies to choose from, our ability to target theoretical and psychosocial determinants of behavior change, to assess adherence to technology components, and to objectively evaluate behavior change and health outcomes has never been greater. Current and emerging technologies offer an abundance of opportunities to integrate functions, test multicomponent behavioral interventions that use a hybrid of technologies, and deliver and capture data through multiple modes of delivery.

REFERENCES

1. Burnett KF, Taylor CB, Agras WS. Ambulatory computer-assisted therapy for obesity: A new frontier for behavior therapy. *Journal of Consulting and Clinical Psychology* 1985; 53(5):698–703.
2. Taylor CB, Agras WS, Losch M, Plante TG, Burnett K. Improving the effectiveness of computer assisted weight loss. *Behavior Therapy* 1991; 22(2):229–236.
3. Ritterband LM, Thorndike F. Internet interventions or patient education Web sites? *Journal of Medical Internet Research* 2006; 8(3):e18; author reply e9.
4. Murray E, Burns J, See TS, Lai R, Nazareth I. Interactive health communication applications for people with chronic disease. *Cochrane Database System Review* 2005; 4:CD004274.
5. Wantland DJ, Portillo CJ, Holzemer WL, Slaughter R, McGhee EM. The effectiveness of Web-based vs. non-Web-based interventions: A meta-analysis of behavioral change outcomes. *Journal of Medical Internet Research* 2004; 6(4):e40.
6. Marks IM, Cavanagh K, Gega L. Computer-aided psychotherapy: Revolution or bubble? *British Journal of Psychiatry* 2007; 191:471–473.
7. Saperstein SL, Atkinson NL, Gold RS. The impact of Internet use for weight loss. *Obesity Review* 2007; 8(5):459–465.
8. Wieland LS, Falzon L, Sciamanna CN, Trudeau KJ, Brodney S, Schwartz JE, et al. Interactive computer-based interventions for weight loss or weight maintenance in overweight or obese people. *Cochrane Database System Review* 2012; 8:CD007675.
9. Davies CA, Spence JC, Vandelanotte C, Caperchione CM, Mummery WK. Meta-analysis of Internet-delivered interventions to increase physical activity levels. *International Journal of Behavior, Nutrition and Physical Activity* 2012; 9:52.
10. Free C, Phillips G, Galli L, Watson L, Felix L, Edwards P, et al. The effectiveness of mobile-health technology-based health behaviour change or disease management interventions for health care consumers: A systematic review. *PLoS Medicine* 2013; 10(1):e1001362.
11. Webb TL, Joseph J, Yardley L, Michie S. Using the Internet to promote health behavior change: A systematic review and meta-analysis of the impact of theoretical basis, use of behavior change techniques, and mode of delivery on efficacy. *Journal of Medical Internet Research* 2010; 12(1):e4.
12. Neve M, Morgan PJ, Jones PR, Collins CE. Effectiveness of Web-based interventions in achieving weight loss and weight loss maintenance in overweight and obese adults: A systematic review with meta-analysis. *Obesity Review* 2010; 11(4):306–321.

13. Arem H, Irwin M. A review of Web-based weight loss interventions in adults. *Obesity Review* 2011; 12(5):e236–243.

14. Riley WT, Rivera DE, Atienza AA, Nilsen W, Allison SM, Mermelstein R. Health behavior models in the age of mobile interventions: Are our theories up to the task? *Translational Behavior Medicine* 2011; 1(1):53–71.

15. Head KJ, Noar SM, Iannarino NT, Grant Harrington N. Efficacy of text messaging–based interventions for health promotion: A meta-analysis. *Social Science Medicine* 2013; 97:41–48.

16. Bennett GG, Herring SJ, Puleo E, Stein EK, Emmons KM, Gillman MW. Web-based weight loss in primary care: A randomized controlled trial. *Obesity* (Silver Spring) 2010; 18(2):308–313.

17. Bennett GG, Warner ET, Glasgow RE, Askew S, Goldman J, Ritzwoller DP, et al. Obesity treatment for socioeconomically disadvantaged patients in primary care practice. *Archives of Internal Medicine* 2012; 172(7):565–574.

18. Haapala I, Barengo NC, Biggs S, Surakka L, Manninen P. Weight loss by mobile phone: A 1-year effectiveness study. *Public Health Nutrition* 2009; 12(12):2382–2391.

19. Hunter CM, Peterson AL, Alvarez LM, Poston WC, Brundige AR, Haddock CK, et al. Weight management using the Internet: A randomized controlled trial. *American Journal of Preventive Medicine* 2008; 34(2):119–126.

20. Morgan PJ, Collins CE, Plotnikoff RC, Cook AT, Berthon B, Mitchell S, et al. Efficacy of a workplace-based weight loss program for overweight male shift workers: The Workplace POWER (Preventing Obesity Without Eating like a Rabbit) randomized controlled trial. *Preventive Medicine* 2011; 52(5):317–325.

21. Patrick K, Raab F, Adams MA, Dillon L, Zabinski M, Rock CL, et al. A text message–based intervention for weight loss: Randomized controlled trial. *Journal of Medical Internet Research* 2009; 11(1):e1.

22. Patrick K, Calfas KJ, Norman GJ, Rosenberg D, Zabinski MF, Sallis JF, et al. Outcomes of a 12-month Web-based intervention for overweight and obese men. *Annals of Behavioral Medicine* 2011; 42(3):391–401.

23. Steinberg DM, Tate DF, Bennett GG, Ennett S, Samuel-Hodge C, Ward DS. The efficacy of a daily self-weighing weight loss intervention using smart scales and e-mail. *Obesity* (Silver Spring) 2013; 21(9):1789–1797.

24. Wylie-Rosett J, Swencionis C, Ginsberg M, Cimino C, Wassertheil-Smoller S, Caban A, et al. Computerized weight loss intervention optimizes staff time: The clinical and cost results of a controlled clinical trial conducted in a managed care setting. *Journal of the American Dietetic Association* 2001; 101(10):1155–1162; quiz 63–64.

25. Cussler EC, Teixeira PJ, Going SB, Houtkooper LB, Metcalfe LL, Blew RM, et al. Maintenance of weight loss in overweight middle-aged women through the Internet. *Obesity* (Silver Spring) 2008; 16(5):1052–1060.

26. Thomas D, Vydelingum V, Lawrence J. E-mail contact as an effective strategy in the maintenance of weight loss in adults. *Journal of Human Nutrtion and Dietetics* 2011 Feb;24(1):32–38.

27. Thorndike AN, Sonnenberg L, Healey E, Myint UK, Kvedar JC, Regan S. Prevention of weight gain following a worksite nutrition and exercise program: A randomized controlled trial. *American Journal of Preventive Medicine* 2012; 43(1):27–33.

28. Werkman A, Hulshof PJ, Stafleu A, Kremers SP, Kok FJ, Schouten EG, et al. Effect of an individually tailored one-year energy balance programme on body weight, body composition and lifestyle in recent retirees: A cluster randomised controlled trial. *BMC Public Health* 2010; 10:110.

29. Dekkers JC, van Wier MF, Ariens GA, Hendriksen IJ, Pronk NP, Smid T, et al. Comparative effectiveness of lifestyle interventions on cardiovascular risk factors among a Dutch overweight working population: A randomized controlled trial. *BMC Public Health* 2011; 11(1):49.

30. Jackson RA, Stotland NE, Caughey AB, Gerbert B. Improving diet and exercise in pregnancy with Video Doctor counseling: A randomized trial. *Patient Education and Counseling* 2011; 83(2):203–209.

31. Kelders SM, Van Gemert-Pijnen JE, Werkman A, Nijland N, Seydel ER. Effectiveness of a Web-based intervention aimed at healthy dietary and physical activity behavior: A randomized controlled trial about users and usage. *Journal of Medical Internet Research* 2011; 13(2):e32.

32. Robroek SJ, Polinder S, Bredt FJ, Burdorf A. Cost-effectiveness of a long-term Internet-delivered worksite health promotion programme on physical activity and nutrition: A cluster randomized controlled trial. *Health Education Research* 2012; 27(3):399–410.

33. Winett RA, Anderson ES, Wojcik JR, Winett SG, Bowden T. Guide to health: Nutrition and physical activity outcomes of a group-randomized trial of an Internet-based intervention in churches. *Annals of Behavioral Medicine* 2007; 33(3):251–261.

34. Mehring M, Haag M, Linde K, Wagenpfeil S, Frensch F, Blome J, et al. Effects of a general practice guided Web-based weight reduction program—results of a cluster-randomized controlled trial. *BMC Family Practice* 2013; 14:76.

35. Morgan PJ, Lubans DR, Collins CE, Warren JM, Callister R. 12-month outcomes and process evaluation of the SHED-IT RCT: An Internet-based weight loss program targeting men. *Obesity* (Silver Spring) 2011; 19(1):142–151.

36. Harvey-Berino J, West D, Krukowski R, Prewitt E, VanBiervliet A, Ashikaga T, et al. Internet delivered behavioral obesity treatment. *Preventive Medicine* 2010; 51(2):123–128.

37. Womble LG, Wadden TA, McGuckin BG, Sargent SL, Rothman RA, Krauthamer-Ewing ES. A randomized controlled trial of a commercial Internet weight loss program. *Obesity Research* 2004; 12(6):1011–1018.

38. Harvey-Berino J, Pintauro S, Buzzell P, DiGiulio M, Casey Gold B, Moldovan C, et al. Does using the Internet facilitate the maintenance of weight loss? *International Journal of Obesity and Related Metabolic Disorders* 2002; 26(9):1254–1260.

39. Svetkey LP, Stevens VJ, Brantley PJ, Appel LJ, Hollis JF, Loria CM, et al. Comparison of strategies for sustaining weight loss: The weight loss maintenance randomized controlled trial. *JAMA* 2008; 299(10):1139–1148.

40. Wing RR, Tate DF, Gorin AA, Raynor HA, Fava JL. A self-regulation program for maintenance of weight loss. *New England Journal of Medicine* 2006; 355(15):1563–1571.

41. Burke LE, Conroy MB, Sereika SM, Elci OU, Styn MA, Acharya SD, et al. The effect of electronic self-monitoring on weight loss and dietary intake: A randomized behavioral weight loss trial. *Obesity* (Silver Spring). 2011; 19(2):338–344.

42. Burke LE, Styn MA, Sereika SM, Conroy MB, Ye L, Glanz K, et al. Using mHealth technology to enhance self-monitoring for weight loss: A randomized trial. *American Journal of Preventive Medicine* 2012; 43(1):20–26.

43. McDoniel SO, Wolskee P, Shen J. Treating obesity with a novel hand-held device, computer software program, and Internet technology in primary care: The SMART motivational trial. *Patient Education and Counseling* 2010; 79(2):185–191.

44. Pellegrini CA, Verba SD, Otto AD, Helsel DL, Davis KK, Jakicic JM. The comparison of a technology-based system and an in-person behavioral weight loss intervention. *Obesity* (Silver Spring) 2012; 20(2):356–363.

45. Polzien KM, Jakicic JM, Tate DF, Otto AD. The efficacy of a technology-based system in a short-term behavioral weight loss intervention. *Obesity* (Silver Spring) 2007; 15(4):825–830.

46. Shay LE, Seibert D, Watts D, Sbrocco T, Pagliara C. Adherence and weight loss outcomes associated with food-exercise diary preference in a military

weight management program. *Eating Behavior* 2009; 10(4):220–227.

47. Shuger SL, Barry VW, Sui X, McClain A, Hand GA, Wilcox S, et al. Electronic feedback in a diet- and physical activity-based lifestyle intervention for weight loss: A randomized controlled trial. *International Journal of Behavioral Nutrition and Physical Activity* 2011; 8:41.

48. Hebden L, Cook A, van der Ploeg HP, King L, Bauman A, Allman-Farinelli M. A mobile health intervention for weight management among young adults: A pilot randomised controlled trial. *Journal of Human Nutrition and Dietetics* 2013; 27(4):322–332.

49. Lombard C, Deeks A, Jolley D, Ball K, Teede H. A low intensity, community based lifestyle programme to prevent weight gain in women with young children: Cluster randomised controlled trial. *British Medical Journal* 2010; 341:c3215.

50. McConnon A, Kirk SF, Cockroft JE, Harvey EL, Greenwood DC, Thomas JD, et al. The Internet for weight control in an obese sample: Results of a randomised controlled trial. *BMC Health Services Research* 2007; 7:206.

51. Spring B, Duncan JM, Janke EA, Kozak AT, McFadden HG, DeMott A, et al. Integrating technology into standard weight loss treatment: A randomized controlled trial. *JAMA Internal Medicine* 2013; 173(2):105–111.

52. Michie S, Ashford S, Sniehotta FF, Dombrowski SU, Bishop A, French DP. A refined taxonomy of behaviour change techniques to help people change their physical activity and healthy eating behaviours: The CALO-RE taxonomy. *Psychological Health* 2011; 26(11):1479–1498.

53. Brindal E, Freyne J, Saunders I, Berkovsky S, Smith G, Noakes M. Features predicting weight loss in overweight or obese participants in a Web-based intervention: Randomized trial. *Journal of Medical Internet Research* 2012; 14(6):e173.

54. Collins CE, Morgan PJ, Hutchesson MJ, Callister R. Efficacy of standard versus enhanced features in a Web-based commercial weight-loss program for obese adults, part 2: Randomized controlled trial. *Journal of Medical Internet Research* 2013; 15(7):e140.

55. Gabriele JM, Carpenter BD, Tate DF, Fisher EB. Directive and nondirective e-coach support for weight loss in overweight adults. *Annals of Behavioral Medicine* 2011; 41(2):252–263.

56. Gold BC, Burke S, Pintauro S, Buzzell P, Harvey-Berino J. Weight loss on the web: A pilot study comparing a structured behavioral intervention to a commercial program. *Obesity* (Silver Spring) 2007; 15(1):155–164.

57. Hersey JC, Khavjou O, Strange LB, Atkinson RL, Blair SN, Campbell S, et al. The efficacy and cost-effectiveness of a community weight management intervention: A randomized controlled trial of the health weight management demonstration. *Preventive Medicine* 2012; 54(1):42–49.

58. Micco N, Gold B, Buzzell P, Leonard H, Pintauro S, Harvey-Berino J. Minimal in-person support as an adjunct to Internet obesity treatment. *Annals of Behavioral Medicine* 2007; 33(1):49–56.

59. Rothert K, Strecher VJ, Doyle LA, Caplan WM, Joyce JS, Jimison HB, et al. Web-based weight management programs in an integrated health care setting: A randomized, controlled trial. *Obesity* (Silver Spring) 2006; 14(2):266–272.

60. Shapiro JR, Koro T, Doran N, Thompson S, Sallis JF, Calfas K, et al. Text4Diet: A randomized controlled study using text messaging for weight loss behaviors. *Preventive Medicine* 2012; 55(5):412–417.

61. Tate DF, Jackvony EH, Wing RR. Effects of Internet behavioral counseling on weight loss in adults at risk for type 2 diabetes: A randomized trial. *JAMA* 2003; 289(14):1833–1836.

62. Tate DF, Jackvony EH, Wing RR. A randomized trial comparing human e-mail counseling, computer-automated tailored counseling, and no counseling in an Internet weight loss program. *Archives of Internal Medicine* 2006; 166(15):1620–1625.

63. Tate DF, Wing RR, Winett RA. Using Internet technology to deliver a behavioral weight loss program. *JAMA* 2001; 285(9):1172–1177.

64. Turner-McGrievy G, Tate D. Tweets, apps, and pods: Results of the 6-month Mobile Pounds Off Digitally (Mobile POD) randomized weight-loss intervention among adults. *Journal of Medical Internet Research* 2011; 13(4):e120.

65. van Genugten L, van Empelen P, Boon B, Borsboom G, Visscher T, Oenema A. Results from an online computer-tailored weight management intervention for overweight adults: Randomized controlled trial. *Journal of Medical Internet Research* 2012; 14(2):e44.

66. van Wier MF, Ariens GA, Dekkers JC, Hendriksen IJ, Smid T, van Mechelen W. Phone and e-mail counselling are effective for weight management in an overweight working population: A randomized controlled trial. *BMC Public Health* 2009; 9:6.

67. Webber KH, Tate DF, Michael Bowling J. A randomized comparison of two motivationally enhanced Internet behavioral weight loss programs. *Behaviour Research and Therapy* 2008; 46(9):1090–1095.

68. Wing RR, Crane MM, Thomas JG, Kumar R, Weinberg B. Improving weight loss outcomes of community interventions by incorporating behavioral strategies. *American Journal of Public Health* 2010; 100(12):2513–2519.

69. Burke LE, Wang J, Sevick MA. Self-monitoring in weight loss: A systematic review of the literature. *Journal of the American Dietetic Association* 2011; 111(1):92–102.

70. Collins CE, Morgan PJ, Jones P, Fletcher K, Martin J, Aguiar EJ, et al. A 12-week commercial web-based weight-loss program for overweight and obese adults: Randomized controlled trial comparing basic versus enhanced features. *Journal of Medical Internet Research* 2012; 14(2):e57.

71. van Wier MF, Dekkers JC, Hendriksen IJ, Heymans MW, Ariens GA, Pronk NP, et al. Effectiveness of phone and e-mail lifestyle counseling for long term weight control among overweight employees. *Journal of Occupational and Environmental Medicine* 2011; 53(6):680–686.

72. Lustria ML, Cortese J, Noar SM, Glueckauf RL. Computer-tailored health interventions delivered over the Web: Review and analysis of key components. *Patient Education and Counseling* 2009; 74(2):156–173.

73. Hawkins RP, Kreuter M, Resnicow K, Fishbein M, Dijkstra A. Understanding tailoring in communicating about health. *Health Education Research* 2008; 23(3):454–466.

74. Krebs P, Prochaska JO, Rossi JS. A meta-analysis of computer-tailored interventions for health behavior change. *Preventive Medicine* 2010; 51(3-4):214–221.

75. Lustria ML, Noar SM, Cortese J, Van Stee SK, Glueckauf RL, Lee J. A meta-analysis of Web-delivered tailored health behavior change interventions. *Journal of Health Communication* 2013; 18(9):1039–1069.

76. Dickinson WP, Glasgow RE, Fisher L, Dickinson LM, Christensen SM, Estabrooks PA, et al. Use of a website to accomplish health behavior change: If you build it, will they come? And will it work if they do? *Journal of the American Board of Family Medicine* 2013; 26(2):168–176.

77. Cavallo DN, Tate DF, Ries AV, Brown JD, DeVellis RF, Ammerman AS. A social media-based physical activity intervention: A randomized controlled trial. *American Journal of Preventive Medicine* 2012; 43(5):527–532.

78. Napolitano MA, Hayes S, Bennett GG, Ives AK, Foster GD. Using Facebook and text messaging to deliver a weight loss program to college students. *Obesity* (Silver Spring). 2013; 21(1):25–31.

79. Valle CG, Tate DF, Mayer DK, Allicock M, Cai J. A randomized trial of a Facebook-based physical activity intervention for young adult cancer survivors. *Journal of Cancer Survival* 2013; 7(3):355–368.

80. Turner-McGrievy GM, Campbell MK, Tate DF, Truesdale KP, Bowling JM, Crosby L. Pounds

Off Digitally study: A randomized podcasting weight-loss intervention. *American Journal of Preventive Medicine* 2009; 37(4):263–269.

81. Turner-McGrievy GM, Tate DF. Weight loss social support in 140 characters or less: Use of an online social network in a remotely delivered weight loss intervention. *Translational Behavior Medicine* 2013; 3(3):287–294.

82. Perri MG, Nezu AM, McKelvey WF, Shermer RL, Renjilian DA, Viegener BJ. Relapse prevention training and problem-solving therapy in the long-term management of obesity. *Journal of Consulting and Clinical Psychology* 2001; 69(4):722–726.

83. Baranowski T, Buday R, Thompson DI, Baranowski J. Playing for real: Video games and stories for health-related behavior change. *American Journal of Preventive Medicine* 2008; 34(1):74–82.

84. LeBlanc AG, Chaput JP, McFarlane A, Colley RC, Thivel D, Biddle SJ, et al. Active video games and health indicators in children and youth: A systematic review. *PLoS One* 2013; 8(6):e65351.

85. Peng W, Crouse JC, Lin JH. Using active video games for physical activity promotion: A systematic review of the current state of research. *Health Education & Behavior* 2013; 40(2):171–92.

86. Hekler EB, Gardner CD, Robinson TN. Effects of a college course about food and society on students' eating behaviors. *American Journal of Preventive Medicine* 2010; 38(5):543–547.

87. Robinson TN, Killen JD, Kraemer HC, Wilson DM, Matheson DM, Haskell WL, et al. Dance and reducing television viewing to prevent weight gain in African-American girls: The Stanford GEMS pilot study. *Ethnicity & Disease* 2003; 13(1 Suppl 1):S65–77.

88. Collins LM, Murphy SA, Strecher V. The multiphase optimization strategy (MOST) and the sequential multiple assignment randomized trial (SMART): New methods for more potent eHealth interventions. *American Journal of Preventive Medicine* 2007; 32(5 Suppl):S112–118.

10

Evidence-Based Approaches to Harnessing Technology to Provide Social-Emotional Support

TIMOTHY BICKMORE

INTRODUCTION

Computerized treatments for mental health disorders such as depression and anxiety are a rapidly emerging area of interest, with dozens of interventions reported in the literature (1,2). Automated interventions have the potential to reach a much wider population than therapist-driven individual or group therapy, given their lower costs and greater convenience. Automated interventions can also help to avoid issues of stigma that may be associated with conventional mental health treatment, by allowing individuals to initiate and receive treatment in the privacy of their homes (3). However, the evidence regarding how well these automated systems actually work has been mixed. Recent meta-analyses and large-scale, randomized controlled trials of Web-based computerized cognitive behavioral therapy systems for anxiety and depression have failed to demonstrate significant outcomes (2,4), and other meta-analyses have indicated that completely automated interventions for depression and anxiety do not perform as well as computer-mediated interventions involving human therapists (5). Although technology is constantly improving and automated behavioral interventions represent a burgeoning area of research and development, these early results indicate that something fundamental may be missing from current systems.

What do conventional computer media, such as text-laden information websites or interactive text modules, lack that a good therapist can provide? One possibility is that conventional media lacks the "human touch" of a therapist: the ability to convey the image of a trusting, compassionate, supportive persona that patients are comfortable working with, relying on, and sharing their most private concerns with. Such trusting relationships are key in healing, whether with a therapist or a wider support network of friends and family. Trusting, supportive relationships with therapists are typically conceptualized as "therapeutic alliance" relationships in the research literature (6), whereas the more generalized perception of having a network of people to rely on is generally referred to as "social support" (7). Given the importance of trust and supportive relationships in therapy, it is important to understand how people build trusting, supportive relationships and how this behavior can be infused into our computerized systems. Increasing patients' trust in computerized therapy systems should increase both adherence to the system's recommendations and treatment retention. Retention in particular has been a significant problem with most automated interventions for depression evaluated to date (2).

This chapter highlights the growing area of technology-based relational agents—computational artifacts designed to build and maintain alliance relationships with patients for the purpose of improving retention and outcomes in automated health behavior change interventions (8,9). Following a discussion of the conceptual framework for development of relational agents, examples of how these technologies have been applied in behavioral healthcare will be described.

TRUST IN THE THERAPIST: THERAPEUTIC ALLIANCE

The therapeutic alliance (also "working alliance") is based on the trust and belief that a therapist and patient have in each other as team members in achieving a desired outcome, and has been hypothesized to be the single common factor underlying the therapeutic benefit of therapies ranging from behavioral and cognitive therapies to psychodynamic therapy (6,10). The working alliance construct has three subcomponents: a goal component, reflecting the degree to which the therapist and client agree on the goals of the therapy; a task component, reflecting the degree to which the therapist and client agree on the therapeutic tasks to be performed; and a bond component, reflecting the trusting, empathetic relationship between the client and therapist (10,11). Relational agents primarily draw upon the bond component of working alliance that focuses primarily on the emotional support component of the relationship.

There is now a significant body of evidence demonstrating the association between a strong alliance and outcomes in psychotherapy (12). One meta-analysis of 190 studies demonstrated a strong, positive effect of therapeutic alliance on outcomes across many types of individual treatment (6), a result consistent with several other meta-analyses (13,14). This association has also been found to hold in computer-mediated therapy in which patients interact remotely with a healthcare professional via e-mail, video conferencing, virtual reality, or chat technology (15). Patients who interacted with their therapists via computer felt that use of the technology allowed their working relationship to develop, and resulted in closer agreement of patient-rated and therapist-rated alliance compared to face-to-face interactions.

Whether face to face or mediated, the impact of alliance on therapy outcomes is at least in part due to improvement in treatment retention. A meta-analytic study demonstrated a strong relationship between weak alliance and dropout in psychotherapy (16), and mental health treatments that are delivered for inadequate durations are ineffective (17). Alliance "ruptures" have been shown to lead to failures in psychotherapy (12), but even subtle fluctuations in the therapeutic relationship have been shown to be impactful. One study that investigated longitudinal changes in alliance and symptoms found evidence for a reciprocal causal model, in which the alliance predicted subsequent changes in symptoms, and prior symptom change also affected the alliance (18).

TRUST IN THE SOCIAL NETWORK: SOCIAL SUPPORT

Social support is the feeling of being cared for and having assistance available from others when needed. There are many kinds of support, including tangible (e.g., shopping for someone), emotional (e.g., nurturance), social network (e.g., introducing one to others), informational (e.g., advice), and companionship (e.g., sense of belonging). In addition to the well-known buffering effect of social support in preventing mental illness (7), social support is an important factor in healing for individuals diagnosed with mental health disorders. For example, family and community social support has been shown to be an important factor in positive outcomes for individuals with schizophrenia (19). One meta-analysis demonstrated that simple befriending as an intervention had a significant positive impact on depressive symptoms (20).

HOW PEOPLE ENGENDER TRUST

Before turning to automated systems, it is useful to first review the specific behaviors that therapists and others use to build trust in face-to-face interaction. People build and maintain relationships primarily in the context of face-to-face interaction, because it is the primal and primary site of human interaction and language use. Several communication studies have demonstrated that when the social aspects of an interaction are especially important, such as in getting-acquainted conversations, the face-to-face interaction is crucial. In a review of studies comparing video- and audio-mediated communication, Whittaker and O'Conaill concluded that video was superior to audio only for social tasks, while there was little difference in subjective ratings or task outcomes for tasks in which the social aspects were less important (21). These researchers found that for social tasks, interactions were more personalized, less argumentative, and more polite when conducted via video-mediated communication; that participants believed video-mediated (and face-to-face) communication was superior to audio-only communication; and that groups conversing via video-mediated communication tended to like each other more, compared to audio-only interactions. Obviously, some nonverbal communication must be responsible for these differences.

Nonverbal behavior can be used to express a wide range of cues, including emotions, interpersonal attitudes, factual information, and self-presentation, and to signal rituals such as greetings (22), in addition to relational cues. Emotional and attitudinal displays are especially important in building relationships and providing support, and these are enacted primarily through facial displays (23). Another type of nonverbal behavior important in building relationships and expressing support is "immediacy behavior," which serves to demonstrate affiliation or liking, and includes cues such as close conversational distance, direct body and facial orientation, forward lean, increased and direct gaze, smiling, pleasant facial expressions and facial animation in general, nodding, frequent gesturing, and postural openness (22,24).

In addition to nonverbal cues, there are many verbal behaviors that supporters can use to engender feelings of trust and companionship. In the literature on working alliance, the relational factor most often mentioned as being crucial in forming and maintaining the alliance is the patient's perception of the therapist's empathy for him or her (10). Empathy can be conveyed both verbally (25) and through facial displays of concern or compassion. In addition to conveying an appropriate amount of empathy, trust and rapport can be developed through social dialogue (26–29), reciprocal deepening self-disclosure (though there are mixed opinions about how much self-disclosure a therapist should do) (30,31), emphasizing commonalities (32), humor (33–35), meta-relational communication (particularly emotional aspects) (34,36), and expressing happiness to see the patient (37). Other relational strategies that could be used to effect increases in trust and the bond dimension of the alliance include talking about the past and future together (38,39), continuity behaviors (appropriate greetings and farewells, and talk about the time spent apart) (40), and reference to mutual knowledge. Specific language constructs that may also be effective include the use of inclusive pronouns (25), and politeness strategies (41,42) and greeting and farewell rituals (43) indicative of a close relationship.

ENGENDERING TRUST IN AUTOMATED SYSTEMS FOR BEHAVIORAL MEDICINE

Given the importance of the alliance and social support for retention and long-term outcomes in psychotherapy, it is no wonder that completely automated interventions that lack human-centered features to promote alliance have not demonstrated the same efficacy as that of person-delivered therapy. Since many of the cues used to build and maintain therapeutic alliance are nonverbal in nature, traditional Web-based media involving text and static imagery is lacking in its ability to convey the relational cues that people use to instill trust, as well as to provide cues that allow patients to personify automated systems in order to feel supported and empathized with. These nonverbal cues are particularly important for establishing the bond dimension of the working alliance, since displays of empathy, compassion, and attentiveness can be significantly enhanced using nonverbal channels such as facial display and voice prosody.

Over the last decade a number of software and robotic systems have been developed to explicitly address the deficiency in attention to therapeutic alliance in traditional computer-mediated interventions, by using animated characters or robots that are humanoid in form and use many of the same behaviors that people use to engender feelings of trust, support, and companionship in their users. The remainder of this chapter provides an overview of this technology and its use in behavioral medicine.

RELATIONAL AGENTS

Relational agents are computational artifacts that are explicitly designed to build and maintain alliance relationships with patients for the purpose of improving retention and outcomes in automated health behavior change interventions, including psychotherapy (8,9). In order to use the same verbal and nonverbal cues that therapists use in face-to-face interaction with patients, relational agents are typically designed to be human in appearance, with animated or robotic faces and bodies (Figure 10.1). Obviously, to display relational nonverbal behavior with fidelity, in a

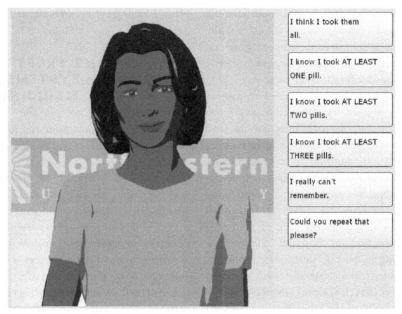

FIGURE 10.1: Example of relational agent for antipsychotic medication adherence.

way that patients will be able to immediately and tacitly understand, requires an anthropomorphic interface: a face to display emotions, and a body to display leaning, for example.

Relational agents can also be designed to provide social support and companionship. Given that computer systems can be personified and given relational behaviors, they are capable of providing almost all types of social support that people can. Computer agents have been developed that provide some forms of tangible, emotional, social network, informational, and companionship support to users.

SYSTEMS DESIGNED TO BUILD THERAPEUTIC ALLIANCE: VIRTUAL COACHES AND COUNSELORS

One of the first automated health counselors designed explicitly to foster a therapeutic alliance with its users was a virtual exercise coach named "Laura." This system was designed to allow experimentation on automated relationship-building behaviors within the context of a longitudinal health behavior change intervention. The system was first used to assist with a relatively simple behavior—walking promotion in older adults—and was later adapted for mental health counseling for college-aged young people.

In a study of counseling to promote well-being and physical activity, Laura was evaluated in a three-condition randomized trial with 101 young adults from the Massachusetts Institute of Technology (MIT) community to test the ability of the agent's relational behavior to foster a sense of therapeutic alliance in study participants over 30 days of brief daily counseling (8). The counseling included behavioral (e.g., positive reinforcement), social cognitive (e.g., problem solving to develop self-efficacy), and cognitive behavioral (e.g., promotion of positive thoughts about exercise) techniques. One group of participants (RELATIONAL) interacted with a version of Laura in which all of her relational behavior (social dialogue, empathy, immediacy, etc.) was enabled, while a second group interacted with the same agent in which these relational behaviors were removed (NON-RELATIONAL). A third group acted as a non-intervention control and simply recorded their daily physical activity (CONTROL). Participants in the RELATIONAL condition reported significantly higher Working Alliance scores on the Bond subscale of the working alliance measure compared with subjects in the NON-RELATIONAL condition, both at 1 week and at the end of the 4-week intervention. Participants in the RELATIONAL and NON-RELATIONAL groups combined, increased the number of days per week that they engaged in at least 30 minutes of moderate or more vigorous physical activity significantly more than subjects in the CONTROL condition. However, there were no significant differences between the RELATIONAL and NON-RELATIONAL groups with respect to gains in physical activity, likely due to the short duration of the intervention (8,44).

Laura was also adapted to provide counseling for adults with schizophrenia, focusing on promoting adherence to antipsychotic medication and increases in moderate exercise (45) (Figure 10.1). The system ran on a laptop computer as a stand-alone system and was designed as a 1-month, daily contact intervention. The agent tracked each patient's medication-taking behavior for a single antipsychotic taken by mouth in pill or capsule form based on self-report, and also reminded patients to take all of their other medications as prescribed.

The agent dialogue and nonverbal behavior were tailored specifically to interact with individuals with schizophrenia. Extended time was spent during orientation and termination phases of the intervention schedule to help patients ease into and out of their working relationship with the agent. The first several days were spent only on relational behavior and visit adherence, before discussions of medication, exercise, and schizophrenia were started. The last several days were spent preparing patients for termination, addressing their feelings about ending their daily conversations with the agent and focusing the counseling on promotion of self-maintenance behaviors. The dialogue scripts were reviewed to ensure that simple, direct language was used throughout by the agent, and its nonverbal behavior was simplified by removing conversational "gaze-aways" that patients may take as a cue of untrustworthiness.

The agent was also designed to promote social support, by suggesting that a particular individual in the user's social network provide them with instrumental support. At enrollment time, the study nurse asked the patient for the given name of and relationship to someone who could help them with their medications. The agent then recommended that the user enlist the aid of this helper when certain conditions arise. Examples included asking the helper to remind the user to take their medications at a particular time, or to fill their prescription if they keep forgetting ("Do you think your sister Sally could remind you?"), or asking the user if the helper could drive them to the pharmacy if they indicate they are having trouble getting their prescription filled because of transportation problems.

A quasi-experimental study was conducted to assess acceptance and use. Twenty participants, aged 19–58, were recruited from a mental health outpatient clinic who met the *DSM-IV-R* criteria for schizophrenia, were on any antipsychotic medication, and had two or more episodes of non-adherence in the 72 hours prior to recruitment. Sixteen participants (80%) completed the study and, of these, one participant developed paranoia and stopped using the agent after a few days.

System logs indicated that participants interacted with the agent an average of 65.8% of the available days, with nine of the participants interacting with the agent at least 25 times during the 30-day intervention. Self-report ratings of satisfaction averaged 4.0 on a 1 ("not at all") to 5 ("very much") scale. Self-reported medication dose adherence was 89%. Satisfaction was rated an average 4.5 on a 1 = "not at all" to 5 = "very much" scale. Although a validated measure of working alliance was not used, participants did rate their trust in the agent an average 4.4 on a 5-point scale (5 = "very much"). These results indicate that the patients with schizophrenia largely accepted and regularly interacted with the agent and were satisfied with their daily counseling conversations (45).

Robotic relational agents have also been developed as automated health counselors. "Autom" is a non-mobile interactive social robot designed to promote diet tracking among overweight users (46). Autom was programmed to use a few of the relational behaviors described earlier in its daily conversation with users, such as appropriate greetings and limited social chat. In a 6-week study, 45 participants who were class I or II obese (BMI range of 25 up to 42) interacted with either the robot or a touch screen computer or used a paper diary to record their eating behavior daily. Participants rated the robot significantly higher on working alliance compared to the touch screen condition. In addition, participants who interacted with Autom continued recording their diet behavior significantly longer than those in the computer or paper diary conditions. There were no significant differences in actual weight loss between the groups (46). These results provide further evidence that patients find anthropomorphic agents more engaging than equivalent systems that are not personified. Whether a robotic embodiment is more effective than an equivalent screen-based animated agent at engaging users or motivating behavior change has yet to be demonstrated.

Another randomized controlled trial directly compared a state-of-the-art website for delivering tailored health behavior change to the same website with the addition of a relational agent counselor (47). The year-long intervention was designed to promote exercise and UV (sunlight) avoidance for cancer prevention. A national sample of 914 participants were randomized to the two conditions, with those in the relational agent group demonstrating higher engagement by completing significantly more interactions per week with the intervention system (0.142 vs. 0.048 average interactions with the Web agent per week).

Several laboratory studies have also been conducted to identify individual agent behaviors that may elicit therapeutic alliance in users or that compared relational agents with other media. One study compared four different media for relational agents on a handheld computer—text messages only, static agent image plus text, animated agent, and animated agent plus speech—and the ability of the agent to establish a therapeutic alliance with a user in a single, brief counseling session (48). Results indicated that animation was key: relative to non-animated versions, the two versions with the animated character resulted in significantly higher user scores on the Working Alliance Inventory, as well as ratings of how caring the agent was (48).

Additional laboratory studies have investigated the ability of conversational agents to comfort users who are distressed, through empathy and other behaviors. The CASPER affect-management agent was demonstrated to provide relief to users experiencing frustration (49). The system interacted with users via text messages and menus, and presented frustrated users with a series of menus that prompted them to describe their emotional state, allowed users to correct the computer's assessment (if necessary), and then provided empathetic and sympathetic text feedback. This agent was found to be significantly better than a venting-only agent (to which users could simply describe how they felt in an open-ended manner without feedback) or an agent that ignored their emotions completely, in relieving frustration, as measured both by self-report measures and by the length of time users were willing to continue working with a computer after a frustrating experience (49). In another series of studies on the ability of conversational agents to comfort users, it was found that the mere presence of an animated relational agent provided a positive change in affect for frustrated users (50), and that a conversational agent that provided empathically accurate feedback provided more comfort than an agent that afforded greater user expressivity about their distress (51).

Finally, a series of studies was conducted exploring the use of physical touch by a relational agent, for comforting users and establishing trust and therapeutic alliance (52). Touch is an important channel for communicating empathic understanding of distress and conveying a message of comfort and caring in human–human interaction, including nurse–patient interaction. One study of 30 critical care nurse–patient dyads in a hospital setting found that caring touch was used by the nurses twice per hour, on average (53). To explore how this haptic communication channel could be used by relational agents, an agent was developed that could gently squeeze users' hands using a computer-controlled air bladder (Figure 10.2). Studies found that use of the haptic channel in comforting conversations with a relational agent resulted in significant increases in working alliance, but only for users who were comfortable being touched by strangers; it had the opposite effect on users who were not comfortable being touched.

SYSTEMS DESIGNED TO PROVIDE SOCIAL SUPPORT: VIRTUAL COMPANIONS

Several automated systems have been developed for the purpose of providing people with automated companions, to increase feelings of social support and decrease loneliness. Loneliness among older adults in particular represents a significant societal problem, and has thus been the target of most technological interventions in this area. Fully 40% of older adults experience loneliness (54), and this has been linked with a variety of health problems, including increased risk of cardiovascular disease and death (55).

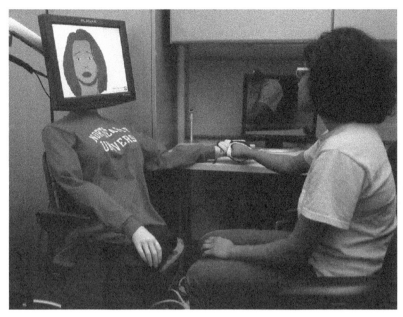

FIGURE 10.2: A relational agent capable of comforting touch.

Some efforts in academia and industry have focused on creating robotic pets for older adults, to provide the companionship and positive effects found in animal-assisted therapy (56). The "mental commit" robots take the form of cute stuffed animals, such as a cat or a harp seal pup (named "paro"), and are designed to foster an attachment with users. One study compared the effects of these robots on older adults in a nursing home with the effects of an identical robot that had a much simpler behavioral repertoire, however, no significant differences were found (57). Another study compared the use of a Sony AIBO robotic dog with that of a stuffed toy dog and a "clothed" AIBO by a group of older adults with severe dementia. This study found that patients actually interacted more with the stuffed toy than with either of the AIBOs, but the differences were not significant (58). Other research in this area involves the use of an animatronic teddy bear as a communication medium between elders and their remote families (59). Turkle also reported several qualitative studies on the use of robotic toys by nursing home residents with mixed results in terms of positive impact (60).

The "AlwaysOn" project also seeks to develop in-home companion agents, specifically to address loneliness in isolated older adults. One series of studies investigated the topics that older adults would like to discuss with an animated companion, using an agent that was remote-controlled by researchers (61). This study found that most participants wanted to talk about their families, wanted to engage in small talk, such as chat about the weather, and wanted the agent to listen to stories they told about their past. A second study compared an autonomous in-home companion agent that participants had to initiate conversations with to the same agent with the added ability to proactively initiate conversation when they walked by (62). Results demonstrated that after a week in participants' homes, the proactive agent resulted in significantly lower reports of loneliness compared to those with the passive agent. Future studies will evaluate an autonomous companion agent capable of a range of social support activities in elders' homes for extended periods of time.

The hospital environment is another context in which companion agents are needed. Despite the fact that dozens of providers and staff may enter and leave an inpatient's room in a day, the patient experience is typically one of extreme isolation, boredom, and disorientation. The "hospital buddy" is being developed as a persistent bedside agent that can provide companionship, health counseling, and many other functions to patients throughout their hospital stay (63) (Figure 10.3). In a pilot study in which the agent was provided to hospital patients for 24 hours each, patients reported high levels of satisfaction with the

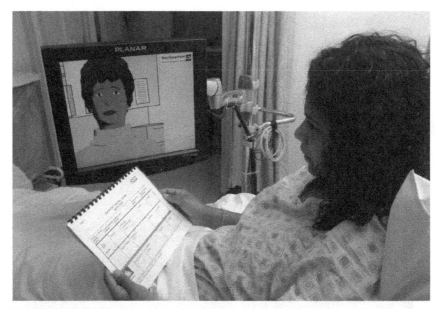

FIGURE 10.3: The hospital buddy companion agent.

system, conducted an average of 17 conversations each with the agent, and volunteered that it was an effective companion ("The best thing about the system, like, you know, when you don't have anyone here with you . . . it was actually nice to have her. I mean it kept me company.").

SYSTEMS DESIGNED TO INCREASE ENGAGEMENT IN BEHAVIORAL INTERVENTIONS

Several studies have investigated specific techniques that relational agents can use to maintain long-term engagement with users in longitudinal health interventions. In one study, the repetitiveness of an agent was manipulated so that users either interacted with a virtual exercise coach that looked the same and used the same language every day, or a variable coach that delivered the same intervention (same semantic content) but using language and visual appearance that was superficially changed daily. In a 141-day longitudinal study with 24 participants, users who were randomized to the variable coach conducted significantly more conversations and expressed a significantly higher desire to continue working with the coach, compared to the non-variable group, although there were no differences in dropout rates between the groups over the fixed duration of the study (64). In a second study, one version of the exercise coach agent told personal stories about its

childhood ("backstories"), and this was compared to an equivalent agent that told the same stories but in third person, as if they were about one of the other users of the system. In a 37-day longitudinal study with 26 participants, those who interacted with the backstory agent conducted significantly more conversations compared to the other group, demonstrating that users are more engaged with agents that present themselves as humans (64).

CONCLUSIONS

There has been significant progress in the design of technologies for boosting user perceptions of trust, therapeutic alliance, and social support in computer systems. To date, only a few of these relational technologies have been evaluated in randomized clinical trials, but results have been generally positive. Perhaps the biggest impact of these systems in behavioral medicine lies in their ability to increase retention in treatment, since system use is generally a prerequisite for positive outcomes, and many automated interventions developed thus far have demonstrated poor retention of users. Although treatment dropout may not be a problem if outcomes are shown to be positive for all patients, regardless of treatment duration, mental health treatments that are delivered for inadequate durations are generally ineffective (17). However, increased perceptions of social support and companionship may have important impacts in their own right, serving to decrease loneliness and accelerate healing. More research is needed to explore the long-term effects of these technologies.

REFERENCES

1. Marks I, Cavanagh K, Gega L. *Hands-on Help: Computer-Aided Psychotherapy.* New York: Psychology Press; 2007.

2. So M, Yamaguchi S, Hashimoto S, Sado M, Furukawa TA, McCrone P. Is computerised CBT really helpful for adult depression? A meta-analytic re-evaluation of CCBT for adult depression in terms of clinical implementation and methodological validity. *BMC Psychiatry* 2013; 13:113.

3. Corrigan P. How stigma interferes with mental health care. *American Psychologist* 2004; 59(7):614–625.

4. Phillips R, Schneider J, Molosankwe I, Leese M, Foroushani PS, Grime P, et al. Randomized controlled trial of computerized cognitive behavioural therapy for depressive symptoms: Effectiveness and costs of a workplace intervention. *Psychological Medicine* 2013; 24:1–12.

5. Spek V, Cuijpers P. Internet-based cognitive behaviour therapy for symptoms of depression and anxiety: A meta-analysis. *Psychological Medicine* 2007; 37(3):319–328.

6. Horvath AO, Del Re AC, Fluckiger C, Symonds D. Alliance in individual psychotherapy. *Psychotherapy* (Chicago) 2011; 48(1):9–16.

7. Lakey B, Cronin A. Low social support and major depression. In Dobson KS, Dozois DJ (Eds.), *Risk Factors for Depression.* New York: Academic Press; 2008, pp. 385–408.

8. Bickmore T, Gruber A, Picard R. Establishing the computer-patient working alliance in automated health behavior change interventions. *Patient Education and Counseling* 2005; 59(1):21–30.

9. Bickmore T, Gruber A. Relational agents in clinical psychiatry. *Harvard Review of Psychiatry* 2010; 18(2):119–130.

10. Gelso C, Hayes J. *The Psychotherapy Relationship: Theory, Research and Practice.* New York: Wiley; 1998.

11. Horvath AO, Greenberg LS. Development and validation of the Working Alliance Inventory. *Journal of Counseling Psychology* 1989; 36(2):223–233.

12. Muran JC, Barber JP. *The Therapeutic Alliance: An Evidence-Based Guide to Practice.* New York: Guilford; 2010.

13. Martin DJ, Garske JP, Davis ML. Relation of the therapeutic alliance with outcome and other variables: A meta-analytic review. *Journal of Consulting and Clinical Psychology* 2000; 68(3):438–450.

14. Shirk SR, Karver M. Prediction of treatment outcome from relationship variables in child and adolescent therapy: A meta-analytic review. *Journal of Consulting and Clinical Psychology* 2003; 71(3):452–464.

15. Sucala M, Schnur JB, Constantino MJ, Miller SJ, Brackman EH, Montgomery GH. The therapeutic relationship in e-therapy for mental health: A systematic review. *Journal of Medical Internet Research* 2012; 14(4):e110.

16. Sharf J, Primavera LH, Diener MJ. Dropout and therapeutic alliance: A meta-analysis of adult individual psychotherapy. *Psychotherapy* (Chicago). 2010; 47(4):637–645.

17. Edlund MJ, Wang PS, Berglund PA, Katz SJ, Lin E, Kessler RC. Dropping out of mental health treatment: Patterns and predictors among epidemiological survey respondents in the United States and Ontario. *American Journal of Psychiatry* 2002; 159(5):845–851.

18. Falkenström F, Granström F, Holmqvist R. Therapeutic alliance predicts symptomatic improvement session by session. *Journal of Counseling Psychology* 2013; 60(3):317–328.

19. Randolph ET. Social networks and schizophrenia. In Mueser KT, Tarrier N (Eds.), *Handbook of Social Functioning in Schizophrenia.* Boston: Allyn & Bacon; 1998.

20. Mead N, Lester H, Chew-Graham C, Gask L, Bower P. Effects of befriending on depressive symptoms and distress: Systematic review and meta-analysis. *British Journal of Psychiatry* 2010; 196(2):96–101.

21. Whittaker S, O'Conaill B. The role of vision in face-to-face and mediated communication. In Finn KE, Sellen AJ, Wilbur SB (Eds.), *Video-Mediated Communication.* Mahway, NJ: Erlbaum Associates; 1997, pp. 23–49.

22. Argyle M. *Bodily Communication* (2nd ed.). New York: Methuen & Co.; 1988.

23. Ekman P. Facial expression and emotion. *American Psychologist* 1993; 48(4):384–392.

24. Richmond V, McCroskey J. *Immediacy. Nonverbal Behavior in Interpersonal Relations.* Boston: Allyn & Bacon; 1995, pp. 195–217.

25. Havens L. *Making Contact: Uses of Language in Psychotherapy.* Cambridge, MA: Harvard University Press; 1986.

26. Malinowski B. The problem of meaning in primitive languages. In Ogden CK, Richards IA (Eds.), *The Meaning of Meaning.* London: Routledge & Kegan Paul; 1923.

27. Schneider KP. *Small Talk: Analysing Phatic Discourse.* Marburg: Hitzeroth; 1988.

28. Laver J. Communicative functions of phatic communion. In Kendon A, Harris R, Key MR (Eds.),

The Organization of Behavior in Face-to-Face Interaction. The Hague: Mouton; 1975, pp. 215–238.

29. Bickmore T, Cassell J. Relational agents: A model and implementation of building user trust. *Proceedings of the SIGCHI Conference on Human Factors in Computing Systems*, Seattle, Washington. 365304: ACM; 2001, pp. 396–403.

30. Altman I, Taylor D. *Social Penetration: The Development of Interpersonal Relationships.* New York: Holt, Rinhart & Winston; 1973.

31. Moon Y. Intimate self-disclosure exchanges: Using computers to build reciprocal relationships with consumers. Cambridge, MA: Harvard Business School, 1998, Working paper 99-059.

32. Gill D, Christensen A, Fincham F. Predicting marital satisfaction from behavior: Do all roads really lead to Rome? *Personal Relationships* 1999; 6(3):369–387.

33. McGuire A. Helping behaviors in the natural environment: Dimensions and correlates of helping. *Personality and Social Psychology Bulletin* 1994; 20(1):45–56.

34. Stafford L, Canary D. Maintenance strategies and romantic relationship type, gender and relational characteristics. *Journal of Social and Personal Relationships* 1991; 8(2):217–242.

35. Cole T, Bradac JJ. A lay theory of relational satisfaction with best friends. *Journal of Social and Personal Relationships* 1996; 13(1):57–83.

36. Dainton M, Stafford L. Routine maintenance behaviors: A comparison of relationships type, partner similarity and sex differences. *Journal of Social and Personal Relationships* 1993; 10(2):255–271.

37. Okun BF. *Effective Helping: Interviewing and Counseling Techniques* (5th ed.). Pacific Grove, CA: Brooks/Cole Publishing; 1997.

38. Planalp S, Benson A. Friends' and acquaintances' conversations I: Perceived differences. *Journal of Social and Personal Relationships* 1992; 9(4):483–506.

39. Planalp S. Friends' and acquaintances' conversations II: Coded differences. *Journal of Social and Personal Relationships* 1993; 10(3):339–354.

40. Gilbertson J, Dindia K, Allen M. Relational continuity constructional units and the maintenance of relationships. *Journal of Social and Personal Relationships* 1998; 15(6):774–790.

41. Brown P, Levinson SC. *Politeness: Some Universals in Language Usage.* New York: Cambridge University Press; 1987.

42. Lim T. Facework and interpersonal relationships. In Ting-Toomey S (Ed.), *The Challenge of Facework: Cross-Cultural and Interpersonal Issues.* Albany, NY: State University of New York Press; 1994, pp. 209–229.

43. Laver J. Linguistic routines and politeness in greeting and parting. In Coulmas F (Ed.), *Conversational Routine.* The Hague: Mouton; 1981, pp. 289–304.

44. Bickmore T, Picard R. Establishing and maintaining long-term human-computer relationships. *ACM Transactions on Computer Human Interaction* 2005; 12(2):293–327.

45. Bickmore T, Puskar K, Schlenk E, Pfeifer L, Sereika S. Maintaining reality: Relational agents for antipsychotic medication adherence. *Interacting with Computers* 2010; 22(4):276–288.

46. Kidd CD. *Engagement in Long-Term Human-Robot Interaction.* Cambridge, MA: MIT; 2007.

47. Velicer W, Reading CA, Blissmer B, Babbin SF, Paiva A, Bickmore T, et al. Using relational agents in tailored interventions for multiple risk factors: Preliminary 12 month results. Paper presented at the Society of Behavioral Medicine 2013 Annual Meeting, March 22, 2013; San Francisco.

48. Bickmore T, Mauer D. Modalities for building relationships with handheld computer agents. *CHI '06 Extended Abstracts on Human Factors in Computing Systems*, Montreal. 1125567: ACM; 2006. pp. 544–549.

49. Klein J, Moon Y, Picard RW. This computer responds to user frustration: Theory, design, results, and implications. *Interacting with Computers* 2002; 14(2):119–140.

50. Bickmore T, Schulman D. The comforting presence of relational agents. *CHI '06 Extended Abstracts on Human Factors in Computing Systems*, Montreal. 1125568: ACM; 2006, pp. 550–555.

51. Bickmore T, Schulman D. Practical approaches to comforting users with relational agents. *CHI '07 Extended Abstracts on Human Factors in Computing Systems*; San Jose, CA. 1240996: ACM; 2007. pp. 2291–2296.

52. Bickmore TW, Fernando R, Ring L, Schulman D. Empathic touch by relational agents. *IEEE Transactions on Affective Computing* 2010; 1(1):60–71.

53. Schoenhofer SO. Affectional touch in critical care nursing: A descriptive study. *Heart & Lung* 1989; 18(2):146–154.

54. Dickens AP, Richards SH, Greaves CJ, Campbell JL. Interventions targeting social isolation in older people: A systematic review. *BMC Public Health* 2011; 11:647.

55. Perissinotto CM, Stijacic Cenzer I, Covinsky KE. Loneliness in older persons: A predictor of functional decline and death. *Archives of Internal Medicine* 2012; 172(14):1078–1083.

56. Banks M, Banks W. The effects of animal-assisted therapy on loneliness in an elderly population in long-term care facilities. *Journals of Gerontology*

Series A: Biological Sciences and Medical Sciences 2002; 57(7):M428–M32.

57. Wada K, Shibata T, Saito T, Tanie K, editors. Effects of robot assisted activity to elderly people who stay at a health service facility for the aged. *Proceedings of 2003 IEEE/RSJ International Conference on Intelligent Robots and Systems (IROS)*, October 27–31, 2003.

58. Tamura T, Yonemitsu S, Itoh A, Oikawa D, Kawakami A, Higashi Y, et al. Is an entertainment robot useful in the care of elderly people with severe dementia? *Journals of Gerontology Series A: Biological Sciences and Medical Sciences* 2004; 59(1):83–85.

59. Stiehl WD, Lieberman J, Breazeal C, Basel L, Cooper R, Knight H, et al. (Eds.). The huggable: A therapeutic robotic companion for relational, affective touch. *Consumer Communications and Networking Conference*, 2006 3rd IEEE, January 8–10, 2006.

60. Turkle S. *Alone Together: Why We Expect More from Technology and Less from Each Other.* New York: Basic Books; 2012.

61. Vardoulakis LP, Ring L, Barry B, Sidner CL, Bickmore T. Designing relational agents as long-term social companions for older adults. In Nakano Y, Neff M, Paiva A, Walker M (Eds.), *Intelligent Virtual Agents. Lecture Notes in Computer Science* Heidelberg: Springer; 2012 pp. 289–302.

62. Ring L, Barry B, Totzke K, Bickmore T. Addressing loneliness and isolation in older adults: Proactive affective agents provide better support. Paper presented at the International Conference on Affective Computing and Intelligent Interaction (ACII), September 2–5, 2013, Geneva, Switzerland.

63. Bickmore T, Bukhari L, Vardoulakis L, Paasche-Orlow M, Shanahan C. Hospital Buddy: A persistent emotional support companion agent for hospital patients. Paper presented at the International Conference on Intelligent Virtual Agents, September 12–14, 2012, Santa Cruz, CA.

64. Bickmore T, Schulman D, Yin L. Maintaining engagement in long-term interventions with relational agents. *Applied Artificial Intelligence* 2010; 24(6):648–666.

SECTION III

Methods for the Evaluation of Technology-Based Behavioral Healthcare

11

mHealth Analytics

DANIEL M. SMITH AND THEODORE A. WALLS

INTRODUCTION

The broad emergence of technological devices designed for use in daily life has increased tremendously the portability of health information capture, a trend that is most likely still at its very beginning. Mobile technologies include, for example, smartphones (e.g., iPhone, BlackBerry, Android), media players (e.g., iPod), handheld game consoles (e.g., PlayStation Vita, Nintendo DS), personal digital assistants (PDAs), and tablet computers. These types of devices possess some or all of the following features: text messaging (SMS), telephone, Internet access, e-mail, mobile application software, camera (photo and video capture), multimedia messaging (MMS) and playback, voice recognition, global positioning system (GPS), accelerometry, and the ability to connect to peripheral devices such as wearable sensors or other wearable medical instruments. Their increasing mobility, popularity, functionality, and processing speeds make mobile devices efficient and effective means by which to monitor health and deliver health interventions. Not only raw data, but also calculation-based summary data and data from peer or network interactions such as counts of interactions, can be shared among these devices, enabling a higher level dialogue among their consumers. Moreover, this information is accessible in collectively available electronic storage for a variety of stakeholders, ranging from individuals to entire communities, including analysts. In the realm of healthcare and health research, the net of these advances and the platforms aimed at measuring health states and delivering prophylaxis or intervention has been captured recently under the term *mHealth*, an abbreviation for *mobile health* (1,2). For brevity, we will refer to this arena of technology use in health simply as mHealth.

In this chapter, we consider a selection of topics related to mHealth analytics that we feel are most applicable to mHealth studies based on our experience with *intensive longitudinal data* (ILD). The goal of this chapter is to benefit mHealth researchers and practitioners by providing a limited review of design considerations and an overview of basic and some advanced modeling techniques for a range of analytic needs. Most of our commentary is limited to what we know best, albeit relatively static, a posteriori analytic approaches, rather than real-time mHealth analytics to which the field increasingly aspires. We readily acknowledge the inevitability of incomplete coverage in this rapidly evolving area of methods development and hope that the shelf life of our contributions here persists at least a little longer than the current wave of devices producing mHealth data!

We organize our consideration of *mHealth analytics* here as follows. We start with some general comments about the diverse objectives of mHealth analytics and the ILD that mHealth studies generate. Next, we take on a crucial topic in the analysis of mHealth data—that of design. Although almost any scientific design could be deployed in the mHealth arena, we attend to some that are most relevant to the development and evaluation of mHealth interventions and to some of the study design features that may present challenges or opportunities. We then review basic analytical considerations as relevant to most studies, but again focus on techniques that have found traction in ILD and on some important topics such as power, the prevailing multilevel model, time series, and a few other common approaches. We then briefly consider areas in which advanced analytic approaches have been developed that could be used for various mHealth studies. We close with a look to the future, at the trend toward real-time analytics and the data management, expertise, and training needs that we expect to emerge alongside advances in the field of mHealth analytics.

Diverse Data Analytic Objectives for mHealth

There are diverse analytic objectives for data resulting from mHealth projects. For population-level monitoring, for example, the objective may be as simple as improving estimates of public health, such as by monitoring more patients at more times on crucial ambulatory measures such as blood pressure or heart rate. Analytical advances in this case may be limited to simply calculating well-known values with more data, perhaps with adjusted confidence intervals as needed for serial data. Other objectives may be analytic, but quite rudimentary in nature, such as triggering an alert when a value exceeds a threshold. However, clearly such computations, though highly valuable and potentially life-saving, are not necessarily the ones that come to mind most frequently when stakeholders consider the richness of mHealth data in the many forms that it takes. More detailed hypotheses about a phenomenon tend to be of paramount interest, for example, tracking the relationship between health indicators before and after a major disaster, and studying the contexts in which they may have greatest effects or studying their potential causes (see, for example, reference 3). Hence, inferential efforts aimed at deriving more detailed information from participants, their naturalistic behavior, and their response to varied interventions, all in an increasingly information-rich environment with computation-savvy players, are what mHealth studies demand.

mHealth Studies Generate Intensive Longitudinal Data

As mentioned earlier, intensive longitudinal data are typically generated by mHealth studies. When Walls and Schafer (4) developed this term in the early 2000s, they saw it as an attractive term because the word *intensive* could refer to high dimensionality over time points and also other dimensions, such as a large number of repeated measures, persons, and/or variables. This term was intended to capture databases being generated within several areas of human science that included more than several occasions of measurement. At that time, these authors also recognized

that the change in databases generated by mobile devices was universal, affecting all dimensions of measurement and their interaction. Inferences can be drawn from not only the time dimension as individual characteristics are tracked over time on many variables but also, for example, the subjects' dimension, as when there are measured interindividual differences that allow analysts to group people meaningfully. As such, the currently popularized notion of "big data" can be applauded for both its recent ubiquity, mainly in business realms, and for what we can do with data. Amidst the evolution of mHealth data as a space to which we turn for scientific and clinical meaning, one thing is certain: A thirst for understanding grows in the presence of more data, rather than being quenched by it.

The recent emergence of mHealth to encompass a range of behavioral and physical health applications, extending electronic measurement and integrating mobile interventions, brings the production of voluminous and increasingly complicated databases to yet new levels. These data are distinct from those found in traditional health studies in many respects—from the sheer number of things that can be tracked; to the number of participants typically involved; to the sometimes extremely complicated protocols that elicit layered, network, interactive, or aggregated data, to name just a few features. But what draws many to these data is the fact that inherent to the opportunity to impart change via mobile devices is the basic idea of measuring health aspects before, during, and after key events, such as life changes or health interventions. In order to measure change, we need baseline measurements and surveillance throughout subsequent epochs, such as during and after treatment regimes. Hence, a core opportunity in analyzing mHealth data, regardless of their complexity, is to take advantage of intensive longitudinal measurements to measure the course of change over time, as diverse individuals manifest change differentially along rich panels of variables. When we refer to mHealth analytics, we mean inferential techniques used to obtain parameter estimates with accompanying confidence intervals from data collected via mobile health applications and devices, used either in real time or a posteriori. When we refer to these techniques, we mean those in which parameter estimates are derived from the actual sampling of health data, rather than data that reflect the entire population of persons or time points, simulation-based data, or data from techniques used to affect decisioning of computer programs in networks or among users. That is, we are working from core assumptions in statistical modeling in our data analytic frame of reference.

BASIC APPROACHES

As in any research, mHealth investigations begin with basic science questions, which drive the design of interventions, study protocols, and subsequent data analysis. In general, mHealth analytics can help to characterize human behavior, informing the development and delivery of *momentary interventions*, defined as interventions that respond in real time to physical or psychological symptoms or contextual risk factors occurring in individuals' natural, real-world settings (5). Moreover, mHealth analytics are used to evaluate the effectiveness of interventions throughout various phases of project development. In the early stages, the priority is to determine what intervention components, and in what combination, sequence, and amount, are most effective. Additional questions might address user engagement (e.g., "Specifically, how did participants interact with the intervention materials?", "How did they direct their attention?") and overall evaluation of the intervention (e.g., "How long did it take participants to reach a specified goal?", "How was progress toward a goal related to baseline predictor variables?", "Did particular subgroups show similar courses of progress?"). Of course, each of these forms of inquiry requires attention to considerations for collecting and later analyzing the rich, fine-grained, temporal data sets that mHealth studies generate.

Design Considerations

In any longitudinal research problem, a well-articulated theoretical model of change is needed to drive the design of a longitudinal protocol that gives a clear view of the process or phenomenon in question (6; see Chapter 2 in this volume). In the context of mHealth, existing theory pertaining to social context, psychological state, physiological state, environment, and biomechanics provides the basis for intervention and algorithm design. Following the identification of a target group, target behaviors, variables, and potential treatment arms, three design considerations are particularly relevant in the realm of mHealth: overall protocol size, reactivity and intrusiveness, and instrumentation.

Overall protocol size includes the number of participants, variables, treatment arms, and number, spacing, and frequency of time points. Shiffman (7) provides a guide to event-based and time-based assessment approaches. In general, event-based approaches are best suited to sampling discrete phenomena (e.g., seizures, sexual intercourse, meals, panic attacks). Depending on available technology, a defined event can be identified by an algorithm (e.g., sensing technology that detects smoking movement) or by the participant (e.g., subject makes an entry after smoking). The study of continuous experience such as heart rate, blood glucose level, mood, and self-efficacy lends itself to time-based sampling, which can occur at regularly, variably, or randomly spaced intervals.

Beyond the theoretical model, the practical issues of *reactivity* and *intrusiveness* bear directly on the frequency, number, and spacing of measurements. Some modes of data collection (e.g., wearable sensors and smartphone sensors) might operate relatively seamlessly within an individual's daily routine, while others can be relatively more intrusive, burdensome, and prone to reactivity (8). For measurements that require some action on the part of participants, intrusiveness can be thought of as a function of frequency of observation and time to complete measures (i.e., response burden). When data are collected by sensor technologies, intrusiveness is related to the level of discomfort or inconvenience of wearing or carrying the device and/or sensors. Intrusive, burdensome protocols can cause user fatigue, a risk that would need to be weighed against the analytical benefits of more frequent assessment.

Reactivity, the degree to which participants change their behaviors simply because they know they are being watched, can vary as a function of intrusiveness (9,10). That is, relatively frequent or burdensome observational techniques make the knowledge of being watched more salient to the participant, increasing reactivity. A priming effect, an initial rise or fall in the mean response, might occur as participants familiarize themselves with a protocol and settle into a routine. Over time, diminished within-subjects variation might result as participants become indifferent, favor a certain response, or neglect to respond. Assessing participants in various places and at different times of day can also influence reactivity. It is very difficult to isolate the effects of reactivity through a design or later analysis, so researchers must be particularly aware of its potential effects on data.

Another design consideration is the specific type of *instrumentation*. In mHealth research, data can be collected by prompting subjects to record information via text messaging or a smartphone application, by remote patient monitoring (RPM), and through other on-board, wearable, or peripheral sensing technologies. Measurement can consist of physiological and environmental indices, spatial positioning, performance on a task, and self-report. Biomolecular and bioelectric sensing, mobile microscopy, and imaging technologies can collect data about physiological states (e.g., blood pressure, heart rate, body temperature, trace gases in human breath, biomarkers in body fluids, sleep status) and environmental conditions (e.g., noise level, presence of airborne allergens). Task performance could include cognitive tasks (e.g., memory, speed, verbal fluency), physical tasks (e.g., jumping, running), and others. Self-report requires that participants respond when prompted or initiate data input to provide their observations, feelings, perceptions, and behaviors. Spatial positioning data can be collected using GPS, wifi, radio-frequency tracking, and accelerometers, which detect movements (e.g., exercise, driving, tooth brushing, falls). Bussmann and Ebner-Priemer (11) classify ambulatory instruments of movement behavior as activity counters (e.g., pedometers, step counters), actometers (accelerometers that only measure when a person is active), and multichannel ambulatory devices. Multichannel ambulatory movement sensor devices assess activity, posture, and motion patterns continuously, are capable of detecting different types of postures and movements, and can represent features of movements such as balance and symmetry (12). There is also the possibility to collect data through more than one of these pathways simultaneously. For example, the use of social networking as an intervention component provides the opportunity for network-enabled sampling and signaling to, from, and among participants, data that are crucially relevant in the evaluation of the program's effectiveness.

Basic Designs

In this section, we briefly consider designs most relevant to the creation and implementation of mHealth projects. Please see Chapter 12, by Dallery, Nahum-Shani, and Riley in this volume for a more detailed discussion on research designs for evaluating technology-based behavioral health interventions. As we mentioned earlier, development of mHealth interventions follows a logical progression, and selection of a research design depends to some extent on this. In the early stages, single-subject or small-n studies, which typically employ pre-test, post-test, or time series elements, are useful to assess feasibility and gain knowledge about potentially efficacious intervention components (13,14). Naturalistic time series designs may help to establish baseline patterns of health over time prior to intervention. ABAB designs involve assessment at baseline (A), following treatment (B), upon return to baseline (A), and again following treatment (B). The return to baseline step allows the researcher to observe any extinction in an outcome following removal of the treatment. This enables the researcher to plausibly attribute changes in the outcome to the treatment and not to other factors. Using an ABAB design, multiple treatment groups can be used to compare the relative efficacy of interventions or intervention components. Similarly, repeated trials designs can be used to make comparisons using a between-subjects factor (e.g., intervention component) across a within-subjects factor (e.g., multiple trials). Such smaller scale studies are also useful to rule out software or hardware flaws before moving to larger scale studies.

Recent scholarship has focused on how knowledge of the intervention components derived from pilot studies can be influential in informing full factorial or fractional factorial designs (15,16). These designs help to assess the most effective combination, sequence, and dosage of intervention components. In the case of large factorial designs, it may be not be feasible to populate the groups adequately to maintain statistical power. Hence, results from earlier tests can be used to select which cells to include in a fractional factorial design. Adaptive interventions use control systems engineering to assign and adjust treatment dosage and/or type in response to a participant's values on variables that are predicted to moderate the treatment's effect (17,18). In the context of mHealth, these variables, known as tailoring variables, can be monitored frequently by devices, allowing the intervention to adapt periodically or in real time to the needs of the participant. Dynamic models of relationships among tailoring variables, treatment, and dosage inform the creation of decision rules, which determine the appropriate intervention type and dosage to deploy.

Although these innovative and resource efficient strategies have potentially great value, the randomized controlled trial (RCT) remains the prevailing gold standard for clinical trials. Because RCTs can demand many resources, often fewer occasions of measurement are employed than intensive longitudinal designs typically have. However, advances in mHealth instrumentation will likely alleviate burdens to both participants and investigators, increasing the feasibility of RCTs that utilize the rich, time-graded information inherent to ILD.

Interrupted time series (ITS) is a methodologically strong quasi-experimental approach for investigating the effect of an intervention longitudinally. It involves capturing a sequence of repeated measures with one or more discontinuities in measurement present in the series. Typically, the approach to analyzing ITS data involves looking at differences in intercept and slope parameters before and after a time point that marks a naturally occurring or experimentally introduced change in the series (e.g., segmented regression analysis; see reference 19). That is, these designs can be naturalistic or experimental. In the former case, naturally occurring conditions (e.g., relapse into alcohol use) mark time points around which the change in trajectory can be analyzed. In the latter, the discontinuity represents the introduction of an experimental manipulation such as an mHealth intervention. Pre-intervention observations act as a control for the post-intervention segment so single-group designs can be methodologically rigorous for studying intervention effects. Seasonal effects can be assessed by including a control group, detrending the data, and/or including additional dependent variables that are not influenced by the intervention but would respond to validity threats in the same way as the primary outcome variables.

Time-scale-dependent longitudinal designs (TDLD), which evolve from the basic ITS design, involve discontinuity of measurement on two or more time scales (e.g., days and months). Time scale decisions demand careful attention to theory or empirical evidence about how a phenomenon is optimally captured (20). Using time scales that capture an appropriate degree of granularity, there is the potential to reveal patterns within a larger trajectory and to detect discrete events that disrupt the course of the trajectory. Time points should be selected with appropriate frequency (daily, hourly, many times per hour, etc.) and spacing (regular or irregular) in order to optimally capture the phenomenon in question. This requires attention to theory or prior research about the speed and shape with which the change is likely to occur. When possible, working to define the measurement timing for the period in which a phenomenon may reflect features of interest can help to ensure both resource efficiency and optimal analytical results (21). When little prior knowledge exists regarding the measurement timing for variables of interest, if possible, it is prudent to err on the side of more frequent, regularly spaced measurement in order to avoid missing interesting patterns of change. In the case of technology-enabled measurement, this is often feasible with little increase in resource consumption. However, as this efficiency enables a larger protocol size, the practical issues of capacity and architecture of back-end data storage and battery life of portable devices need to be considered.

TDLD offer a number of benefits. First, they enable the examination of a long period of time intensively without obtaining intensive measures continuously over the entire course of the study. Second, they allow integration of data that is specific to different time scales of measurement. For example, data aggregated by day and week can give complementary insights into the process under investigation. Third, they can help illuminate the likely speed, peak level, and stability of behavior change based on exposure to a favorable environment or set of conditions, thus informing the planning of an intervention. Within TDLD, many designs are possible. The intervention can be implemented within the higher or lower time scale. Spacing of measurements can be fixed or uneven (i.e., event driven or randomized). Additionally, it is possible to examine more than two levels of time, compare more than two groups, and intervene on multiple time scales (22).

Basic Analytical Considerations

As in any data analysis, the fundamental questions are, in the case of a hypothesis-driven study, what are those hypotheses, how have the design and measures been operationalized to sample information on units of analysis for the study, and what specific analytical approach or battery of approaches will lead to the best tests of those hypotheses? In the case of exploratory or naturalistic measurement, which techniques separate the possibly large amount of noise in mHealth studies from signals of interest? In selecting an approach, there are three primary considerations.

First, will the inferences to be drawn correspond well with the study design so that study stakeholders will believe that informational value has been generated and the core motivating questions have been tackled? This is a particularly important, and often overlooked, consideration. In mHealth studies researchers are usually interested in making new and more informative claims about the data than simple averages produce. Yet, many analysts revert to the simplicity and routine of simple averages and difference tests, often because consumers demand concrete and easy-to-consume articulation of findings. Although meeting this demand can be essential for consideration of many hypotheses, and key findings are often encapsulated in these simple statistics, they are rarely satisfactory on their own given the voluminous data that everyone knows is there, and persistent intuition that there could be richer descriptions. Substantive stakeholders will also need to become increasingly literate about mHealth analytics. It is also possible to go to the other extreme in adopting an approach that is comprehensible by such a small community of specialists that institutional stakeholders, such as funders or policy makers, cannot realize a return on their investment.

Second, there is a substantial amount of preprocessing needed to reduce the data to either a manageable or appropriately structured set of values. For example, Varkey, Pompili, and Walls (23) and Raiff, Karatas, Pompili, and Walls (24) employed machine learning approaches to combine signals from about 10 devices placed in several locations on the body to detect movements associated with cigarette smoking. In these examples, the raw data that result when these devices detect smoking movement need to be organized into quantities that are meaningful in the context of smoking research.

Third, naturally, the expertise of analysts to handle the extensive programming needed to set up mHealth studies, to manage increasingly large and complex datasets that result, and to deploy and summarize analyses in thoughtful, creative ways is crucial. Given this, we now focus on some possible ingredients that could lead to success, including typical modeling frameworks, data visualization, multilevel models, and time-oriented models.

Typical Modeling Frameworks

For the moment, many mHealth applications collect data, albeit with many ambulatory devices, interconnected processing and storage servers and multiple data interfaces, and conduct analyses on static multivariate, longitudinal data, or ILD. Basic approaches to analysis include all of the typical biomedical analyses, such as calculating the probability of a behavior occurring in a given context (e.g., at home or at work) using a range of regression techniques. For example, if a study tracks duration of sleep for a random sample of individuals over several time points, the researcher might collapse all of the data into a z-test or t-test of means. If the study involves multiple condition groups, a one-way ANOVA can be used to make between-group comparisons. Another simple approach would be to average within-subject scores for between-subject analyses using traditional regression techniques. These approaches are best for generating some coarse interpretations about a phenomenon, but they are often limited in terms of more complicated hypotheses or in accounting for error variance due to design, instrumentation, and, especially, nesting of hierarchical effects. The most prevalent approaches to this analysis have been survival models (inclusive of multilevel versions) for event type responses (discrete or ordinal) and multilevel models for continuous outcomes (25–28).

Several introductory resources have been developed for these types of models (9,10,25,29,30). We will discuss these models in limited detail below, but typically they involve partitioning of between-subject and within-subject variation of the dependent variables in relation to some clustering guideline, such as group membership or time trends, and simultaneous regression of resulting random coefficients on key predictors such as treatment or gender. The objective of this model is to account for within-cluster variability (such as within-person) before deploying estimates at the second level of the model. In some limited cases, time series models have been deployed at the first level to describe the stability of processes, rather than trends or mean levels (30–32).

Across these modeling frameworks, there are some overarching logic systems that may impact selection of an analytical approach. One logic system is to attend to one dimension at the expense of another dimension. For example, collapsing all cigarettes smoked over 50 days and using this single proxy variable underattends to time-related possibilities but may allow greater focus on a set of predictor variables. Benefits of this approach are speed and apparent simplicity, but the risk of oversimplification is high. Another approach is to work from the spirit of the hypotheses and fundamental research questions—be they oriented toward treatment effects, population statistics, endogenous dynamics of a system, or exogenous influences on a set of entities or units. In fact, many mHealth studies provide a rich repository of data that may serve to study many questions, so multiple analyses of the same database have routinely been generated (33).

Data Visualization

Certainly, every student in statistical analysis has engaged in plotting data both for data exploration and reporting. For longitudinal data, typical plots include bar charts for missing data, plots of residuals in regression analyses, and various depictions of raw trend information so as to inform parameterization of shape through profile plots, panel plots, and other line graphs. However, in the last few years, the increase in computational power and graphic capabilities in software has given rise to a new field called *data visualization*, which refers to special graphical efforts to make data interpretation more functional and accessible, and sometimes more elegant (34–36).

This field is at the intersection of data reporting and visual design and graphic arts. For example, recent scholarship by members of the Broad Institute, IBM work groups, and many other industry–academic collaborations have focused on developing new concepts for describing data

and developing a better knowledge base for what kinds of lines, symbols, and other features tend to convey certain types of information well (37,38). A representative paper by Krzywinski and Wong (39) regarding scatter plots covers ways to improve these plots for better interpretability. Recent work in the software program R on data visualization includes innovation in lattice plots, which display information on the same distribution in many panels, and the ggplot function, which can be used to colorize and layer many forms of data. Representative of the many recent titles on these features are Springer titles by Sarkar (40) and Wickham (41). This is a very active area of research with players from many sectors, and it promises to become both normative and expected by many information consumers that certain types of data will be displayed in certain ways, in increasingly high-quality formats. Interactive formats such as those inherent to 3D visualization tools, in which users can rotate multicolored images of data in order to look at them from various vantage points, are also very interesting. The likely confluence of these tools with real-time data streaming akin to what we have seen in ultrasound and MRI imagery is already close at hand.

In mHealth, the possible applications of data visualization are many. It can be used to represent the association between variables (e.g., air quality and asthma, environmental toxicants and cancer, noise exposure and hypertension) over geographic areas on a map, for example. Such a geographic representation showing regional differences in the implementation or effectiveness of an mHealth intervention would also be valuable to researchers and healthcare providers, perhaps especially so in developing countries. Participants involved in an mHealth study might view progress toward a behavioral goal (e.g., smoking cessation, physical activity, healthy eating, adherence to medication, etc.) via functional, accessible graphics. One simple example of this is a calendar showing a measure of the behavior for each day of the last month. Another example is a graphic showing the social or environmental conditions in which the participant is most likely to engage in a behavior such as smoking. If the study involves social networks, participants might also view their own data relative to others in their social network, and study investigators would also benefit from graphical representations of behavioral data among persons within a network (see "Social Network Analysis," below).

Multilevel Models

One concentration of models is easily found in the realm of multilevel modeling and its extensions. Multilevel models (also known as hierarchical linear models, nested models, mixed models, random effects models, and random coefficients models) are models of parameters that vary at more than one level. Central to multilevel modeling is the use of random effects at various levels to account for the hierarchical or clustered structure of the data. Data are collected from units that are nested within higher levels such as groups (e.g., students within classes, classes within schools, etc.). Likewise, repeated observations over time can be nested within persons, who are analogous to groups in the above example. These can be thought of as an elaboration on the growth curve model, with the first level being the within-subjects, or measurement occasions, level. More extensive pedagogical and conceptual discourse on multilevel models is available (42–48).

Multilevel models have several key advantages that have resulted in their pervasive application to ILD, and their relevance to mHealth data is equally high. The first is that they allow the modeling of heterogeneity of individual and group intercepts and growth curves. Traditional regression techniques, including ANOVA, rely on fixed group values for the intercept and slope. Thus, one set of values is used to characterize the growth pattern of all individuals in a sample. In multilevel models, individual intercepts and slopes are computed and their variances are introduced into higher levels of the model. These models frequently include fixed or time-varying covariates to predict the heterogeneity of intercepts and slopes between subjects, allowing each individual growth pattern to be described by one's own set of values. Second, the multilevel model is flexible in that quantities resulting from a range of other modeling frameworks can be incorporated (see reference 9). Third, multilevel models are conducive to analyzing data collected on both contextual influences and mechanisms potentially operating within the unit of analysis of interest (e.g., person, dyad, etc.; see Chapter 13 in this volume). These models have been used routinely for the study of ILD from a range of mHealth sources, such as patient records,

ambulatory measurements, and cardiac care (see, for example, reference 49).

Time-Oriented Models

Coverage of the many data analytic tools that can be employed when data are collected over time cannot be achieved within the confines of this chapter. Introductory texts on time series analysis, such as the classic text by Box and Jenkins (50), and innumerable introductory texts on the topic, such as that by Chatfield (51), are easily found. Advanced techniques range from autocorrelation approaches, to single subject analysis, to state space models (which make it easier to consider multivariate processes with various underlying processes being estimated), to control systems and other dynamic models. As a family, these approaches are used for inferences that involve illuminating difficult-to-observe temporal patterns that underlie a phenomenon. Although somewhat more difficult to learn and deploy, these approaches have been used extensively in a range of health applications and remain among our chief tools to study large longitudinal databases.

Power Considerations

Before we proceed with more advanced modeling topics, in this section we highlight an important challenge facing researchers who work with the ILD that mHealth studies produce. This consideration applies to the calculation of statistical power, and specifically to the way correlation patterns in a series of many repeated measures (which is often the case in mHealth studies) are modeled. This is a crucial topic in mHealth analytics because power analyses are important both for determination of sufficient sample sizes and for numbers of occasions.

In general, the calculation of statistical power is based on the particular statistical model that is selected for the analysis. A number of software packages have been developed for determining power for specific models, such as the multilevel model (52). In keeping with this, Bolger and Laurenceau (29) discuss statistical power for longitudinal designs and employ a standard power calculation for multilevel models. The formula comprises a within-subjects part and a between-subjects part. Bolger and Laurenceau note that increasing the number of subjects (N) reduces both parts of the sampling variance of the slope, while increasing the number of time points (T) reduces only the within-subjects term. Hence, all else held constant, adding subjects typically boosts power more than adding time points.

On the other hand, assuming an unautocorrelated level-1 error variance for a series of data may be problematic. To illustrate this point, suppose a study involves the ambulatory assessment of an individual's mood over the course of a day. These data are likely to show serial dependence (53). That is, a person's mood at the first time point is most closely related to mood at the second time point, less so with mood at the third time point, and decreasingly so with each subsequent measurement as the day goes on. Serial dependence is likely to be observed in many variables of interest to mHealth researchers, including physiological and environmental indices, spatial positioning, task performance, and self-report of feelings, perceptions, and behaviors (see discussion of instrumentation above for examples of variables).

Hence, a future challenge for researchers working with mHealth data is to refine assumptions about how the covariance structure should be incorporated in power analyses. Assuming no autocorrelation when little is known about the covariance structure of the phenomenon under investigation may be among the safer alternatives, but it is unlikely to be the most accurate if something about the phenomenon is known. Although some current software packages adopt basic assumptions about the covariance structure, these may result in inaccurate power analyses (56). With many repeated measures, mitigating this problem is not as simple as knowing the covariance structure. Data that may reflect monotonic variances could be based on one estimate of covariance, while cases where the simple error covariance should be structured require either specific covariance estimates or ordered patterns. With a large number of repeated measures relative to sample size, there may not be enough degrees of freedom present in the model to pursue this effectively. Linear exponent autoregressive (LEAR) patterns assume that correlations between repeated measures decline exponentially. Guo, Logan, Glueck, and Muller (54) posit that the flexibility of LEAR patterns might currently be the best compromise vs. more basic assumptions, some of which may falsely inflate the Type I error rate or require

more parameters than models can estimate. Badly needed are simulation-based models in which careful attention to covariance structure is given to the development and validation of power analysis methods for large mHealth studies with very intensive longitudinal data.

AREAS OF ADVANCED MODELING
Multivariate Shape Models

Extending from substantial scholarship in the realm of functional data analysis, several specialized models for the consideration of long multivariate series with covariates and complex shapes of the response have been developed (30,55,56). Recent advances within this modeling framework, including time-varying effect models (TVEM), have been introduced as a novel approach for analyzing ILD. When collecting data about a covariate and a response, both at frequent intervals and when theory suggests an active interplay of the two, the model may help show differential levels of association at discrete times over a series, such as against baseline (57). In essence, by creating splines of both variables of varying complexity (as reflected by the number of estimated knots), the model reflects momentary associations of the responses well. In general, functional models utilize nonparametric estimation approaches to investigate the association between time-varying covariates and outcomes without imposing assumptions about the shape of temporal trajectories. This can be very useful when the shape of change is not linear, quadratic, or cubic or is unknown a priori. For example, Tan, Shiyko, Li, Li, and Dierker (57) illustrate the application of TVEM using ILD from a clinical smoking cessation trial that monitored smoking behavior and explored time-varying associations between negative affect and self-efficacy. In the realm of mHealth, TVEM could be applied to a wide range of behaviors (e.g., physical activity, alcohol use, smoking, eating, sleeping, medication adherence, etc.) and time-variant covariates (e.g., mood, stress, affect, urges, self-efficacy, attitude, location or other contextual factors, physiological states, etc.). Moreover, like any mixed model, they can be used to investigate the effect of time-invariant covariates such as an intervention by illuminating changes in the intervention's impact over time.

Another approach that has proven very useful in the study of ILD from behavioral health studies is the family of location-scale models developed by Hedeker, Berbaum, and Mermelstein (58). These models are used when the level of measurement of the response is not continuous, but ordinal. Since many studies involve reports on Likert scales for moods or have other scales of measurement with limited range and fixed intervals, these models have come to be quite routinely used in a fairly short time. Easily deployed using readily available SAS code, extensions have been developed to allow for the effects of covariates and for parameterizing variances in appropriate ways. Some researchers have experimented with the inclusion of different parameters at the first level of multilevel models, such as time series estimates (59,60), and refining the estimation of derivatives at multiple time scales to reflect dynamics toward multilevel implementations (61). Others have used a range of related modeling frameworks involving state space methods and latent variable models, including structural equation models reflecting change and dynamics (9,62–65).

Engineering Control Models

People can be thought of as systems whose complex combination of inputs (e.g., psychological and physiological states, external and contextual influences, etc.) interact to influence various outputs, such as behaviors. In our daily lives, we often experience departures from a desired state (e.g., negative affect, lack of exercise, heightened nicotine cravings), requiring the development of feedback loops to reach a more desirable setpoint. This model of controlling our behavior is akin to the control of many systems in the realm of engineering and biology (e.g., heating and cooling, cruise control, homeostasis). Ramsay (66) offers a summary of how control technology can be applied to the study of human behavior. Control systems engineering uses dynamic models to develop algorithms that enable the control of system variables. In a control model, for example, a setpoint for a given variable, such as urge to smoke, may be posited. Inputs to the system may have the effect of controlling the setpoint, acceleration or other parameters of this quantity, and exogenous variables that may influence the whole system (67,68). In general, in control systems modeling, theoretical models of behavior change can be expressed

as a system of differential equations, designed to reflect a diversity of theories. An example of this kind of model is a dynamical model of weight loss that incorporates physiological factors and the theory of planned behavior presented by Navarro-Barrientos, Rivera, and Collins (69).

Models Considering Groups

In addition to the typical multilevel model and its extensions, several recent modeling frameworks focus on the delineation of groups that share common features. These include latent class and transition models (70), cluster algorithms (71), and the broad family of mixture models (for a review, see reference 72). In addition, pattern recognition models also achieve the goal of clustering similar information together to form groups (73; see Chapter 3 in this volume). Because mHealth data often contain signals that are very diverse and there is a need for data reduction toward consideration of homogenous groups of units, such as people, geographic tracts, times of day, and so on, this modeling framework will have continued and increased relevance. For example, in cases where a unique group can be identified based on similar properties, further analyses of temporal effects and multivariate predictions can be run within-group. Various types of finite mixture models enable these kinds of predictive models across obtained groups, allowing consideration of differential effects, although review of these models is beyond the scope of this chapter.

Social Network Analysis

Finally, social network (or simply network) models emerge as high on the list of models likely to be employed increasingly in the next several years, because they parameterize the very interesting interchanges among members of a community, often as these interchanges evolve over time. Network models typically examine characteristics such as *centrality*, a measure of one's influence within the network; *density*, the ratio of an individual's direct connections to the total number; and *reach*, the degrees of separation to which one's influence extends. A number of studies have used network models to examine a range of behaviors, including health-related behaviors. Christakis and Fowler (74,75) investigated network phenomena in obesity and smoking cessation, finding, for example, that clusters of smokers became nonsmokers in a large social network, and reach extended to three degrees of separation.

One methodological challenge in network analysis is *homophily*, the notion that individuals are connected through similarities (76). Latent homophily and shared environmental factors confound social contagion. For example, a group of friends might become more physically active in part due to a predisposition on which the friendship is based (e.g., interest or participation in a sport), in part due to a shared environmental factor (e.g., advertisements promoting activity), and in part due to influence on each other. Sensitivity analysis has been used to explain away the effects of latent homophily and environmental factors (77).

In mHealth, we anticipate growth in the use of network modeling due to three major shifts. First, through the rise of social networking websites, interaction between contacts occurs increasingly online and on mobile devices. Second, many health and wellness programs (e.g., workplace-based physical activity initiatives) attempt to harness social influences on health behavior within networks. Third, a number of mHealth smartphone applications (e.g., Fitbit, Endomondo, Fitocracy) incorporate social networking as a primary feature, encouraging users to find their friends, join virtual communities, and share their progress on other platforms. Data visualization is particularly relevant here. For example, one element of an intervention might be to display visually meaningful summaries of participants' own and friends' progress toward a goal. Likewise, social network analysts benefit from well-designed graphical representations of networks. As interventions are designed intentionally to connect participants, interesting new opportunities to analyze the spread of behaviors through networks will continue to materialize.

CONCLUSIONS

In this chapter, we have reviewed several design topics that bear high relevance to mHealth, reviewed basic analyses in the field, and described areas in which advanced modeling options can be found. Research and practice in mHealth yield ILD, which call for designs that demonstrate careful consideration to number, spacing, and frequency of measurements, reactivity, and the

many instrumentation types available now and in the near future. We see a trend in the development and use of resource-efficient designs that utilize the rich, fine-grained, time-stamped data that we now have the capability of capturing with increasingly ubiquitous mobile technologies. These data emerge from carefully developed research designs and take special forms that require innovative visualization and analytical strategies.

The rate at which design variations and statistical models that bear relevance has proceeded is incredibly fast, and the opportunities are great, both for practitioners of design and analysis, and also for the science that drives mHealth. Investigators may wish to consider where to invest their own energies in training or staffing for mHealth studies with respect to mHealth analytics. Certainly a key initial question to consider is whether any one analyst is likely to have command of the burgeoning frameworks of models that bear relevance, and we suspect that the answer to that question is ultimately no. Core expertise in statistics and computing is essential, but the dexterity in model deployment needed to realize maximal benefit from analyses is probably housed most frequently in those who specialize in a given framework. Hence, we can expect multiple analysts to play roles in mHealth analytics, passing data from one modeling environment to another as parameters are extracted, groups are determined, and preliminary conclusions are drawn.

Another interesting question, as mentioned earlier, is the extent to which real-time analyses can be leveraged in mHealth studies. Such real-time analyses are essential to leveraging mHealth in harm prevention in some areas such as cardiac monitoring, suicidality, falls in the elderly, and other serious life threats (78,79). Hence, we have started to see a temporal merging of what is typically considered to be prelaunch instrumentation and programming with inferential techniques. A key difference between mHealth and traditional health studies is the desire for immediately available information that has developed both in general in society and in relation to devices. Just as we have all used search engines as memory aids, our expectations for quick answers increase when we know that mobile technologies have archived information that we are interested in. Similarly, there is a tendency for stakeholders to want analyses of mHealth data to be ready almost as rapidly as the data were collected. Unlike in past research epochs in health behavioral science, in which weeks to months of data entry cleaning and preprocessing were needed before analyses could be completed, investigators often wish to seize on inferential efforts as soon a data are uploaded. Already now and into the future, researchers may even want analyses to be formulated and programmed into devices so that results roll out in real time, from cloud servers to investigators, stakeholders, or even research participants (see, for example, reference 80). Such a trend forces us to distinguish between *static,* a posteriori deployed analyses and *real-time* implementations. Current analytical frameworks tend to stop short of these real-time implementations, especially for very advanced approaches. However, at least basic techniques, those with little to no incremental analytical judgment required, could be deployed in real time, provided the source variables are sufficiently suited for given analyses.

To elaborate, borrowing from the spirit of fractional factorial designs, in which pilots can be used to determine cells of likely greatest importance, it is possible that continuous feeds of mHealth data can enable essentially continuously running experiments that iterate and update users, much as we might expect analytics in financial markets or military applications to assure. In other words, is a key part of the future of mHealth analytics real-time monitoring and analysis aimed at risk assessment, harm reduction and prevention, and rapid intervention? Will there be obtained "latent" or second-order variables reflecting overall system functioning that we can monitor in real time and work to control? As such, it seems as though we can expect a melding not only of statistical analytic expertise but also of whole team abilities, from substantive knowledge of a health issue to behavioral inputs to software-driven tooling of electronically mediated intervention, all woven together.

Real-time data capture and analytics also create data management issues such as storage and processing demands and data privacy and security. Indeed, collaborating with professionals who possess technical computing expertise will be critical in not only finding solutions but also ensuring that research teams and practitioners can make the most of available technology (e.g., cloud computing, sharing data across mHealth applications). Currently, mobile intervention in the form of text messages, online experiences, and e-mail communication is in its infancy. As information about location, time in an electronic medium, performance on learning or gaming modules, and network attributes are increasingly aggregated, the fusion of the inferential opportunities reflected by the above areas of advanced modeling can be anticipated and is in fact already happening. In light of these changes, we foresee the emergence of new fields for training analysts, perhaps in mHealth analytics proper. We anticipate several workshop formats for training to be available to meet this need from a variety of sources, including through our own and affiliated universities and centers. Individuals who wish to specialize in mHealth analytics can expect exciting and challenging new opportunities as analytical models and mHealth applications continue to evolve, both in technology and scope of use, and improve health outcomes worldwide.

REFERENCES

1. Laxminarayan S, Istepanian RSH. UNWIRED E-MED: The next generation of wireless and internet telemedicine systems. *IEEE Transactions on Information Technology in Biomedicine* 2000; 4(3):189–193.

2. Istepanian RSH, Jovanov E, Zhang YT. Guest editorial introduction to the special section on m-Health: Beyond seamless mobility and global wireless health-care connectivity. *IEEE Transactions on Information Technology in Biomedicine* 2004; 8(4):405–414.

3. Gerin W, Chaplin W, Schwarz JE, Holland J, Alter R, Wheeler R, et al. Sustained blood pressure increase after an acute stressor: The effects of the 11 September 2001 attack on the New York City World Trade Center. *Journal of Hypertension* 2005; 23(2):279–284.

4. Walls TA, Schafer JL. Introduction: Intensive longitudinal data. In Walls TA, Schafer JL (Eds.), *Models for Intensive Longitudinal Data* (pp. ix–xi). New York: Oxford University Press; 2006.

5. Heron KE, Smyth JM. Ecological momentary interventions: Incorporating mobile technology into psychosocial and health behaviour treatments. *British Journal of Health Psychology* 2010; 15(1):1–39.

6. Collins LM. Analysis of longitudinal data: The integration of theoretical model, temporal design, and statistical model. *Annual Review of Psychology* 2006; 57:505–528.

7. Shiffman S. Designing protocols for ecological momentary assessment. In Stone AA, Shiffman S, Atienza AA, Nebeling L (Eds.), *The Science of Real-Time Data Capture* (pp. 27–53). New York: Oxford University Press; 2007.

8. Goodwin MS. Passive telemetric monitoring: Novel methods for real-world behavioral assessment. In Mehl MR, Conner TS (Eds.) *Handbook of Research Methods for Studying Daily Life.* (pp. 251–266). New York: Guilford Press; 2012.

9. Walls TA, Schafer JL. *Models for Intensive Longitudinal Data.* New York: Oxford University Press; 2006.

10. Walls TA. Intensive longitudinal data. In Little TD (Ed.), *The Oxford Handbook of Quantitative Methods in Psychology: Vol. 2 Statistical Analysis* (pp. 432–440). New York: Oxford University Press; 2013.

11. Bussmann JBJ, Ebner-Priemer UW. Ambulatory assessment of movement behavior: Methodology, measurement, and application. In Mehl MR, Conner TS (Eds.), *Handbook of Research Methods for Studying Daily Life* (pp. 235–250). New York: Guilford Press; 2012.

12. Chang T-Y, Su T-C, Lin S-Y, Jain R-M, Chan C-C. Effects of occupational noise exposure on 24-hour ambulatory vascular properties in male workers. *Environmental Health Perspectives* 2007; 115(11):1660–1664.

13. Barlow D, Nock M, Hersen M. *Single Case Research Designs: Strategies for Studying Behavior Change.* New York: Allyn and Bacon; 2008.

14. Dallery J, Cassidy RN, Raiff BR. Single-case experimental designs to evaluate novel technology-based health interventions. *Journal of Medical Internet Research* 2013; 15(2):e22.

15. Collins LM, Baker TB, Mermelstein RJ, Piper ME, Jorenby DE, Smith SS, et al. The multiphase optimization strategy for engineering effective tobacco use interventions. *Annals of Behavioral Medicine* 2011; 41:208–226.

16. Resnicow K, Strecher V, Couper M, Chua H, Little R, Nair V, et al. Methodologic and design issues in patient-centered e-health research. *American Journal of Preventive Medicine* 2010; 38(1):98–102.

17. Rivera DE, Pew MD, Collins LM. Using engineering control principles to inform the design of adaptive interventions: A conceptual introduction. *Drug and Alcohol Dependence* 2007; 88S:S31–S40.

18. Collins LM, Murphy SA, Bierman KL. A conceptual framework for adaptive preventive interventions. *Prevention Science* 2004; 5(3):185–196.

19. Wagner AK, Soumerai SB, Zhang F, Ross-Degnan D. Segmented regression analysis of interrupted time series studies in medication use research.

Journal of Clinical Pharmacy and Therapeutics 2002; 27:299–309.

20. Bertenthal BI. Dynamical systems: It's about time. In Boker SM, Wenger MJ (Eds.), *Data Analytic Techniques for Dynamical Systems* (pp. 1–24). Mahwah, NJ: Erlbaum; 2007.

21. Fairlie AM. *Measurement timing in growth mixture modeling of alcohol trajectories* (Doctoral dissertation, University of Rhode Island); 2012. Retrieved from http://digitalcommons.uri.edu/dissertations/AAI3522627

22. Walls TA, Barta WD, Stawski RS, Collyer C, Hofer SM. (2011). Time-scale-dependent longitudinal designs. In Laursen BP, Little TD, Card NA (Eds.), *Handbook of Developmental Research Methods* (pp. 46–64). New York: Guilford Press; 2011.

23. Varkey JP, Pompili D, Walls TA. (2011). Human motion recognition using a wireless sensor-based wearable system. *Personal and Ubiquitous Computing* 2011; 16(7):897–910.

24. Raiff B, Karatas C, Pompili D, Walls TA. Laboratory validation of inertial body sensors to detect cigarette smoking arm movements. *Electronics* 2014;3: 87–110.

25. Walls TA, Hoeppner BB, Goodwin MS. Statistical issues in intensive longitudinal data analysis. In Stone A, Shiffman S, Atienza A, Nebelling L (Eds.), *The Science of Real-Time Data Capture* (pp. 338–360). New York: Oxford University Press; 2007

26. Therneau TM, Grambsch PM. *Modeling Survival Data.* New York: Springer; 2001.

27. Yau KK. Multilevel models for survival analysis with random effects. *Biometrics* 57(1):96–102; 2001.

28. SAS Institute, Inc. *The GLIMMIX Procedure.* Cary, NC: SAS Institute; 2009.

29. Bolger N, Laurenceau J-P. *Intensive Longitudinal Methods: An Introduction to Diary and Experience Sampling Research.* New York: Guilford Press; 2013

30. Walls TA, Jung H, Schwartz J. Multilevel models and intensive longitudinal data. In Walls TA, Schafer JL (Eds.), *Models for Intensive Longitudinal Data* (pp. 3–37). New York: Oxford University Press; 2006.

31. Hoeppner B, Goodwin MS, Velicer WF, Heltshe J. An applied example of pooled time series analysis: Cardiovascular reactivity to stressors in children with autism. *Multivariate Behavioral Research* 2007; 42(4):707–727.

32. Dierker L, Stolar M, Richardson E, Tiffany S, Flay B, Collins L, for the Tobacco Etiology Research Network. Tobacco, alcohol and marijuana use among first-year U.S. college students: A time series analysis. *Substance Use and Misuse* 2008; 43(5):680–699.

33. Shiffman S, Ferguson SG, Gwaltney CJ. Immediate hedonic response to smoking lapses: Relationship to smoking relapse and effects of nicotine replacement therapy. *Psychopharmacology* 2006; 184:608–618.

34. Van Wijk JJ, Van Selow ER. Cluster and calendar based visualization of time series data. In *Information Visualization, 1999 IEEE Symposium on Information Visualization* (pp. 4–9); 1999.

35. Tufte ER. *The Visual Display of Quantitative Information* (2nd ed.). Cheshire, CT: Graphics Press; 2001

36. Few S. *Now You See It: Simple Visualization Techniques for Quantitative Analysis.* Analytics Press; 2009.

37. Wong B. Visual representation of scientific information. *Science Signaling* 4(160); 2011.

38. Viegas FB, Wattenberg M, Van Ham F, Kriss J, McKeon M. Manyeyes: A site for visualization at internet scale. *IEEE Transactions on Visualization and Computer Graphics* 2007; 13(6):1121–1128.

39. Krzywinski M, Wong B. Points of view: Plotting symbols. *Nature Methods* 2013; 10:451.

40. Sarkar D. *Lattice: Multivariate Data Visualization with R.* New York: Springer; 2008.

41. Wickham H. *ggplot2: Elegant Graphics for Data Analysis.* New York: Springer; 2009.

42. Fitzmaurice GM, Laird NM, Ware JH. *Applied Longitudinal Analysis.* New York: Wiley; 2004.

43. Goldstein H. *Multilevel Statistical Models* (3rd ed.). New York: Oxford University Press; 2003.

44. Hox JJ. *Multilevel Analysis: Techniques and Applications.* Mahwah, NJ: Erlbaum; 2002.

45. Kreft IGG, de Leeuw J. *Introducing Multilevel Modeling.* London: Sage; 1998.

46. Raudenbush SW, Bryk AS. *Hierarchical Linear Models: Applications and Data Analysis Methods.* Thousand Oaks, CA: Sage; 2002.

47. Snijders TAB, Bosker RL. *Multilevel Analysis: An Introduction to Basic and Advanced Multilevel Modeling.* Thousand Oaks, CA: Sage; 1999.

48. Singer JD, Willett JB. *Applied Longitudinal Data Analysis.* New York: Oxford University Press; 2003.

49. Chang T-Y, Su T-C, Lin S-Y, Jain R-M, Chan C-C. Effects of occupational noise exposure on 24-hour ambulatory vascular properties in male workers. *Environmental Health Perspectives* 2007; 115(11):1660–1664.

50. Box GEP, Jenkins GM. *Time Series Analysis: Forecasting and Control.* Oakland, CA: Holden-Day; 1976.

51. Chatfield C. *The Analysis of Time Series: An Introduction* (6th ed.). Boca Raton, FL: Chapman & Hall; 2003.

52. Snijders TAB. Power and sample size in multilevel modeling. In Everitt BS, Howell DC (Eds.), *Encyclopedia of Statistics in Behavioral Science* (Vol. 3, pp. 1570–1573). Chichester: Wiley; 2005.

53. Matyas TA, Greenwood KM. Serial dependency in single-case time series. In Franklin RD, Allison DB, Gorman BS (Eds.), *Design and Analysis of Single-Case Research* (pp. 215–243). Hillsdale, NJ: Erlbaum; 1996.

54. Guo Y, Logan HL, Glueck DH, Muller KE. Selecting a sample size for studies with repeated measures. *BMC Medical Research Methodology* 2013; 13:1–8.

55. Ramsay J, Hooker G, Graves S. *Functional Data Analysis with R and MATLAB.* New York: Springer; 2009.

56. Fok CCT, Ramsay J. Fitting curves with periodic and nonperiodic trends and their interactions with intensive longitudinal data. In Walls TA, Schafer JL (Eds.), *Models for Intensive Longitudinal Data* (pp. 109–123). New York: Oxford University Press; 2006.

57. Tan X, Shiyko MP, Li R, Li Y, Dierker L. A time-varying effect model for intensive longitudinal data. *Psychological Methods* 2012; 17(1):61–77.

58. Hedeker D, Berbaum M, Mermelstein R. Location-scale models for multilevel ordinal data: Between- and within-subjects variance modeling. *Journal of Probability and Statistical Science* 2006; 4(1):1–20.

59. Harvey A, Ruiz E, Shephard N. Multivariate stochastic variance models. *Review of Economic Studies* 1994; 61(2):247–264.

60. Rovine MJ, Walls TA. Multilevel autoregressive modeling of interindividual differences in the stability of a process. In Walls TA, Schafer JL (Eds.), *Models for Intensive Longitudinal Data* (pp. 127–147). New York: Oxford University Press; 2006.

61. Deboeck PR, Montpetit MA, Bergeman CS, Boker SM. Using derivative estimates to describe intraindividual variability at multiple time scales. *Psychological Methods* 2009; 14(4):367–386.

62. Chow S-M, Ho M-HR, Hamaker EL, Dolan CV. Equivalence and differences between structural equation modeling and state-space modeling techniques. *Structural Equation Modeling* 2010; 17(2):303–332.

63. Ho M-HR, Shumway R, Ombao H. The state space approach to modeling dynamic processes. In Walls TA, Schafer JL (Eds.), *Models for Intensive Longitudinal Data* (pp. 148–175). New York: Oxford University Press; 2006.

64. Levy JA, Elser HE, Knobel RB. (2012). The promise of the state space approach to time series analysis for nursing research. *Nursing Research* 2012; 61(6):388–394.

65. Nesselroade JR, McArdle JJ, Aggen SH, Meyers JM. Dynamic factor analysis models for representing process in multivariate time-series. In

Moskowitz DS, Hershberger SL (Eds.), *Modeling Intraindividual Variability with Repeated Measures Data* (pp. 235–265). Mahwah, NJ: Erlbaum; 2002.

66. Ramsay J. The control of behavioral input/output systems. In Walls TA, Schafer JL (Eds.), *Models for Intensive Longitudinal Data* (pp. 176–194). New York: Oxford University Press; 2006.

67. Riley WT, Rivera DE, Atienza AA, Nilsen W, Allison SM, Mermelstein R. Health behavior models in the age of mobile interventions: Are our theories up to the task? *Translational Behavioral Medicine* 2011; 1(1):53–71.

68. Walls TA, Rivera DE. Control engineering-based approaches to modeling substance abuse data. In *17th Annual Meeting of the Society for Prevention Research*. Washington, DC, May, 2009.

69. Navarro-Barrientos J-E, Rivera DE, Collins LM. A dynamical model for describing behavioural interventions for weight loss and body composition change. *Mathematical and Computer Modelling of Dynamical Systems* 2011; 17(2):183–203.

70. Collins LM, Lanza ST. *Latent Class and Latent Transition Analysis: With Applications in the Social, Behavioral, and Health Sciences*. New York: Wiley; 2010.

71. Everitt BS, Landau S, Leese M, Stahl D. *Cluster Analysis* (5th ed.). New York: Wiley; 2011.

72. Melnykov V, Maitra R. Finite mixture models and model-based clustering. *Statistics Surveys* 2010; 4:80–116.

73. Pratima D, Nimmakanti N. Pattern recognition algorithms for cluster identification problem. *International Journal of Computer Science and Informatics* 2012; 2(1):25–32.

74. Christakis NA, Fowler JH. The spread of obesity in a large social network over 32 years. *New England Journal of Medicine* 2007; 357:370–379.

75. Christakis NA, Fowler JH. (2008). The collective dynamics of smoking in a large social network. *New England Journal of Medicine* 2008; 358:2249–2258.

76. McPherson M, Smith-Lovin L, Cook JM. Birds of a feather: Homophily in social networks. *Annual Review of Sociology* 2001; 27:415–444.

77. VanderWeele TJ. Sensitivity analysis for contagion effects in social networks. *Sociological Methods and Research* 2011; 40(2):240–255.

78. Lo BPL, Wang JL, Yang G-Z. From imaging networks to behavior profiling: Ubiquitous sensing for managed homecare of the elderly. In *Adjunct Proceedings of the 3rd International Conference on Pervasive Computing*, 2005: 101–104. Available online at: http://www.pervasive.ifi.lmu.de/adjunct-proceedings/demo/p101-104.pdf

79. Minutolo A, Sannino G, Esposito M, De Pietro G. A rule-based mHealth system for cardiac monitoring. In *Biomedical Engineering and Sciences (IECBES), 2010 IEEE EMBS Conference* (pp. 144–149); 2010.

80. Viswanathan H, Chen B, Pompili D. Research challenges in computation, communication, and context awareness for ubiquitous healthcare. *IEEE Communications Magazine* 2012; 50(5):92–99.

12

Research Designs to Develop and Evaluate Technology-Based Health Behavior Interventions

JESSE DALLERY, WILLIAM T. RILEY, AND INBAL NAHUM-SHANI

INTRODUCTION

Digital and information technologies hold unique opportunities to deliver efficacious behavioral interventions, as well as to obtain empirical evidence that can inform the development of high-quality behavioral interventions. Technology enables frequent assessment of the ebb and flow of health behavior in naturalistic contexts. This fine-grained analysis can enhance understanding of how behavioral and psychological processes unfold over time. For example, frequent, mobile-phone-based assessment of smoking behavior can be tied to dynamic changes in craving, mood, and other variables that are also assessed using the mobile phone. Technology also permits automated treatment delivery, which can enhance treatment fidelity, efficiency, and the ability to rapidly adapt the timing and the type of the treatment based on ongoing assessment of behavior. These new advances in technological tools may be ushering in "a new paradigm for evidence generation in health research" (1).

Technology also poses some challenges in designing research studies regarding the development of technology-based behavioral interventions. For example, because of the rapid pace of change in technology, the technology used during a traditional randomized controlled trial (RCT) may be relatively obsolete by study completion (1,2). In addition, researchers may encounter logistical issues in testing new treatments. If the assessment or treatment is delivered via a new special-purpose device (e.g., newly developed sensor), the researcher may have only a limited number of prototypes available

for testing. Finally, technology-based interventions often include multiple components, from the mode of delivery (computer, mobile phone), to the nature of what is delivered (reminders, feedback, incentives, skills training, etc.), to strategies for re-engagement and for enhancing long-term maintenance (3). The relative contribution of these components and their combinations is often unclear (4). Fortunately, many of these challenges may be obviated by use of alternative and, in some cases, more efficient research designs compared to RCTs.

In this chapter, we describe the nascent literature on research designs that can inform the development of efficacious technology-based interventions and that are synergistic with the unique features of technology-based tools. First, we discuss research designs that permit researchers to optimize and evaluate technology-based interventions in the process of developing an intervention (i.e., prior to its dissemination). Second, we discuss scientific and design considerations pertaining to the use of RCTs in evaluating technology-based interventions, as well as how technology can be used to improve the scientific yield obtained via an RCT. Third, we describe additional alternatives to RCTs that may be more relevant to evaluation efforts as interventions are disseminated and implemented in real-world contexts. Although our discussion of methods is organized by different phases of the intervention lifecycle (development to dissemination), we should note that the methods within each phase are not exclusive to that phase and could also be used during other phases.

OPTIMIZING AND EVALUATING DURING THE DEVELOPMENT PHASE

Technology-based interventions to promote health behavior are expanding rapidly. In many cases, interventions are outpacing the ability of careful, scientific studies to establish their acceptability, efficacy, and sustainability. This is especially true for commercial products. In part, the rapid pace of development is due to economic contingencies and the desire of many companies to simply get their product to market. Thus, many commercial products do not have adequate scientific support (5,6). Another factor may be the perceived difficulty in conducting rigorous, efficient studies to optimize and/or evaluate the intervention. In this section, we describe a set of methods that can be used to optimize interventions during the development phases of technology-based interventions.

Single-Case Designs

Assessments of the feasibility, acceptability, and preliminary efficacy of a novel technology-based treatment are important first steps in development. Methods to assess feasibility and acceptability (i.e., social validity), which are critically important during development efforts, are described elsewhere (7–11). Here, we focus on how single-case designs can be used to assess preliminary efficacy. *Preliminary efficacy* can be defined as clinically significant improvement in behavior or symptoms over the course of treatment (12). One way to establish preliminary efficacy is to use one of several single-case research designs. We describe here several examples of single-case designs. We should also note that there have been several advances in the design and analysis of single-case designs. There are new quality control design standards for single-case designs (13), structured criteria for performing visual analysis of the graphically displayed data (13), and a plethora of new statistical techniques to supplement visual analysis (including effect size measures and techniques to perform meta-analysis) (13–16). Also noteworthy are recent efforts to combine single-case designs using Bayesian methods, to enable population-level claims about the merits of different intervention strategies (15).

Single-case designs include a family of methods in which each case serves as his, her, or its own control. A "case" does not have to be an individual—it could be any unit of analysis such as different healthcare agencies, group homes, hospitals, or communities. In a typical study, some behavior or self-reported symptom is measured repeatedly during control (baseline) and intervention conditions for all cases (hereafter "participants," for clarity and convenience). The researcher systematically introduces and withdraws control and intervention conditions, and then assesses effects of the intervention on behavior or symptoms across replications of these conditions within and across participants. The main characteristics of these studies include repeated, frequent assessment of behavior, experimental manipulation of the independent variable, and replication of effects within and across participants. Clinically meaningful improvement in behavior can be revealed by changes in health-related behavior from baseline to treatment, and the cause(s) of these changes can be verified via replications within and across participants.

One common concern in single-case research is the issue of establishing generality of treatment effects. In the context of single-case designs, generality of treatment effects is achieved through a series of systematic replications. In systematic replications, the methods from previous studies are used in a new setting or population, or they are applied to a new target behavior (17). By carefully choosing the characteristics of the individuals, settings, or other relevant variables in a systematic replication, the researcher can help identify the conditions under which a treatment works. One advantage of a single-case approach to establishing generality is that a series of strategic studies can be conducted with some degree of efficiency. See Dallery, Cassidy, and Raiff (10) for a further discussion of generality and single-case research.

Examples of Single-Case Designs

Some common single-case designs—and those that are most relevant to technology-based interventions—are presented in Table 12.1. The table also presents some procedural information, as well as advantages and disadvantages for each design. These designs permit inferences about causal relations between independent and dependent variables (observations of behavior, self-reports of symptoms, etc.).

TABLE 12.1. COMMON SINGLE-CASE DESIGNS: GENERAL PROCEDURES, ADVANTAGES, AND DISADVANTAGES

Design	Procedure	Advantages	Disadvantages
Reversal	Baseline is conducted, treatment is implemented, and then treatment is removed.	Within-subject replication; clear demonstration of an intervention effect in one subject	Not applicable if behavior is irreversible, or when removing treatment is undesirable
Multiple-Baseline	Baseline is conducted for varying durations across participants; then treatment is introduced in a staggered fashion.	Treatment does not have to be withdrawn.	No within-subject replication. Potentially more subjects needed to demonstrate intervention effects than when using reversal design.
Changing Criterion	Following a baseline phase, treatment goals are implemented. Goals become progressively more challenging as they are met.	Demonstrates within-subject control by levels of the independent variable without removing treatment; useful when gradual change in behavior is desirable	Not applicable for binary outcome measures—must have continuous outcomes

In a *reversal design*, a treatment is introduced after the baseline period. The number of data points in the treatment condition must be sufficient to predict behavior if treatment were to continue (e.g., stable performance and no trends toward baseline levels of the dependent variable). If there is a trend in the direction of the anticipated treatment effect during baseline, the ability to detect a treatment effect will be limited. Thus, stability, or trend in the direction *opposite* the predicted treatment effect, is desirable. There are no universally agreed-upon rules about the extent to which baselines must be stable, but there are several metrics available to measure and report the degree of stability (18,19). Following the treatment period, the baseline period is reintroduced, hence the "reversal" in this design. Three is the minimum number of alternations to document experimental control in a reversal design. Using only two conditions, such as a pre-post design, is not considered sufficient to demonstrate experimental control because other sources of influence over behavior cannot be ruled out (20). For example, a smoking cessation intervention could coincide with a price increase in cigarettes. By returning to baseline conditions, we can assess and possibly rule out the influence of the price increase on smoking. (The reversals also rule out other rival hypotheses about the sources of behavior change, such as regression to the mean, effects of repeated assessment, or maturation). Researchers also often employ a subsequent "reversal" to the treatment condition. Thus, the experiment ends during a treatment period, not a baseline period. This may be desirable not only from the participant's perspective but also from the researcher's perspective, in that it provides a replication of the main variable of interest—the treatment (21,22).

Figure 12.1 displays a hypothetical, four-condition reversal design, and each panel shows data from a different participant (an ABAB design, where "A" indicates baseline and "B" indicates treatment; as described in reference 10). For the purposes of illustration, assume the treatment conditions represent a text-based intervention to decrease smoking. Although all participants were exposed to the same four conditions (two baseline conditions and two treatment conditions), the duration of the conditions differed because of trends in the conditions. Assume the dependent variable is number of cigarettes smoked per day. For example, for Participant 1, the beginning of the first baseline condition displays a consistent downward trend in smoking behavior (in the same direction as the expected text-message treatment effects). If we were to introduce the smoking cessation–related texts after only five or six baseline sessions, it would be unclear if the decrease in smoking was a function of the independent variable. Therefore, continuing the baseline condition until there is no visible trend helps build confidence about the causal role of the treatment when it is introduced.

The immediate decrease in the level of smoking for Participant 1 when the treatment is introduced also suggests that treatment was responsible for the change. Similar patterns, which also illustrate differences in the magnitude and variability of the effects, can be seen for Participants 2–4. Overall, Figure 12.1 illustrates a reliable, replicated change in behavior as a function of treatment.

Reversal designs have been used to provide evidence of treatment efficacy (23,24). For instance, Raiff and Dallery (24) assessed whether an Internet-based incentive program could increase adherence to blood glucose testing for four teenagers diagnosed with type 1 diabetes. Teens monitored glucose levels with a glucometer during a 5-day, stable baseline condition. During a 5-day treatment condition, participants earned incentives for adhering to blood glucose testing recommendations (i.e., four tests per day). After the treatment condition, participants monitored blood glucose just as they did during the first baseline condition for 5 days, without the possibility of earning incentives. Participants submitted a mean of 1.7 and 3.1 blood glucose tests per day, respectively, during the baseline and return-to-baseline conditions, compared to 5.7 tests per day during the treatment condition. More relevant than the averaged changes to detect treatment effects were the replicated changes in behavior within and across participants. A limitation of reversal designs is the potential for carryover effects of the treatment after it has been withdrawn. If skills are taught during the treatment, for instance, these learned skills cannot be "withdrawn" after treatment, thereby producing continued treatment effects that are not reversible. Therefore, reversal designs are best used when the treatment effects are short-lived and expected to end soon after the treatment has been withdrawn (e.g., medications with short half-lives, incentive-based interventions).

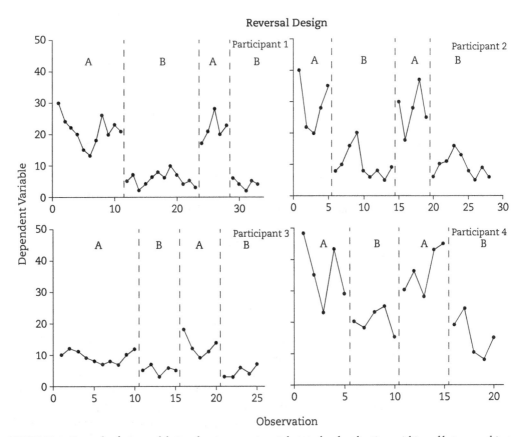

FIGURE 12.1: Example of a reversal design showing experimental control and replications within and between subjects. Each panel represents a different participant, each of whom experienced two baseline and two treatment conditions. Reprinted from Dallery et al. (10).

In a *multiple-baseline design*, the durations of the baselines vary systematically for each participant, or for multiple and independent targeted behaviors within a participant, in a "staggered" fashion. For example, one participant may start treatment after 5 baseline days, another after 7 baseline days, then 9, and so on. The precise number should be determined on the basis of observation of trends and variability in the data, so these numbers are merely examples. Alternatively, multiple behaviors can be targeted by the intervention in a staggered fashion (e.g., dietary feedback after 7 days of baseline, physical activity feedback after 14 days of baseline) within participants. After baseline, treatment is introduced and remains until the end of the experiment (i.e., there are no reversals).

The rigor of these designs is derived from demonstrating that change occurs when, and only when, the intervention is directed at a particular participant or behavior (or whatever the unit of analysis happens to be) (25). The influence of other factors, such as idiosyncratic experiences of the individual or self-monitoring (e.g., reactivity), can be ruled out by replicating the effect across multiple individuals. As replications are observed across individuals, and behavior changes when and only when treatment is introduced, confidence that behavior change was caused by the treatment increases. These designs are also useful for technology-based interventions that teach new skills, where behavior would not be expected to "reverse" to baseline levels. Multiple-baseline designs also obviate the ethical concern that participants in control conditions in a between-group design are not exposed to the active treatment, as all participants are exposed to the (potentially) active treatment with multiple-baseline designs. Although all participants in a reversal design also receive the treatment, the treatment must be withdrawn to assess treatment effects.

Figure 12.2 illustrates a simple, two-condition multiple-baseline design replicated across four participants. Similar to the reversal design, treatment should be introduced only when the data appear stable. The durations of the baseline conditions are staggered for each participant, and the dependent variable increases when, and only when, the independent variable is introduced for all participants. Figure 12.2 suggests reliable increases in behavior, and that the treatment was responsible for these changes. (See "Interrupted Time Series Designs" and "Stepped Wedge Designs" later in the chapter for discussion of research designs that are very similar to multiple-baseline designs.)

There are several examples of multiple-baseline designs to test technology-based interventions (26,27). For example, Cushing, Jensen, and Steele (27) investigated the ability of a mobile device, used to measure adherence to a self-monitoring intervention, to improve weight management with a multiple-baseline design. Overweight adolescents ($n = 3$) were given weekly self-monitoring goals based on recording their meals and activity levels. During baseline, self-monitoring was completed with a traditional pencil-and-paper method, and goal attainment was measured for 4, 5, and 9 weeks for each successive participant. Following baseline, participants were instructed to use mobile devices with automated software to input their daily health information. Goal attainment increased reliably when the mobile device was used, and the staggered presentation of the independent variable demonstrated that the mobile device increased self-monitoring of food intake and activity levels.

In some cases, a technology-based intervention may seek to reduce or produce a behavior gradually over time (e.g., gradual reductions in smoking, gradual increases in physical activity). The *changing criterion design* can be used to evaluate such interventions. In a changing criterion design, a baseline is conducted until stability is attained. Then, a treatment goal is introduced, for example, an increase in activity by 1,000 steps relative to baseline (as measured by an accelerometer). Once the goal is met for 3 out of 5 days (for example), the next criterion is established, which could be a further increase of 1,000 steps. Thus goals are made systematically and progressively more difficult. Behavior should change in accord with changes in the criteria; that is, it should follow or "track" the introduction of each goal. Such tracking demonstrates control by the level of the intervention (19,25). Kurti and Dallery (28) used a changing-criterion design to increase activity in six sedentary adults using an Internet-based contingency management program to promote walking. Weekly step count goals were gradually increased across 5-day blocks. The step counts for all six participants increased reliably with each increase in the goals.

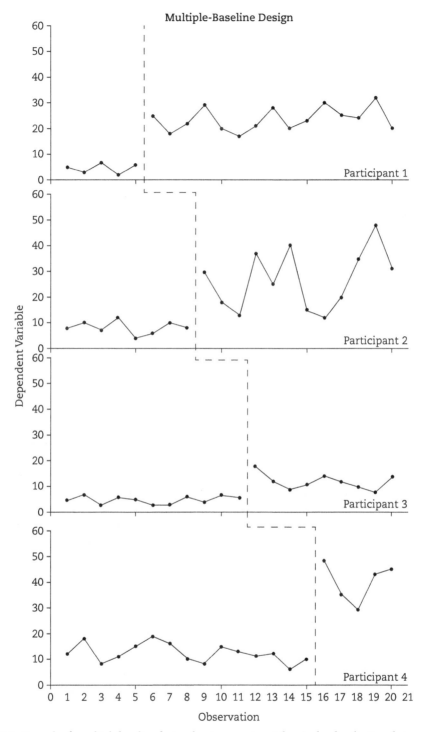

FIGURE 12.2: Example of a multiple baseline design showing experimental control and replications between subjects. Each row represents a different participant, each of whom experienced a baseline and treatment. The baseline durations differed across participants. Reprinted from Dallery et al. (10).

Component and Parametric Analysis

A *component analysis* is "any experiment designed to identify the active elements of a treatment condition, the relative contributions of different variables in a treatment package, and/or the necessary and sufficient components of an intervention" (29). Single-case research designs, in particular reversal and multiple-baseline designs, may be used to perform a component analysis. The essential experimental ingredients, regardless of the method, are that the components (both singly and combined) are systematically introduced and/or withdrawn, combined with replication of effects within and/or between subjects. Thus, component analysis may allow for an efficient way to optimize treatment during early development phases.

There are two main types of component analyses: the dropout and add-in analyses. In a dropout analysis, the full treatment package is presented following a baseline phase, and then components are systematically withdrawn from the package. A limitation of dropout analyses is when components produce irreversible behavior change (i.e., learning a new skill). Instead, in add-in analyses, components can be assessed individually and/or in combination before the full treatment package is assessed. Add-in designs "provide the most powerful and complete analysis of the active components of a treatment package because they reduce potential confounding from the effects of component combinations" (29). Of course, the possibility of sequence effects should be considered, and researchers could address such effects through counterbalancing, brief "washout" periods, or explicit investigation of these effects (30).

To our knowledge, there are no published reports of optimizing technology-based health interventions using a component analysis, despite the fact that most technology-based packages can be dismantled into distinct components. Thus, we provide two hypothetical component analyses in Figure 12.3. In the left panel, one component, labeled X, is presented in isolation following an initial baseline phase. Following a replication of the baseline phase the second component, labeled Y, is presented. For the purposes of illustration, assume that the goal of the intervention is to decrease smoking, and that X is a text message support system and Y is access to computer-based videos of peer success stories. The data paths suggest that both components produce some reduction in the smoking relative to baseline. When both components are combined, labeled XY, they produce an additive effect and smoking is reduced further. The panel on the right shows a different pattern for two different hypothetical components, again labeled X and Y. The pattern reveals a synergistic relation: The components must be combined to achieve a meaningful decrease in behavior. The sequences of introducing the individual components and their combinations in both panels are arbitrary. In practice, they would be chosen on the basis of characteristics of the intervention and/or behavior under study (see Ward-Horner and Sturmey [29] for more details).

Parametric analysis is similar to component analysis, but rather than manipulating different components, different parameters of a single treatment are manipulated. For example, text-based prompts can be delivered at different frequencies,

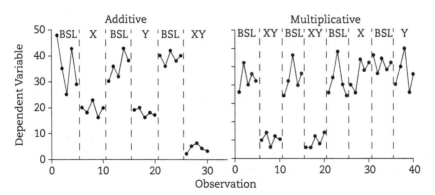

FIGURE 12.3: Two examples of possible results from a component analysis. BSL = baseline, X = first component, Y = second component. The panel on the left shows an additive effect of components X and Y, and the panel of the right shows a multiplicative effect of components X and Y. Reprinted from Dallery et al. (10).

incentives can be delivered at different magnitudes and frequencies, physical activity can occur at different frequencies and intensities, engagement in a Web-based program can occur at different levels, medications can be administered at different doses and frequencies, and all of the interventions could be delivered for different durations. The goal of a parametric analysis is to identify the optimal value (or values) that produces a behavioral outcome, as well as to identify general patterns of behavior engendered by a range of values of the independent variable (30,31). Parametric analysis can detect effects that may be missed using a standard group design with only one or two values of the independent variable. Guyatt and colleagues (32) provide an excellent discussion about how parametric analysis can be used to optimize an intervention. For the nascent field of technology-based interventions, parametric analyses provide an efficient method for determining the optimal doses of text messages, alerts, data recording, feedback, and other treatment parameter decisions during application development.

Other Types of Experimental Designs for Optimizing Multicomponent Interventions

As noted earlier, technology-based interventions often involve multiple components, where a component corresponds to any aspect of the intervention that can be reasonably separated for investigation (3). These include the content of the intervention, modes of delivery, the dose or intensity of the intervention, and tactics used to promote compliance, adherence, and long-term maintenance. Many technology-based interventions are conceptualized as black-box interventions because it is unclear (i.e., there is insufficient empirical evidence and/or theoretical basis to determine) which intervention component is effective, how well the components work together, and how best to sequence and adapt the intervention components over time. Here, we discuss how two experimental approaches—factorial designs (FD) and the sequential multiple assignment randomized trials (SMART)—can be used to efficiently address important scientific questions concerning the optimal selection, sequencing, and adaptation of intervention components. While the focus of this section is on the use of FDs and SMART to optimize technology-based interventions,

these designs can also be used in other phases in the process of developing a technology-based intervention.

Factorial Designs

Factorial designs can efficiently address scientific questions about the selection of intervention components, as well as their most effective level or intensity (see references 3,33). Factorial designs are randomized trials that include more than one factor and in which the levels of the factors vary systematically; that is, the two factors are "crossed" (33). For example, assume an investigator is interested in developing a 12-week mobile-based intervention that targets heavy-episodic drinking among college students (this example is loosely based on reference 34). The investigator considers three intervention modules: 1) personalized normative feedback (PNF), which includes information targeting descriptive normative misperceptions about alcohol; 2) protective behavioral strategies (PBS), which includes recommendations such as limiting the number of drinks consumed per hour, alternating alcoholic drinks with nonalcoholic drinks, and using a designated driver; and 3) information about drinking (IAD), which includes educational messages focusing on the negative consequences of drinking. To build an optimized intervention, the investigator needs to decide which intervention module should be included in the intervention.

A factorial design can be used to efficiently test the efficacy of each of the three individual intervention components (i.e., intervention modules). This design will involve three factors, each corresponding to one of the intervention components under consideration. We assume that each factor has two levels: ON (i.e., when the component is active; e.g., the participant receives PNF via the mobile device) or OFF (i.e., when the component is not active; e.g., PNF is not offered to the participant). The investigator might consider a 2×2×2 factorial design, in which the two levels of each factor are "crossed" with the levels of the other factors. This *complete* factorial design (i.e., a factorial design that includes all possible combination of the levels of the factors) will involve eight experimental conditions (described in Table 12.2). Throughout this example, we assume that the investigator has resources to conduct a trial with 400 participants. Hence (assuming participants are equally randomized to the eight

TABLE 12.2. EFFECT CODING FOR A 2×2×2 FACTORIAL DESIGN
IN THE MOBILE-BASED INTERVENTION EXAMPLE

Condition	Components	IAD	PBS	PNF	IAD × PBS	IAD × PNF	PBD × PNF	IAD × PBS × PNF
Conditions in the factorial design:								
1 (N = 50)	Untreated	−1	−1	−1	+1	+1	+1	−1
2 (N = 50)	PNF only	−1	−1	+1	+1	−1	−1	+1
3 (N = 50)	PBS only	−1	+1	−1	−1	+1	−1	+1
4 (N = 50)	PNF and PBS	−1	+1	+1	−1	−1	+1	−1
5 (N = 50)	IAD only	+1	−1	−1	−1	−1	+1	+1
6 (N = 50)	IAD and PNF	+1	−1	+1	−1	+1	−1	−1
7 (N = 50)	IAD and PBS	+1	+1	−1	+1	−1	−1	−1
8 (N = 50)	All three	+1	+1	+1	+1	+1	+1	+1

IAD, information about drinking; PBS, protective behavioral strategies; PNF, personalized normative feedback.

experimental conditions in Table 12.1), we expect that 50 participants will be assigned to each of the eight experimental conditions (see Table 12.2).

To clarify how the design described in Table 12.2 can be used to efficiently inform the selection of intervention components, consider how data from this factorial experiment can be used to test the efficacy of each of the three intervention modules under consideration. The efficacy of the first module (i.e., PNF) can be investigated by testing the main effect of PNF, namely by estimating the difference between the ON and OFF levels of PNF, averaged over the levels of the other factors. This can be done by comparing the mean outcome across all the experimental conditions in which PNF was set to ON (conditions 2, 4, 6, and 8 in Table 12.2; N = 200) and the mean outcome across all the conditions in which PNF was set to OFF (cells 1, 3, 5, and 7 in Table 12.2; N = 200). Similarly, the efficacy of the second module (i.e., PBS) can be investigated by comparing the mean outcome across all the experimental conditions in which PBS was set to ON (conditions 3, 4, 7, and 8 in Table 12.2; N = 200) and the mean outcome across all the conditions in which PBS was set to OFF (cells 1, 2, 5, and 6 in Table 12.1; N = 200). Finally, the efficacy of the third module (i.e., IAD) can be investigated by comparing the mean outcome across all the experimental conditions in which IAD was set to ON (conditions 5, 6, 7, and 8 in Table 12.2; N = 200) and the mean outcome across all the conditions in which IAD was set to OFF (cells 1, 2, 3, and 4 in Table 12.2; N = 200).

Notice that the efficacy of each of these three modules can be tested by pooling outcome information from all study participants (N = 400). This is known as the "recycling" feature of factorial designs, namely the reuse of participant information for addressing more than one scientific question concerning the selection of intervention components (or their level/intensity). Collins and colleagues (33,35) discuss this property in detail, demonstrating the efficiency of factorial designs compared to relevant alternatives (e.g., individual experiments). They also discuss fractional factorial designs (i.e., factorial designs which involve a special, carefully chosen subset of the experimental conditions in a complete factorial) and their utility when the implementation of a complete factorial experiment is not feasible due to resource or practical limitations.

Beyond the efficiency of factorial designs for addressing scientific questions concerning the selection of intervention components, data from these designs can also be used to gain insights concerning the potential mediators by which each intervention component (or specific combinations of intervention components) exerts its effect on the outcome (36). A *mediator* is a variable that is responsible for (i.e., that explains) the change in the outcome. For example, an intervention or component (X) may produce changes in a mediator (M) that in turn produces changes in the outcome (Y). Relative to data from a standard RCT, data from factorial designs studies enable the investigation of more complex mediational processes.

Specifically, data from a standard RCT can be typically used to investigate whether and the extent to which a specific variable or a set of variables mediate the effect of the intervention package as a whole. For example, a mobile-based intervention package consisting of all the three intervention modules noted earlier (i.e., personalized normative feedback, protective behavioral strategies, and information about drinking), may produce changes in heavy-episodic drinking by improving self-regulation capabilities. However, data from a factorial design study can be used to investigate and identify which variables mediate the effect of specific intervention components and/or their combinations. For example, the particular component that increases (or that is most useful in increasing) self-regulatory capabilities in the mobile-based intervention could be identified (e.g., protective behavioral strategies). Such investigation has the potential to inform behavioral theory and intervention development, by shedding light on why specific components work well while others do not.

The Sequential, Multiple Assignment, Randomized Trial (SMART)

SMART is an experimental trial design that was developed specifically to help investigators address critical questions concerning the sequencing and adaptation of intervention components (37). A SMART includes multiple stages of randomization; each corresponds to a critical question or a critical decision concerning the sequencing and

adaptation of the intervention. To make the discussion more concrete, consider the mobile-based example described earlier, and assume the investigator is interested in addressing the following three critical questions:

1. Which intervention module should be offered first, PNF (i.e., feedback) or IAD (i.e., information)?
2. What is the best maintenance strategy for participants who respond well to the intervention (e.g., those who do not engage in heavy episodic drinking at 4-week follow-up)? Is it better to offer a booster session or not?
3. What is the best subsequent intervention tactic for participants who do not respond well to the intervention (e.g., those who engage in heavy episodic drinking at 4-week follow-up)? Is it better to continue with the same intervention modality (i.e., the same mobile-based intervention) or enhance the intensity of the intervention (e.g., by adding telephone coaching sessions)?

The hypothetical SMART design described in Figure 12.4 can be used to efficiently address all three questions. During the initial phase of this design, participants are randomized (with 0.5 probability) to two initial intervention options, to either IAD as the initial module, or PNF. Then (e.g., at week 4), participants who are classified

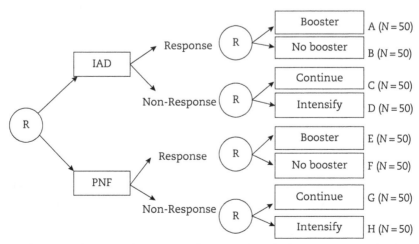

FIGURE 12.4: A hypothetical SMART design. IAD, information about drinking; PNF, personalized normative feedback. See text for details.

as non-responders are re-randomized to two sub-sequent tactics, to either CONTINUE with the same intervention modality, or INTENSIFY the intensity of the intervention by adding phone sessions. Participants who are classified as responders at week 4 are re-randomized to two maintenance tactics, to either receive a booster session or receive no booster session.

The SMART in Figure 12.4 includes three factors (i.e., independent variables), as it is designed to investigate three intervention components simultaneously: 1) the initial module; 2) the maintenance strategy for responders; and 3) the subsequent tactic for non-responders. Each factor includes two levels, and similar to a factorial design, the levels of the factors are 'crossed'. However, a SMART design might differ from a typical factorial design in three main respects First, the intervention components under investigation in a SMART vary in terms of the timing of their provision. For example, in Figure 12.4, Component #1 is delivered first, and Components #2 and #3 are delivered later (e.g., at a 4-week follow-up). Second, the randomization in a SMART is sequential, corresponding to the order of the intervention components under investigation. For example, in the SMART example above, participants are first randomized to the initial module (i.e., Factor 1), and only 4 weeks later are they re-randomized to the maintenance strategies for responders (i.e., Factor 2) and to the subsequent tactics for non-responders (Factor 3). Finally, in a SMART design, the levels of the factors might be crossed in a restricted manner. For example, in Figure 12.4 the levels of Factor 1 are crossed with the levels of Factor 2; the levels of Factor 1 are crossed with the level of Factor 3; but the levels of Factors 2 and 3 are not crossed. This is because the re-randomization to the subsequent tactics (i.e., continue vs. intensity) is restricted to non-responders, and re-randomization to the maintenance strategies (i.e., booster vs. no-booster) is restricted to responders. In other words, response/non-response is a tailoring variable (i.e., information concerning the participant that is used to make treatment/intervention decision) that is embedded in this SMART design, that is, different intervention components are considered for responders vs. non-responders.

Despite these differences, SMART, like a factorial design, is designed such that information from the same participant can be "recycled" (i.e., reused) to address more than one scientific question concerning the optimal sequencing and adaptation of an intervention. To better appreciate this, assume again that the investigator has resources to conduct a trial with 400 participants. Assuming that the rate of non-response at week 4 is 50%, each individual experimental condition in Figure 12.4 will include 50 participants. The first scientific question (about the initial module) can be addressed by testing the main effect of Factor 1. This can be done by comparing the mean outcome across all the experimental conditions in which participants received IAD initially (i.e., A–D; $N = 200$) and the mean outcome across all the conditions in which participants received PNF initially (i.e., E–H; $N = 200$). Notice that information from all study participants can be used to address this scientific question.

The second question (about the maintenance strategies for responders) can be addressed by testing the main effect of Factor 2. This can be done by comparing the mean outcome across all the experimental conditions in which responders received a booster session (i.e., A and E; $N = 100$) and the mean outcome across all the conditions in which responders did not receive a booster session (i.e., B and F; $N = 100$). Similarly, the third question concerning the subsequent tactics for non-responders can be addressed by testing the main effect of Factor 3. This can be done by comparing the mean outcome across all the experimental conditions in which participants received the continue tactic (i.e., C and G; $N = 100$) to the mean outcome across all the conditions in which participants received the intensify tactic (i.e., D and H; $N = 100$).

Notice that for both questions 2 and 3, because of the restricted randomization (described earlier), information from half of the study participants (responders only in the case of Factor 2, and non-responders only in the case of Factor 3) can be used for inference. Nonetheless, this experimental design is efficient, compared to other alternatives, because information from each participant can be used to address two critical questions concerning the optimized intervention. More specifically, information from non-responders can be used to address two questions (1 and 3) and information from responders can be used to address two questions (1 and 2).

In sum, SMART designs can be used to efficiently address scientific questions concerning the sequencing and adaptation of intervention components. Nahum-Shani and colleagues (38) further discuss the efficiency of SMART designs compared to that of alternatives (e.g., standard factorial designs, and multiple separate experiments). Beyond main effects, data from SMART studies can also be used to address other important scientific questions concerning (a) the comparisons of sequences of intervention options that are embedded in a SMART design (38) and (b) the construction of more deeply tailored sequences of intervention options, beyond those embedded in a SMART study (39).

EVALUATION USING STANDARD RANDOMIZED CONTROLLED TRIALS

The standard RCT will remain an indispensible tool to evaluate technology-based interventions. In this section, we discuss two issues in conducting an RCT of a technology-based intervention: choosing appropriate comparison groups and choosing relevant outcome variables. We highlight how technology may help with recruitment and retention and may aid in evaluating potential mediators of treatment outcomes.

The first question in conducting an RCT of a technology-based intervention, or any intervention, is selecting the appropriate comparison group. If the technology-based intervention fills a gap where no other intervention exists, then a no-intervention condition may be appropriate. The no-intervention condition may include access to the technology (e.g., mobile phones) and perhaps delivery of relatively "neutral" content (e.g., general, supportive text messages). The timing of access to the neutral content can be matched to the timing of access to the active intervention (e.g., theory-based text messages to assist in smoking cessation). If the intervention is intended to supplement an existing intervention, then an additive design in which the existing intervention is compared to the existing intervention plus the technology-based intervention would be appropriate. If the technology-based intervention is intended to replace an existing in-person, equivalent intervention, then the in-person

delivery of the same intervention or content may be the appropriate comparison condition.

The second question concerns the choice of outcome variables. For example, in cases where the technology-based intervention is intended to supplement or replace the existing intervention, it is critical to ask in what way(s) the technology-based intervention is hypothesized to be better than the existing interventions. It may not be the case that the technology-based approach is expected to produce better outcomes; rather, the intervention may be hypothesized to provide comparable outcomes at a lower cost. As a result, a cost-per-unit change may be a better outcome for many technology-based interventions. In addition, a technology-based intervention may be more acceptable or accessible relative to an in-person intervention; as such, constructs like acceptability, satisfaction, helpfulness, and engagement should also be measured and compared to the existing intervention.

Although RCTs are indispensable, they typically require considerable time to complete. Riley, Glasgow, Etheredge, and Abernethy (2) estimated that randomized trials take approximately 7 years from grant application submission to publication. This time frame is substantially longer than typical technology development and commercialization business cycles, and often results in the published results of dated technologies. Fortunately, mobile and Internet technologies can be used to streamline the RCT process. Information technology can be used to recruit participants rapidly and to conduct the trial remotely. For example, Rodgers and associates (40) recruited participants (smokers) and conducted the study remotely across New Zealand. By recruiting with a text message to mobile phone users, the researchers were able to make the study convenient for participants (e.g., no travel for in-person visits) and to reduce study costs (e.g., fewer research staff and facilities were required). As a validity check of the data, the researchers scheduled in-person visits with 10% of the participants to obtain biochemical measures of smoking status. The frequent longitudinal assessments and the automated reminder prompts to complete the study assessments also potentially reduced missing data and the number of participants needed to detect the hypothesized effect.

Technology may also aid in assessing potential mediators of intervention outcomes in the context of an RCT (41). Temporal precedence—that the mediator effects occurred before the outcome effect—must be established in any mediation analysis. Thus, assessing mediators to establish temporal precedence can be accomplished by using longitudinal, technology-based data capture. As noted by Baralidi, Wurpts, MacKinnon, and Lockhart (in Chapter 13, this volume), "mediation is a process that necessities the use of longitudinal data due to its emphasis on the causal relations between variables."

One way to collect the longitudinal data necessary to establish temporal precedence is to use technology-based methods, such as ecological momentary assessment (EMA). McCarthy and colleagues (42) used EMA to assess potential mediators (i.e., withdrawal, negative/positive affect, and craving) of the effects of bupropion on smoking outcomes. EMA was performed up to 7 times per day for 2 weeks preceding and 4 weeks following a quit attempt using bupropion. In addition to frequent EMA, participants completed a battery of retrospective measures, including craving measures, each evening. McCarthy et al. found that bupropion's effects were not due to withdrawal but were partially mediated by reduced cigarette cravings and increased positive affect. Furthermore, whether craving was a mediator depended on the measurement interval: Craving was not a significant mediator of bupropion when measured in the evening and retrospectively, but it was when craving was measured frequently using EMA. These findings suggest that even daily assessments may be inadequate to detect certain behavioral mechanisms. Intensive, technology-enabled assessment of potential mediators of outcomes may be necessary to better identify mechanisms, which will also aid in designing future studies to target these mechanisms.

EVALUATING DURING IMPLEMENTATION

A controlled experiment to establish the efficacy of a technology-based intervention is often a crucial step before disseminating and implementing the intervention, but controlled trials of technology-based interventions are not always feasible to conduct before the intervention is made publicly or commercially available. Some interventions are developed to address a pressing public health need, necessitating rapid deployment. Ministries of health, nongovernmental organizations, and other public health entities may not have the time or resources to support a controlled trial, or they may not want to randomize participants to a group that does not receive the intervention (43). Commercial entities have development and commercialization timelines that often cannot accommodate a controlled trial and risk having their product become dated or even obsolete by the time an RCT can be completed (2).

As a result, much of the mobile health (mHealth) evidence to date is in the form of small pilot trials (e.g., single-arm, pre-post designs), which can be conducted rapidly but offer little in the way of robust evidence (5). There are, however, a number of quasi-experimental designs that can be employed to evaluate a technology-based intervention while it is being implemented (6). Often, these designs are more externally valid than RCTs since the intervention is evaluated in naturalistic, real-world contexts, and, if well designed, the internal validity of these designs approaches the validity achieved by RCTs (44). The frequent longitudinal assessments often integrated into technology-based interventions can be leveraged to perform automated evaluations of the intervention while it is being disseminated and implemented using these designs. The following examples of designs to evaluate the implementation of interventions in vivo show that dissemination of a technology-based intervention should not represent the end of the research process.

Interrupted Time Series Designs

The interrupted time series design has been used to analyze the effects of interventions on not only single subjects but also single systems. Interventions delivered at the school, community, or hospital level are often evaluated using interrupted time series because it is impractical to randomize a sufficient number of these entities to treatment vs. control (45). For example, Kim and colleagues (46) used an interrupted time series to assess the effect of radio-frequency identification (RFID) tracking of emergency department staff, patients, and equipment, to improve workflow and reduce waiting times. Results from this study are presented in Figure 12.5.

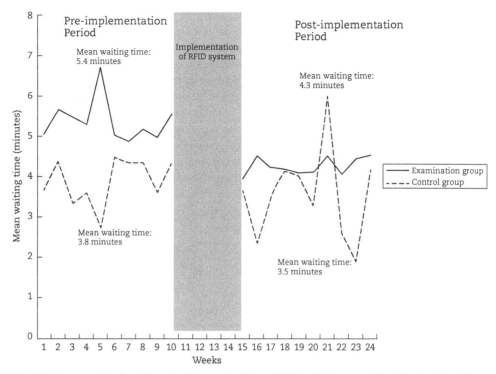

FIGURE 12.5: An example of an interrupted time series design. RFID, radiofrequency identification. From Kim et al. (46), reprinted with permission.

The basis of the interrupted time series design is a sequence of successive data points in time, typically at regular time intervals, from the same source. Time series analyses can be used for many purposes, but in the context of interrupted time series, the value of time series data is the ability to predict future data points in the series (both point estimate and confidence interval) from the prior data points. Time series forecasting is commonly used to predict financial markets, and this market-driven use has provided considerable impetus for continued improvements and refinements of these time series analyses (47). A time series can be influenced or "interrupted" by numerous events, including an intervention, and if the actual time series values of the dependent or outcome variable following the intervention exceed the confidence interval of the predicted values based on the prior time series, then this provides evidence that the intervention likely influenced the outcome.

The inferences from an interrupted time series can be strengthened in a number of ways:

1. *Stable baseline*: Similar to single-case designs, the greater the variability of the time series prior to the intervention, the more difficult it will be to find an effect because the confidence intervals around the future predicted values will be higher. Therefore, noise or measurement error limits the potential to find an effect. In cases in which the dependent variable of interest truly varies substantially over time (e.g., emotional states, heart rate), longer or more frequent baseline measurements may be needed to produce reasonable confidence intervals for future (post-intervention) data points.

2. *No trends in baseline data*: Although time series analyses will account for secular trends, it is preferable to have data that either do not trend or trend in the opposite direction of the hypothesized intervention effect. If the pre-intervention data trend in the direction of the intervention effect, which is commonly the case from self-monitoring data,

then it is more difficult to find an effect. Therefore, less reactive data collection methods are preferred for interrupted time series analyses.

3. *Lags in intervention effect*: While an immediate effect from the intervention is preferable, there are many cases in which the outcome is not expected until some period after the intervention is initiated (e.g., dietary intervention and weight loss). An a priori hypothesis of when the intervention effect is expected allows one to censor the post-intervention data that are not expected to change and evaluate the intervention only for the time series that begins after the intervention effect is expected.

4. *Control time series*: Finding an interrupted time series effect is strengthened if no effect is found for a similar individual, group, or system that did not receive the intervention during the same time period. If a similar effect on control is found, then some other phenomena shared by both the intervention and control condition likely produced the effect (e.g., cyclical or seasonal effects). To adjust for differences between the intervention and control conditions, propensity score weightings can be applied (48).

5. *Multiple and staggered interrupted time series*: Like single-case designs, nothing prohibits a researcher from conducting multiple interrupted time series with different individuals, groups, or systems. If these interrupted time series are staggered such that the intervention is delivered at different times to each experimental unit (individual, group, or system), then this decreases the likelihood that an event other than the intervention produced the observed changes in the time series.

Ramsey and colleagues (49) assessed the methodological quality of interrupted time series from two systematic reviews (mass media interventions, practice-based treatment guideline dissemination and implementation) based on the following criteria: (a) intervention occurred independently of other changes over time, (b) intervention was unlikely to affect data collection, (c) primary outcome was assessed blindly or was measured objectively, (d) primary outcome was reliable or was measured objectively, (e) composition of the data set at each time point covered at least 80% of the total number of participants in the study, (f) shape of the intervention effect was prespecified, (g) rationale for the number and spacing of data points was described, and (h) study was analyzed appropriately using time series techniques. They reanalyzed the data from 33 of the 58 studies reviewed and, although all studies concluded that the intervention tested was effective, approximately half showed no significant effect upon reanalysis. Clearly, the inferences possible from interrupted times series analyses are predicated on conducting a sound, methodological, rigorous study that attends to these criteria.

Technology-based health behavior interventions are uniquely suited for interrupted time series analyses. Many technology-based interventions collect baseline data for a period of time before initiating the intervention and continue to collect these data throughout the intervention period. Technology-based interventions designed to regularly collect precise measures of the target outcome, that do so in a manner that minimizes missing data (e.g., passive sensor data, recording reminder prompts), and that precede the intervention initiation with a period of baseline data collection are well positioned to utilize interrupted time series to assess the effect of the intervention. Longer and more intensive baseline data collection is more likely to produce a stable baseline and find a significant effect from the intervention, but this must be balanced with the potentially negative motivational effect to the user of delaying the intervention. The baseline period also can be adjusted for each user and shortened when the stability of the user's baseline data is sufficient to detect a minimally clinically significant post-intervention outcome. With some forethought, any technology-based intervention that regularly collects data on the primary outcome and that includes a baseline data collection period can evaluate the effect of the intervention on all users via interrupted time series analyses.

Stepped Wedge Design

During beta and early commercial release, technological applications are often rolled out in a

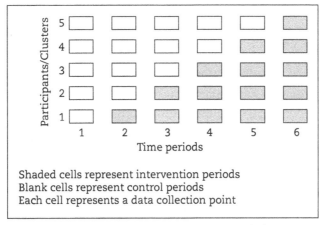

FIGURE 12.6: An example of a stepped wedge design. From Brown and Lilford (50).

limited and staggered fashion, often in select markets or with select users. This limited release allows the developers to detect remaining programming bugs and user interface problems, and to gradually gear up distribution, marketing, and customer service for the new product before making it widely available. This limited and gradual rollout is consistent with a stepped wedge design. The stepped wedge design rolls out the intervention in a staggered or sequential manner to individuals or clusters of individuals over a number of assessment periods (see Figure 12.6, which is reproduced from Brown and Lilford [50], for a graphical representation of this design). This design is particularly appropriate if (a) there are well-defined, independent cohorts (i.e., communities, schools) that are unlikely to share the intervention with other cohorts before they are scheduled to receive the intervention, (b) data on the targeted outcome can be obtained regularly across all of the cohorts, and (c) there are ethical or political reasons not to withhold the intervention from any of the cohorts, especially if there are also insufficient resources to introduce the intervention to all of the cohorts at once. These cohorts can be naturally occurring (e.g., schools, hospitals, communities) or artificial (e.g., user names beginning A-F, G-L, M-R, S-Z), as long as the cohorts can be defined a priori and can be randomized to the order in which they will receive the intervention.

Although existing surveillance data from registries and hospital records are often used for stepped wedge designs (51), data can be collected from users via the technology-based intervention if the intervention and its effects are short enough and data collection procedures are minimally burdensome for the last cohort to tolerate the wait until they receive the intervention. For example, a technology-delivered workplace program to prompt activity and reduce sedentary behavior would be anticipated to have a rapid effect on sedentary behavior (e.g. within 1 week) and can be monitored passively via accelerometers. In such a design, the workplaces could all receive accelerometers to monitor employee sedentary behavior, each step would need to be only 1 week in length, and such a study across five workplaces would require the last workplace to wait only 5 weeks to receive the intervention.

Analysis of stepped wedge data can be within each cohort (pre- vs. post- intervention for each cohort group) or between cohorts (comparison of cohorts who have or have not yet received the intervention at each step period). Handley, Schillinger, and Shiboski (52) give a more detailed description of the stepped wedge design and analysis approaches. It should be noted that the stepped wedge design is not without detractors, who argue that the cluster randomized design can achieve many of the benefits of the stepped wedge design while also being a controlled trial that can more definitively infer causality (53). While there is no question that the cluster randomized design is more rigorous than the stepped wedge design, the stepped wedge design provides speed and flexibility that some technology-based intervention evaluations require.

Regression Discontinuity Design

Perhaps one of the least utilized but most rigorous quasi-experimental designs is the regression discontinuity design. This design assigns participants to intervention on the basis of a cutoff variable and analyzes the change in slope or intercept at the cutoff between those who receive and those who do not receive the intervention. This design is often used when only those deemed more in need or at risk are provided the intervention. For example, if a health maintenance organization wants to provide a technology-based weight management program but has the funds to provide the program only to its obese members (BMI >30), the weights of the full range of overweight (BMI of 25 to 29.9) and obese members can be regularly monitored but the intervention provided only to those who meet the BMI >30 cutoff. The intervention can then be evaluated by comparing those receiving or not receiving the intervention, by analyzing differences in the prediction of outcome (weight after the intervention period) from the continuous variable (e.g., BMI) used as the basis for the cutoff score. The term *regression discontinuity* refers to the break or shift of the regression line from those below the cutoff (who did not receive the intervention) to those above the cutoff (who received the intervention). It is critical in the regression discontinuity design that the cutoff criteria remain unchanged throughout the study (see reference 44 for discussion of other assumptions that must be met). Any variation in referral cutoff based on the risk score will introduce bias. Performed rigorously, the regression discontinuity design is comparable to RCTs in controlling for research confounds and biases (44,54).

CONCLUSIONS

This chapter has illustrated the rich and maturing array of research designs that can be applied to evaluate technology-based health interventions. These designs can and should be used during all phases of development and deployment, from preliminary efficacy testing, to optimizing treatment, to evaluating treatments as they are disseminated and implemented in real-world contexts. A variety of factors will influence the choice of research design, and there is no set of decision rules to inform which design should be used in a particular scenario. There are trade-offs between internal validity and external validity, efficiency, cost, acceptability, and feasibility. The choice of an experimental design should be primarily motivated by the scientific questions that investigators wish to address, as well as by practical considerations and resource constraints. What is clear from the discussion in this chapter is that technology has opened a door to a range of both old and new research designs that can be used to inform the development of more efficacious technology-based behavioral interventions.

REFERENCES

1. Kumar S, Nilsen WJ, Abernethy A, Atienza A, Patrick K, Pavel M, et al. Mobile Health Technology Evaluation: The mHealth Evidence Workshop. *American Journal of Preventive Medicine* 2013; 45(2):228–236.
2. Riley WT, Glasgow RE, Etheredge L, Abernethy AP. Rapid, responsive, relevant (R3) research: A call for a rapid learning health research enterprise. *Clinical and Translational Medicine* 2013; 2(1):10.
3. Collins LM, Murphy SA, Strecher V. The Multiphase Optimization Strategy (MOST) and the Sequential Multiple Assignment Randomized Trial (SMART): New methods for more potent ehealth interventions. *American Journal of Preventive Medicine* 2007; 32(5):S112-S118.
4. Strecher VJ, McClure JB, Alexander GL, Chakraborty B, Nair VN, Konkel JM, et al. Web-based smoking-cessation programs: Results of a randomized trial. *American Journal of Preventive Medicine* 2008; 34(5):373–381.
5. Tomlinson M, Rotheram-Borus MJ, Swartz L, Tsai AC. Scaling up mHealth: Where is the evidence? *PLoS Medicine* 2013; 10(2):e1001382.
6. Mohr DC, Cheung K, Schueller SM, Hendricks Brown C, Duan N. Continuous evaluation of evolving behavioral intervention technologies. *American Journal of Preventive Medicine* 2013; 45(4):517–523.
7. Foster SL, Mash EJ. Assessing social validity in clinical treatment research: Issues and procedures. *Journal of Consulting and Clinical Psychology* 1999; 67(3):308–319.
8. Winett RA, Moore JF, Anderson ES. Extending the concept of social validity: Behavior analysis for disease prevention and health promotion. *Journal of Applied Behavior Analysis* 1991; 24(2):215–230.
9. Schwartz IS, Baer DM. Social validity assessments: Is current practice state of the art? *Journal of Applied Behavior Analysis* 1991; 24(2):189–204.
10. Dallery J, Cassidy RN, Raiff BR. Single-case experimental designs to evaluate novel technology-based

health interventions. *Journal of Medical Internet Research* 2013; 15(2).

11. Devito Dabbs A, Song MK, Hawkins R, Aubrecht J, Kovach K, Terhorst L, et al. An intervention fidelity framework for technology-based behavioral interventions. *Nursing Research* 2011; 60(5):340–347.

12. Rounsaville BJ, Carroll KM, Onken LS. A stage model of behavioral therapies research: Getting started and moving on from stage I. *Clinical Psychology: Science and Practice* 2001; 8(2):133–142.

13. Kratochwill TR, Hitchcock JH, Horner RH, Levin JR, Odom SL, Rindskopf DM, et al. Single-case intervention research design standards. *Remedial and Special Education* 2013; 34(1):26–38.

14. Duan N, Kravitz RL, Schmid CH. Single-patient (n-of-1) trials: A pragmatic clinical decision methodology for patient-centered comparative effectiveness research. *Journal of Clinical Epidemiology* 2013; 66(8 Suppl):S21–28.

15. Zucker DR, Ruthazer R, Schmid CH. Individual (N-of-1) trials can be combined to give population comparative treatment effect estimates: Methodologic considerations. *Journal of Clinical Epidemiology* 2010; 63(12):1312–1323.

16. Jenson WR, Clark E, Kircher JC, Kristjansson SD. Statistical reform: Evidence-based practice, meta-analyses, and single subject designs. *Psychology in the Schools* 2007; 44(5):483–493.

17. Valentine JC, Biglan A, Boruch RF, Castro FG, Collins LM, Flay BR, et al. Replication in prevention science. *Prevention Science* 2011; 12(2):103–117.

18. Killeen PR. Stability criteria. *Journal of the Experimental Analysis of Behavior* 1978; 29(1):17–25.

19. Kazdin AE. *Single-Case Research Designs: Methods for Clinical and Applied Settings* (2nd ed.). New York: Oxford University Press; 2011.

20. Risley TR, Wolf, MM. Strategies for analyzing behavioral change over time. In Nesselroade J, Reese HW (eds.), *Life Span Developmental Psychology: Methodological Issues*. New York: Academic Press; 1972, p. 175.

21. Cooper JO. *Applied Behavior Analysis*. Upper Saddle River, NJ: Pearson/Merrill-Prentice Hall; 2007.

22. Barlow DH, Hersen M. Single-case experimental designs: Uses in applied clinical research. *Archives in General Psychiatry* 1973; 29(3):319–325.

23. Dallery J, Glenn IM, Raiff BR. An Internet-based abstinence reinforcement treatment for cigarette smoking. *Drug and Alcohol Dependence* 2007; 86(2-3):230–238.

24. Raiff BR, Dallery J. Internet-based contingency management to improve adherence with blood glucose testing recommendations for teens with type 1 diabetes. *Journal of Applied Behavior Analysis* 2010; 43(3):487–491.

25. Barlow DH, Nock MK, Hersen M. *Single Case Experimental Designs: Strategies for Studying Behavior Change* (3rd ed.). Boston: Allyn & Bacon; 2009.

26. Meredith SE, Grabinski MJ, Dallery J. Internet-based group contingency management to promote abstinence from cigarette smoking: A feasibility study. *Drug and Alcohol Dependence* 2011; 118(1):23–30.

27. Cushing CC, Jensen CD, Steele RG. An evaluation of a personal electronic device to enhance self-monitoring adherence in a pediatric weight management program using a multiple baseline design. *Journal of Pediatric Psychology* 2011; 36(3):301–307.

28. Kurti AN, Dallery J. Internet-based contingency management increases walking in sedentary adults. *Journal of Applied Behavior Analysis* 2013; 46(3):568–581

29. Ward-Horner J, Sturmey P. Component analyses using single-subject experimental designs: A review. *Journal of Applied Behavior Analysis* 2010; 43(4):685–704.

30. Sidman M. *Tactics of Scientific Research*. Oxford: Basic Books; 1960.

31. Branch MN, P HS. Generality and generalization of research findings. In Madden GJ, Duke WV, Hackenberg TD, Hanley GP, Latal KA (eds.), *APA Handbook of Behavior Analysis*. Washington, DC: American Psychological Association; 2011:151–175.

32. Guyatt GH, Heyting A, Jaeschke R, Keller J, Adachi JD, Roberts RS. N of 1 randomized trials for investigating new drugs. *Controlled Clinical Trials* 1990; 11(2):88–100.

33. Collins LM, Dziak JJ, Li R. Design of experiments with multiple independent variables: A resource management perspective on complete and reduced factorial designs. *Psychological Methods* 2009; 14(3):202–224.

34. Witkiewitz K, Desai SA, Bowen S, Leigh BC, Kirouac M, Larimer ME. Development and evaluation of a mobile intervention for heavy drinking and smoking among college students. *Psychology of Addictive Behaviors* 2014, Jul 7.

35. Dziak JJ, Nahum-Shani I, Collins LM. Multilevel factorial experiments for developing behavioral interventions: Power, sample size, and resource considerations. *Psychological Methods* 2012; 17(2):153–175.

36. Smith RA, Coffman DL, Collins LM. Multivariate mediation: Investigating competing theorized mediators of message conditions on stigmatization via a factorial experiment. Under review.

37. Murphy SA. An experimental design for the development of adaptive treatment strategies. *Statistical Medicine* 2005; 24(10):1455–1481.

38. Nahum-Shani I, Qian M, Almirall D, Pelham WE, Gnagy B, Fabiano GA, et al. Experimental design and primary data analysis methods for comparing adaptive interventions. *Psychological Methods* 2012; 17(4):457–477.

39. Nahum-Shani I, Qian M, Almirall D, Pelham WE, Gnagy B, Fabiano GA, et al. Q-learning: A data analysis method for constructing adaptive interventions. *Psychological Methods* 2012; 17(4):478–494.

40. Rodgers A, Corbett T, Bramley D, Riddell T, Wills M, Lin RB, et al. Do u smoke after txt? Results of a randomised trial of smoking cessation using mobile phone text messaging. *Tobacco Control* 2005; 14(4):255–261.

41. Collins LM, MacKinnon DP, Reeve BB. Some methodological considerations in theory-based health behavior research. *Health Psychology* 2013; 32(5):586–591.

42. McCarthy DE, Piasecki TM, Lawrence DL, Jorenby DE, Shiffman S, Baker TB. Psychological mediators of bupropion sustained-release treatment for smoking cessation. *Addiction* 2008; 103(9):1521–1533.

43. Bastawrous A, Armstrong MJ. Mobile health use in low- and high-income countries: An overview of the peer-reviewed literature. *Journal of the Royal Society of Medicine* 2013; 106(4):130–142.

44. Shadish WR, Galindo R, Wong VC, Steiner PM, Cook TD. A randomized experiment comparing random and cutoff-based assignment. *Psychological Methods* 2011; 16(2):179–191.

45. Biglan A, Ary D, Wagenaar AC. The value of interrupted time-series experiments for community intervention research. *Prevention Science* 2000; 1(1):31–49.

46. Kim JY, Lee HJ, Byeon NS, Kim HC, Ha KS, Chung CY. Development and impact of radio-frequency identification-based workflow management in health promotion center: Using interrupted time-series analysis. *IEEE Transactions on Information Technology in Biomedicine* 2010; 14(4):935–940.

47. Tsay RS. *Analysis of Financial Time Series* (2nd ed.). Hoboken, NJ: Wiley; 2005.

48. Linden A, Adams JL. Applying a propensity score-based weighting model to interrupted time series data: Improving causal inference in programme evaluation. *Journal of Evaluation in Clinical Practice* 2011; 17(6):1231–1238.

49. Ramsey CR, Matowe L, Grilli R, Grimshaw JM, Thomas RE. Interrupted time series designs in health technology assessment: Lessons from two systematic reviews of behavior change strategies. *International Journal of Technology Assessment in Health Care* 2003; 19:613–623.

50. Brown CA, Lilford RJ. The stepped wedge trial design: A systematic review. *BMC Medical Research Methodology* 2006; 6:54.

51. The Gambia Hepatitis Study Group. The Gambia Hepatitis Intervention Trial. *Cancer Research* 1987; 47:5782–5787.

52. Handley MA, Schillinger D, Shiboski S. Quasi-experimental designs in practice-based research settings: Design and implementation considerations. *Journal of the American Board of Family Medicine* 2011; 24(5):589–596.

53. Kotz D, Spigt M, Arts IC, Crutzen R, Viechtbauer W. The stepped wedge design does not inherently have more power than a cluster randomized controlled trial. *Journal of Clinical Epidemiology* 2013; 66(9):1059–1060.

54. Linden A, Adams JL, Roberts N. Evaluating disease management programme effectiveness: An introduction to the regression discontinuity design. *Journal of Evaluation in Clinical Practice* 2006; 12(2):124–131.

13

Evaluating Mechanisms of Behavior Change to Inform and Evaluate Technology-Based Interventions

AMANDA N. BARALDI, INGRID C. WURPTS,
DAVID P. MACKINNON, AND GINGER LOCKHART

INTRODUCTION

In prevention and treatment research, a mediation framework helps researchers understand how an intervention changes an outcome by first changing a mediating variable (1). Mediation analysis is an important component in evaluating technology-based interventions, as it can provide evidence of how an intervention achieved its effects. This understanding of the mechanisms of change between an intervention and an outcome is essential for designing effective and efficient technology-based interventions. Once evidence of mediating variables is established, mediation analysis can also be used in designing interventions. In this context, a researcher develops an intervention to target a mediating variable that is hypothesized or previously demonstrated to change the desired outcome. Not only does mediation analysis provide a check of whether the intervention changed the outcomes it was designed to change, it also provides a check of whether the targeted mediators are actually related to the outcomes. In this way, mediation analysis is important in both discovering how interventions work and designing optimally effective interventions.

In a mediation model, the antecedent variable (X) causes a change in the mediating variable (M), which in turn causes a change in the outcome variable (Y). Thus, mediation describes how three (or more) variables in a causal chain are related. Examples of theoretical mediating processes are how childhood disadvantage leads to inaccurate interpersonal perceptions that increases aggressive behavior (2), how smoking cessation reduces

craving to reduce relapse (3), and how exposure to an Internet intervention "Guide to Health" based on social cognitive theory increases self-efficacy to reduce obesity (4). In one example of a technology-based intervention, a home telemedicine intervention provided home televisits with a dietician or nurse educator to recommend lifestyle and medication changes. The intervention increased diet and exercise knowledge, which in turn decreased waist circumference (5). Further examples of mediation in technology-based interventions include a Web-based intervention that aimed to simultaneously increase mindfulness and decrease procrastination, which in turn decreased stress (6), as well as a clinical trial in which Internet training and phone conversations were used to increase the mediators of autonomy, competence, and relatedness, which in turn increased quality of life among newly diagnosed breast cancer patients (7).

The purpose of this chapter is to describe how mediation analysis can be incorporated into technology-based research. We begin by providing a broad overview of mediation that applies to both technological and non-technological contexts. Later, we discuss issues particular to mediation with technology-based interventions. We start with the cross-sectional mediation model for data collected from each participant at only one timepoint during a study. As an example of a cross-sectional mediation study, consider an intervention for test anxiety. The intervention or control procedure (X) is delivered immediately prior to a test. At the same time as delivery of the

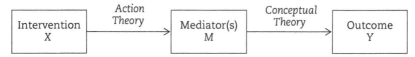

FIGURE 13.1: Action and conceptual theory for an intervention model.

test, researchers also collect a measure of anxiety (M), which is thought to mediate the relationship between the intervention and the outcome, test performance (Y). Mediation analysis addresses whether the intervention improved test performance, and whether decreases in anxiety mediated the effect. We then describe the multilevel longitudinal mediation model, where measurement of X, M, and/or Y occurs at multiple points in time. Using the test anxiety example, the intervention may be enrollment in a special English class that includes anxiety program components, with the control being a normal English class (X), and anxiety (M) and test performance (Y) may be measured monthly over a school year. Because the values of M and Y may vary over time, the data require longitudinal mediation analyses. We focus on a type of multilevel mediation model specific to the case of repeated measures of the intervention (X), the mediating variable (M), and the dependent variable (Y). Finally, we describe how the longitudinal mediation model can answer questions using technology-based tools such as ecological momentary assessment and ecological momentary intervention. Our overall goals are to provide an overview of mediation in technology-based interventions, and to encourage researchers to apply these models to understand mediation processes in their research studies.

OVERVIEW OF THE MEDIATION MODEL

The mediation model includes two important theoretical components (8). The first component, action theory, represents a theory about the relation between the intervention and the mediating variable. For example, in a technology-based Internet intervention program for weight loss, the action theory represents how the behavioral intervention condition changes dietary practices (9). The second component, conceptual theory, represents the relation between the mediating variable and the outcome. In the weight loss intervention example, the conceptual theory

refers to how dietary practices affect weight loss. Figure 13.1 shows how the action and conceptual theory relate to an intervention mediation model.

Both action and conceptual theory are important for the design and evaluation of an intervention. Generally, there must be significant effects of action theory and conceptual theory for the intervention to have an effect on the outcome. If an intervention does not produce a change in the outcome variable, this may be due to a failure of either the action theory, the conceptual theory, or both. Examining both theoretical components of the mediation model may suggest changes needed to enhance an intervention. A nonsignificant action theory component suggests that the intervention itself may need to be improved to more strongly affect the mediator, or that the mediator may need to be measured more accurately. A nonsignificant conceptual theory suggests the possibility of needing to target a different mediator, or that program effects may occur later in time (10). If both action and conceptual theory relations are nonsignificant, then a revised mediation theory must be considered.

For an example of action and conceptual theory in intervention research, perhaps a mobile phone application providing reminders to exercise is successful in increasing the amount of teenagers' physical activity. Investigators may want to know if there were any mediating variables: Did the intervention work because it decreased the teenagers' time in sedentary activity, such as watching television, which in turn increased physical activity, such as engaging in recreational sports or riding their bikes? Alternatively, did the intervention increase their motivation to be physically active, which then increased their physical activity? Identifying the causal chain underlying an observed effect may lead to a more refined intervention that focuses solely on the mediators that produce a change in the desired outcome.

THE CROSS-SECTIONAL MEDIATION MODEL

The basic mediation model, $X \rightarrow M \rightarrow Y$ for cross-sectional data, can be estimated with three regression equations, as shown in Figure 13.2, using notation widely used in the social sciences (1). Equation 1 estimates the effect of the independent variable X on the outcome Y, not accounting for any mediated effects. In terms of the previous technology-based Internet weight loss intervention, this would be a simple estimate of how the membership in the experimental conditions predicts post-intervention body mass index (BMI).

$$Y = i_1 + cX + e_1 \tag{1}$$

In Equation 1, c represents the effect of X on Y. Equation 2 estimates the effect of the independent variable X and the mediator M on the outcome Y.

$$Y = i_2 + c'X + bM + e_2 \tag{2}$$

In Equation 2, c' represents the effect of X on Y, accounting for M. In the example, this would be the effect of the intervention on BMI, accounting for dietary changes. The b coefficient in Equation 2 gives the effect of M on Y, accounting for X. This would be the effect of dietary changes on BMI, accounting for the intervention. Equation 3 estimates the effect of X on M. The coefficient a in this equation estimates the effect of the intervention on dietary changes. The i coefficients and e coefficients in Equations 1–3 represent the intercepts and residual variances, respectively.

$$M = i_3 + aX + e_3 \tag{3}$$

The mediated effect can be estimated by multiplying a and b or by subtracting c minus c' (11).

Choosing Mediators

As described earlier, the informed choice of possible mediators is based on action and conceptual theory. Typically, conceptual theory is based on prior research that provides information about the relation between a potential mediator and the outcome of interest. However, action theory can also inform the selection of mediators, based on what variables can be changed by experimental manipulation or intervention. The choice of approach largely depends on the available information in a particular research domain (1). When there exists substantial prior research on a topic, a theory-driven approach based on empirical results may be used (8,12,13). Mediators may be chosen on the basis of an established theoretical framework in the research area, literature detailing prior mediation analysis, or pilot studies or data. When there exists little prior research to guide the selection of mediator variables (as in newly developing areas of research), less scientifically driven approaches must be used, including determining

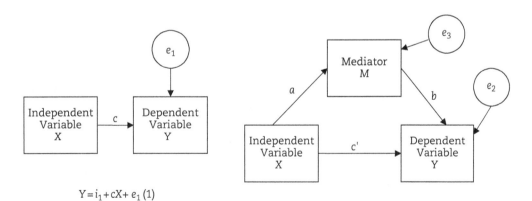

FIGURE 13.2: Single-mediator model in cross-sectional design.

Ms. Baraldi has no disclosures to report.

Ms. Wurpts has no disclosures to report.

Dr. Mackinnon has no disclosures to report.

Dr. Lockhart has no disclosures to report.

mediators on the basis of common sense or a researcher's informed judgment.

In the technology-based health intervention literature, mediators can include variables such as self-efficacy, social norms, and knowledge (of nutrition, exercise, etc.). For example, a Web-based stress reduction intervention was designed to increase mindfulness and decrease procrastination, which in turn decreased stress (6). In this study, mindfulness was examined as a mediator based on previous literature showing the general effectiveness of mindfulness-based stress reduction interventions (14). Procrastination was examined as a mediator because it is a hypothesized cause of stress (15). In both cases, mindfulness and procrastination were targeted on the basis of previous literature that suggested these constructs have an effect on stress. According to action and conceptual theory, the intervention would increase participants' mindfulness and decrease their procrastination, which would lead to reduced stress. In fact, the intervention was successful in decreasing stress, with significant indirect effects through both mindfulness and procrastination (6).

Assumptions of the Mediation Model

Although the basic mediation model provides a framework for testing the mechanism by which X transmits a relation to Y, it has several challenging assumptions. Each regression equation in the single-mediator model requires satisfying the usual assumptions of regression analysis. For instance, the modeled relations must be of the correct functional form, there should be no omitted influences, and the variables should consist of accurate and reliable measures (1,16). Because the mediation model is more complex than standard linear regression, problems resulting from violation of these assumptions may be particularly acute. Furthermore, there are several important assumptions of the single-mediator model beyond the assumptions inherent to regression analysis (1). One of these assumptions is temporal precedence for the $X \to M \to Y$ relation. In other words, X precedes M in time and M precedes Y. Temporal precedence is necessary for inference of causal relationships. A cross-sectional study does not provide convincing evidence for temporal precedence, and researchers must provide evidence for temporal relations from theory or previous empirical research. If X represents randomization

to conditions, then temporal precedence for X to M and X to Y is obtained. However, temporal precedence for the M-to-Y relation is a substantial challenge of mediation analysis, as the mediator often cannot be manipulated prior to measuring Y. Another important assumption is sequential ignorability (17,18). Sequential ignorability holds that the relation between X and M (Sequential Ignorability A), and the relation between M and Y (Sequential Ignorability B), is unaffected by other third variables (such as covariates, confounders, or moderators). Randomizing participants to levels of X satisfies the assumption of Sequential Ignorability A, because randomization balances potential third variables between levels of X (given a large enough sample size). In practice, the assumption of Sequential Ignorability B is met rarely, as participants typically self-select their value of M; it is not randomly assigned to them. A final related assumption is that there are no variables that are affected by the independent variable that subsequently confound the M-to-Y relation.

Causal Inference and the Mediation Model

The mediation model is a causal model, yet the data collected from research studies often do not provide easy causal conclusions. In many research scenarios, X represents randomization to one of two treatment conditions. In the case where X is a randomly assigned condition, the coefficients b and c' in Equation 2 represent adjusted, or conditional, relations. Even though there is random assignment to experimental groups, the b and c' coefficients do not have a clear interpretation as causal effects because participants select their own value of the mediating variable and are therefore susceptible to confounding. This ambiguity of self-selection to the value of the mediator is a primary focus of modern causal inference approaches to mediation. Random assignment to the levels of X is common in many mediation studies, but a second random assignment to the value of M (called double randomization) is rare and often difficult for ethical or logistical reasons. In double-randomization studies, one randomized study evaluates the X-to-M relation and a second randomized study evaluates the M-to-Y relation, adjusting for X (1,19,20).

Two other designs, blockage designs and enhancement designs, can also address the issue of causality in mediation. In blockage designs, a manipulation is used to block or prevent the mediation process, thereby demonstrating that the mediator was crucial (1,21). If the blocking manipulation removes the mediation relation, this provides support for a mediational process. As an example of a blockage design, consider a scenario in which all high school freshmen are provided with access to an Internet resource page to help support them during their freshman year. One feature of this resource page is access to counselors and tutors providing support electronically. The intervention website (X) is thought to increase access to emotional and academic support (M) and thus increase GPA (Y). Using a blockage design, participants may be assigned to a blocking treatment condition where the amount of online emotional support available was limited. If support is a mediator of the relationship between the Internet resource page and GPA, then participants in the blockage treatment condition should not show as large a mediated effect as participants in the control condition because the mediating process was blocked. Closely related is the enhancement design, the aim of which is to enhance (rather than eliminate, as in the blockage design) the mediated effect in the treatment group. In this design, those in the enhancement intervention group would use a resource page that provided a deeper level of support (e.g., 24/7 resources, video calling, more types of resources). In an enhancement design, participants in the enhancement treatment condition ideally show larger mediated effects than participants in other conditions. For other examples, see MacKinnon (1); Maxwell, Bashook, and Sandlow (22); and Klesges, Vasey, and Glasgow (23).

When randomization of X and/or M is not possible, there are ways to strengthen causal arguments. For one, researchers may include measures of confounding variables that may explain the X-to-M and M-to-Y relations and thereby obtain estimates adjusted for the relations. Researchers may also use measures of possible confounders in modern causal analysis methods such as propensity score methods; these methods incorporate measures of confounders in weighted analysis to obtain unbiased estimates (24). Covariates may also be used in principal strata methods; these methods analyze data on the basis of different types of responses to the intervention (25,26). To investigate the sensitivity of research conclusions to potential omitted variables, there are methods that estimate the size of a confounder effect and determine if it is plausible that the confounder influenced the mediated effect (27–29). Furthermore, variations on experimental design (such as blockage and enhancement designs) and follow-up research focusing on testing the consistency and specificity of mediation relations across different contexts, subgroups, and measures of the mediating and outcome variables can further enhance causal inference (19).

EXPANDING THE BASIC MEDIATION MODEL TO LONGITUDINAL DESIGNS

We now expand the discussion to intervention designs with longitudinal data. When investigating mediational relations, longitudinal models can help explicate the mediating process. Furthermore, as will be explored later, the increasingly popular methods of ecological momentary assessment and intervention necessitate analyses that take into account how daily (or hourly, weekly, etc.) measures are nested within participants.

There are three benefits of using longitudinal data (1). First, longitudinal data can provide more information regarding the temporal precedence among the independent variables, mediators, and outcomes. In fact, technically, mediation is a process that necessitates the use of longitudinal data because of its emphasis on the causal relations between variables. Rather than relying on prior research and theory, a longitudinal model can elucidate whether changes in X occur prior to changes in M and whether changes in M occur prior to changes in Y. Second, longitudinal data, unlike cross-sectional data that only assess differences among individuals, permit examination of changes both within and between individuals. This is particularly important, because the nature of the changes within individuals may be different from the changes between individuals. Third, longitudinal data help to reveal some alternative explanations of cross-sectional mediated effects. Because each participant's own score on repeated measures can serve as a control, longitudinal data remove some of the potential omitted variable explanations found in cross-sectional data.

Details of the Longitudinal Mediation Model

There are two general frameworks for longitudinal mediational models: (1) the multilevel framework and (2) the multilevel structural equation modeling (MSEM) framework. This chapter will focus on the multilevel framework, as it is more easily understood by those without a strong SEM background; mediation in the MSEM framework has been explained further in other literature (30,31).

Before delving into the mediation aspect of the multilevel modeling approach for repeated measures observations, it is important to understand basic multilevel equations; for a full treatment of multilevel modeling, see Raudenbush and Bryk (32). In any given study, researchers may assess measures repeatedly across time—time varying—and measures that vary between individuals—time invariant. In a multilevel model with repeated observations within participants, the time-varying variables (i.e., variables that could potentially differ at each measurement occasion) are included in an individual growth model. To add context, time-varying predictors might include daily caloric intake, weekly systolic blood pressure, or daily number of social media posts. This level 1 growth model, which expresses a time-varying outcome variable as a function of the time-varying variable(s), is expressed as:

$$Y_{ti} = \beta_{0i} + \beta_{1i} X_{ti} + \varepsilon_{ti} \ (\text{Level-1}) \tag{4}$$

where subscript i denotes the ith participant in the sample and subscript t denotes time (i.e., measurement occasion). Thus, Y_{ti} denotes the value of person i's outcome variable at time t, β_{0i} denotes person i's intercept (i.e., value of Y at $t = 0$), and β_{1i} denotes a person's linear coefficient (i.e., slope). The final term, ε_{ti}, indicates each person's residual error at time t. Stated differently, the residual represents the difference between the predicted scores and the observed scores for each person at each value of time. In basic terms, the level 1 model applies a separate regression equation to each individual's set of scores. As an example, X might be daily level of anxiety and Y might be number of calories consumed. Equation 4 models each individual's relation between anxiety and caloric intake. If growth over time is predicted, as is often hypothesized in educational or developmental

research, then the model also includes the variable that measures time.

Next, the level 2 model, expressed in multiple equations, quantifies between-person differences.

$$\beta_{0i} = \gamma_{00} + \gamma_{01}Z + \zeta_{0i} \tag{5}$$

$$\beta_{1i} = \gamma_{10} + \gamma_{11}Z + \zeta_{1i} \tag{6}$$

In Equations 5 and 6, Z is a time invariant predictor. In other words, Z is a variable that remains stable across all waves (e.g., gender and ethnicity do not change over time). Note that the dependent variables in Equations 5 and 6 are the intercept and slope parameters from Equation 4. Equation 5 predicts the level 1 intercepts (β_{0i}) and slopes (β_{1i}) as a function of the level 2 variable, Z. Both of the level 2 equations include a residual term denoted by ζ_i. These residual terms denote individual deviations from the group predicted intercept and slope values.

Now that we have reviewed the general multilevel model, we turn to a multilevel mediation model. Recall that these models may include both variables that are measured repeatedly across time (i.e., time varying) and variables that vary between individuals (i.e., time invariant). To expand the single-mediator model from a cross-sectional design in Equation 1 to a longitudinal design, one must consider whether X, M, and Y are time varying and belong in the level 1 equation or time invariant and belong in the level 2 equation(s). A longitudinal single-mediator model is composed of any combination of time-varying and time-invariant variables, and the nuances of such an analysis depend on the nature of X, M, and Y. Table 13.1 is adapted from Card (31) and provides all possible combinations for a single-mediator model.

To illustrate substantively how various mediation models might consider X, M, and Y at varying levels, consider a study evaluating daily nutritional intake. An example of a 1-1-1 mediation model might be that high daily anxiety levels (X) increase daily caloric intake (M), which in turn increases daily feelings of negative self-worth among a sample of participants with binge-eating disorder (Y). In a 2-2-1 model, a nutritional intervention given at the beginning of measurement (level 2) may increase overall knowledge

TABLE 13.1. POSSIBLE COMBINATIONS OF TIME-VARYING AND TIME-INVARIANT VARIABLES FOR A MEDIATION MODEL

Model	X	M	Y
1-1-1	Time varying (level 1)	Time varying (level 1)	Time varying (level 1)
1-1-2	Time varying (level 1)	Time varying (level 1)	Time invariant (level 2)
1-2-1	Time varying (level 1)	Time invariant (level 2)	Time varying (level 1)
1-2-2	Time varying (level 1)	Time invariant (level 2)	Time invariant (level 2)
2-1-1	Time invariant (level 2)	Time varying (level 1)	Time varying (level 1)
2-1-2	Time invariant (level 2)	Time varying (level 1)	Time invariant (level 2)
2-2-1	Time invariant (level 2)	Time invariant (level 2)	Time varying (level 1)

Note. Adopted from Card (31). Model 2-2-2 was not included because in a two-level data structure, a 2-2-2 model is actually a cross-sectional model as described at the beginning of this chapter.

of nutrition (level 2), which then predicts an increase in daily fruit and vegetable consumption (level 1). Likewise, in a 2-1-1 model, a nutritional intervention (level 2) may decrease the number of times a participant chooses unhealthy snacks each day (level 1), which then may increase fruit and vegetable consumption (level 1). Virtually any combination of level 1 and level 2 models may be incorporated into the mediation model framework (although a 2-2-2 model is just the basic mediator model from Equations 1–3). In this chapter we will focus primarily on the 1-1-1 model. For information on other types of longitudinal mediation models, please see Card (31) or MacKinnon (1). For purposes of this chapter, we have limited the discussion to models with only two levels: repeated measures nested within participants. These models can be expanded to three (or even more) levels. For example, a research study might have repeated measures (level 1) nested within students (level 2) nested within classrooms or schools (level 3). Alternatively, in the case of ecological momentary assessment data (discussed later), observations may be nested within days (level 2), which are then nested within individuals (level 3).

Multilevel Mediation Models for 1-1-1 Design

The multilevel mediation model for 1-1-1 designs (MLM 1-1-1) has been discussed extensively in several places (33–36). If *X*, *M*, and *Y* are all measured at level 1, then two sets of multilevel equations are used to evaluate mediation. The first set of equations quantifies the *a* path and is the multilevel analogue to Equation 3 predicting *M* from *X*.

$$M_{ti} = \beta_{0i} + \beta_{1i}X_{ti} + \beta_{2i}M_{ti} + \varepsilon_{ti} \tag{7}$$

$$\beta_{0i} = \gamma_{00} + \zeta_{0i} \tag{8}$$

$$\beta_{1i} = \gamma_{10} + \zeta_{1i} \tag{9}$$

In these equations, γ_{10} corresponds to the *a* path. Any additional time-invariant (level 2) variables can be added to Equations 8 and 9. Likewise, Equation 7 may include any time-varying (level 2) covariates, just as in Equation 3.

The second set of equations used to address mediation in the MLM 1-1-1 model regress *Y* on *M*, controlling for *X*. The next set of equations quantifies the *b* and *c′* paths and is analogous to Equation 1 in the basic mediator model.

$$Y_{ti} = \beta_{0i} + \beta_{1i}X_{ti} + \beta_{2i}M_{ti} + \varepsilon_{ti} \tag{10}$$

$$\beta_{0i} = \gamma_{00} + \zeta_{0i} \tag{11}$$

$$\beta_{1i} = \gamma_{10} + \zeta_{1i} \tag{12}$$

$$\beta_{2i} = \gamma_{20} + \zeta_{2i} \tag{13}$$

Here, γ_{20} corresponds to the *b* path. The estimate of the mediated effect is the product of γ_{10} from Equation 9 and γ_{20} from Equation 13. To illustrate, consider an example where participants receive a daily motivating text. Participants in the treatment group (*X* = 1) receive information on the benefits of healthy food choices, and participants in the control group $(X = 0)$ receive a generic inspirational message. Participants are also measured on their daily desire to eat healthy food, M, and amount of junk food consumption, Y. The set of equations above can be used to estimate the mediated effect and determine if the program decreases junk food consumption mediated by desire to consume health food. Note that there are some nuanced decisions in such an analysis, including whether or not the slopes (β's) may vary across individuals. For more discussion on this, see Bauer, Preacher, and Gill (33), or Kenny, Korchmaros, and Bolger (35).

TECHNOLOGY-BASED DATA AND INTERVENTIONS

So far, we have discussed mediation analysis in the context of testing intervention programs—*any* intervention program. The next question to ask is, "What might be different when the data collection methods or interventions are technologically based?" From an analytical standpoint, there is nothing different. Assuming the technological intervention targets some mediator, M, which is then theorized to change some outcome, Y, a straightforward cross-sectional technology prevention program can be evaluated like any prevention program—technology or otherwise. From a theoretical or substantive standpoint, the nature of the technological intervention informs action theory. Recall from the earlier discussion of choosing mediators that a researcher must consider what the prior literature suggests regarding action and conceptual theory for an outcome targeted for change. Because some forms of technology are newer, there may not be a lot of existing literature to aid in making these decisions. Relations may be inferred from non-technical interventions, but researchers should consider the nuanced effect of the technology on action theory.

Another theoretical issue in technology-based interventions is that similar interventions delivered via technological means instead of conventional means may have different mediators linking the same intervention to the same desired outcome. For example, consider an intervention to increase efficacy to make healthy snack choices. Delivered in a weekly support group, this intervention may result in group camaraderie and personal attention from the leader (mediators), which in turn increase participants' efficacy to make healthy snack choices. The same intervention delivered via technological means may also be effective, but the effects may occur through different mediators. Delivered regularly via text, the intervention may increase mindfulness about eating (mediator) during times and situations when people choose snacks, which then increases efficacy to make healthy snack choices. An intervention delivered via weekly support group may not have an effect on the mindfulness mediator, and an intervention delivered via text may not have an effect on group camaraderie. The differences in mechanisms of action between technologically based interventions and traditional interventions illustrate why a thorough understanding of action theory is so important in intervention research.

In addition, while many interventions take place in a clinical or laboratory environment, technological interventions and their subsequent data are increasingly delivered and collected in a naturalistic environment (ecological) and in real time (momentary). Ecological momentary assessment (EMA) and ecological momentary interventions (EMI) are becoming increasingly popular now that technology is less expensive and more easily accessed by research participants. These methods often provide large data sets that are rich in potential information but potentially cumbersome in analysis. EMI can result in personalized adaptive interventions that result in more complex action theory than a traditional intervention. For example, each person may have a distinctive set of targeted mediators.

ECOLOGICAL MOMENTARY ASSESSMENT TO IDENTIFY MEDIATORS

EMA data are characterized by the repeated collection of real-time data (37,38). Although methods for collecting data vary and are not necessarily limited to technological means of assessment, most applications of EMA rely on the use of technology to collect data. The benefit of EMA research is the reduction of recall bias and the ability to study processes over time. One of the most common methods uses electronic diaries and questionnaires. With the increasing abundance of participant-owned smartphones, EMA is becoming even easier, because a smartphone application can often replace the need for a researcher-provided device.

Schwartz and Stone (39) have outlined a series of questions that can be answered by real-time momentary data. Many of these questions can be adapted to identify potential mechanisms of an intervention that are illustrated here with data from an EMA study designed to identify mechanisms for an intervention. Grenard and colleagues (40) evaluated the cues associated with eating behavior in a group of adolescents. In this study, participants between the ages of 14 and 17 years self-reported their food consumption and responded to a variety of questions identifying their location, who they were with, their mood, and what they ate. These same questions were also prompted randomly to assess similar information when participants were not eating. Daily summaries regarding mood, stress, and food availability were collected once a day. Additionally, demographic information and other presumably stable measures were collected on each participant, such as physical characteristics (height, weight, measure of pubertal development), basic demographics, self-reported food consumption, family environment, and physical activity. For purposes of illustration, we ignore the day level and consider two levels of variables: 1) the level 1 time-varying momentary assessments with many observations per participant, and 2) the level 2 time-invariant variables (e.g., demographics and one-time surveys) measured once per participant. Using this data structure, we will illustrate the ways that Schwartz and Stone's questions may inform development of interventions and a greater understanding of the mechanism of an intervention.

Question 1: Is this intervention worth doing? By asking this question, the researcher can determine if there are variations in behaviors of interest between participants. For example, we can determine if there are between-subject differences in sweet-snack cravings. In other words, do adolescents differ in their average level of sweet-snack cravings? This question can be answered by the unconditional multilevel model:

$$Cravings_{ti} = \beta_{0i} + \varepsilon_{ti} \,(\text{Level-1}) \tag{14}$$

$$\beta_{0i} = \gamma_{00} + \zeta_{0i} \,(\text{Level-2}) \tag{15}$$

In Equation 14, β_{0i} is the participant's mean, and the residual term, ε_{ti}, is the deviation from the individual's mean. In Equation 15, γ_{00} is the grand mean, and ζ_{0i} denotes a person's mean deviation from the grand mean.

Question 2: Is there a particular group that needs the intervention more than another group? In terms of the obesity research example, a question could be "Do cravings vary by gender?" Again, this question can be answered by specifying a set of multilevel models:

$$Cravings_{ti} = \beta_{0i} + \varepsilon_{ti} \,(\text{Level-1}) \tag{16}$$

$$\beta_{0i} = \gamma_{00} + \gamma_{01} \, GENDER_i + \zeta_{0i} \,(\text{Level-2}) \tag{17}$$

The coefficient γ_{01} provides information regarding whether the time-invariant variable gender predicts mean levels of cravings. A significant γ_{01} indicates that gender is a predictor of cravings.

Question 3: Are there malleable predictors or cues that can be targeted by the intervention? Here we consider time-varying predictors and are looking to see if one variable is related to another variable. For example, are increases in embarrassment related to increases in sweet-snack cravings? To answer this question, we add embarrassment as a level 1 predictor model. Thus our set of predictive equations is:

$$Cravings_{ti} = \beta_{0i} + \beta_{1i} Embarass + \varepsilon_{ti} \,(\text{Level-1}) \tag{18}$$

$$\beta_{0i} = \gamma_{00} + \zeta_{0i} \,(\text{Level-2}) \tag{19}$$

$$\beta_1 = \gamma_{10} \,(\text{Level-2}) \tag{20}$$

Note that Equation 20 does not include a residual term. The lack of a residual term treats the slope of the relation between embarrassment and cravings as a fixed effect and assumes the effect is the same for all participants. By adding a residual term, we can answer the next question.

Question 4: Do these malleable predictors vary across individuals?

$$Cravings_{ti} = \beta_{0i} + \beta_{1i} Embarass_{ti} + \varepsilon_{ti} \,(\text{Level-1}) \tag{21}$$

$$\beta_{0i} = \gamma_{00} + \zeta_{0i} \,(\text{Level-2}) \tag{22}$$

$$\beta_1 = \gamma_{10} + \zeta_{1i} \text{ (Level-2)} \qquad (23)$$

Note that Equations 21 and 22 are identical to Equations 18 and 19. The variation of the equation to answer this question lies in the residual term in Equation 23. By adding this term, the slope relating embarrassment and cravings is a random effect, allowing this relation to vary within person. This addresses potential individual differences in the relation between cravings and embarrassment.

Question 5: Are there particular individuals who benefit most from changing these malleable predictors or cues that can be targeted for the intervention? For example, the researcher might theorize that differences in the relation of embarrassment and cravings are associated with gender. To address this question, GENDER is added to the equation predicting the level 1 intercept (Equation 22 turns into Equation 25) and potentially added to the equation predicting the level 1 slope (Equation 23 turns into Equation 26).

$$Cravings_{ti} = \beta_{0i} + \beta_{1i} Embarass_{ti} + \varepsilon_{ti} \text{ (Level-1)} \quad (24)$$

$$\beta_{0i} = \gamma_{00} + \gamma_{01} Gender_i + \zeta_{0i} \text{ (Level-2)} \qquad (25)$$

$$\beta_{1i} = \gamma_{10} + \gamma_{11} Gender_i + \zeta_{1i} \text{ (Level-2)} \qquad (26)$$

By including GENDER in Equation 26, we are now evaluating a cross-level interaction. This can be observed by combining Equations 24–26 into one model, by replacing β_{0i} and β_{1i} in Equation 24 with the expressions in Equations 25 and 26.

$$
\begin{aligned}
Cravings_{ti} = {} & \gamma_{00} + \gamma_{01} Gender + \zeta_{0i} \\
& + (\gamma_{10} + \gamma_{11} Gender + \zeta_{0i}) \\
& \times Embarass + \varepsilon_{ti}
\end{aligned} \qquad (27)
$$

With algebraic manipulation, the resulting combined equation can be expressed as:

$$
\begin{aligned}
Cravings_{ti} = {} & \gamma_{00} + \gamma_{01} Gender_i + \zeta_{0i} \\
& + \gamma_{10} Embarass_{ti} \\
& + \gamma_{11} Gender_i \times Embarass_{ti} \\
& + \zeta_{0i} Embarass_{ti} + \varepsilon_{ti}
\end{aligned} \qquad (28)
$$

The coefficient, γ_{11}, quantifies this cross-sectional interaction effect, which addresses the question of whether the relation between embarrassment and cravings is moderated by gender. Just as in a cross-sectional interaction, it is advisable to compare a main-effect-only model (GENDER not included in Equation 26) with the cross-level interaction (GENDER included in Equation 26) to assess the extent to which adding the interaction improves the model.

EMA data are rich information. Typically, participants provide information many times on each variable, resulting in a complex, but bountiful, data structure. The number of research questions that may be addressed are extensive. Fortunately, the multilevel framework provides a way to answer these questions. Furthermore, these questions may be addressed in more complex multilevel models. For example, in the nutrition research example, moments are nested within days, which are nested within participants. The questions and equations above can be expanded to a model in which observations are a level 1 variable, daily responses are at level 2, and participant-level attributes are level 3 variables. In an educational study, observations (level 1) are often nested within students (level 2), which are nested within classrooms (level 3) and subsequently nested within schools (level 4). For additional resources on multilevel models, see Raudenbush and Bryk (32).

ECOLOGICAL MOMENTARY INTERVENTIONS AND ADAPTIVE INTERVENTIONS

Ecological momentary interventions are interventions that, like EMA, are delivered to people as they go about their daily lives. These interventions can be delivered in natural settings when the intervention is most needed. Because EMI can provide treatment in real-world settings, people have instantaneous opportunity to practice skills learned in the intervention, which makes the effects of intervention programs more generalizable (41). EMI are typically delivered via mobile electronic devices, such as handheld computers or personal digital assistants, which allow the intervention to be delivered at any time. EMI are by definition delivered to people in their natural environment and at specific moments of everyday life, but they can take on further ecological validity if they include elements of adaptive interventions that are specifically tailored to individual needs.

As an example of EMI, a smoking cessation intervention was delivered via text message to smokers in New Zealand using an automated system, and the messages were individualized to the participant (42). This individualization of health messages has shown effectiveness for smoking cessation, consumption of dietary fat and fruits and vegetable, mammography, and physical activity (43). Not only can the content of an intervention be tailored to the individual, but the timing of the intervention can be tailored to when each individual is most in need of support (41). The use of EMI enables the possibility of using technology to implement adaptive interventions. Interventions that are tailored as needed—adaptive interventions—more closely resemble a clinical administration in that there is potential for different "dosages" of different intervention components to be delivered on different administration questions in response to the needs of the individual (44).

What Is an Adaptive Intervention?

An adaptive intervention adapts the intervention to the needs of the individual in real time, based on the current state of the individual. Rather than a fixed dosage, schedule, and program as for most interventions, adaptive interventions are tailored to be the best response based on the individual's current state (Chapter 12) (44). Decision rules are used to link characteristics of a person to different program components. For example, a decision rule might state that any people with stage 1 hypertension will receive a message instructing them to eat only 1,500 milligrams of sodium per day each time that they eat. Importantly, these methods can be developed using modern causal inference techniques to address some of the assumptions of mediation mentioned earlier—especially the role of confounding variables. Murphy (45) advocates using sequential multiple assignment randomized trials (SMART) to develop adaptive intervention strategies. The use of randomized experimentation supports the ability to make valid inferences about adaptive interventions. For further information on the use of SMART methodology in adaptive interventions, including detailed examples, see additional resources (46–49).

An adaptive intervention is not necessarily technology based, but the advent of EMI-administered data opens up a new frontier for implementation of an intervention that is not only adaptive based on the individual, but adaptive in terms of program delivery over time. In future

research, EMA analyses may be combined with EMI adaptive interventions. Mediators targeting the outcomes may be identified in an initial EMA study, and interventions may be fine-tuned to address person-specific mediators or be delivered at person-specific time intervals during the course of an adaptive EMI protocol. Furthermore, interventions may be tailored in real time such that a person's response at one time will serve as a tailoring variable for the intervention they receive the next time.

Intensive Longitudinal Data

EMA and EMI studies generally involve many repeated measures (38). There is a varying intensity of assessment, with some studies implementing a dense schedule of assessment (50) over a period of days or perhaps only once a day for a period as long as a year (51). As a result, researchers typically obtain intensive longitudinal data. According to Bolger and Laurenceau (34), intensive longitudinal data may be defined as "any study with enough repeated measurements to model a distinct change process for each individual." The exact definition of this largely depends on the phenomena being evaluated and the length of the change process, but Bolger and Laurenceau (34) recommend a minimum of five observations, as these are enough data points to descriptively and graphically provide information of change for a given participant. In other words, in intensive longitudinal data, it would be possible to analyze trends and growth curves for each participant as separate entities. Methods for evaluating intensive longitudinal data are important and can determine whether causal processes actually occur in real-world settings. Fortunately, evaluating a mediation method with intensive longitudinal data is no different than implementing the 1-1-1 model previously discussed. The added data points increase the power to detect the mediated effect. For more information on within-subject mediation analysis for intensive longitudinal data, see Chapter 9 in Bolger and Laurenceau (34).

CONCLUSIONS

This chapter combined traditional mediation models (commonly used in intervention studies) with longitudinal mediation methods useful for technology-based interventions such as EMI and EMA. EMA studies collect data in real time and in a natural environment. Similarly, EMIs can be delivered to participants in real time and in natural settings. Generally, these methods rely on mobile technology to collect data and deliver interventions. This allows for data and interventions to achieve high levels of ecological validity, as EMA and EMI take place in real-world settings, rather than clinical settings such as a therapist's office. Such interventions can achieve even more ecological validity, by adapting the intervention to person-specific needs. Mediators collected from EMA studies may be used to further tailor interventions. Overall, technology-based interventions and assessment methods provide unique opportunities to further understand the theoretical mechanisms of change.

REFERENCES

1. MacKinnon DP. *Introduction to Statistical Mediation Analysis*. Mahwah, NJ: Lawrence Erlbaum Associates; 2008.

2. Dodge KA. Social-cognitive mechanisms in the development of conduct disorder and depression. *Annual Review of Psychology* 1993; 44:559–584.

3. Li X, Hartwell KJ, Owens M, Lematty T, Borckardt JJ, Hanlon CA, et al. Repetitive transcranial magnetic stimulation of the dorsolateral prefrontal cortex reduces nicotine cue craving. *Biological Psychiatry* 2013; 73(8):714–720.

4. Anderson-Bill ES, Winett RA, Wojcik JR, Williams DM. Aging and the social cognitive determinants of physical activity behavior and behavior change: Evidence from the Guide to Health Trial. *Journal of Aging Research 2011*; 2011: 505928. Retrieved from http://www.hindawi.com/journals/jar/2011/505928/abs/

5. Izquierdo R, Lagua CT, Meyer S, Ploutz-Snyder RJ, Palmas W, Eimicke JP, et al. Telemedicine intervention effects on waist circumference and body mass index in the IDEATel project. *Diabetes Technology & Therapeutics* 2010; 12(3):213–220.

6. Drozd F, Raeder S, Kraft P, Bjørkli CA. Multilevel growth curve analyses of treatment effects of a Web-based intervention for stress reduction: Randomized controlled trial. *Journal of Medical Internet Research* 2013; 15(4):e84.

7. Hawkins RP, Pingree S, Shaw B, Serlin RC, Swoboda C, Han J-Y, et al. Mediating processes of two communication interventions for breast cancer patients. *Patient Education and Counseling* 2010; 81(Supplement 1):S48–S53.

8. Chen H. *Theory-Driven Evaluations*. Newbury Park, CA: Sage; 1990.

9. White MA, Martin PD, Newton RL, Walden HM, York-Crowe EE, Gordon ST, et al. Mediators of weight loss in a family-based intervention presented over the internet. *Obesity Research* 2004; 12(7):1050–1059.

10. MacKinnon DP, Fairchild AJ, Fritz MS. Mediation analysis. *Annual Review of Psychology* 2007; 58(1):593–614.

11. Mackinnon DP, Dwyer JH. Estimating mediated effects in prevention studies. *Evaluation Review* 1993; 17(2):144–158.

12. Lipsey MW. Theory as method: Small theories of treatments. *New Directions in Program Evaluation* 1993; 57:5–38.

13. Sidani S, Sechrest L. Putting program theory into operation. *American Journal of Evaluation* 1999; 20(2):227–238.

14. Chiesa A, Serretti A. Mindfulness-based stress reduction for stress management in healthy people: A review and meta-analysis. *Journal of Alternative & Complementary Medicine* 2009; 15(5):593–600.

15. Stead R, Shanahan MJ, Neufeld RWJ. "I'll go to therapy, eventually": Procrastination, stress and mental health. *Personal and Individual Differences* 2010; 49(3):175–180.

16. Cohen J, Cohen J. *Applied Multiple Regression/Correlation Analysis for the Behavioral Sciences*. Mahwah, NJ: Lawrence Erlbaum Associates; 2003.

17. Imai K, Keele L, Tingley D. A general approach to causal mediation analysis. *Psychological Methods* 2010; 15(4):309–334.

18. Lynch KG, Cary M, Gallop R, Have TRT. Causal mediation analyses for randomized trials. *Health Services Outcomes Research Methodology* 2008; 8(2):57–76.

19. MacKinnon DP, Pirlott AG. Statistical approaches for enhancing causal interpretation of the M to Y relation in mediation analysis. *Personality and Social Psychology Review* 2014; pii: 1088868314542878.

20. Spencer SJ, Zanna MP, Fong GT. Establishing a causal chain: Why experiments are often more effective than mediational analyses in examining psychological processes. *Journal of Personal and Social Psychology* 2005; 89(6):845–851.

21. Robins JM, Greenland S. Identifiability and exchangeability for direct and indirect effects. *Epidemiology* 1992; 3(2):143–155.

22. Maxwell, JA, Bashook PG, Sandlow CJ. Combining ethnographic and experimental methods in educational research: A case study. In Fetterman DM, Pitman MA (eds.), *Educational Evaluation: Ethnography in Theory, Practice, and Politics*.Thousand Oaks, CA: Sage Publications; 1986, pp. 121–43.

23. Klesges RC, Vasey MM, Glasgow RE. A worksite smoking modification competition: Potential for public health impact. *American Journal of Public Health* 1986; 76(2):198–200.

24. Coffman DL. Estimating causal effects in mediation analysis using propensity scores. *Structural Equation Modeling* 2011; *18*(3):357–369.

25. Jo B. Causal inference in randomized experiments with mediational processes. *Psychological Methods* 2008; *13*(4):314–36.

26. Jo B, Stuart EA, MacKinnon DP, Vinokur AD. The use of propensity scores in mediation analysis. *Multivariate Behavioral Research* 2011; *46*(3):425–452.

27. Cox MG, Miocevic M, MacKinnon DP. Sensitivity plots for confounder bias in the single mediator model. *Evaluation Review* 2013; *37*(5):405–431.

28. Imai K, Keele L, Yamamoto T. Identification, inference and sensitivity analysis for causal mediation effects. *Statistical Science* 2010; *25*(1):51–71.

29. VanderWeele TJ. Bias formulas for sensitivity analysis for direct and indirect effects. *Epidemiology* 2010; *21*(4):540–551.

30. Preacher KJ, Zyphur MJ, Zhang Z. A general multilevel SEM framework for assessing multilevel mediation. *Psychological Methods* 2010; *15*(3):209–233.

31. Card NA. Multilevel mediation analysis in the study of daily lives. In Mehl MR, Conner TS (eds.), *Handbook of Research Methods for Studying Daily Life.* New York: Guilford Press; 2012, pp. 479–494.

32. Raudenbush SW, Bryk AS. *Hierarchical Linear Models: Applications and Data Analysis Methods.* Thousand Oaks, CA: Sage Publications; 2002.

33. Bauer DJ, Preacher KJ, Gil KM. Conceptualizing and testing random indirect effects and moderated mediation in multilevel models: New procedures and recommendations. *Psychological Methods* 2006; *11*(2):142–163.

34. Bolger N, Laurenceau J-P. *Intensive Longitudinal Methods: An Introduction to Diary and Experience Sampling Research.* New York: Guilford Press; 2013.

35. Kenny DA, Korchmaros JD, Bolger N. Lower level mediation in multilevel models. *Psychological Methods* 2003; *8*(2):115–128.

36. Jose PE. *Doing Statistical Mediation and Moderation.* New York: Guilford Press; 2013.

37. Stone AA, Shiffman S. Ecological momentary assessment (EMA) in behavorial medicine. *Annals of Behavioral Medicine* 1994; *16*(3):199–202.

38. Shiffman S, Stone AA, Hufford MR. Ecological momentary assessment. *Annual Review of Clinical Psychology* 2008; *4*:1–32.

39. Schwartz, JE, Stone AA. The analysis of real-time momentary data: A practical guide. In Stone A, Shiffman S, Atienza A, Nebeling L (eds.), *The Science of Real-Time Data Capture: Self-Report in Health Research.* New York: Oxford University Press; 2007, pp. 76–113.

40. Grenard JL, Stacy AW, Shiffman S, Baraldi AN, MacKinnon DP, Lockhart G, et al. Sweetened drink and snacking cues in adolescents. A study using ecological momentary assessment. *Appetite* 2013; *67*:61–73.

41. Heron KE, Smyth JM. Ecological momentary interventions: Incorporating mobile technology into psychosocial and health behaviour treatments. *British Journal of Health Psychology* 2010; *15*(1):1–39.

42. Rodgers A, Corbett T, Bramley D, Riddell T, Wills M, Lin R-B, et al. Do u smoke after txt? Results of a randomised trial of smoking cessation using mobile phone text messaging. *Tobacco Control* 2005; *14*(4):255–261.

43. Kreuter MW, Strecher VJ, Glassman B. One size does not fit all: The case for tailoring print materials. *Annals of Behavioral Medicine* 1999; *21*(4):276–283.

44. Collins LM, Murphy SA, Bierman KL. A conceptual framework for adaptive preventive interventions. *Prevention Science* 2004; *5*(3):185–196.

45. Murphy SA. An experimental design for the development of adaptive treatment strategies. *Statistical Medicine* 2005; *24*(10):1455–1481.

46. Almirall D, McCaffrey DF, Ramchand R, Murphy SA. Subgroups analysis when treatment and moderators are time-varying. *Prevention Science* 2013; *14*(2):169–178.

47. Collins LM, Murphy SA, Nair VN, Strecher VJ. A strategy for optimizing and evaluating behavioral interventions. *Annals of Behavioral Medicine* 2005; *30*(1):65–73.

48. Collins LM, Murphy SA, Strecher V. The multiphase optimization strategy (MOST) and the sequential multiple assignment randomized trial (SMART): New methods for more potent eHealth interventions. *American Journal of Preventive Medicine* 2007; *32*(5, Supplement):S112–S118.

49. Murphy SA, Lynch KG, Oslin D, McKay JR, TenHave T. Developing adaptive treatment strategies in substance abuse research. *Drug and Alcohol Dependence* 2007; *88*(Supplement 2):S24–S30.

50. Shapiro D, Jamner LD, Davydov DM, James P. Situations and moods associated with smoking in everyday life. *Psychology of Addictive Behavior* 2002; *16*(4):342–345.

51. Jamison RN, Raymond SA, Levine JG, Slawsby EA, Nedeljkovic SS, Katz NP. Electronic diaries for monitoring chronic pain: 1-year validation study. *Pain* 2001; *91*(3):277–285.

14

Economics Analysis of Technology-Based Behavioral Healthcare Systems

DANIEL POLSKY

INTRODUCTION

The concept of technology-based behavioral healthcare systems (that employ Web and mobile tools) has an economic appeal among various actors in the healthcare system, including patients, providers, and insurers. For patients, there is an appeal to taking control of one's own health with the aid of technology. This can reduce the costs of healthcare through fewer direct interactions with the healthcare system, which can be painful, time consuming, and expensive. For providers, off-loading the management of self-care to technology can free up resources to provide higher level care that is more appropriate for the level of training of the provider. For insurers, there is a desire to incentivize the use of technology-based behavioral healthcare systems if they can be leveraged to sufficiently reduce downstream care that can be more expensive than the implementation of the use of these technology-based systems.

But the reality is that there are trade-offs between the costs of these systems and their benefits. Thus, the ultimate decision to implement a technology-based behavioral healthcare system will involve determining whether the benefits outweigh the costs. This decision is made more complex by the fact that those that benefit from these systems are not necessarily bearing the costs. As a result, it is entirely possible that even systems that have benefits that far outweigh the costs would not be implemented and systems that do not have benefits that would outweigh the costs would be implemented.

The goal of an economic analysis of technology-based behavioral healthcare systems is first to determine if the intervention is economically beneficial from a societal perspective. The second aim is to identify barriers to adoption, by determining which stakeholders benefit and which ones face the cost burden, so that economic incentives can be created to reduce the barriers to adoption of economically beneficial systems.

ECONOMIC TAXONOMY OF TECHNOLOGY-BASED BEHAVIORAL SYSTEMS

As presented in this content of this book, a technology-based behavioral healthcare system can take many forms and be implemented at various levels of the healthcare system. The economic consequences will depend heavily on which type of system is implemented and at which level of the healthcare system. For the purpose of this chapter I will describe here a simple taxonomy of systems.

The systems that we will consider are those technology-based systems that aim to improve interactions. These interactions can be between providers and patients, between providers and other providers, and between a patient and his or her body. For interactions between providers and patients, there is a traditional aspect, which is based on how the provider interacts toward the patient. These aspects can be enhanced by technology, but the novel aspect of technology here is improving how the patient can interact with the provider, as it enables the provider to monitor the patient outside of the traditional healthcare system and receive feedback about the patient that is automated and potentially actionable. For interactions between providers, technology-based behavioral healthcare systems are generally used to improve care coordination and potentially medication adherence. For interactions between patients and themselves, these are the systems that focus on self-monitoring and self-management. There are two subcategories here. One is where the patient system is linked to a provider, managed by a provider, or initiated by a provider. The other is where the patient is really a consumer and acts entirely outside of the healthcare system to engage in wellness or self-improvement.

When considering an economic analysis, it is important to understand how the technology system fits into the larger healthcare system, as this will drive the potential economic costs and savings. At its core, a technology-based behavioral healthcare system can act as an economic substitute or an economic complement. Economics has a formal definition of goods that are substitutes or complements (1). Consider two goods. The two goods are complements when the greater use of one good leads to a greater use of the second good. For example, peanut butter and jelly are complements. If the price of peanut butter goes down, not only do people buy more peanut butter, they also buy more jelly. The two goods are substitutes when greater use of one good leads to a reduction in the use of the other good. For example, tea and coffee are substitutes.

Some systems are aimed at having the technology replace at least a portion of direct clinical contact. In this case, the system acts as a substitute for clinical care. The clinical argument for this substitution is that it can produce better outcomes through increased fidelity in a scalable way, it provides just-in-time access, and it may increase service capacity. Other tools act as a complement by improving coordination between providers or sharing of information with the provider that can lead to more effective monitoring and direct clinical intervention. This distinction is important for understanding the source of the economic savings. Substitutes can produce direct savings from reduced direct per-patient clinical contact, while complements do not produce this source of savings. In fact, direct costs of clinical care may rise if the technology tool leads to greater access to providers. However, if either the substitute or the complement is effective, there is an opportunity for indirect savings from the potential for downstream savings of healthcare resources. For example, there could be fewer hospitalizations if the technology leads to improved adherence to medication therapy.

PAYING FOR TECHNOLOGY-BASED BEHAVIORAL SYSTEMS

Under payment systems that reward provision of traditional clinical services, such as the fee-for-service model, providers may not be properly incentivized to adopt technology-based systems. If the technology itself does not have a specific reimbursement code from which to receive direct payment, the economic incentive to provide the service would depend on whether the provider paying for the system would be able to sufficiently reduce its operational costs and not its revenue. This is unlikely to occur in a strict fee-for-service system where the reduction in cost is often from a reduction in services provided. If these services are services that have fees attached, the savings themselves do not accrue to the provider that paid for the technology-based system. Systems that substitute for the care of the clinical provider that is in control of the technology are the systems that are most directly faced with this economic barrier. What incentive does a counselor have to reduce counseling time if this would reduce his or her revenue? Now if the counselor was exceedingly busy, then the counselor could see more patients enhanced by the efficiency of technology. But if the opportunity for greater patient flow were not in place, then the substitution of time away from revenue-producing time would not sufficiently incentivize the provider to adopt the new technology.

Incentive challenges also exist for all of these technologies if the savings from improved effectiveness and reduced downstream costs are not at least partially captured by the provider paying for the technology service. It is common to hear about new technologies that make sense for the healthcare system as a result of evidence that these technologies can avoid downstream hospitalizations or other costly health events. It is also common for these beneficial technologies to be underutilized. There is an economic explanation for underutilization. If the provider being asked to invest and adopt the new technology does not receive the economic returns from the downstream savings, these downstream savings will not be factored into the calculation as to whether it would be worth the economic investment in the technology. Systems to improve behavioral health often fall into this category, because improved health behaviors are a major risk factor for developing or exacerbating expensive chronic conditions. As a result, innovations in payment that allow for the user of these technologies to capture downstream savings may be necessary for adequate utilization of technology-based behavioral healthcare systems.

This problem of underinvestment in interventions that may lead to downstream healthcare savings is not limited to technology-based behavioral healthcare systems. As a result, there are a number of healthcare delivery systems that are experimenting with new models of payment that are specifically designed to share some of the potential downstream healthcare expenditure savings between insurers and providers. These payment models are often being developed within accountable care organizations (ACOs). ACOs offer the opportunity to provide the right kind of incentives for adoption of these services.

While the definition of ACOs is evolving, it can be thought of as a voluntarily formed group of doctors, hospitals, and other healthcare providers who organize in some way to deliver more coordinated care. These organized groups then seek to tie their reimbursement to improved quality of care delivery and lower overall healthcare expenses among a population of patients. It is the sharing of savings achieved by these organizations that will induce providers to invest in these behavioral health technologies. The payment models that are being adopted by ACOs are not only sharing savings; others involve risk to the organization if their performance is below expectation, and still others may take the form of capitation. The key to these organizations is that they become accountable for the quality of care delivered to the patients.

Ultimately, barriers to adoption are driven by who pays for the technology. As discussed earlier, if the provider of direct clinical care pays for the service, the cost of the technology is unlikely to be captured by the purchaser of the technology. If the insurer is willing to pay for the technology, they can capture the downstream savings because they are typically the beneficiaries of reduced service use. However, because the provider is typically needed to institute the technology-based service, the payer would still need to create sufficient incentives for the provider to offer this service. They could either adopt a fee-for-service model for the technology itself or consider alternative

payment models to incentivize the provider, such as those being considered by ACOs. When the patient pays, insurance can act as a barrier to adoption. If insurance only covers traditional healthcare services and not technology-based behavioral healthcare systems, the patient would prefer the traditional service because insurance would reduce the out-of-pocket costs for the traditional service and not for the technology-based service. However, if the system is a consumer-oriented system that incentivizes wellness and acts outside of the healthcare system, the myriad of barriers erected by the healthcare system are not present, and the system would be purchased for those who derive sufficient benefit from the system and for those who can afford to pay for the system.

DEVELOPING THE ECONOMIC CASE: ECONOMIC EVALUATIONS OF TECHNOLOGY-BASED BEHAVIORAL INTERVENTIONS

Economic evaluations involve not only assessing the incremental costs of an intervention but also expressing those costs in relation to the effectiveness of an intervention. A great number of effective interventions cost more than any downstream savings they may produce. If the focus is on costs alone, worthwhile interventions may not be adopted. There is a willingness to spend additional dollars to get improved health. But given limited resources, this willingness is not limitless. The cost-effectiveness ratio is an expression of the additional costs of an intervention divided by the additional effectiveness of that intervention. This ratio expresses the trade-off between spending more and getting more in return. There are other ways of expressing this trade-off, such as cost-benefit analysis (2), but the focus here, as in most of the medical literature, will be on cost-effectiveness.

Ideally, there would be an opportunity to conduct an economic evaluation alongside the randomized, clinical trial of the technology-based behavioral intervention, because trial-based economic evaluation offers several advantages over an economic evaluation based on modeling of existing data. First, there is a one-time opportunity to conduct an economic evaluation that would produce results at the time the clinical findings on efficacy or effectiveness are released. This timeliness can be essential in providing needed information to entities when making adoption and reimbursement decisions. Second, the internal validity made possible by randomization applies to economic evaluations as well. An economic model based on data from non-randomized studies suffers from the same internal validity problems that lead one to conduct a clinical trial in the first place. Third, economic evaluations based on clinical trials offers a level of transparency in methods that are lacking in models. Fourth, the cost of a separate retrospective economic evaluation can be much greater than the incremental cost of adding an economic aim to an existing trial.

The design of an economic trial involves four main items: identifying relevant perspective, measurement of benefits, enumeration of costs, and consideration of issues of time horizon and sample size. The perspective from which the study will be conducted should be constructed on the basis of an understanding of who will eventually utilize the findings of the economic investigation. For example, a trial done from a payer's perspective could highlight how much a new treatment will cost for reimbursement purposes, but also how much it could save in terms of reduced downstream medical costs. Once the appropriate perspective(s) is defined, then design can turn to determining which benefits and costs are appropriate to capture and how to measure them. Finally, the time horizon and sample size become critical last items, because these will often differ from the clinical trials time horizon or sample size. Each of these factors will be described in more detail below.

Identifying Relevant Perspective

An economic study's perspective needs to account for the likely set of decision-makers that will be called upon to use the economic findings to make meaningful policy decisions. Conducting an economic evaluation that can provide information relevant for the perspective of the various potential decision makers would be ideal. The perspectives of economic evaluations typically are those of payers, providers, clients, and society as a whole.

Payers and other third parties, such as employers, have a need to determine how to allocate funds and advocate for programs based on potential benefits. Providers may wish to understand the direct financial impact of implementing a program. For the patient or client level, economic evaluations can help to highlight the importance of these programs to the individual, as well as identify potential economic barriers to successful treatment in the real world. The broadest perspective is that of society as a whole. This perspective is necessary for the decision to determine the best allocation of limited resources. This perspective combines the costs and benefits among all stakeholders.

Insurance companies typically need some understanding of the cost implications of a new treatment before authorizing reimbursement for services by providers. An economic evaluation can be an effective tool for helping insurers understand short- and long-term costs and savings for implementing a technology-based service. For example, an initial increase in costs associated with its implementation may lower long-term costs due to decreased utilization of downstream medical care. The rationale for economic studies is strongest for interventions that are expensive and/or interventions that have important downstream economic consequences that are critical to payers. There is also an important rationale for interventions that may not have a standard form of reimbursement, such as a technology-based behavioral intervention. If insurance companies do not have standard ways for reimbursing these new and innovative services, making the economic argument to these stakeholders will be essential if reasonable reimbursement mechanisms are to be developed.

At a very granular level, treatment sites and providers may find clinical evidence compelling but may need further understanding of the initial and recurring costs required to implement a successful treatment program. Providers may require a more limited analysis that provides greater detail on the site-specific budget impact of implementation of a technology-bases system. Site directors and providers may wish to understand the required start-up costs and recurring costs that are needed to assure that the results can be replicated in a real-world setting. This will require an economic analysis that breaks down estimated resource utilization so that site directors and providers can impute costs from their own estimated unit costs. Many technologies have considerable up-front fixed costs. The financial impact of these costs on a treatment provider will depend heavily on the way the program is managed. If the fixed costs of the technology can be spread across more patients, this will reduce the per-patient costs of the investment. Spreading costs will depend on the ability to generate take-up of the technology among the panel of patients and the overall size of the program.

The economic studies that capture the client's perspective may enable identification of economic burdens that are directly related to initiation, adherence, and maintenance of the technology-based system. Clinical trials may find positive effects of an intervention, but those findings may be implicitly conditional upon clients initiating and adhering to a treatment program. Real-world costs, such as the opportunity cost of time or reliance on caregiver's time, may reduce the actual effectiveness of an intervention. This particular effect could be large if treatments require large resource utilization by clients and caregivers that is not captured in the clinical trial. A well-executed economic evaluation may provide insight into potential barriers to initiation, adherence, and maintenance of treatment in an environment that is more representative of actual constraints.

Society has a limited set of resources that can be dedicated to different types of activities. In its broadest sense, economic evaluations are intended to inform this decision such that society will get the largest "bang per buck." The societal perspective takes into account costs borne by all stakeholders, including providers, payers, patients, and the community. Often patients face considerable costs during treatment. The societal perspective will include these costs. For technology-based behavioral interventions, this may involve treatment outside of the healthcare system. Using technologies in this manner may save the patient resources that would otherwise be devoted to travel to providers. Ignoring these costs may prevent a full understanding of the value of technology-based interventions.

Measuring Benefits

How benefits are measured is a crucial component of economic evaluation. There are two types of cost-effectiveness assessments: one measures benefits using clinical benefits, and the other measures effectiveness in a standard way using quality-adjusted life years (QALY). By clinical benefits, the effectiveness measure can vary from study to study. For example, depending on the study, the effectiveness measures could be reduced hospitalizations, depression-free days, or opioid-free days. A cost-effectiveness analysis that has benefits denominated in a clinical outcome, such as hospitalizations avoided, does allow for direct comparisons between interventions that avoid hospitalizations. This may be highly relevant and understandable to other researchers and providers aiming to reduce hospitalizations, but it will not capture the full societal impact of an intervention, nor will it allow for translation across behaviors for a more comprehensive behavioral healthcare system.

Cost-effectiveness analysis that uses a standardized measure for benefits, such as QALYs, is occasionally referred to as *cost-utility analysis*. The QALY is a broad measure that captures both the quality and the duration of life. The use of QALY makes it possible to compare interventions across diseases because this is a broad and standard measure and allows comparisons to other types of medical treatments and to rules of thumb regarding maximum willingness to pay for a QALY. Such comparisons are useful to discussions at the highest policy levels on the relative importance of funding treatment for technology-based behavioral interventions vs. other behavioral and medical interventions.

Cost-benefit analysis may best capture benefits beyond the medical sector such as gains in productivity or crime avoided. However, the choice between these various ways of measuring benefits is not obvious, because economic studies denominated by broader outcomes, such as QALYs, may lose relevance to providers and behavioral specialists who are used to dealing with more direct outcomes.

Once the denominator of the final outcome is chosen, it is critical to integrate appropriate measurement of the outcome into clinical data collection. For example, it may be necessary to add quality-of-life measures. There are a number of tools that can facilitate the collection of QALYs, such as the EQ-5D (3) and the MOS 36-item Short-Form Health Survey (SF-36) (4). These are general health survey instruments that are implemented to estimate a client's quality of life while in a certain state or condition. While they differ in their methods of measurements and reported dimensions, they allow for quantifying quality of life in a way that can be compared across diseases.

Costs: Resource Use and Unit Costs

In terms of costs, tabulation typically involves tracking resource use and applying an estimate of the unit costs for each of those resources. Costs for economic evaluation in clinical trials are typically estimated by the resource costing method. Costs for each patient are calculated by finding the amount of each resource used, multiplied by its unit cost, and then summing across all of the resource costs used by the patient. Resources that should be tracked prospectively during the clinical trial include inputs that are needed as part of the treatment intervention, medical services obtained by the clients outside of the treatment intervention, and relevant nonmedical services. The resources that are tracked will depend on the perspective taken in the trial, so they may include resources relevant to the provider, patient, and other affected caregivers, like families. Because behavioral interventions can improve retention in a single arm of a trial, it is important to capture resources involved in standard care and not just the resources involved in the differences in service use between clients in different arms of the trial that might occur on a given day in a treatment center.

For the costs of each unit of service, the objective is to estimate a "price" that reflects the opportunity cost of the resources being monitored. The resources that are critical to the intervention itself may require more detailed data collection from the intervention sites. The SASCAP (Substance Abuse Services Cost Analysis Program) (5) provides a standardized tool to estimate the unit costs of individual services delivered within the intervention site. For client and caretaker unit costs, the DATCAP (Drug Treatment Cost Analysis Program) (6) offers specific client and caretaker data collection tools. External sources may be sufficient for gathering unit costs of non-study services, which typically include the costs of prescription drugs, mental health services, hospitalizations, and physician visits.

It is important for costs to be reflective of those that would occur in a naturalistic setting. For costs to be estimated properly within a clinical trial setting, one should not include activities within a clinical trial setting that would not be undertaken if the intervention was disseminated into the community (such as data collection), as these activities should not be part of the intervention itself. To put it another way, activities that are not part of the intervention should not inform aspects of the clinical care. This is often a challenge.

Sample Size and Timeline

The next step is to determine if the current clinical design is sufficient to meet economic aims. Economic trials often require larger sample sizes; however, there are important exceptions, and formal size and power calculations are recommended. In general, the goal of sample size and power calculations is to identify the likelihood that an experiment will allow one to be confident that a therapy is a good or bad value, based on an assumed decision threshold (7,8). Size will change according to correlation of costs with effects and the level of confidence that investigators deem satisfactory to make statements about the cost-effectiveness of an intervention given a specific threshold. For example, an economic investigator may wish to be sure with 95% certainty that the cost-effectiveness ratio is lower than $100,000 per QALY.

Similarly, economic timelines are typically longer than those in clinical trials, because benefits may be realized beyond the typical length of follow-up for behavioral health clients. Ideally there should be a sufficient time horizon to identify economic outcomes. However, it is common to also consider using proximal markers of longer term economic benefits. In this case, a cost-effectiveness analysis based on the proximal marker over the time horizon of the trial could be supplemented by an economic model of lifetime benefits. Regardless of the duration of follow-up chosen for the design of the trial, it is ideal to collect information for all patients randomized for the entire follow-up period and to minimize attrition from the data collection. Patient selection out of treatment (dropouts) may threaten the underlying assumption that censored observations are missing at random (MAR). This may be minimized through follow-up with clients through linkages to administrative databases, phone interviews, and checks with various administrative systems such as Medicaid and the criminal justice system.

CONCLUSIONS

Technology-based behavioral healthcare systems offer great promise for improving health behaviors and health of populations. However, systems that are found to be highly effective may face great barriers to adoption within our healthcare system. Understanding the economic complexity between various actors within the healthcare system and how a new technology-based system fits into that complexity is an important step in overcoming the barriers that might exist for adoption of systems that may not only be effective but also improve the efficacy of our healthcare system. But this understanding is not sufficient. Quantifying the costs and benefits of interventions under consideration is a critical piece to overcoming barriers. This quantification must start by determining whether the new intervention is of sufficient benefit to society. From an economic point of view, this means that the societal benefits of the intervention are sufficient to justify the societal costs.

But because technology-based systems are often not integrated into existing payment models and because these systems almost always involve the involvement of various stakeholders in the healthcare system, including patients, providers, and payers, it is critical to understand the economic impact of these systems from the perspective of the various stakeholders. Only through understanding that many of these interventions would require an economic loss among the adopters of these programs will it be possible to design appropriate incentives to overcome these economic barriers.

We offer suggestions for how to design an appropriate economic design that will provide estimates of benefits and costs that are of sufficient precision over a relevant time horizon. But these technical aspects of design must be oriented to serve the aims of the analysis. For technology-based behavior healthcare systems, we emphasize that the aims must carefully take into account the potential barriers of adoption and offer economic information that can help overcome those barriers.

REFERENCES

1. Varian HR. *Microeconomic Analysis* (3rd ed.). New York: W.W. Norton; 1992, Chapters 1–6.
2. Drummond M, Sculpher MJ, Torrance GW, O'Brien BJ, Stoddart GL *Methods for the Economic Evaluation of Health Care Programmes* (2nd ed.). Oxford: Oxford University Press; 1997.
3. Brooks R. EuroQol: The current state of play. *Health Policy* 1996; 37:53–72.
4. Ware JE, Jr, Sherbourne CD. The MOS 36-item Short-Form Health Survey (SF-36): I. Conceptual framework and item selection. *Medical Care* 1992; 30:473–483.
5. Zarkin GA, Dunlap LJ, Homsi G. The substance abuse services cost analysis program (SASCAP): A new method for estimating drug treatment services costs *Evaluation and Program Planning* 2004; 27:35–43.
6. French MT, Popovici I, Tapsell L. The economic costs of substance abuse treatment: Updated estimates and cost bands for program assessment and reimbursement. *Journal of Substance Abuse Treatment* 2008; 35:462–469.
7. Al MJ, Van Hout BA, Michel BC, Rutten FFH. Sample size calculation in economic evaluations. *Health Economics* 1998; 7:327–335.
8. Laska EM, Meisner M, Siegel C. Power and sample size in cost-effectiveness analysis. *Medical Decision Making* 1999; 19:339.

SECTION IV

Effective Dissemination
and Implementation

15

Models for Effective Dissemination and Implementation of Technology-Based Therapeutic Approaches to Behavioral Healthcare

SARAH E. LORD

INTRODUCTION

As has been described in chapters throughout this volume, there is a rapidly growing evidence base for technology approaches to healthcare delivery across a range of health conditions and across the care continuum—from education and prevention, to screening and assessment, to treatment and recovery support, to wellness monitoring and chronic disease management. These technology-based tools constitute approaches to care delivered online (e.g., Web-based cognitive behavioral treatment for depression) or by way of mobile devices (e.g., addiction recovery support application), either as stand-alone programs or as augments to care. Studies have consistently demonstrated that technology-based therapeutic approaches work as well as, or better than, traditional therapeutic approaches delivered by trained clinicians (1–3).

Technology-based therapeutic tools have the potential to overcome many of the implementation barriers to traditional evidence-based care and to dramatically expand the reach of services to those who are more disenfranchised or perceive stigma regarding traditional service use. Technology allows for care delivery outside the boundaries of traditional clinics and office settings and can therefore extend care and be accessible when individuals need it the most. Technologies also have the ability to improve channels of communication between patients and providers and between provider team members, increasing potential for continuity and coherence of care. For these reasons, interactive health information technologies are central to the current healthcare reform initiatives in the United States. Under the Patient Protection and Affordable Care Act of 2010, health service organizations are mandated to provide more efficient care, be more accountable for services, and meet the growing demand for behavioral healthcare services in a climate where the demand will likely exceed the supply of care providers. Organizations will be looking for lower cost alternatives to reach broad client populations with evidence-based care. Technology-based care approaches have the potential to meet, at least in part, these demands. Yet, as is the case with most science-based interventions, demonstrated evidence does not ensure that an intervention will be adopted and used; it takes approximately 17 years for an evidence-based intervention to be translated from research to routine care (4,5). More recently, implementation science has focused on identifying strategies for accelerating the process of moving evidence-supported practice into routine care (6,7). There may be opportunities for technology to reduce the translational gap between research and practice.

As highlighted in this volume and elsewhere, the inherent qualities of technology allow for use of innovative methodologies (e.g., single-case and factorial designs) that may have the potential to accelerate the development and evaluation of technology-based interventions (8,9; see Chapter 12, this volume). To complement innovations in development and evaluation, there is also a need for focused attention on implementation science related to translation of technology-based behavioral healthcare approaches into routine care. To effectively translate the science of technology-based care approaches into practice, dissemination efforts must reach the diverse stakeholder and service system audiences, including patients and consumers, practitioners, program directors and administrators, researchers, service payers, and policymakers, with meaningful information and support to optimize potential for program adoption and integration into routine care within and across diverse service systems.

This chapter explores factors associated with the effective dissemination and implementation of technology-based approaches to behavioral healthcare. The chapter begins with a discussion of individual and organizational change and implementation models and how these models inform practice and research agendas regarding technology-based care approaches. Lessons learned from research in the implementation of technology innovations are explored, followed by a description of strategies and existing infrastructure resources that have great potential for facilitating successful translation of technology-based care approaches into routine care.

DIFFUSION OF INNOVATIONS: UNDERSTANDING ORGANIZATIONAL CHANGE

The diffusion of innovations (10) theory is a useful framework to conceptualize translation of technology-based behavioral healthcare approaches to optimize their likelihood of adoption. This model describes the process through which an *innovation*, defined as an idea perceived as new (i.e., technology-based treatment for substance abuse or serious mental illness), spreads over time within a system (10). The model distinguishes between diffusion (passive spread of innovation), dissemination (active and planned efforts to persuade target groups to adopt an innovation), implementation (active and planned efforts to mainstream an innovation within an organization), and sustainability (making an innovation routine) (11). The (passive) diffusion of innovations typically occurs via unplanned, informal, decentralized, and horizontal communication channels (e.g., peer to peer), while active dissemination of an innovation is typically more centralized and likely to occur through vertical communication mechanisms (e.g., patient–provider, provider–program director, administrator–policymaker) (11).

The diffusion of innovations model frames adoption of innovations as a function of characteristics of the innovation, of individual users of the innovation, and of the organizations or systems within which the innovation could be adopted (10). The model posits that the spread of an innovation within and across systems can vary according to the needs or motivations of those adopting the innovation (10,12). Early adopters of an innovation (i.e., technology-delivered therapeutic approach) tend to do so because of a favorable appraisal of the innovation, while subsequent adopters may do so because others have done so or because they feel compelled to do so in order to compete for resources. Late adopters of an innovation are more likely to be influenced by pressure to implement (12).

The model also posits a process of individual adoption of an innovation that includes (a) building awareness about the innovation (knowledge), (b) developing a positive (or negative) attitude about the innovation (persuasion), (c) deciding to try the innovation (decision), (d) learning how to use the innovation (implementation), and (e) incorporating the innovation into routine practice through the experience of repeated success (confirmation) (10). This groundbreaking model has contributed to a greater understanding of behavioral and organizational change and has a broad scope of practical applications for public health (13).

A number of researchers have developed conceptual frameworks building on diffusion of innovations (10) to help guide translational implementation research and practice within health services (11,14–16). The consolidated framework for implementation research (14) presents a unifying framework that summarizes conceptual constructs related to health services intervention implementation in five thematic domains: 1) intervention attributes, 2) characteristics of individuals using the intervention, 3) inner organizational setting, 4) outer organizational setting, and 5) implementation process. Each of these thematic domains is briefly described below and considered in the context of technology-based behavioral health innovations.

Intervention Characteristics

There are a number of characteristics of innovations that increase the likelihood of successful implementation. One characteristic is *relative advantage*, or the extent to which potential end-users perceive a clear advantage for using the innovation, such as better treatment effectiveness, cost-effectiveness, or improved job performance. The more an innovation is perceived as having an advantage over other approaches, the more likely it is to be adopted. The extent to which innovations are *compatible* with intended users' values, norms, and perceived needs is another important characteristic of successful innovations. Strategies to improve feasibility and workability of innovations at both individual and organizational levels can improve chances of successful adoption. The *simplicity* of an innovation, or the extent to which innovations are perceived as easy to use and understand, is another key characteristic of successful innovations, as is *trialability*, the ease with which intended users can try out the innovation and observe its impact on processes and outcomes prior to adoption. Most successful innovations also have *flexibility*, or the ability to be readily integrated into a system's infrastructure and adapted to meet user needs, and clear *knowledge transfer* about how to use the innovation. Finally, most successful innovations have available *support* in terms of technical assistance (e.g., on-demand support, customization, help desk), and acceptable *cost* in terms of time and resources needed to implement (10,11,14).

A promising innovation for rapid adoption would be an evidence-based innovation that has a clear advantage over other practices, is compatible with organization needs and simple to use, and could be tried temporarily, with results readily observable. Technology-delivered therapeutic approaches inherently contain many features shown to improve the likelihood of adoption of innovations within systems. Technology-based solutions offer a number of relative advantages over person-delivered evidence-based interventions by way of time and cost efficiencies, outcomes, and audience reach (17). Many technology-delivered approaches allow complex interventions to be delivered at a low cost, without increasing demands on staff time or training needs. Content is consistently delivered, producing greater fidelity, and services can reach individuals that are unable or unwilling to access traditional treatment settings. In addition, the anonymity afforded by technology-based approaches may be perceived as particularly appealing when addressing sensitive topics, such as substance abuse and other risk behavior. Technology-based interventions also require active responding by users, and use of multimedia can accommodate diverse learning styles and cognitive capabilities (18,19). Further, by offering technology-based interventions as part of a broader array of services, treatment settings can expand their client reach and thus their potential revenues and cost efficiencies.

As highlighted throughout this volume, the use of computers and mobile phones is nearly ubiquitous across age and socioeconomic demographics; such use is highly compatible with integration into service. Well-developed technology-based therapeutic tools are easy to use and include clear, repeatable user instructions (knowledge) and on-demand assistance (support). Given the self-contained nature of many technology-based approaches, the ability to trial these tools, with appropriate training, technical assistance, and resources, is relative easy, and data collection and visualization capabilities can provide readily observable results regarding impact on process and outcomes to inform later initiatives. The nature of computer and mobile technologies lends a good deal of adaptation flexibility to accommodate new information as it becomes available, as well as temporal flexibility, allowing a user to access a program at a time convenient to the user. Finally, technology-based approaches may enable individuals to engage in therapeutic activities for a longer period of time than is possible in a care setting or with a provider, such as to review repetitive but necessary skills training. The provider then has more time to spend on more challenging aspects of care (17).

Characteristics of Individuals

A number of individual-level factors can influence adoption and implementation processes, including demographics (e.g., age) gender, general personality attributes of potential end-users (e.g., openness to new things), and innovation-specific factors, such as knowledge and attitudes about the innovation, motivation to implement the innovation, and self-efficacy or perceived confidence in abilities to successfully use or promote implementation of the innovation.

There is strong consumer desire for technology-based healthcare services (20). Use of online and mobile technologies is increasingly ubiquitous across age, race and ethnicity, and geography (21–23). Increasingly, consumers rely on Internet and smartphone-based tools for health information and tracking (24). For example, in one report a majority of clients with severe mental illness were interested in receiving a variety of mental health services (e.g., reminders about appointments or medications, regular check-ins with provider) via mobile technologies (25).

Potential end-users of technology-based care approaches can include consumer patients, as well as clinicians charged with incorporating a technology into their treatment approach. An understanding of how the array of potential end-users currently use technologies and perceive technology-based therapeutic approaches can facilitate planning and support for integration of the approach in care. For instance, individuals working in a position for a longer period of time or who have a specific treatment orientation may be more resistant to a technology innovation than those newer to the job or who have a more flexible approach to treatment (15).

Optimizing Intervention Attributes and User Experience with Technology

Among potential end-users of technology-based therapeutic tools are consumers, providers that may be charged with supporting the use of a technology-based approach with their patients or with integrating such use into a treatment plan, and organization administrators who may be considering ways to integrate technology care approaches to meet the growing service demands of the organization. Key to ensuring that attributes of a technology-based intervention are engaging to potential end-users is an iterative development process that elicits diverse stakeholder perspectives from the outset and obtains feedback throughout the course of development (26). This user-centered development approach includes use of formative participatory methods to identify stakeholder attitudes and needs and to obtain feedback on iterations of the technology as it is being developed. Iterative user-centered development approaches to technology-based tools help to

optimize the likelihood that the technology-based approach is engaging and acceptable to all end-users and can also improve the likelihood of successful integration into routine care (27–33).

Inner Organizational Setting

Organizational characteristics associated with the adoption of behavioral health treatment innovations include a stable infrastructure with low staff and leadership turnover, and an organizational climate marked by clarity of mission, supportive leadership, staff cohesion and cooperation, open communication between leadership and staff, adaptability, and openness for embracing innovations (10,11,15). Organizational decision-making style can also influence implementation. While mandates can affect short-term adoption of an innovation, a shared decision-making process among all stakeholders can promote more sustained implementation (11).

Organization motivation, or tension, for change can positively influence the adoption of innovations. Such motivation can derive from internal pressures (e.g., clients, staff, administration) or from pressures from external sources (i.e., payers, policies, healthcare reform) (11,15,34). Along with motivation for change, the readiness of an organization for implementation is another key component of success and includes strong leadership committed to prioritizing and supporting the intervention, strong opinion leaders and champions to advocate for use of the intervention, the availability of resources to support and maintain the intervention (i.e., infrastructure changes, budget, physical space and time, workforce development to promote self-efficacy and skills for implementing the innovation, and workflow re-engineering to accommodate the innovation), and access to methods of training and ongoing technical assistance to promote use of the intervention (14,15,35,36).

Consistent and ongoing messages about the relative priority of the intervention within the organization, and reward systems to promote motivation to use the intervention either through explicit rewards or incentives or implicit expectations of performance can all enhance implementation (37). Clear monitoring and measurement of the implementation process is also critical, so that meaningful feedback about implementation impact is given to all stakeholders throughout the process to reinforce implementation (36). Studies of sustainability of evidence-based interventions have demonstrated that maintenance of implementation success is most associated with active leadership to support re-engineering of workflow strategies to promote implementation (36,38) and reinforcement of implementation through measurement and feedback to providers and other stakeholders (36). Importantly, feedback about the impact of an intervention should be developed to clearly highlight the compatibility of the intervention for meeting the needs of all end-user stakeholders, emphasizing not only how the intervention works but also why it works and how it meets the needs of stakeholders (11,12,39). For example, feedback about cost efficiencies of a technology-based care approach may be most relevant for organization administrators, while relevant feedback for providers might be targeted to time efficiencies and the potential for providers to work at their optimal level of training.

Inner Organizational Setting and Technology Approaches

The scientific literature for adoption of innovations in service settings provides directions and targets for planning for, and implementation of, technology-based behavioral healthcare approaches. Whether it is a depression self-management mobile application or a Web-based psychosocial intervention to augment clinician-delivered substance use treatment, a goal is for technology-based care approaches to become a routine part of the menu of services in care settings. As such, providers, case managers, and other staff may be charged with introducing these tools to patients or monitoring their impact as part of a treatment process. An understanding of attitudes about, and skills and experiences with, technologies across potential stakeholders can facilitate implementation planning to promote engagement with a technology-based approach. Further, assessment of the characteristics of service organizations that could support or hinder potential integration of technology solutions can guide organization-level interventions to promote receptivity to these approaches.

There is a growing research base that informs a better understanding of organizational factors associated with adoption and implementation of technology-based care approaches. In a recent survey of 96 substance use treatment counselors, Buti and colleagues found that intention to use

a Web-delivered psychosocial intervention was associated with perceived social norms for using the program (i.e., by opinion leaders), but not with attitudes about Web-delivered interventions (40). In a study of the readiness of healthcare organizations to implement an interactive health communication system, compatibility of the system with institutional goals and resources, and quality of the system and available support for meeting patient user needs were the most important organization-level constructs for predicting implementation readiness (35). Obstfelder, Engeseth, and Wynn (41) described key features of successfully implemented telemedicine applications, including identification of local service delivery problems and clear communication about ways in which telemedicine could positively address the problem, communication about how telemedicine could address broader healthcare delivery policy, collaboration between telemedicine promoters and users (including providers and patients), technical assistance to address organizational and technical needs (i.e., technology infrastructure, resources, workflow re-engineering, standard guidelines), and early identification of sustainability needs (i.e., funding mechanisms, quality improvement protocols, standard guidelines).

To assess readiness of community behavioral healthcare settings to use technology-based approaches to care from the perspective of potential adoption decision-makers, Lord, Lardiere, Ramsey, Greene, and Marsch (42) conducted an online survey of administrators, program directors, and clinical care supervisors from a national network of community behavioral health organizations. While overall perceived readiness to use technology-based care approaches was high, readiness varied in relation to organizational infrastructure and climate. As anticipated, leaders that reported higher levels of use of technology in current care processes, such as e-mail, text messaging, and videoconferencing, indicated more readiness to integrate other technology-based assessment and intervention approaches into care delivery. Also as expected, motivation for organizational change was associated with technology readiness. The more pressures felt from both internal (e.g., clients, staff, supervisors) and external (e.g., funding sources, reimbursement policies, healthcare reform) change forces, the greater the readiness to use technology-based care approaches.

Organizations characterized as having stable staff and leadership, leaders that were supportive of technology-based care approaches, open communication channels, and flexibility regarding innovations were reported as having higher readiness to implement new technologies to enhance client care (42).

A qualitative analysis of perceived barriers to implementation of technology-based therapeutic approaches among potential adoption decision-makers from the same network of community behavioral healthcare settings described above revealed a number of key barriers. These barriers include funding sources and costs associated with technology infrastructure, hardware and software; privacy and security concerns associated with use of computer and mobile technologies; and limited awareness about technology-based care approaches and how these approaches can be used in care delivery. Attitudes regarding adverse effects on client–provider relationship quality, replacement of jobs, or increased time and resources required of providers and agencies are also a factor, as are disparities in accessibility of technologies and connectivity, and reimbursement methods for technology-based care approaches (43). This research highlights important directions for both research and practice with regard to implementation of technology-based therapeutic tools.

Overcoming Barriers to Dissemination and Implementation of Technology-Based Therapeutic Tools

As discussed in Chapter 21 this volume, U.S. federal policy and regulations regarding reimbursement of technology-based care delivery models are powerful "outer organization" forces that will ultimately guide how technologies can be integrated into behavioral healthcare delivery models. These policies should be driven by good science, and, as such, it is imperative to clearly demonstrate the added value and short- and long-term cost savings of integrating innovative technology-based tools into care delivery by way of rigorous comparative and cost-effectiveness studies. Such research should include clear metrics of value and efficiency for providers (i.e., improved workflow, increased client reach, more time to focus on high-need clients, improved client outcomes) as well as organizations (i.e., return on investment). Demonstration

trials of technology-based approaches using different payer models may help to identify reimbursement models that maximize outcome in relation to fiscal impact. In all cases, research results should be communicated to healthcare agencies, payers and policymakers, organization leadership, and providers in ways that are accessible, relevant, and meaningful to the array of stakeholders, so as to promote adoption and integration of these approaches into routine care.

Prior research has also documented high levels of public concern regarding privacy and security of personal health information amidst growing use of electronic health records (EHR) and other health technologies (44). These privacy concerns can act as a substantial barrier to consumer acceptance of health technology implementation and may delay adoption of technology use for some providers (45). To address implementation barriers associated with concerns about privacy and security with technology-based therapeutic approaches, the healthcare field must collectively work to ensure that technology-based therapeutic are developed in ways to ensure compliance with regulatory guidelines and protection of client end-users. Technology literacy can also be developed through provision of clear and comprehensive education about ways that individuals can protect themselves when using different technologies. Such initiatives to promote technology literacy and develop clear risk-management strategies may promote both comfort and confidence among organization administrators, managers, providers, and consumers with regard to use of technology care approaches.

There is also a growing need for broad dissemination of information and education about available evidence-based technological tools, accessible and thorough training in the use of these technology-based tools within (and outside of) different systems of care, and ongoing technical assistance to help consumers and provider stakeholders build the skills and confidence to successfully use these tools as part of standard care. To alleviate barriers associated with beliefs regarding fears of compromised client care, increased work load, or job loss, implementation support and technical assistance can frame messaging regarding the use of these tools as a way to enable providers to work at their highest level of training with their clientele and to focus on the most high-need issues. Carefully planned demonstration pilots can help specify implementation processes that align with workflow and preserve the important role of client–provider relationships. These demonstrations also allow for first-hand experience of technology-based approaches by organization stakeholders, including providers and consumers, which can foster acceptance and adoption of the technology-based care approach. Careful attention to fostering key organizational capacity and climate elements prior to demonstration trial of a technology-based therapeutic approach can facilitate overall implementation.

While disparities do still exist in the United States with regard to accessibility of technologies and the Internet, access to mobile phones and Internet access continues to grow (22). Additionally, many public and healthcare settings (i.e., libraries, hospitals, community centers, treatment settings) offer computer and Internet capabilities. Connectivity and service issues are still primary impediments to the provision of technology-delivered services within rural areas. While wireless network coverage is slowly expanding, other technology-related strategies can be implemented in rural areas, such as mobile applications that include full offline capabilities and telemedicine approaches. Federal initiatives to promote technology infrastructure in the United States will influence the potential dissemination of mobile and Internet-based behavioral healthcare approaches in more rural settings.

Outer Organizational Setting

External factors that influence organizational implementation processes include the social network within with organizations exist (i.e., agency networks, professional networks), as well as policies, regulations, and incentives that could influence dissemination and implementation of treatment innovations (11,14,15). Professional organizations and local and state organizations can be social systems for change and can have a positive feedback effect in terms of moving motivation toward increased adoption of interventions (12). Policies, regulations, and incentives that promote the use of an intervention can also facilitate its adoption and translation into practice. What follows is a description of some of the external influences currently in play for influencing broad dissemination and implementation

of technology-based behavioral healthcare approaches.

External Characteristics and Technology-Based Care Approaches

Federal U.S. and state policy initiatives associated with healthcare reform under the Patient Protection and Affordable Care Act (PPACA) of 2010 offer an extraordinary opportunity for facilitating translation of technology-based behavioral healthcare approaches into routine care. The PPACA expands affordable health insurance and healthcare coverage to nearly 32 million Americans (46). Provisions of the Act also mandate inclusion of substance abuse and mental health services as essential services that state insurance exchanges offer (47). PPACA provisions aim to reduce healthcare costs, through emphasis on prevention and wellness; promotion of evidence-based and integrated care, including coordination of substance abuse and mental health services with general medical care; accountability regarding patient outcomes; implementation of health information technology (i.e., EHR) and expanded data collection systems; and use of technology-based treatment approaches to foster efficiencies in care delivery (48). The potential for demand for behavioral healthcare services to exceed provider resource capacity is high, particularly within community care systems with already limited resources (49). Offering a "toolkit" of technology-based therapeutic approaches for behavioral healthcare holds great promise for meeting increasing service demands (48).

Electronic health records, personal health records (PHR), and interactive health information exchanges are central components of the technology infrastructure espoused by the ACA to build efficiencies and quality of healthcare. This technology infrastructure is intended as a platform for engaging consumer patients in self-management, enhancing coordination, continuity, and integration of care across settings and over time, and facilitating performance and outcome measurement and monitoring (50). These technologies could serve as platforms for access to technology-based therapeutic tools. To foster full integration with care, ready exchange of information between these therapeutic tools and electronic health or personal records will be important. Exchange of behavioral healthcare information is made more complex by federal and state regulations associated with exchange of health information related to mental health and substance use treatment (e.g., 42 CFR Part 2). Attention to these regulations when developing technology-based therapeutic tools will be important to facilitate ready integration of these tools with developing models of care and thereby foster more widespread dissemination and implementation of technology-based approaches to care delivery.

A review of uptake and dissemination of EHR and PHR in mental healthcare settings and among those receiving mental healthcare found that rates of uptake and use of these systems in general medical settings are low; rates are even lower within specialty behavioral healthcare settings (50). Incorporation of end-users into the development and rollout of these technologies can help foster uptake. In a recent study, an electronic PHR was adapted to improve relevance and applicability to mental health consumers, based on iterative feedback from consumers (50). To promote implementation, consumers were provided with computer training to overcome health and technology literacy barriers, and with technical assistance by nurse practitioners to enter and maintain record information. Strategies were also provided for finding and securely logging into the system from computers in public access locations, such as public libraries. In a demonstration pilot to evaluate quality of medical care in a community mental health setting, having a PHR resulted in significantly improved quality of care and increased use of medical services, particularly outpatient preventive services (33).

Another example of a powerful external influence is the 2009 Health Information Technology for Economic and Clinical Health (HITECH) Act, which provides economic incentives to federally qualified health centers (FQHCs) to support technology infrastructure for integration and meaningful use of health information technologies in care delivery. However, current legislation excludes most community behavioral health organizations from this incentive plan. As such, these organizations are reliant on limited, and potentially decreasing, funding sources to implement a technology infrastructure, and many do not. Federal and state policy initiatives to extend incentives to community behavioral

health organizations may help these organizations to achieve parity with other health systems and position the organizations to be more ready to use technologies to efficiently increase access to, and provide quality behavioral healthcare for, individuals most in need.

While the discussion to this point has focused on U.S. federal and state initiatives that influence dissemination and implementation of technology-based behavioral healthcare approaches, international initiatives similarly can impact broad-based diffusion of technology approaches for care. Penetration of mobile technologies worldwide is 90% in developed countries, and mobile phones are used more than any other modern technology in developing countries (more than 35%) (51). The potential for broad dissemination and implementation of mobile applications for behavioral healthcare is tremendous (52,53). A systematic review of eHealth implementations in developing countries found that systems that improve communication between treatment providers and institutions, assist in ordering and managing of medications, and help to monitor and detect patients at risk for not following up on care demonstrated particular promise (52). Yet, there has been little rigorous evaluation of the health outcome impact and cost efficiencies of eHealth systems in developing countries. Funding priorities are needed to support implementation research on the deployment and impact of eHealth systems on patient outcomes, provider workflow, and quality of care.

In summary, there are a number of factors external to organizations that can influence the ultimate adoption and integration of evidence-based technology approaches to behavioral healthcare to diverse care settings. What is clear is that new technologies will need to be useful, and usable, across patients and provider workforces and across multiple platforms and systems if they are to be adopted more widely in behavioral healthcare. Accelerating the adoption of health technologies will likely require public–private partnerships to foster broad awareness of the potential of these technologies and support development of infrastructure, regulations to ensure protection of end-user privacy and security, and new policies to address reimbursement issues and incentives for use of technologies in care delivery (52,54).

IMPLEMENTATION ROAD MAPS: CHARTING A COURSE FOR IMPLEMENTATION

Regardless of the nature of a technology-based therapeutic tool, be it a mobile symptom self-management application or a mobile recovery support program to augment clinical care, research on how these types of tools can be integrated into the fabric of care is critical. In the next section, a model for the implementation process is outlined, and implications for effective dissemination and implementation of technology-based therapeutic approaches are highlighted.

There are four essential activities of the implementation process across organizational change models: planning, engaging, executing, and evaluating and reflecting (14). Instead of these activities being viewed in a linear model, each can be revisited throughout implementation in an iterative, recursive process.

Planning

Planning focuses on development of a specific course of action to promote implementation by building capacity for an intervention, at both individual and organizational levels. Planning includes activities to gain an understanding of diverse stakeholder needs and perspectives, workflow processes, as well as external and internal organizational characteristics that could facilitate or hinder implementation, and developing concrete strategies for overcoming potential barriers. Careful and intentional planning provides the foundation for successful implementation (14).

Planning for implementation of a technology-based intervention in a health services setting might include a needs and capacity assessment regarding current service; observational research and surveys of stakeholders to gather insight about organizational structure and climate, technology literacy, attitudes about technology-based care approaches and compatibility with existing values and treatment philosophy; and evaluations of workflow to identify ways that technology could be seamlessly integrated into work process, and of the workforce landscape to identify key supporters.

Engagement

Engagement involves establishing the support team for the implementation—the team that is going to promote implementation buy-in and drive the implementation process. There are a number of implementation change agents, each having a role in fostering implementation success (11,14,55). Opinion leaders are individuals in an organization that influence the attitudes and beliefs of colleagues regarding a new intervention. Opinion leaders may exert influence through expertise, authority, or status (experts) or through their representativeness and credibility among colleagues (peers) (14). Opinion leaders typically lead through example and are usually distinct from champions, or those charged with actively promoting, marketing, and supporting the intervention within the organization. Finally, external change agents, such as the program developers or research team, can provide the necessary training and technical assistance for the intervention.

A solid support team for implementation of technology-based therapeutic approaches should include administrator and provider champions who have a good understanding of technology and its potential for healthcare, and who can support implementation of the technology at both administrative and front-line care delivery levels. Where appropriate, consumer and client champions can also help the implementation process with their peer end-users. Opinion leaders that use the technology at each of these levels can help to build buy-in from others.

Execution

Carefully planned demonstrations are invaluable for optimizing implementation process to maximize outcomes and increase potential for translation of interventions into routine care. Dearing (12) describes two types of demonstration projects, both central to optimizing implementation. Experimental demonstrations are field tests of interventions carried out to assess external validity across different settings, target populations, or intervention protocols. Such demonstrations can provide valuable information not only about ways to improve an intervention for real world deployment but also about strategies to optimize implementation at individual (client and/or provider) and organizational levels and methods to assess and report outcomes. Experimental demonstrations pave the way for exemplary implementation demonstrations or full-scale naturalistic deployment of an intervention with all processes and supports in place and clear indicators of cost-effectiveness. Exemplary demonstrations are intended to showcase interventions and influence adoption decisions (12). Mixed-purpose demonstrations, that is, efforts to optimize implementation outcomes in a full-scale deployment to also assess system and client outcomes, can lead to interest in an intervention but not adoption (12).

The nature of most technology-based therapeutic approaches positions them as excellent candidates for demonstration trials once necessary hardware and software needs are met. Experimental implementation demonstrations technology-based care approaches can yield important information about how to use the given technology tool when naturally deployed, and about ways to refine the implementation plan and evaluation metrics before moving to full-scale exemplary trials.

Evaluation and Reflection

Measurement and feedback in demonstrations are key to heighten visibility and observability of impact. Consistent with rapid-cycle quality improvement models derived from business and engineering frameworks (i.e., Plan, Do, Study, Act; PDSA) (56), demonstration trials of technology-based therapeutic approaches should include collection of key metrics to evaluate implementation success, such as penetration of the technology across potential end-users, acceptability of the technology, compatibility of the technology with workflow, and cost impact. To promote consensus and implementation, results of demonstration trials should be communicated to all end-user stakeholders with messages that are relevant and meaningful to each stakeholder group.

PROMOTING TRANSLATION OF EVIDENCE-BASED TECHNOLOGY APPROACHES TO BEHAVIORAL HEALTHCARE

Momentum for promoting evidence-based behavioral healthcare approaches has grown tremendously in the past decade. Many federal funding agencies, such as the Substance Abuse and Mental Health Services Administration (SAMHSA), the Center for Substance Abuse Treatment (CSAT), and the Center for Disease Control and Prevention (CDC), require use of evidence-based

interventions for organizations to receive funding. The efforts of the National Institute on Drug Abuse (NIDA) and SAMHSA/CSAT to bridge the gap between research and practice have yielded important initiatives, including the Clinical Trials Network (CTN: NIDA), Addiction Technology Transfer Centers (ATTC: CSAT/NIDA), and Treatment Improvement Protocols (TIP: SAMHSA/CSAT). Each of these avenues offers promising potential for providing support, training, technical assistance, and knowledge transfer for implementation of technology-based behavioral healthcare treatments such as those highlighted in this volume. There are also a number of other assistance resources specifically focused on promotion of technologies in delivery of healthcare. What follows is a brief description of the support resources offered by each of these federal initiatives, and suggestions for ways that technology-based approaches could be readily integrated into their support practices and services.

Addiction Technology Transfer Centers (CSAT/NIDA)

The ATTC network, funded by SAMHSA and CSAT since 1993, is a national network of 14 regional centers and a national office charged with facilitating the systematic translation of research-based practices into treatment settings across the process of adoption, implementation, and sustainability (57). ATTC staff work with researchers and intervention developers to create training and technical assistance resources, or translation packages, to support building of organization workforce knowledge, attitudes, and skills to implement the evidence-based intervention or practice. Translation packages should include all of the requirements needed for successful implementation of an innovation, including the requisite materials for promotion to clients and providers, and resources for implementation and sustainability, such as organizational needs (e.g., policy, staffing), training (e.g., materials, equipment, cost, accountability for loss of billable time), and strategies for assessing fidelity.

For a technology-based intervention, such as a mobile depression management application, a resource package could include hardware and software requirements for clients and providers, requisite training for use of the program, and identification of metrics for evaluating implementation success, including client- and provider-level acceptability, adoption, appropriateness, feasibility, fidelity, cost, penetration, and sustainability, as well as service and client outcomes.

NIDA/SAMHSA Blending Initiative

The NIDA/SAMHSA Blending Initiative is a related federal effort to promote the translation of science to practice for substance use and co-occurring mental health disorders (58). Blending Teams, consisting of ATTC Network staff, NIDA researchers, and community treatment providers from NIDA's Clinical Trials Network (CTN), work together to develop user-friendly awareness kits and training packages to introduce providers to evidence-based treatment approaches that have been evaluated through the CTN. Blending Team products have been created for buprenorphine treatment and its use in short-term opioid withdrawal and with young adults, treatment planning, supervisory tools for motivational interviewing, and motivational incentives (58).

A Blending Product is currently under development for Therapeutic Education System (59), an Internet- and mobile-based psychosocial substance abuse intervention demonstrated to be effective for reducing substance use and related risk behaviors (59, 60). To the best of our knowledge, this is the first technology-based behavioral intervention to be a target of the Blending Initiative. It provides the framework for support of other technology-based care initiatives with demonstrated evidence.

Treatment Improvement Protocol (TIP)

Treatment Improvement Protocols are best practice guidelines for the treatment of substance abuse. A publication of SAMHSA/CSAT, TIPS are developed in concert with consensus panels of clinical, research, and administrative experts in a given area and are distributed to a growing number of facilities and individuals across the country. Each TIP provides hands-on practical guidance on how to implement a given practice, as well as a comprehensive list of resources and references to support the empirical basis of the target practice. A TIP on technology-based therapeutic tools targeting behavioral health was developed with input

of two consensus panels of clinical and administrative experts, including the editors of this volume (Marsch, Lord). This publication includes a comprehensive compendium of empirical research as well as implementation guidelines, user-friendly tips, and practical scenarios to demonstrate strategies for how technology-based tools can be successfully incorporated into workflow to promote client outcomes across a variety of care settings.

Quality Improvement Collaboratives (QIC)

Quality improvement collaboratives, or learning collaboratives, are another common strategy for promoting best practices in a given area of care. Learning collaboratives typically consist of a multidisciplinary team of experts and peers that works together to facilitate and guide best practices and improvement in delivery of care in a specified area. Grounded in business management and organizational quality improvement models, common structural and process components of learning collaboratives related to healthcare include in-person learning sessions, phone meetings and email or Web-based support, data reporting, feedback, and training in quality improvement methods (61).

A recent meta-analysis of QIC targeting healthcare found that while there is good evidence that collaboratives can improve the process of care delivery (workflow), the results with regard to effect on provider and client outcomes are inconsistent (61). Among features of a collaborative that participants found most useful were input from expert faculty, the sharing of ideas and experiences, training and support in implementation of data-driven quality improvement processes, and a collaborative Internet discussion forum (62). While there is considerable research to be done to better understand the cost-benefit value of learning collaboratives, they provide a model for supporting sustained implementation of technology-based behavioral healthcare by building capacity for addressing client, provider, and organization implementation barriers; improving knowledge, skills, and self-efficacy for implementation steps; and using a collective forum for training, utilization, and sharing of data as well as feedback to inform improvement initiatives.

Technology can also be used to support implementation of learning collaboratives to promote broader reach of support services for technology-based therapeutic tools. For example, by way of videoconferencing learning sessions or through online discussion boards, stakeholders can share strategies for overcoming implementation barriers and gather advice from others, locally, nationally, and internationally. Mobile and cloud technologies also enable ready collection of quality improvement initiatives (indeed, even real time via mobile ecological momentary assessment) and display of data to provide contextually relevant feedback to stakeholders relevant to their implementation efforts.

The Network for the Improvement of Addiction Treatment (NIATx) is a learning collaborative comprised of addiction treatment centers focused on process improvement in drug and alcohol treatment (56). NIATx provides technical assistance and toolkit supports to help treatment settings with change initiatives, according to five process improvement principles: 1) understand and involve the customer, 2) focus on fixing key problems or barriers, 3) pick a powerful change leader who can effectively guide a change team, 4) get ideas from outside the organization, and 5) use rapid cycle testing to execute and evaluate trials of the innovation to obtain feedback for implementing the desired change. In a case study evaluation, most organizations were able to follow the principles and affect improvements in clinic service delivery (56). Current efforts focus on working with organizations to prepare for healthcare reform and technological advances.

Health Information Technology Workforce Program

Training represents another powerful mechanism for promoting dissemination and implementation of technology-based approaches to behavioral healthcare. The Health Information Technology Workforce Program of the HITECH Act provides incentives for a number of training initiatives aimed at building health information technology literacy among the next-generation health service workforce (45). Examples of incentive strategies include funding of a community college consortium to educate students to become health information technology professionals (i.e., practice workflow and information management redesign specialists,

implementation support specialists or managers, technical/software support specialists), assistance to 4-year universities to establish or expand health information technology programs that require university-level training (i.e., health information privacy and security specialists, research, and development scientists), and funding to support curriculum development and competency examinations for these higher education initiatives. In addition to federal initiatives, providers can now receive specialized training in health informatics, enabling them to become implementation specialists and change agents to promote technologies within systems of care (63).

Center for Technology and Behavioral Health (CTBH)

Just as important as the need to train the clinical workface, to build awareness and capacity for integrating technology advances in behavioral healthcare, is the need to train the researcher workforce, to advance the evidence base for technology-delivered approaches to behavioral healthcare. The Center for Technology and Behavioral Health (CTBH) is a P30 Center for Excellence, established in 2010 and funded by the NIDA, that serves as a national and international resource to promote evidence-based development, evaluation, dissemination, and implementation of technology delivery solutions for behavioral healthcare. Based at the Geisel School of Medicine at Dartmouth College, CTBH is led by a nationally represented interdisciplinary core faculty and advisory network representing anthropology, computer science, engineering, graphic design, health economics, internal medicine, psychology, psychiatry, pediatrics, statistics, and primary care. A central mission of CTBH is to promote awareness about, and use of, technology-based therapeutic approaches among consumer clients, practitioners, researchers, and policymakers. Activities to support this mission include a seminar series to highlight the work of innovators in the field of technology and behavioral healthcare (i.e., technologists, researchers, data analytic experts, game developers, human factor experts, user interface design professions); local and national workshops, presentations, and consultations to practitioners, researchers, and policymakers to promote awareness about evidence-based technology approaches and implementation strategies; and a pilot program to encourage innovation among researchers to seed the way for larger research projects. CTBH currently supports a number of postdoctoral fellows and early faculty to develop programs of research targeting technology-based behavioral healthcare approaches.

Additionally, the CTBH website includes an interactive toolkit with resources to foster awareness of scientifically supported, technology-based therapeutic tools and to promote effective implementation of technology-based approaches in systems of care, a compendium of up-to-date research literature regarding technology-based care approaches, and a blog and social media presence to highlight innovations in the field. Since its launch in 2010, CTBH has been successful in fostering awareness about evidence-based technology approaches to behavioral healthcare. From March 2013 through August 2014 alone, the CTBH website had 16,297 visits, representing 11,138 new visitors and 5159 return visitors from the United States and abroad. These numbers reflect the explosion of interest in technology-based approaches to healthcare.

CONCLUSIONS

Technology has tremendous potential for transforming delivery of behavioral healthcare and for reaching broad, and often disenfranchised, consumer populations with evidence-based care. There is an impressive emerging science base for Internet and mobile behavioral health treatment approaches, and there is tremendous opportunity for programs of implementation science research to determine strategies for successfully integrating these approaches into standard care. A number of directions for practice and research in this area are highlighted in this chapter. For example, more research is needed to understand consumer and provider attitudes about different technology-based behavioral healthcare approaches and how best to promote use of these technologies. Implementation research is also needed to identify best practices and optimal payer models for sustainable integration of technology-based approaches into diverse systems of care.

REFERENCES

1. Barak A, Hen L, Boniel-Nissim M, Shapira N. A comprehensive review and a meta-analysis of the effectiveness of Internet-based psychotherapeutic interventions. *Journal of Technology in Human Services* 2008; 26(2-4):109–160.
2. Noar SM, Black HG, Pierce LB. Efficacy of computer technology-based HIV prevention interventions: A meta-analysis. *AIDS* 2009; 23(1):107–115.
3. Marsch LA. Leveraging technology to enhance addiction treatment and recovery. *Journal of Addictive Diseases* 2012; 31(3):313–318.
4. Balas EA, Weingarten S, Garb CT, Blumenthal D, Boren SA, Brown GD. Improving preventive care by prompting physicians. *Archives of Internal Medicine* 2000; 160(3):301–308.
5. Green LW, Ottoson JM, Garcia C, Hiatt RA. Diffusion theory and knowledge dissemination, utilization, and integration in public health. *Annual Review of Public Health* 2009; 30:151–174.
6. Proctor EK, Landsverk J, Aarons G, Chambers D, Glisson C, Mittman B. Implementation research in mental health services: An emerging science with conceptual, methodological, and training challenges. *Administration and Policy in Mental Health* 2009; 36(1):24–34.
7. Chambers DA. Advancing the science of implementation: A workshop summary. *Administration and Policy in Mental Health* 2008;35(1-2):3–10.
8. Dallery J, Raiff BR, Grabinski MJ. Internet-based contingency management to promote smoking cessation: A randomized controlled study. *Journal of Applied Behavior Analysis* 2013; 46(4):750–764.
9. Nahum-Shani I, Qian M, Almirall D, Pelham WE, Gnagy B, Fabiano GA, et al. Experimental design and primary data analysis methods for comparing adaptive interventions. *Psychological Methods* 2012; 17(4):457–477.
10. Rogers EM. *Diffusion of Innovations* (5th ed.). New York: Free Press; 2003.
11. Greenhalgh T, Robert G, Macfarlane F, Bate P, Kyriakidou O. Diffusion of innovations in service organizations: Systematic review and recommendations. *The Milbank Quarterly* 2004; 82(4):581–629.
12. Dearing JW. Applying diffusion of innovation theory to intervention development. *Research on Social Work Practice* 2009; 19(5):503–518.
13. Haider M, Kreps GL. Forty years of diffusion of innovations: Utility and value in public health. *Journal of Health Communication* 2004; 9(Suppl 1):3–11.
14. Damschroder LJ, Aron DC, Keith RE, Kirsh SR, Alexander JA, Lowery JC. Fostering implementation of health services research findings into practice: A consolidated framework for advancing implementation science. *Implementation Science* 2009; 4:50.

15. Lehman WE, Greener JM, Simpson DD. Assessing organizational readiness for change. *Journal of Substance Abuse Treatment* 2002; 22(4):197–209.

16. Glasgow RE, Klesges LM, Dzewaltowski DA, Estabrooks PA, Vogt TM. Evaluating the impact of health promotion programs: Using the RE-AIM framework to form summary measures for decision making involving complex issues. *Health Education Research* 2006; 21(5):688–694.

17. Marsch LA, Lord S. Applying technology to the assessment, prevention, treatment, and recovery support of substance use disorders: Opportunities for new service delivery models. In el-Guebaly N, Galanter M, Carra G (eds.), *The Textbook of Addiction Treatment: International Perspectives.* Calgary, Canada: International Society of Addiction Medicine (ISAM); (in press).

18. Lieberman DA, Linn MC. Learning to learn revisited: Computers and the development of self-directed learning skills. *Journal of Research on Computing in Education.* 1991; 23(3):373–395.

19. Shavinina LV. Interdisciplinary innovation: Psychoeducational multimedia technologies. *New Ideas in Psychology* 1998; 16(3):189–204.

20. Patient choice an increasingly important factor in the age of the "Healthcare Consumer": Harris Interactive; 2012. Retreived from http://www.harrisinteractive.com/NewsRoom/HarrisPolls/tabid/447/mid/1508/articleId/1074/ctl/ReadCustom%20Default/Default.aspx

21. Duggan M, Smith A. Cell Internet usage 2013: Pew Research Center; 2013. Retrieved from http://www.pewinternet.org/2013/09/16/cell-internet-use-2013/

22. Smith A. Smartphone ownership 2013: Pew Research Center; 2013. Retrieved from http://www.pewinternet.org/2013/06/05/smartphone-ownership-2013/

23. Zickuhr K, Smith A. Home broadband 2013: Pew Research Center; 2013. Retrieved from http://www.pewinternet.org/2013/08/26/home-broadband-2013/

24. Fox S, Duggan M. Health online 2013: Pew Research Center; 2013. Retrieved from http://www.pewinternet.org/2013/01/15/health-online-2013/

25. Ben-Zeev D, Davis KE, Kaiser S, Krzsos I, Drake RE. Mobile technologies among people with serious mental illness: Opportunities for future services. *Administration and Policy in Mental Health* 2013; 40(4):340–343.

26. van Velsen L, Beaujean DJ, van Gemert-Pijnen JE. Why mobile health app overload drives us crazy, and how to restore the sanity. *BMC Medical Informatics and Decision Making* 2013; 13:23.

27. Brunette MF, Ferron JC, Drake RE, Devitt TS, Geiger PT, McHugo GJ, et al. Carbon monoxide feedback in a motivational decision support system for nicotine dependence among smokers with severe mental illnesses. *Journal of Substance Abuse Treatment* 2013; 45(4):319–324.

28. Lord SE, Trudeau KJ, Black RA, Lorin L, Cooney E, Villapiano A, et al. CHAT: Development and validation of a computer-delivered, self-report, substance use assessment for adolescents. *Substance Use & Misuse* 2011; 46(6):781–794.

29. Veinot TC, Campbell TR, Kruger DJ, Grodzinski A. A question of trust: User-centered design requirements for an informatics intervention to promote the sexual health of African-American youth. *Journal of the American Medical Informatics Association: JAMIA* 2013; 20(4):758–765.

30. LeRouge C, Wickramasinghe N. A review of user-centered design for diabetes-related consumer health informatics technologies. *Journal of Diabetes Science and Technology* 2013; 7(4):1039–1056.

31. McCurdie T, Taneva S, Casselman M, Yeung M, McDaniel C, Ho W, et al. mHealth consumer apps: The case for user-centered design. *Biomedical Instrumentation & Technology* 2012; 46(s2):49–56.

32. Henderson VA, Barr KL, An LC, Guajardo C, Newhouse W, Mase R, et al. Community-based participatory research and user-centered design in a diabetes medication information and decision tool. *Progress in Community Health Partnerships: Research, Education, and Action* 2013; 7(2):171–184.

33. Druss BG, Ji X, Glick G, von Esenwein SA. Randomized trial of an electronic personal health record for patients with serious mental illnesses. *American Journal of Psychiatry* 2014; 171(3):360–368

34. Simpson DD, Flynn PM. Moving innovations into treatment: A stage-based approach to program change. *Journal of Substance Abuse Treatment* 2007; 33(2):111–120.

35. Wen KY, Gustafson DH, Hawkins RP, Brennan PF, Dinauer S, Johnson PR, et al. Developing and validating a model to predict the success of an IHCS implementation: The Readiness for Implementation Model. *Journal of the American Medical Informatics Association: JAMIA* 2010; 17(6):707–713.

36. Torrey WC, Bond GR, McHugo GJ, Swain K. Evidence-based practice implementation in community mental health settings: The relative importance of key domains of implementation activity. *Administration and Policy in Mental Health* 2012; 39(5):353–364.

37. Weiner BJ. A theory of organizational readiness for change. *Implementation Science* 2009; 4:67.

38. Flanagan ME, Ramanujam R, Doebbeling BN. The effect of provider- and workflow-focused strategies for guideline implementation on provider acceptance. *Implementation Science* 2009; 4:71.

39. Gustafson DH, Sainfort F, Eichler M, Adams L, Bisognano M, Steudel H. Developing and testing a

model to predict outcomes of organizational change. *Health Services Research* 2003; 38(2):751–776.

40. Buti AL, Eakins D, Fussell H, Kunkel LE, Kudura A, McCarty D. Clinician attitudes, social norms and intentions to use a computer-assisted intervention. *Journal of Substance Abuse Treatment* 2013; 44(4):433–437.

41. Obstfelder A, Engeseth KH, Wynn R. Characteristics of successfully implemented tele-medical applications. *Implementation Science* 2007; 2:25.

42. Lord S, Lardiere M, Ramsey A, Greene MA., & Marsch, L.A. Taking a pulse on tech: Readiness for technology-based care approaches in community behavioral health care organizations. *Administration and Policy in Mental Health and Mental Health Services Research.* 2014 (Manuscript under review).

43. Ramsey A, Lord S, Torrey J, Marsch L, Lardiere M. Paving the way to successful implementation: Identifying key barriers to use of technology for delivery of behavioral health care. *Journal of Behavioral Health Services & Research* 2014 (In Press).

44. Hiller J, McMullen MS, Chumney WM, Baumer DL. Privacy and security in the implementation of health information technology (electronic health records): U.S. and EU compared. *BUJ Science & Technology Law* 2011; 17(1):1–39.

45. Williams C, Mostashari F, Mertz K, Hogin E, Atwal P. From the Office of the National Coordinator: The strategy for advancing the exchange of health information. *Health Affairs* 2012; 31(3):527–536.

46. Garfield RL, Zuvekas SH, Lave JR, Donohue JM. The impact of national health care reform on adults with severe mental disorders. *American Journal of Psychiatry* 2011; 168(5):486–494.

47. Buck JA. The looming expansion and transformation of public substance abuse treatment under the Affordable Care Act. *Health Affairs* 2011; 30(8):1402–1410.

48. Pating DR, Miller MM, Goplerud E, Martin J, Ziedonis DM. New systems of care for substance use disorders: treatment, finance, and technology under health care reform. *Psychiatric Clinics of North America* 2012; 35(2):327–356.

49. Thomas KC, Ellis AR, Konrad TR, Holzer CE, Morrissey JP. County-level estimates of mental health professional shortage in the United States. *Psychiatric Services* 2009; 60(10):1323–1328.

50. Druss BG, Dimitropoulos L. Advancing the adoption, integration and testing of technological advancements within existing care systems. *General Hospital Psychiatry* 2013; 35(4):345–348.

51. Sanou B. *The World in 2013: ICT Facts and Figures.* Geneva, Switzerland: International Telecommunication Union; 2013. Retrieved from http://www.itu.int/ITU-D/ict/publications/world/world.html

52. Blaya JA, Fraser HS, Holt B. E-health technologies show promise in developing countries. *Health Affairs* 2010; 29(2):244–251.

53. Kahn JG, Yang JS, Kahn JS. 'Mobile' health needs and opportunities in developing countries. Health Affairs 2010; 29(2):252–258.

54. Goldzweig CL, Towfigh A, Maglione M, Shekelle PG. Costs and benefits of health information technology: New trends from the literature. *Health Affairs* 2009; 28(2):w282–293.

55. Rogers EM. Lessons for guidelines from the diffusion of innovations. *The Joint Commission Journal on Quality Improvement* 1995; 21(7):324–328.

56. Hoffman KA, Green CA, Ford JH, 2nd, Wisdom JP, Gustafson DH, McCarty D. Improving quality of care in substance abuse treatment using five key process improvement principles. *Journal of Behavioral Health Services & Research* 2012; 39(3):234–244.

57. Addiction Technology Transfer Center (ATTC) Network Technology Transfer Workgroup. Research to practice in addiction treatment: Key terms and a field-driven model of technology transfer. *Journal of Substance Abuse Treatment* 2011; 41: 169–178.

58. Martino S, Brigham GS, Higgins C, Gallon S, Freese TE, Albright LM, et al. Partnerships and pathways of dissemination: The National Institute on Drug Abuse-Substance Abuse and Mental Health Services Administration Blending Initiative in the Clinical Trials Network. Journal of Substance Abuse Treatment 2010; 38(Suppl 1):S31–43.

59. Marsch LA, Guarino H, Acosta M, Aponte-Melendez Y, Cleland C, Grabinski M, et al. Web-based behavioral treatment for substance use disorders as a partial replacement of standard methadone maintenance treatment. *Journal of Substance Abuse Treatment* 2014; 46(1):43–51.

60. Campbell AN, Nunes EV, Miele GM, Matthews A, Polsky D, Ghitza UE, et al. Design and methodological considerations of an effectiveness trial of a computer-assisted intervention: An example from the NIDA Clinical Trials Network. *Contemporary Clinical Trials* 2012; 33(2):386–395.

61. Nadeem E, Olin SS, Hill LC, Hoagwood KE, Horwitz SM. Understanding the components of quality improvement collaboratives: A systematic literature review. *The Milbank Quarterly* 2013; 91(2):354–394.

62. Nembhard IM. Learning and improving in quality improvement collaboratives: Which collaborative features do participants value most? *Health Services Research* 2009; 44(2 Pt 1):359–378.

63. Rojas CL, Seckman CA. The Informatics Nurse Specialist role in electronic health record usability evaluation. *Computers, Informatics, Nursing: CIN* 2014;. 32(5):214–220

16

Privacy, Security, and Regulatory Considerations as Related to Behavioral Health Information Technology

PENELOPE P. HUGHES AND MELISSA M. GOLDSTEIN

INTRODUCTION

As exemplified in chapters throughout this compendium, the potential for technology-based therapeutic tools to enhance behavioral healthcare is great. Yet, the use of information technology within behavioral healthcare also presents a number of challenges. This chapter focuses on one of the most complex—the evolving privacy and security regulatory environment. For the purpose of this chapter, *privacy* is defined as an individual's ability to have control over access to, and use of, his or her personal information (1). *Security* refers to the tools and technologies used to prevent inappropriate access to an individual's personal information (1).

The legal environment governing the privacy and security of behavioral health information is complicated, with a variety of state and federal statutes and regulations that apply to health information generally, in addition to those that apply solely to particular types of health information, such as information related to mental health or substance abuse treatment. In addition, as the use of information technology in behavioral healthcare grows more widespread and sophisticated, the number of entities involved in managing behavioral health information—including storing and/or transmitting this information electronically—and the statutes and regulations governing them, also grow.

To understand this complexity, it is helpful to examine first the variety of entities potentially involved in storing and sharing behavioral health information. For example, consider a mobile phone application (app) developed to provide cognitive behavioral therapy for depression that collects, shares, and analyzes video and audio recordings from a patient's phone, as well as photos, text messaging data, data from sensors (including GPS sensors and accelerometers), and data from connected tools such as sleep monitors (2). At each data collection point, and wherever data are stored or shared, entities such as device manufacturers, mobile network operators, app developers, data storage companies, or data analytics companies may be accessing the patient's information and presenting potential privacy and security issues.

In this chapter, we will discuss the history of health information privacy statutes and regulations, focusing in particular on behavioral health information. We will then examine the statutes and regulations protecting the privacy and security of health information generally, and behavioral health information specifically, as well as those developed to address the growing ecosystem of health information technology entities that gain access to health information when their technology is implemented. Finally, the future regulatory environment, including regulatory trends and potential upcoming activity that will affect the privacy and security of behavioral health technologies, will be discussed.

Because of the breadth of the issues involved, we have limited our discussion to issues surrounding the health information of adults; privacy rights and other issues related to minors (as defined by relevant state and federal law) are beyond the scope of this chapter. Further, our discussion does not constitute legal advice regarding any particular factual circumstance. Such interpretations depend on the specific circumstances involved and should be discussed within an institution's policy structure and in concert with counsel.

Finally, while our focus in this chapter is on U.S. domestic laws and policies related to the privacy and security of health information and information technology, the international policy context is also relevant to the transfer of personal information, including health information, across international borders. For example, data protection regulations such as those favored in Europe generally would allow the transfer of personal information only to countries where equally strong data protections are in place (2). In addition, work is ongoing internationally on consumer data policy frameworks to facilitate interoperable privacy regimes, such as the Safe Harbor Frameworks developed between the United States, the European Union (EU), and Switzerland that allow companies to certify that they comply with the EU Data Protection Directive and transfer data from the EU to the United States (3).

THE HISTORICAL UNDERPINNINGS OF PRIVACY AND SECURITY

In the United States, individual privacy has long been viewed as a fundamental and firmly held right, with both constitutional and common law (the law made by judges and courts) origins. The Fourth Amendment to the U.S. Constitution's "right of the people to be secure in their persons, houses, papers and effects, against unreasonable searches and seizures" (4) provides the underpinning of this right, and common law recognizes and reinforces it (5). For example, the common law tort of invasion of privacy, recognized in almost every state, allows individuals to bring civil lawsuits for harms including intrusion on an individual's privacy, unreasonable publicity, appropriation of another person's name or likeness, and publicity placing someone in a false light (6).

Historically, advancements in technology have often driven the need and desire for privacy protections. As illustrated by Samuel Warren and Louis Brandeis in the law review article, "The Right to Privacy," new technology can have unexpected consequences, such as when the development of "instantaneous photography" in the late 1800s enabled individuals' images to be captured quickly, without long exposure times and also without their knowledge, creating a new threat to the sense of privacy and the right "to be left alone," along with an urgency to guard against that threat

(7). This is no less true today in the context of information technology than it was in 1890 when the highly influential article was published.

In response to the rapid development of information technology in the late 1960s and the accompanying increase in electronic government databases, the Privacy Rights Act of 1974 was passed to provide protections for individual information collected and stored by the federal government (8). The Act emphasizes the importance of following Fair Information Practice Principles (FIPPS) when collecting data.[1] These principles, which have since become engrained in the concept of consumer privacy protections and adapted by a number of federal agencies and foreign nations, include transparency and notice regarding the collection and use of personally identifiable information; individual consent for the collection and use of such information; purpose specification, or a description of the exact purposes for which the information is going to be used; data minimization, or the collection of only the data necessary to accomplish the intended purpose; use limitation, or use of the information only for the stated purpose; data integrity, which involves ensuring the accuracy and completeness of the data; use of appropriate security safeguards for the information; and auditing, which includes ensuring compliance with all of the principles (9).

Despite the presence of this strong foundation for privacy regulation, the United States has not created an overarching federal privacy law. Instead, the FIPPS have been incorporated to varying degrees in privacy laws addressing different stakeholders and sectors of the economy, such as the federal government, the finance sector, the health sector, or the commercial activity space more generally. Some analysts emphasize that these laws generally promote the concept of privacy as the ability to control the use of one's own data, placing the consumer at the center of decisions about his or her own information and focusing on requirements to inform consumers about how their data are used and shared (10). For example, these laws might require companies to give notice to the consumer of the disclosure of his or her data to third parties, and/or to provide the option to opt out of sharing information with certain types of entities, such as marketing companies.

The FIPPS also form the basis of the Obama Administration's Consumer Privacy Bill of

Rights, which was released in 2012 and outlines the privacy rights that consumers should be able to expect, as well as those that companies should commit to protecting in the commercial Internet environment (3). The statement emphasizes the importance of building consumer trust and ensuring that companies access and use personal information only in ways that are within the context of the consumer's initial interaction with a company—that is, ways that are appropriate given the consumer's relationship with the company and that were disclosed to the consumer clearly at the time he or she originally released personal information, or that would be obvious to the consumer, such as when online retailers provide a customer's name and address to a shipper to fulfill an order (3). Additionally, when releasing the Consumer Privacy Bill of Rights, the Administration encouraged Congress to pass legislation applying its key principles to commercial sectors not covered by existing federal privacy laws (3).

Health Information Privacy

The concept of individual privacy rights extends naturally to health information. In fact, there is a long history in the United States of protecting the privacy and security of health information as a public health priority, in part due to the harm that can occur when such information is disclosed or shared inappropriately (11). Discrimination, in particular by employers or insurers, along with stigma and embarrassment, are all serious potential consequences related to disclosure of sensitive health information (12). It is also well documented that patients may engage in harmful privacy-protective behavior when fearful that their health information will not be kept secure or confidential, such as choosing not to reveal information to a provider or avoiding care altogether (13,14). In the area of behavioral health treatment and interventions in particular, studies have found that privacy concerns can be a significant barrier to accessing treatment (15).

Principles of personal autonomy and bioethics have also driven the need to focus on and protect the privacy of health information (16). Personal autonomy in the medical context encompasses the right of the patient to make informed decisions regarding treatment, including decisions about access to his or her health information (16). Given this interaction between privacy and consent, autonomy has been described as the "accepted rationale" for ensuring the privacy, security, and confidentiality of patient health information (17).

Recent advancements in technology that enable health information to be stored and transmitted electronically, instead of in paper format, have made concerns about the privacy and security of health information even more pressing (18). While acknowledging the value of health information technology, consumers consistently express serious concerns about the privacy and security of their health information when it is exchanged or stored electronically (13,19). In order for patients to participate fully in behavioral health interventions that make use of information technology, the privacy and security of patient health information must be adequately addressed.

HEALTH INFORMATION PRIVACY AND SECURITY LAW
Health Insurance Portability and Accountability Act (HIPAA)

The Health Insurance Portability and Accountability Act of 1996 (HIPAA) is the primary federal law protecting the privacy and security of health information (20). HIPAA sets a privacy floor, or minimum level of privacy protections, and preempts less stringent state laws. However, any state laws that provide greater privacy protections and limit disclosure of health information more strictly than HIPAA remain in force (21).

The HIPAA Privacy and Security Rules (the regulations promulgated pursuant to the statute) (22) address the circumstances under which a patient's protected health information[2] (PHI) can be disclosed by the holder of the information, as well as the types of security measures that holders of health information should have in place. The Privacy and Security Rules apply only to "covered entities" (23), which are defined as health plans, healthcare clearinghouses, and healthcare providers that transmit health information electronically for specific purposes, including those related to healthcare claims and health plans (23). Because of this limited application, products that are not offered by covered entities, but that still collect or access health information, such as free-standing electronic personal health records or mobile health applications marketed directly to the consumer and not offered by a provider, do not have to comply with HIPAA's Privacy and Security Rules. This creates a regulatory gap that would have to be covered by other agencies, including the Federal Trade Commission (FTC) and potentially the Food and Drug Administration (FDA) in the case of mobile health applications, as described later in the chapter.

A. Privacy Rule

Generally, the Privacy Rule allows for the disclosure of a patient's PHI without the patient's consent or permission, for the purposes of treatment, payment, or healthcare operations (24), a category that includes activities such as quality assessments or compliance audits. Additionally, a covered entity is permitted to disclose a patient's PHI in certain other circumstances specified by the Rule, including disclosures for public health purposes or to comply with state or federal laws (25).

While a broad array of disclosures are permissible under the Privacy Rule, any disclosure not permitted or required[3] must have the patient's authorization (26). Also, HIPAA explicitly requires a patient's authorization in several circumstances, including for marketing or sale of a patient's PHI (with some exceptions) as well as for most disclosures of a patient's psychotherapy notes (27). The latter restriction in particular would be important in the case of any behavioral health therapeutic tool that might expose notes recorded by a therapist when treating a patient to disclosure.

Another important aspect of the Privacy Rule is the exception for de-identified information. Any health information that has been de-identified in a way sanctioned by the Privacy Rule is not considered PHI and can be disclosed without restrictions (28). For example, a covered entity could disclose aggregated data that meet the Rule's requirements for de-identification to a third party for analysis of user characteristics or for private marketing studies. For such information to qualify as de-identified, the Privacy Rule requires either that a scientific method[4] be used to render the information incapable of being tied to a particular individual (29), or that a list of 18 specific identifiers be removed in a way that makes it impossible to identify the individual associated with the information (30). This latter method is known as the "safe harbor" method, and identifiers that must be removed include information such as names, telephone numbers, e-mail addresses, dates (except year), and account numbers (30). Under the "safe harbor" method, if the covered entity has knowledge that an individual can be re-identified using the de-identified data, either alone or in combination with other information, the data will not be considered de-identified.

In addition to restricting the use and disclosure of health information, the Privacy Rule requires that all covered entities provide a notice of privacy practices to patients that states how the covered entity may use and disclose a patient's information, what rights the patient may have regarding that information, and the organization's legal duties to protect that information (31). Importantly, where a covered entity does not follow the practices stated in its notice, the FTC could take action if it finds unfair or deceptive trade practices on the part of the covered entity (described below) (32).

B. Security Rule

The Security Rule requires that covered entities implement security protections to prevent a patient's electronic PHI from being accessed or shared improperly (33). These protections include administrative, technical, and physical safeguards. More specifically, covered entities must "ensure the confidentiality, integrity, and availability" of any electronic PHI they create or handle; identify and guard against threats to this information or impermissible uses or disclosures; and ensure that their workforce complies with the Rule (34).

The Security Rule is designed to be scalable and flexible, enabling covered entities of all sizes to comply. The Rule generally does not dictate specific security measures that a covered entity must implement, but it allows organizations to analyze their own security needs and implement appropriate protections. That is, the Rule consists of some "required" specifications that must be implemented, such as the use of unique user identifications (35), as well as a number of "addressable" specifications that the entity can implement as it sees fit, provided those decisions are documented in writing. One especially important "required" specification of the Security Rule is the requirement to conduct a security risk analysis and to mediate "unacceptable" risks to patient data (36). When conducting the required risk analysis, covered entities should identify and document potential threats to electronic health information in their systems, considering both the likelihood and potential impact of each threat; quantify the level of risk associated with each threat; and identify what mitigation is appropriate for each level of risk. Entities are encouraged to rely on this security risk analysis in their approach to the "addressable" specifications described above (34).

C. Breach Notification Rule

An additional key component of HIPAA is the Breach Notification Rule, which requires covered entities to notify the Department of Health and Human Services (HHS) as well as all individuals affected whenever a breach of unsecured PHI has occurred (37,38). According to the Rule, a "breach" is any impermissible use or disclosure of PHI, unless the covered entity or business associate[5] (an organization acting on behalf of a covered entity, discussed in more detail below) (39) can demonstrate that there is a low probability that the PHI was compromised (40). For example, if a covered entity proves that a stolen laptop containing PHI was never opened and the information never accessed or viewed, such factors might prevent an incident from being deemed a breach under the Rule. Meanwhile, "unsecured" PHI refers to information that has not been made unreadable through the use of prescribed technology, including encryption (40). Thus, for example, even if information is impermissibly disclosed and a breach occurs, as long as it is encrypted in accordance with guidance issued by the Office of Civil Rights (OCR) (41), the division of HHS that enforces HIPAA, notification is not necessary because the information is not "unsecured PHI" (40).

Where PHI is held in a personal health record (PHR) that is not covered by HIPAA, the FTC's Breach Notification Rule, which closely mirrors the HIPAA rule, would instead apply to any breach of the information (42). A PHR is defined as an electronic record of an individual's health information that can collect and combine health information from various sources and that is managed either by, or on behalf of, the patient (43). Generally, if a PHR is provided to a patient by a healthcare provider, health plan, or other HIPAA-covered entity, the PHR will be subject to HIPAA (44). However, if the PHR is a stand-alone commercial product that the patient elects to use to store and share his or her PHI, it will likely be subject to regulation by the FTC (44).

D. Business Associates

Contractors and other organizations that conduct business on behalf of covered entities and that create, receive, maintain, or access PHI are considered business associates (BAs) and must comply with all provisions of the Security Rule and most provisions of the Privacy Rule (22). Thus, entities that gain access to patient health information as information technology is adopted, such as mobile app software vendors, may be considered BAs if they act on behalf of covered entities and therefore be responsible for complying with HIPAA's requirements.

Under HIPAA, when a vendor or other third-party entity is considered a BA, a Business Associate Agreement (BAA) must be in place between the covered entity and the BA (45). According to guidance issued by OCR, the agreement must, among other things, define the uses and disclosures of PHI the BA is permitted or required to make and require the BA to use appropriate safeguards to protect PHI, including the requirements in the HIPAA Security Rule (46). Cloud computing services are one type of organization that may be considered a BA under HIPAA. While the issue has not yet been directly addressed by HHS to date, key considerations when determining if a cloud service provider would be required to follow HIPAA's requirements are whether the cloud vendor acts on behalf of a covered entity and whether the service provided by the vendor requires access to PHI on a regular basis. If the answers to these questions are yes, it is more likely that the cloud provider qualifies as a BA under HIPAA and will need to comply with the regulations.

42 Code of Federal Regulations (CFR) Part 2

Some behavioral health information is also subject to restrictions on disclosure pursuant to 42 CFR Part 2 (Part 2)[6] (47), federal regulations that address the disclosure of personal information related to substance use treatment. Part 2 applies to entities holding themselves out as substance use treatment providers who receive support from the federal government, which could include receiving federal funding or qualifying for federal tax-exempt status (48). Part 2 protects any information from a Part 2 program that indicates directly or indirectly that a patient is a participant in a Part 2 program or has a current or past drug or alcohol problem (49).

With very limited exceptions (an emergency, for example) (50), a patient's written consent is required to release information related to Part 2 treatment, and whenever such information is released, a statement that re-release of the information is prohibited must accompany the disclosure (51). In addition, the regulation requires that third parties that contract with Part 2 programs to perform services use a special type of contract to allow access to patient data[7] and also requires Part 2 programs to take certain security precautions with regard to patient data (52). These stringent requirements, which go beyond HIPAA, were implemented because of the great sensitivity of substance use treatment information, the stigma frequently associated with such treatment, and the strong public health interest in not discouraging individuals with substance use issues from seeking treatment (53).

Thus, where a provider subject to Part 2 uses a technology-based therapeutic tool in treating a patient and transmits information regarding the patient to a third party (e.g., another provider), the Part 2 provider would need to ensure (a) that the patient has given consent for data to be released to that particular third party, and (b) that a prohibition on re-disclosure accompanies the data when they are transmitted. Additionally, any third parties involved in the flow of that information (e.g., a data center storing and analyzing the patient's information as part of the tool's functionality) should have appropriate contracts with the Part 2 organization.

Health Information Technology for Economic and Clinical Health Act (HITECH)

With the passage of HITECH (54), Congress not only enhanced HIPAA privacy protections by, for example, placing new limits on the sale of PHI (55), but also created what is commonly referred to as the "meaningful use" program, whereby eligible providers can receive incentive payments for using electronic health records (EHR) (56). In order to receive the incentive payments, providers must use EHRs in particular ways (57) and must meet certain requirements, some of which also enhance privacy and security, such as the requirement to conduct a security risk analysis, described earlier (58). Additionally, providers must use certified technology that meets the criteria set by certification rules (59) issued by the Office of the National Coordinator for Health Information Technology (ONC) within HHS. Under HITECH, ONC was charged with setting up a certification program to ensure that EHRs used by providers as part of the incentive program meet certain minimum requirements (59). These requirements also include a number of privacy and security specifications, for example, the requirement to use authentication and access controls in order to be sure that individuals accessing health information electronically are who they claim to be (60).

Most behavioral health providers, however, are explicitly excluded from the incentive program. Generally, only psychiatrists or psychiatric nurse practitioners who serve a certain percentage of Medicaid or Medicare patients are eligible (61), although ONC has issued guidance to encourage the development and certification of EHR for use by other behavioral health providers as well (62). This guidance includes privacy- and security-related criteria such as authentication and access controls, automatic log-off, or, shutting off use of a system after a set amount of inactivity in order to prevent inappropriate access, and encryption, that is, rendering data unreadable without a special key to decode the information (62).

Use of Health Information for Research

If data collected as part of a behavioral health intervention are intended for use in research, certain laws and privacy protections may apply. The Federal Policy for the Protection of Human Subjects, or "Common Rule," (63) provides protections for human subjects participating in federally funded research projects. Prior to allowing "individually identifiable"[8] (64) data to be used for research, the Common Rule requires that researchers obtain informed consent from each research participant (65) as well as have the research protocol reviewed and approved by an Institutional Review Board (IRB) (66), which must ensure that the research plan has adequate privacy and data confidentiality protections (67). Meanwhile, HIPAA allows data to be disclosed for research purposes without individual authorization in certain limited circumstances, such as when the research has been approved by an IRB (68). Outside of these circumstances, HIPAA allows data to be disclosed for research purposes with the individual's authorization; however the authorization must satisfy specific requirements set forth in the Privacy Rule (69).

Other Department of Heath and Human Services (HHS) Activity

In addition to (and to some degree because of) the laws described above, the federal government, and in particular HHS, has sponsored and encouraged innovative technological solutions to support the exchange of behavioral health information in a way that protects patient privacy (70). These efforts include the Behavioral Health Data Exchange Consortium, an ONC-sponsored effort that piloted interstate electronic exchange of behavioral health records and created draft policies and procedures, and a joint Substance Abuse and Mental Health Services Administration and Health Resources and Services Administration effort to create a 42 CFR Part 2–compliant consent form that could be used in an electronic health information exchange environment (71). Additionally, the Data Segmentation for Privacy Initiative (DS4P), led by the ONC, sponsors pilot projects whose goal is to demonstrate ways to share information protected by 42 CFR Part 2, including electronic transmission of the prohibition on re-disclosure that must accompany disclosures of patient data pursuant to the law (72). ONC has also released a Program Information Notice providing guidance on electronic health information exchange to the beneficiaries of certain federal health information technology programs that emphasizes the importance of providing meaningful choice to patients when their health information is exchanged, as well as other privacy and security recommendations (73).

Other HHS activity addresses the variety in state health information laws (described below) that can complicate the exchange of health information among entities in different states. For example, as part of the implementation of HITECH, ONC established Regional Extension Centers (RECs) across the country to assist providers in utilizing health information technology, including for the purpose of health information exchange (74). The work of the RECs relies in part on earlier efforts of the Health Information Security and Privacy Collaboration (HISPC), which was created in part to assess privacy

and security challenges arising from state laws and identify practical solutions (75). As part of HISPC's efforts, multistate collaborative organizations were formed to help address privacy and security challenges to electronic health information exchange.

State Laws

States also have a variety of laws protecting different types of health information, including, for example, mental health information and substance use treatment information. While these laws vary widely, most prohibit the holder of the information from disclosing it without appropriate authorization (76). While HIPAA would allow disclosure of a patient's health information for treatment, payment, and healthcare operations purposes, for example, some state laws are stricter and may not even allow disclosure in the case of an emergency (77).

In addition, some state laws address various aspects of health information technology directly. For example, in the area of telehealth, which is defined for the purpose of this chapter as the use of information and telecommunications technologies to support long-distance clinical healthcare (78), a 2010 review of state laws and regulations by the American Psychological Association found that several states have enacted laws that generally include informed consent requirements mandating that information related to the privacy and security of the service is given to patients via notices (79).

LAWS IMPACTING MOBILE OR WEB-BASED TECHNOLOGIES

In addition to laws addressing the privacy and security of health information generally, there is growing activity at both the state and federal levels addressing the use of information technology in consumer products and services, including mobile health apps, health-related websites and Web-based services, portable sensors that connect to mobile devices, and other similar products. The primary regulatory actors in this arena include the FTC, the FDA, the National Telecommunications and Information Administration (NTIA), the Federal Communications Commission (FCC), and some states. The various agencies involved have taken different approaches in the past few years as regulators have attempted to keep pace with rapid advances in technology. In general, these efforts have been guided by the FIPPS and the Consumer Privacy Bill of Rights, with an emphasis on industry self-regulation and transparency. Key themes in agency approaches have emerged, such as enabling informed consumer choice through the provision of appropriate notice, expanding the definition of personally identifying information that should be protected, and focusing on the collection of consumer data by third parties, including the communication of such activity to consumers.

Federal Trade Commission (FTC)

Under Section 5 of the Federal Trade Commission Act, the FTC has the authority to prevent "unfair or deceptive" acts related to commercial activity (80). An act is considered "unfair" if it causes, or is likely to cause, substantial injury to a consumer that the consumer is not reasonably able to avoid, and which is not outweighed by benefits to the consumer (81,82). An act is considered "deceptive" if it involves a practice or representation that is likely to mislead a consumer acting reasonably and is also material to the consumer—that is, the practice or representation is likely to have kept the consumer from using the product had it not been misrepresented (82).

A. Enforcement

The FTC relies on investigations and enforcement actions to address unfair and deceptive practices (83). In order to understand how the FTC Act might apply to the privacy and security of behavioral health technologies, it is instructive to examine recent FTC enforcement activities related to mobile devices and apps. Generally, FTC enforcement actions addressing "deceptive" acts have emphasized the importance of following stated privacy policies, including policies and practices described in privacy notices posted on an entity's website, for example, as well as user manuals (84,85). Violation of voluntary codes of conduct that an entity claims to follow could also lead to a deceptive practice enforcement action (86).

As an example, in a February 2013 complaint and consent order against HTC, America, Inc., the FTC's first enforcement action against the maker of a mobile device, the FTC articulated its position that a misrepresentation of security measures, in this case failure to employ the security controls

and permissions described in the user manual, may constitute a deceptive business practice (85). In addition, the "covered information" that the FTC indicated should be secured is broadly defined in the complaint and consent order to include cookies, Internet Protocol (IP) addresses (unique numbers that can be used to identify a computer or device accessing the internet), device IDs (unique device identification numbers used to identify a smartphone or other wireless device), contact lists, e-mails, text messages, and most information either stored on or transmitted by the device—perhaps indicating willingness on the part of the agency to base future enforcement actions on similarly broadly defined categories of information (87).

Regarding "unfair" acts, recent FTC enforcement activities have focused on the security measures that entities employ to protect consumer information, as well as the manner in which entities allow third parties to access and use consumer information (88). In the HTC complaint described above, for example, the FTC alleged an unfair act in HTC's failure to implement reasonable security measures, including secure programming practices, security audits, and privacy and security training for staff (85). Similarly, in a complaint against LabMD, the FTC stated that, among other inappropriate security practices, the use of a peer-to-peer file-sharing network to store personal information about consumers created a significant security risk and enabled unauthorized exposure of a consumer's personal data to third parties, thus constituting an unfair act (89). LabMD's challenge to the complaint was scheduled to be heard in April, 2014 (89,90).

B. Guidance

In addition to enforcing the FTC Act, the FTC has also issued privacy guidance for mobile apps and app developers. The guidance, based on recommendations made in the FTC's March 2012 report, *Protecting Consumer Privacy in an Era of Rapid Change: Recommendations for Businesses and Policymakers* (91), focuses on mobile app privacy disclosures and the process of marketing mobile apps. Regarding disclosures, the guidance stresses the importance of "just-in-time" notices and obtaining affirmative consent when sensitive information (such as health-related information) is being collected by an app or is being shared with third parties (92). "Just-in-time" notices would prompt consumers at the time personal information is about to be collected and ask for permission to use the information. In theory, this process allows consumers to consider the time, place, and exact circumstances in which their personal information is being collected and enables meaningful choice.

The FTC guidance on disclosures also urges app developers to improve coordination with third parties that may have access to consumer data in order to understand what data they collect and how they may be using it, and to facilitate appropriate communication of that information to consumers (92). As the guidance notes, it is common for app developers to include code-enabling data to be shared with third parties for analytics or behavioral advertising[9] without fully understanding, or communicating to the consumer, exactly what information the third party is accessing and how it is being used (92). In fact, a 2013 study of health apps indicated that 39% of free apps and 30% of paid apps were sending data to undisclosed third parties (93).

The FTC guidance on the process of marketing mobile apps and similar technologies emphasizes the importance of adopting "privacy by design" (94), or the concept of building privacy and security features into products from the beginning of product development. These features include, for example, data security measures, limitations on the amount of information collected, appropriate data retention and disposal practices, and data accuracy (94). The guidance also encourages transparency regarding data collection and recommends collecting sensitive information only with affirmative consent (94).

Food and Drug Administration (FDA)

Under the Food, Drug and Cosmetic Act (FD&C Act), the FDA regulates devices that are intended for medical use, including software and hardware, for safety and efficacy (95). Whether or not a product is considered a medical device subject to FDA regulation depends primarily on how the product is intended to be used, including how it is marketed. Generally, products intended for the diagnosis, cure, treatment, mitigation, or prevention of a medical condition are considered medical devices (95).

Recent FDA guidance, which is non-binding but represents the agency's current thinking on the topic, clarifies which types of health apps the FDA will regulate and emphasizes that most would likely not be regulated. According to the guidance, the FDA would only consider an app to fall under its authority if it functions as a medical device— that is, it meets the definition of a device and either it is used as an accessory to a regulated medical device or it transforms a mobile platform into a regulated medical device, and it could pose a risk to patient safety if it did not function as intended (96). For example, the FDA might consider an app that analyzes electrocardiogram or other sensor data to detect heart problems to fall under its authority. The FDA considers such apps to be "mobile medical apps" (96). With regard to enforcement, the FDA has stated that it does not intend to enforce requirements under the FD&C Act for certain types of apps, including mobile apps that serve as videoconferencing portals, apps that help patients with psychiatric conditions through delivery of messages or tips to improve coping skills, or apps that provide education, reminders, or motivation to patients recovering from addiction (96).

Finally, the FDA is currently engaged in a multi-agency effort to explore creation of a non-duplicative regulatory environment for mobile medical apps. The Food and Drug Administration Safety and Innovation Act of 2012 (FDASIA) called for the FDA, along with a diverse federal workgroup that includes the FCC and ONC, to make recommendations for a risk-based regulatory framework for health information technology, including mobile health apps, that protects patient safety and does not duplicate other regulatory efforts (97). With respect to privacy and security issues, the agencies involved in this process have emphasized the importance of examining and considering network security risks and compliance with security standards as part of any resulting regulatory framework (98).

National Telecommunications and Information Administration (NTIA)

The NTIA, a federal agency responsible for advising the administration on telecommunications issues, engaged in a multi-stakeholder collaboration process to develop a draft voluntary code of conduct for mobile app developers that was released to the developer community for testing in July, 2013 (99).

The draft code is focused on notice and choice, and provides guidelines on creating "short-form" notices that consumers can review quickly and use to understand the type of personal information that is being collected by a mobile app and with whom the app shares that data (99). The draft code requires apps to provide this information on a single screen if possible and in "nutrition label" format (99). This means that, for a specified set of categories of information, including health, medical, and therapy information, the notice must indicate whether the app does or does not collect consumer data. In addition, for a specified set of third parties, including ad networks and data analytics companies, the notice must indicate whether or not data are shared (99). Notably, the draft code does not focus on "just-in-time" notices, nor does it require any particular type of notice to be used for sensitive data.

Federal Communications Commission (FCC)

The FCC has a long history of activity in the area of wireless communications, including wireless medical technology, which would extend to the use of mobile devices, sensors, and other wireless communications in behavioral health technology. In particular, the FCC established a mobile health (mHealth) task force to provide recommendations on improving healthcare delivery through wireless health technologies. Although the recommendations of the task force did not focus directly on the privacy and security aspects of mHealth, they did recognize the importance of these issues to mHealth and to the safe and acceptable use of wireless technologies (100). With respect to using wireless technologies to communicate health information, the recommendations support the use of "standards-based means of sending authenticated messages and encrypted health information directly to known, trusted recipients" (100). This would include, for example, the use of standards developed as part of the ONC's Direct Project, or other standards that ensure information is encrypted and is securely delivered to the intended recipient (100).

State Efforts Impacting Mobile and Web-Based Technologies

As discussed earlier, there is no all-encompassing federal privacy law providing baseline privacy protections to individuals, and in the absence of any movement toward federal consumer privacy legislation, even after this was encouraged with release of the Consumer Privacy Bill of Rights, states have begun to take steps by passing a number of laws to protect the privacy of consumers. California has been one of the most active states in the area of consumer privacy, illustrating the role states may play in regulating or influencing behavioral health technologies. The California Online Privacy Protection Act (CalOPPA), for example, requires websites and online services to disclose their data collection and use practices, including disclosure of how third parties may use consumer data (101). CalOPPA also addresses the format these disclosures must take, requiring them to be "conspicuously posted" (102). As an initial indication of California's commitment to enforcing these regulations, the state has created an enforcement unit and has sent warning letters to a number of mobile app companies (103).

Additionally, the California Attorney General has released privacy recommendations specifically designed for mobile apps (104). These recommendations are based on the FIPPS and focus on notice practices, with a strong emphasis on the importance of "just-in-time" notices (104). The guidance encourages use of such notices prior to the collection of sensitive consumer data as well as whenever an app collects consumer data in an unexpected way or allows third-party access to the data. This guidance also includes security recommendations such as encryption of personal information, including device ID, while in transit or in storage (104).

Industry Self-Regulation

In addition to the NTIA efforts described earlier, several voluntary industry codes of conduct have been developed that could impact behavioral health technologies, in particular those relying on mobile devices and apps. As one example, Happtique, a commercial online mobile health app marketplace, launched a certification program to identify apps that contain credible data, use reasonable safeguards, and function as intended (105). As part of this program, Happtique released certification standards that include privacy and security standards, as well as operability and content standards. The privacy standards include a number of requirements reflecting the FIPPS, such as obtaining affirmative express consent prior to collecting sensitive information or providing data to third parties (105). The security standards reference HIPAA, and where the app is collecting protected health information according to the HIPAA definition, the requirements call for full compliance with HIPAA as well as the incentive program certification and standards described earlier (105).

CONCLUSIONS

Several themes have emerged from this review that indicate the direction this area of regulatory activity may take in the future. First, regulations that directly address behavioral health information specifically tend to focus on disclosure restrictions and notice requirements and generally require that reasonable security measures are in place to protect sensitive health data. Various policy efforts have been and are being made to make notices understandable; however, these efforts are rarely enshrined in the regulations themselves, which tend to be general in nature to allow for such flexibility in practice. That is, a regulation might state "notice is required," then leave it up to researchers to study and policymakers to implement. Because compliance with these regulations can be technologically challenging, in particular regarding requirements for disclosure, the results of ongoing pilot projects related to data segmentation and other technical solutions may provide direction for developers as well as influence future policy.

Second, state and federal activity addressing consumer use of information technology more generally has focused on notice and security requirements, without including restrictions on disclosure or requirements for authorization. Increasingly, guidance and enforcement actions have promoted the concept of "just-in-time" notices, or contextual notice, and have required description of third-party access to the data. In addition, this activity has begun to expand the type of data that would be considered individually identifiable information and that must be addressed in notices and protected through reasonable security measures. For example, guidance has begun to include data such as the content of text messages sent by a mobile device, or the contact list stored on a mobile device, as information

that should be discussed in a notice of privacy practices and adequately secured.

On the other hand, agencies have also recognized a need to encourage innovation regarding the use of information technology and have expressed interest in minimizing regulatory impact through adoption of risk-based regulatory schemes that will help avoid unnecessary or duplicative regulation. Government activity in this space also indicates a preference toward industry-driven solutions and self-regulation, supporting the development of voluntary codes of conduct and encouraging industry adoption of privacy-by-design concepts, which require industry consideration of privacy and security issues at each stage of product development. The extent to which industry embraces codes of conduct and/or privacy and security best practices in the near future will help determine the need for more active government involvement.

While health information technology privacy and security regulations can be complex, several key principles have emerged that are useful in interpreting these issues within the context of behavioral healthcare information. These principles include understanding and abiding by legal restrictions on certain disclosures of health information, in particular those involving sensitive health information, such as mental health and/or substance abuse treatment; providing adequate notice and choice to patients regarding disclosure of their health information, including disclosures to third parties; and ensuring appropriate security safeguards are in place to protect health information. Additionally, it is important to follow industry self-regulation efforts and emerging best practices with respect to privacy and security protections. Embracing these core principles can not only help navigate the complex regulatory environment, but will also help enable the use of information technology within behavioral healthcare in a way that protects the privacy and security of sensitive health information and inspires patient trust.

NOTES

1. Fair Information Practice Principles (FIPPS) have their origin in the U.S. Department of Health, Education and Welfare's 1973 report "Records, Computers and the Rights of Citizens" and were advanced through the Privacy Rights Act of 1974.

2. Protected health information is defined in the HIPAA regulations as "individually identifiable health information" (45 C.F.R. § 164.103).

3. 45 C.F.R. 164.502 (a)(2) requires disclosure to individuals when requested or when required by the Secretary of the Department of Health and Human Services in order to investigate compliance.

4. Scientific method refers to a method by which a person with scientific knowledge and understanding of statistical methods applies such methods to de-identify a data set, or remove data that can be used to identify someone, such as a complete zip code or phone number, and determines that the risk of re-identifying an individual from the de-identified data set is very small (45 C.F.R. § 164.514(b)(1)).

5. Business associate is defined as a person who, on behalf of a covered entity, creates, receives, maintains, or transmits protected health information (45 C.F.R. § 160.103).

6. These regulations were promulgated pursuant to the Comprehensive Alcohol Abuse and Alcoholism Prevention, Treatment and Rehabilitation Act of 1970, Pub. L. No. 91-616, 84 Stat. 1848, and the Drug Abuse Office and Treatment Act of 1972, Pub L. No. 92-255, 86 Stat. 65. The rulemaking authority granted by both statutes relating to confidentiality of records can now be found at 42 U.S.C. § 290dd-2 (2006).

7. Third-party organizations providing services to a Part 2 program (such as data-processing or other professional service) and which enter into a "qualified service organization agreement" (QSOA) with a Part 2 program are known as "qualified service organizations," or QSOs. QSOs may share a patient's information without the patient's consent as needed to perform their services, but they are bound by the QSOA to resist any efforts to obtain patient records except as permitted by regulations (42 CFR § 2.11).

8. According to the Common Rule, information is considered "individually identifiable" if "the identity of the subject is or may readily be ascertained by the investigator or associated with the information" (45 C.F.R. § 46.102).

9. Online behavioral advertising refers to the practice of collecting information about an individual's online behavior and using that data to serve ads or content relevant to that individual. See http://www.truste.com/consumer-privacy/about-oba/.

REFERENCES

1. Privacy and confidentiality in the nationwide health information network. Washington, DC: National Committee on Vital and Health Statistics (US); 2006 (June).

2. Patient privacy in a mobile world: A framework to address privacy law issues in mobile health. London: Thomson Reuters Foundation (UK); 2013 (June).

3. Consumer data privacy in a networked world: A framework for protecting privacy and promoting innovation in the global digital economy. Washington, DC: The White House; 2012. Retrieved from www.whitehouse.gov/sites/default/files/privacy-final.pdf

4. U.S. Constitution, Amend. 4.

5. Mariner W. Medicine and public health: Crossing legal boundaries. *Journal of Health Care Law & Policy* 2007; 10:121–151.

6. Post R. The social foundations of privacy: Community and self in the common law tort. *California Law Review* 1989; 77(5):957–1010.

7. Warren S, Brandeis L. The right to privacy. *Harvard Law Review* 1890; 4(5):193–196.

8. The Privacy Act of 1974. Pub.L. 93-579, 88 Stat. 1896 (Dec. 31, 1974), codified at 5 U.S.C. § 552a (2000).

9. National strategy for trusted identities in cyberspace. Washington, DC: The White House; 2011. Retrieved from http://www.whitehouse.gov/sites/default/files/rss.../NSTICstrategy_041511.pdf

10. Schwartz P. Privacy and democracy in cyberspace. *Vanderbilt Law Review* 1999; 52:1610–1701.

11. Beckerman J, Pritts J, Goplerud E, Leifer J, Borzi, P, Rosenbaum, S, et al. A delicate balance: Behavioral health, patient privacy, and the need to know. California HealthCare Foundation; 2008. Retrieved from http://www.chcf.org/resources/download.aspx?id=%7BA5615804-853B

12. Gostin L, Hodge J, Valdiserri R. Informational privacy and the public's health: The model state public health privacy act. *American Journal of Public Health* 2001; 91(9):1388–1392.

13. Agaku A, Adisa A, Ayo-Yusuf O, Connolly G. Concern about security and privacy, and perceived control over collection and use of health information are related to withholding of health information from healthcare providers. *Journal of the American Medical Informatics Association* 2013. Retrieved from http://jamia.bmj.com/content/early/2013/08/23/amiajnl-2013-002079.full.pdf+html

14. Consumers and health information technology: A national survey. California HealthCare Foundation; 2010. Retrieved from http://www.chcf.org/publications/2010/ 04/consumers-and-health-information-technology-a- national-survey

15. Rapp R, Xu J, Carr C, Lane T, Wang J, Carlson R. Treatment barriers identified by substance abusers. *Journal of Substance Abuse Treatment* 2006; 30(3):227–235.

16. Goldstein MM. Health information technology and the idea of informed consent. *Journal of Law & Medical Ethics* 2010; 38(1):27–35.

17. Terry NP, Francis LP. Ensuring the privacy and confidentiality of electronic health records. *University of Illinois Law Review* 2007; 2007(2):681–736.

18. Goldstein M, Rein A. Data segmentation in electronic health information exchange: policy considerations and analysis. Washington, DC: U.S. Department of Health and Human Services, Office of the National Coordinator for Health Information Technology; 2010 (Sept.). Retrieved from http://healthit.hhs.gov/ portal/server.pt/ gateway/ PTARGS_0_11673_950145_0_0_18/ gwu-data-segmentation-final.pdf

19. Making it meaningful: How consumers value and trust health it. National Partnership for Women and Families; 2012. Retrieved from http://go.nationalpartnership.org/ site/ PageServer?pagename= issues_health_IT_survey

20. Health Insurance Portability and Accountability Act of 1996 (HIPAA), P.L. No. 104-191, 110 Stat. 1938 (1996).

21. 45 C.F.R. § 160.203.

22. 45 C.F.R. § 160, 164.

23. 45 C.F.R. § 164.103.

24. 45 C.F.R. § 164.506.

25. 45 C.F.R. § 164.512.

26. 45 C.F.R. § 164.508(a)(1).

27. 45 C.F.R. § 164.508(a)(2).

28. 45 C.F.R. § 164.514.

29. 45 C.F.R. § 164.514 (b)(1).

30. 45 C.F.R. § 164.514 (b)(2)(i).

31. 45 C.F.R. § 164.520.

32. Office for Civil Rights (US). CVS pays $2.25 million and toughens practices to settle hipaa privacy case. Washington, DC: U.S. Department of Health and Human Services; 2009. Retrieved from http://www.hhs.gov/news/press/2009pres/02/20090218a.html

33. 45 C.F.R. § 164.302.

34. 45 C.F.R. § 164.306.

35. 45 C.F.R. § 164.312(a)(2)(i).

36. 45 C.F.R. § 164.308(a)(1)(ii)(A), (B).

37. 45 C.F.R. § 164.404.

38. 45 C.F.R. § 164.408.

39. 45 C.F.R. § 160.103.

40. 45 C.F.R. § 164.402.

41. 45 C.F.R. § 164.304.

42. 16 C.F.R. § 318.

43. 16 C.F.R. § 318.2(d).

44. Health Breach Notification Rule; Final Rule. 74 Fed. Reg. 42964 (Aug. 25, 2009).

45. 45 C.F.R. 164.504(e).

46. Office for Civil Rights (US). Sample business associate agreement provisions. Washington, DC: U.S. Department of Health and Human Services; 2013 (January). Retrieved from http://www.hhs.gov/ocr/privacy/hipaa/ understanding/coveredentities/ contractprov.html

47. 42 U.S.C. § 290dd-2.

48. 42 C.F.R. § 2.11.

49. 42 C.F.R. § 2.12.

50. 42 C.F.R. § 2.51.

51. 42 C.F.R. § 2.3.

52. 42 C.F.R. § 2.16.

53. 42 C.F.R. § 2.3(b)(2).

54. Health Information Technology for Economic and Clinical Health (HITECH) Act, Title XIII, Division A of the American Recovery and Reinvestment Act (ARRA), Pub. L. No. 111-5, §§ 13001-13424, 123 Stat. 115, 228-279 (2009).

55. HITECH § 13405.

56. HITECH § 3011.

57. 42 C.F.R. § 495.6(d).

58. 42 C.F.R. § 495.6.

59. HITECH § 3001(c)(5).

60. 45 C.F.R. §§ 170.314(d).

61. HITECH § 1861(r).

62. Certification guidance for EHR technology developers serving health care providers ineligible for medicare and medicaid ehr incentive payments. Washington, DC: U.S. Department of Health and Human Services, Office of the National Coordinator for Health Information Technology; 2013. Retrieved from http://www.healthit.gov/sites/ default/files/generalcertexchangeguidance_final_9-9-13.pdf

63. 45 C.F.R. § 46.

64. 45 C.F.R. § 46.102.

65. 45 C.F.R. § 46.116.

66. 45 C.F.R. § 46.103.

67. 45 C.F.R. § 46.111.

68. 45 C.F.R. § 164.512(i)(1).

69. 45 C.F.R. § 164.508.

70. Issue brief: Behavioral health and health IT. Washington, DC: Department of Health and Human Services, Office of the National Coordinator for Health Information Technology; 2013. Retrieved from http://www.healthit.gov/sites/default/files/ bhandhit_issue_brief.pdf.

71. Office of the National Coordinator for Health Information Technology (US). Behavioral health

data exchange/primary care and behavioral health integration. Washington, DC: U.S. Department of Health and Human Services; 2013. Retrieved from http://www.healthit.gov/ policy-researchers-implementers/ behavioral-health-data-exchange

72. Office of the National Coordinator for Health Information Technology (US). Consent management. Washington, DC: U.S. Department of Health and Human Services; 2013. Retrieved from http://www.healthit.gov/ policy-researchers-implementers/ consent-management

73. Privacy and security framework requirements and guidance for the state health information exchange cooperative agreement program. Washington, DC: U.S. Department of Health and Human Services, Office of the National Coordinator for Health Information Technology; 2012. Retrieved from http://www.healthit.gov/sites/ default/files/ hie.../onc-hie-pin-003-final.pdf

74. Regional extension centers (recs). Washington, DC: U.S. Department of Health and Human Services, Office of the National Coordinator for Health Information Technology; 2013. Retrieved from http://www.healthit.gov/providers-professionals/ regional-extension-centers-recs

75. Policymaking, regulation and strategy. Washington, DC: U.S. Department of Health and Human Services, Office of the National Coordinator for Health Information Technology; 2013. Retrieved from http:// www.healthit.gov/ policy-researchers-implementers/ federal-state-health-care-coordination

76. Pritts J, White J, Daniel J, Posnack S. Privacy and security solutions for interoperable health information exchange: Report on state law requirements for patient permission to disclose health information. Washington, DC: U.S. Department of Health and Human Services, Office of the National Coordinator for Health Information Technology; 2009 (Aug.). Retrieved from http://www.healthit. hhs.gov/portal/ server.pt/gateway/PTARGS_0_ 10741_910326_0_0_18/ DisclosureReport.pdf

77. See, e.g., Maine, ME. REV. STAT. ANN. tit. 5, § 19203, and Massachusetts, MASS GEN LAWS ch. 111, § 70F, which prohibit disclosure of HIV testing results even in an emergency.

78. Health Resources and Services Administration (US). Telehealth. Washingtion, DC: U.S. Department of Health and Human Services; 2012. Retrieved from http://www.hrsa.gov/ruralhealth/ about/telehealth/

79. American Psychological Association Practice Organization. Telehealth: Legal basics for psychologists. *Good Practice* 2010; 41:2–7.

80. 15 U.S.C. § 45(a)(1),(2).

81. 15 U.S.C. § 45(n).

82. 15 U.S.C. §45(a)(4)(A).

83. 15 U.S.C. §45(b).

84. FTC v. Toysmart.com, LLC, 2000 WL 34016434 (D. Mass. July 21, 2000).

85. In the Matter of HTC America Inc., FTC File No. 122 3049 (2013) (Complaint), http://ftc.gov/os/ caselist/1223049/130702htccmpt.pdf

86. In the Matter of Google, Inc., a corporation. FTC File No. 102 3136 (2011) (Complaint), available at http://www.ftc.gov/os/caselist/1023136/index. shtm

87. In the Matter of HTC America Inc., FTC File No. 122 3049 (2013) (Agreement containing Consent Order), available at http://ftc.gov/os/ caselist/1223049/130222htcorder.pdf

88. In the Matter of Ceridian Corporation, a corporation. FTC File No. 102 3160 (2011) (Complaint), available at http://www.ftc.gov/os/caselist/1023160/ index.shtm

89. In the Matter of LabMd, Inc. a corporation. FTC File No. 102 3099 (2013) (Complaint), available at http://ftc.gov/opa/2013/08/labmd.shtm

90. Respondent LabMDs answers and defenses to administrative complaint. In the Matter of LabMD, Inc., a corporation. Before the Federal Trade Commission Office of the Administrtive Law Judges. Docket No. 9357. Sept. 17, 2013.

91. Protecting consumer privacy in an era of rapid change: recommendations for businesses and policymakers. Washington, DC: Federal Trade Commission; 2012. Retrieved from http://www. ftc.gov/os/2012/03/120326privacyreport.pdf

92. Mobile privacy disclosures: Building trust through disclosures. Washington, DC: Federal Trade Commission; 2013. Retrieved from http://www.ftc. gov/os/2013/02/130201mobileprivacyreport.pdf

93. Ackerman L. Mobile health and fitness applications and information privacy. San Diego, CA: Privacy Rights Clearinghouse; 2013 (July). Retrieved from https://www.privacyrights.org/mobile-medical-a pps-privacy-alert

94. Marketing your mobile app. Washington, DC: Federal Trade Commission; 2012. Retrieved from http:// business.ftc.gov/documents/bus81-marketing-y our-mobile-app

95. Federal Food, Drug and Cosmetic Act (FD&C Act). 21 USC 321 §201(h).

96. Mobile medical applications: Guidance for industry and Food and Drug Administration staff. Washington, DC: Food and Drug Administration; 2013. Retrieved from http://www.fda.gov/medicaldevices/ product-sandmedicalprocedures/ connectedhealth/mobile-medicalapplications/ default.htm

97. Food and Drug Administration Safety and Innovation Act of 2012 (FDASIA) Pub L 112–144. 126 Stat 993 (2012) § 618.

98. Bates D. FDASIA committee report. Washington, DC: Food and Drug Administration Safety and Innovation Act Committee; 2013. Retrieved from http://www.healthit.gov/facas/calendar/2013/09/04/hit-policy-committee

99. Short form notice code of conduct to promote transparency in mobile app practices. Washington, DC: National Telecommunications and Information Administration; 2013. Retrieved from http://ntia.doc.gov/files/ntia/publications/july_25_code_draft.pdf.

100. mHealth Task Force findings and recommendations. Washington, DC: Federal Communications Commission; 2012. Retrieved from http://www2.itif.org/2012-mhealth-taskforce-recommendations.pdf

101. The California Online Privacy Protection Act, Business and Professions Code (CALOPPA) § 22575 (a)—(b).

102. CALOPPA § 22577 (b).

103. California Department of Justice (US). Attorney General Kamala D. Harris notifies mobile app developers of non-compliance with california privacy law. Sacramento, CA: California Department of Justice; 2012 (Oct.). Retrieved from http://oag.ca.gov/news/press-releases/attorney-general-kamala-d-harris-notifies-mobile-app-developers-non-compliance

104. Privacy on the go: Recommendations for the mobile ecosystem. Sacramento, CA: California Department of Justice; 2013. Retrieved from http://oag.ca.gov/sites/all/files/pdfs/privacy/privacy_on_the_go.pdf

105. Health app certification program, certification standards. New York, NY: Happtique; 2013. Retrieved from http://www.happtique.com/app-certification/

17

Harnessing mHealth in Low-Resource Settings to Overcome Health System Constraints and Achieve Universal Access to Healthcare

GARRETT MEHL, LAVANYA VASUDEVAN, LIANNE GONSALVES,
MATT BERG, TAMSYN SEIMON, MARLEEN TEMMERMAN, AND
ALAIN LABRIQUE

INTRODUCTION

Health is critical to social and economic development in low- and middle-income countries (LMICs), and donors and governments alike are investing increasing resources to accelerate achievement of national and international development goals, particularly in reproductive, maternal, newborn, and child health (RMNCH) (1,2). Rural and underserved populations in LMICs suffer disproportionately high maternal and infant mortality rates due to inefficient health systems and disparities in the quality and utilization of preventive and curative RMNCH services (3). In LMICs, mHealth solutions have been embraced in the form of pilot, proof-of-principle projects for their potential to address gaps in the health system, particularly the RMNCH continuum (4,5). Still, this field is recognized as being nascent, and robust evaluations are underway globally to assess the degree to which mHealth strategies may impact processes and outcomes. In this chapter we detail common health system challenges, and ways in which mHealth is being used to effect improvements at each level of the health system.

CURRENT SITUATION OF RMNCH IN LMICS

Despite substantial advances in health indicators globally, nearly 300,000 women die annually from causes directly related to maternal health (6). The majority of these deaths are attributed to preventable obstetric complications prior to, during, and following delivery, with developing countries carrying the vast majority (99%) of the burden (7). Additionally, although mortality for children under 5 years of age has decreased from 12.6 million annually in 1990, to 6.6 million annually in 2012, the burden of these deaths now falls primarily in LMICs, and most of these deaths are from preventable causes (8). Unmet family planning (FP) need, defined as the percentage of women who could become pregnant but do not want to become pregnant, and who are not using any method of contraception, ranges in LMICs from 10% in Morocco to 45.6% in Samoa, with the vast majority of high prevalence of unmet need for FP (>15%) occurring in sub-Saharan Africa and South and Southeast Asia (9).

Despite numerous efforts to strengthen health intervention delivery using a variety of mechanisms such as financial incentives, training schemes, and task shifting,[1] gaps persist in coverage and quality of RMNCH service delivery globally (10). Low rates of skilled birth attendance, postpartum care, and contraceptive use underlie high rates of unintended pregnancies, short birth intervals, and maternal and newborn mortality (3). Challenges in closing these gaps are compounded by inefficient reporting systems that have grown more burdensome and underutilized, even with the increasing need for rapid and reliable information to enhance coverage, quality, and equity of services. Efforts to scale up the delivery of interventions of known efficacy that address maternal, neonatal, and infant morbidity and mortality will either require additional investment or need to optimize current program performance and increase efficiencies of existing community-based and clinical care providers.

United Nations Millennium Development Goals

Since 2001, governments, donors, global development agencies, and civil society have been mobilized to action by the universally ratified United Nations Millennium Development Goals (MDGs) (11). These eight ambitious objectives, established to improve quality of life across the globe, include three specific health objectives (MDGs 4, 5, 6) with others—such as the eradication of poverty and hunger and the promotion of gender equality—that are clearly necessary to enable significant improvements in health outcomes. National health system–strengthening initiatives and multi-country and multisectoral programs were funded and launched to accelerate progress toward the MDGs by the 2015 target date (11).

Adoption of Mobile Technologies in LMICs

As a serendipitous backdrop to these development efforts, the new millennium also witnessed

the emergence of another groundbreaking revolution: mobile telephony, a leapfrog solution to the challenge of expanding wired telecommunication networks to remote populations around the globe. The mobile phone revolution, characterized by exponential growth in voice and data network coverage and access, afforded by rapidly declining costs and innovations like prepaid credit, has fundamentally transformed the concept of population "connectedness," even in remote areas with low population densities and limited resources.

As illustrated by the typical growth of mobile phone subscribers in India between 2000 and October 2013 (Figure 17.1), this changing reality has stimulated transformations in every development sector, from agriculture to education and health (12). At its most basic level, the simple ability to affordably communicate rapidly with anyone at any time began to impact how individuals within a population interact, from Bangladesh to Botswana, across dimensions of personal life, business, political interactions, and even health. Mobile devices have become ubiquitous in everyday life, affecting how people communicate with others and receive information. Phones are empowering individuals, families, and communities; they have

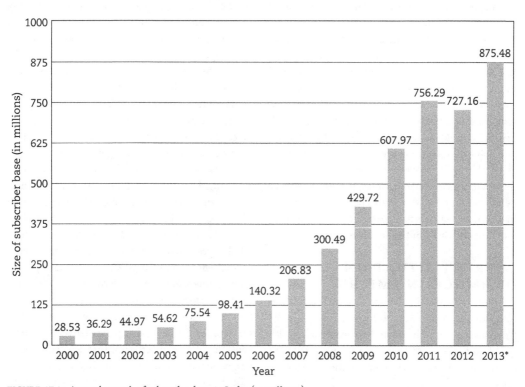

FIGURE 17.1: Annual growth of subscriber base in India (in millions).

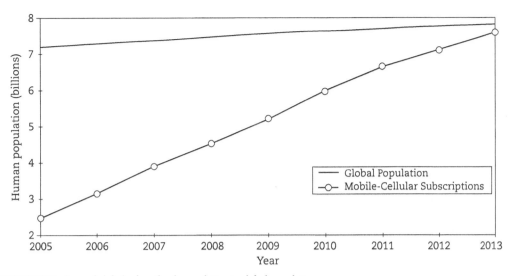

FIGURE 17.2: Annual global subscriber base relative to global population.

the potential to improve health and human development with far-reaching implications.

Figure 17.2 illustrates that over the past 5 years, the penetration of mobile wireless access has reached near saturation levels in many populations—even those where global development and health indicators remain among the lowest globally. In 2013, the number of mobile connections globally was nearly equivalent to the population of humans on the planet, with over half of these connections concentrated in the Asia-Pacific Region (13). The Asian region shares with the African continent the greatest global burden of maternal mortality, creating the opportunity to explore whether this transformative technology may have the potential to further contribute to health MDG target achievement.

Leveraging Technology Innovations to Accelerate Achievement of Health Goals

Over the past decade, and consistent with the spirit of the MDGs, the pursuit of improvements in global health has gone far beyond seeking to eradicate disease or infirmity, extending to prevention, diagnosis, and treatment—distinct phases that require clients to be knowledgeable and demand services, providers to be competent and accountable, and health systems to be supportive and responsive.

In seeking to achieve such national and global development goals, ministries of health are caught at the crossroads, faced with severe budget constraints that limit their ability to adequately finance health services, retain and strengthen the health workforce, purchase commodities, acquire and maintain key health equipment, and ensure that essential services are universally accessible to clients. Among 45 countries in the African region, only 23 are able to finance health at a minimal target of at least US\$44 per capita recommended by the World Health Organization (WHO) (14). All are faced with health system challenges that minimize the potential impact of health services in their populations; all seek to identify approaches that strengthen the ability of severely constrained health systems to improve quality and coverage of existing services.

Understandably, ministries of health tend to be risk-averse when weighing the adoption of innovations, including mHealth solutions. From their perspective, innovations need to promise significant health gains, or equivalent health benefits at reduced cost, or increased population access to the health system, before they commit to invest in and institutionalize their use. Providers of care to populations, whether public- or private-sector agencies, invest in a core selection of essential health interventions for low-resource settings (15,16): contraceptive availability, skilled birth attendance, prevention of mother-to-child transmission, vaccinations, and integrated management of childhood illnesses. Health decision-makers consider investments in innovations based on the extent to which they improve the coverage or quality of existing health interventions at reduced cost by overcoming health system challenges or constraints, and ultimately, save lives (17,18).

The ubiquity of mobile phones and their increasing embeddedness into the daily lives of even the most remote and marginalized populations—including health providers and their beneficiary populations—have provided a launching pad for innovators targeting pervasive health system challenges. Even in the absence of structured mHealth interventions, health system actors have used mobile devices to improve communications across the developing world (19,20).

MHEALTH AS HEALTH SYSTEM CATALYST TO ADDRESS HEALTH SYSTEM CHALLENGES

For decision-makers and implementers working on resolving health constraints in low-resource settings, framing mHealth solutions as mechanisms to address health system constraints that threaten the potential for effective coverage of interventions of known efficacy is helpful to refocus attention on the processes being modified, rather than the underlying technology itself (Figure 17.3). In most cases, mHealth strategies in low-resource settings serve as catalysts to existing

validated health interventions, not as interventions themselves.

Recently in LMICs, mobile wireless technologies have expanded the ability of providers and patients alike to communicate and exchange information. Mobile text messaging, data exchange, and audio and video capabilities are being used to overcome obstacles of distance, in attempts to enhance quality of care and to extend the reach and impact of traditional healthcare services. LMIC governments and other national or global health agencies have been deploying mHealth tools—initially as proof-of-principle projects and more recently as scaled programs—in service of critical health needs ranging from vital registration, client tracking, maintaining medicine stocks, remote diagnostics, point-of-care support and health information dissemination, and behavior change promotion.

mHealth solutions generally take one of three primary approaches, focusing on (a) the *health system* (S)—strengthening supply chain reporting, aggregate performance monitoring, or ensuring quality of service delivery within a health vertical; (b) the *provider* (P)—assisting with workflow management, activity tracking and record-keeping, clinical decision support, or clinical documentation; or (c) the *client or patient* (C)—empowering them with access to information about preventive

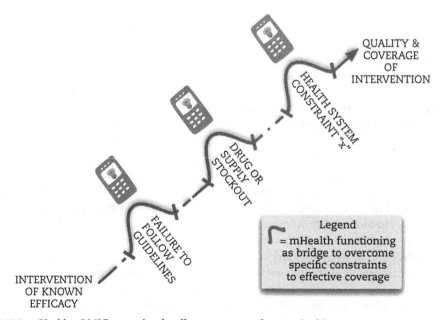

FIGURE 17.3: mHealth in LMICs as catalyst for effective coverage of existing health interventions.

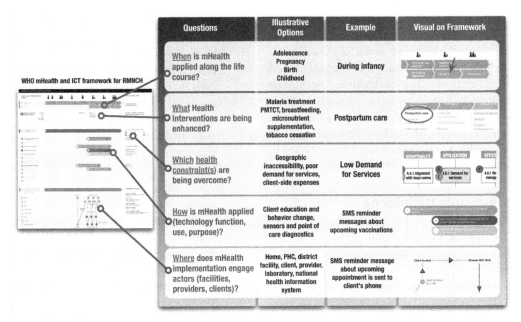

FIGURE 17.4: Components of the WHO mHealth framework for RMNCH.

or curative care, reminders about drug adherence, or motivation to change behaviors (21).

The recognition that mHealth is not monolithic and includes a wide diversity of approaches—which have been difficult to articulate to a general audience—has prompted the development of language and frameworks appropriate for explaining particular mHealth implementations (22).

Figure 17.4 is a simplified schematic representing the components of the mHealth and ICT (information and communication technology) Framework for RMNCH,

WHEN: details the time period (e.g., pregnancy) along the RMNCH continuum in which an mHealth solution is focused.

WHAT: details the specific health interventions for which mHealth serves as a catalyst improving quality and/or coverage.

WHICH HEALTH CONSTRAINTS: refer to the challenges and barriers that impede optimal health promotion, diagnosis, and care, at which mHealth strategies are targeted.

HOW: describes the specific mHealth strategies—mobile technology functions and usage—are employed to improve health.

WHERE: details the information flow deployed in the mHealth implementation,

visualizing the interactions ("touch points") between actors at different levels of the health system through use of the mHealth applications.

The mHealth and ICT Framework for RMNCH (component parts are represented in Figure 17.4) is a tool developed by WHO, UNICEF, Johns Hopkins University Global mHealth Initiative (JHU GMI), and frog design for describing the potential value of mHealth solutions in strengthening health systems--and particularly the delivery of validated essential interventions—across the RMNCH continuum (22). It was developed to aid those in the mainstream health sector to understand the constituent parts and objectives of mHealth implementations (22). These concepts are fundamental to understanding how mHealth is being applied to address health challenges in LMICs.

Health System Constraints Taxonomy

The constraints component of the framework is drawn from a more comprehensive taxonomic classification system developed by members of the WHO Technical and Evidence Review Group on mHealth for RMNCH (mTERG) as a standard way to systematically classify mHealth implementations and, at a meta-level, identify areas with extensive mHealth activity and associated evidence and to detect gap areas (23). After a description of the health system constraints area of the taxonomy, and its constituent parts and definitions, we will use it in the following discussion as a way to structure the discussion about the diversity of uses of mHealth in low-resource settings and their collective potential. These constraints were compiled from a number of published syntheses of Health System constraints, and further key informant input was solicited by the mTERG (24–26).

Constraints Definitions

Under this framework, *constraints* are barriers that impede optimal health promotion, diagnosis, and care. In examining mHealth implementations, the framework and taxonomy prove valuable for addressing the questions "Which constraint(s) does this mHealth strategy address?" or "What improvements result from the application of this mHealth strategy?" mHealth strategies specifically target one or more of the constraints described below and in Figure 17.5. In the figure, constraint areas that are specific to the health system, the provider, and the client are denoted with (S), (P), and (C), respectively.

As illustrated in Figure 17.5, the primary constraint categories within the WHO mTERG mHealth taxonomy include the following:

Information—is the availability of high-quality health-relevant data on clients, populations, health, and vital events, and where and when it is needed. As a constraint category, items include the absence of data to enable unique identification of clients or services provided; poor quality of data; the absence or delay in timing of individual or aggregate level data; challenges in communication between health system, providers or clients; and difficulties accessing needed data or information relevant to health service provision or use.

Availability—is having the right type of care available to those who would need it, as well as having the appropriate type of service providers and materials (27). As a constraint, items in this category focus on barriers that may limit both supply- and user-side availability of health goods and services.

Cost—includes the direct cost of treatment and informal payments, and also indirect costs that deter individuals from seeking treatment. As a constraint, items include direct and indirect financial barriers associated with the provision of, or access to, specific health interventions or behaviors.

Efficiency—accessing or providing appropriate health services in a timely manner and with minimal expenditure of effort. As a constraint category this refers to barriers that impede a person's or a health system's ability to accomplish a given goal, job, or task with minimal time and effort expenditure.

Quality—the technical ability of health services to positively affect people's health (27). Constraints within this category include barriers that impede a healthcare system from functioning optimally and providing individuals and patient populations with healthcare that improves desired health outcomes.

Acceptability—is the alignment of health services with individual, social, and cultural norms, and with expectations of quality. Constraints in this category include social and cultural barriers to the individual in accessing services or continuing treatment, and factors negatively affecting providers' ability to provide specific types of services, or their ability to provide services to specific categories of people on the basis of their ethnicity, health status, age, or sex.

Utilization—Constraints in this category impede an individual's or group's use of a particular health service or treatment—for example, low demand for services; poor transportation infrastructure or geographic distance to needed health services; poor understanding of the treatment regimen; poor provider skills; financial barriers among patients.

Health system constraints span client, provider, and system "competence"—these differ between populations and within populations and across

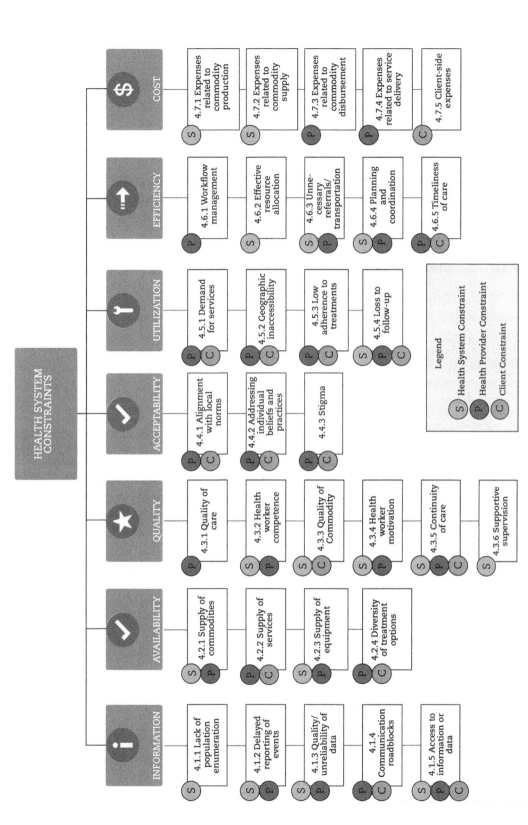

FIGURE 17.5: Health Constraints of the WHO mHealth taxonomy by type.

health domains. mHealth use in LMICs will be further described next using these concepts, detailing which mHealth strategies are used, how they are used, with whom they are used, and when along the continuum, to effect improvements in quality or coverage of health interventions, using concepts represented in Figure 17.4.

MHEALTH STRATEGIES AS DISRUPTIVE HEALTH INNOVATIONS

In LMICs, mHealth approaches may be regarded as disruptive innovations, strategies that deliver fundamental changes to established ways of operating by strengthening the delivery of existing validated health interventions (28). In other words, in LMICs, mHealth approaches as disruptive innovations "do things better," displacing current ways of doing things (systems that support the provision of essential health services), rather than "doing better things" (e.g., new medical interventions) for health. Table 17.1 provides illustrative examples of these disruptive innovations for the health system, provider, and client.

These disruptive innovations supplant conventional health system modalities for delivering essential interventions to more efficiently and effectively respond to the health needs of client populations. In early implementations, mHealth solutions were cumbersome, limited, and poor performing; however, early adopters recognized the promise of approaches that would become faster,

and more accessible and able to provide previously unattainable information. Within RMNCH, the mHealth innovations detailed below are striving to reduce barriers to accessing services, delivering improved quality at reduced cost, and making critical services or timely information more accessible, and/or improving the efficiency and effectiveness of health providers who deliver essential health interventions.

MHEALTH INNOVATIONS THAT OVERCOME HEALTH SYSTEM BARRIERS

The taxonomy of health system–specific constraints is represented as (S) in Figure 17.5. To provide quality services, health systems must be able to uniquely identify and track all beneficiaries, plan and implement programs based on areas of need, ensure availability of medications and other essential health supplies, and deliver services through a cadre of well-trained health workforce in accordance with international medical standards and guidelines. We use the example of Kwame, a district-level health manager, to illustrate the constraints (specific constraints from the taxonomy are denoted in italic bold numbers, e.g., *4.2.1*) faced by health systems in low-resource settings, and provide examples of how mHealth innovations may overcome these constraints.

Kwame is kept busy as a district-level health manager in a densely populated peri-urban region around the capital. He is in charge of the government-run

TABLE 17.1. ILLUSTRATIVE WAYS THAT MHEALTH DISRUPTS CURRENT MODALITIES IN LMICS

Health System Layer	Health Systems Constraint	Conventional Modalities	mHealth Disruptive Innovation
System	Communication roadblocks	Motorcycle couriers to deliver laboratory results	Real-time electronic transfer of lab results to provider and automated notification reminders sent to clients to reduce loss-to-follow-up.
Provider	Workflow management	Paper registers to manage clients and record health events	Electronic registers of clients within provider catchment areas with automated alerts reminding providers of upcoming and overdue health services specific to client needs.
Client	Lack of Access to Information	Flipcharts used by providers to educate clients	Client subscriptions to mobile messaging services that deliver personalized health information, on demand IVR systems, and multimedia content delivered by providers

health facilities in his area, which cover a population of about 500,000 people. Kwame is a jack-of-all-trades and often finds himself trying to juggle quality of health statistics data collection in his area, drug usage and stockouts, staff distribution among clinics, and supervision of health services and care provided. Funding for his district is limited, and he must use the information that he has to direct finances to specific parts of his district and health system that need strengthening.

Kwame has a difficult time putting together a timely and accurate account of births and deaths, due in no small part, he acknowledges, to a traditional preference to give birth at home. **4.1.1** Additionally, he is under pressure from his superiors at the Ministry of Health to ensure that there are functioning systems that provide statistics on disease incidence, vaccination rates, and maternal and child health. **4.1.2/5** Generating performance statistics takes a lot of his health facility staff's time, he knows, but the information is crucial for him to be able to demonstrate regional performance and secure adequate budget and resource support for his facilities. **4.6.2**

Client Registration and Vital Events

Population enumeration through birth registration is a critical function of civil registration and vital statistics (CRVS) systems and facilitates the rights to a name, nationality, as well as social and health services (29). CRVS systems link to health systems to achieve high coverage of births and deaths; these vital statistics allow governments to allocate resources efficiently, based on population size and areas of greatest need. They also enable planning and implementation of health services such as immunization campaigns. Traditional paper-based registration systems have notoriously slow transmission of data; they are also inefficient at capturing births and deaths that occur outside health facilities. As a consequence, unregistered children may be overlooked, their rights may be denied, and statistics may not be available in a timely fashion for public planning and policy making (29). In addition, cause-of-death data may not be captured accurately (14).

Mobile phones have been successful in extending the reach of civil registration systems to rural and remote areas (14). Electronic data collection through mobile phones supports the timely enumeration, registration, and unique identification of all clients in the population. For instance,

several African countries, including Ethiopia, Ghana, Kenya and Rwanda, are members of the MOVE-IT initiative (Monitoring of Vital Events through leveraging innovations and Information Technology advances), while Uganda uses the mobile Vital Registration System (VRS) for community-based birth registration (30,31). In mobile registration initiatives, community-based volunteers use text messages or other mobile phone channels such as USSD to notify the district office of the registrar about new births. The district office verifies the information for completeness and accuracy and then issues birth certificates.

Mobile phone–mediated birth registration has also been integrated with maternal and child health programs. In ChildCount+, implemented by the Millennium Villages Project, community health workers (CHWs) use text messaging to enumerate and register all children under 5 years of age and their mothers (32). Doing so allows the CHWs to monitor health services provided to mothers and children and ensure that life-saving interventions such as vaccinations are up to date. In Bangladesh's mTikka system, a test project being implemented by the Ministry of Health and international partners, local health assistants register new births using digital forms loaded onto smartphones, to create and coordinate vaccination schedules for the infants. The DRISTHI mHealth system in India builds upon the Mother and Child Tracking System (MCTS) implemented by the National Rural Health Mission and registers all beneficiaries across the RMNCH continuum (33,34). The registration information, collected by accredited nurse midwives (ANMs) via digital forms loaded on tablets, is used to assist existing service provision through a suite of mHealth tools on tablets. These range from using multimedia content to strengthen counseling for contraceptive choice for couples of reproductive age, to the use of alerts for providers and reminder messages to clients to increase timely antenatal care (ANC) for pregnant women and improve coverage rates of vaccinations for children.

Kwame is frustrated by the fractured lines of communication and supply chain management that exist between his offices and the clinics he manages. Clinic stockouts occur frequently, especially for antimalarial drugs, which the clinics provide free of charge. **4.2.1** With no way for his office to monitor the supply in the clinics, with and inconsistent reporting of *their distribution, Kwame struggles to anticipate and prevent stockouts at facilities. Although he processes restock requests as soon as he gets them, he worries about the days-long lag time that it takes for clinics to receive their new supply. Kwame worries about tracking diseases as well—malaria season always brings a chaotic uptick in activity from facilities across his district, and with no timely way to monitor the outbreak as it crosses the district, coordinating responses with his facilities is a challenge. 4.6.4*

Supply Chain Management

The availability of medical supplies and commodities is crucial for successful delivery of health services and campaigns such as malaria or HIV prevention. Delays in reporting stockouts using paper forms raises several barriers to effective resource allocation, including unavailability of timely stock level information for decision-making by supply managers and inadequate supply of commodities and equipment to health facilities that need them the most. Inefficient allocation of supplies may also, in turn, raise the costs associated with commodities and spur the distribution of poor-quality health commodities (e.g., counterfeit medicines).

Mobile phones have been used successfully to track stocks of essential commodities and supplies and reduce the turnaround time for restocking them in health centers (35). Real-time availability of electronic data on commodity stocks and usage is advantageous for planning appropriate allotment to health facilities with greatest need.

In the SMS4Life initiative to prevent stockouts of antimalarials in Tanzania, Kenya, and the Democratic Republic of Congo, a stock request is sent to registered mobile phones of health facility workers (HFWs) once a week. HFWs can respond to this query in standard text message format using a free short code. Reminders are issued to HFWs who do not reply to the stock request, while those responding in time receive a monetary incentive. The system notifies the district management office of the various health facilities' stock status (35); a Web-based reporting tool allows the visualization of the geolocations of stockouts, communication statistics, and facilities' stock history. A pilot study showed that the implementation of this supply chain management system reduced stockouts of antimalarials from 79% to less than 26% in three districts in Tanzania (35).

Similarly, Dimagi's CommTrack supply management platform offers the ability for health workers to use text messages for reporting stockouts (36). Using CommTrack, commodity managers can track supplies, create reports, and manage delivery of essential medical supplies. CommTrack has been deployed in Tanzania (ILSGateway), Ghana (Early Warning System), and Malawi (cStock). cStock has doubled the availability of healthcare commodities in Malawi (37). Stockout reporting by health surveillance assistants (HSAs) increased to 80% in most districts from 43% at baseline due to implementation of cStock (37).

Data Collection and Reporting

Mobile phone–based strategies have been used to enable real-time disease surveillance and reduce delays in the identification of and response to outbreaks (38). A syndromic surveillance system was implemented in Madagascar to track malaria, influenza-like illness, and arbovirus infection (38). Health practitioners reported cases using text messages—86.7% of the data were received within 24 hours (38)—and data on daily and weekly disease trends, along with any increase in the number of disease cases, could in turn be shared with the Ministry of Health (38). IICD's Ma Sante program in Mali and Senegal uses data reported via mobile phones to monitor the geographic incidence of malaria cases, issuing alerts to CHWs in case of a suspected outbreak (39).

Possibly the most difficult part of Kwame's job is in supervising his clinic staff. Kwame is a medical doctor by training and is meant to be a resource to the frontline health workers staffing his clinics. However, he is generally too busy with the logistical side of maintaining his group of facilities to be able to provide any practical supervision or decision-making support. 4.3.6 Monitoring health worker competency and performance is a patchwork effort, achieved through a combination of sporadic field visits and scanning incoming data on services provided. Kwame would like to be able to provide in-service education and training programs for his health workers as well as more targeted feedback, but he never has enough timely information to develop a complete understanding of what service delivery looks like on the ground and who would be best served by additional training. 4.3.2

Governments aggregate health data from weekly, monthly, or quarterly reports from individual providers, as well as from local and district health facilities, to monitor the implementation of national programs and measure progress toward the national and global development goals. These data are further used to facilitate planning for training, investments into new areas, and coordination of human resources and commodities for implementation. Delays in aggregation of data collected through paper-based systems make information-driven decision-making challenging. This may result in a mismatch between treatment options and population needs, inadequate support and supervision for health providers, inappropriate or poorly targeted training, and, ultimately, low competency of the health workforce.

Human Resource Management and Supportive Supervision

Data collected electronically using mobile devices are less error-prone and are faster and cheaper than paper-based systems (40). Electronic databases can be linked, minimizing the need for duplication of data. Real-time data flows from service delivery and client response feed dashboard mechanisms that support planning to match service options with needs. Real-time data streams on provider performance can also be used for constructive data-informed feedback by supervisors. For instance:

- Rwanda MOH's mUbuzima system allows CHWs to enter data into the community health information system using mobile phones. These data are used to evaluate individual CHW performance as well as overall progress toward maternal and child health program indicators.
- The Last 10 Kilometers (L10K) program in Ethiopia allows field coordinators to collect program performance data using mobile phones during supportive supervisory visits, increasing the data-based decision-making capacity for district-level managers and reducing delays in making decisions (41).
- The Society for Elimination of Rural Poverty in India uses a Web-based dashboard to track performance scorecards of its nutritional daycare centers at the village, block, and district levels. Exception reports are generated automatically when services are missed and alerts are sent to

the phones of community-based health assistants. In addition, digital reports are used to track monthly health savings and the provision of health risk funding in case of emergencies.
- Dimagi's Active Data Management tool summarizes CHW performance into easy-to-read reports for managers, establishing follow-up actions and goals for the CHW, and allowing the manager to track the status of the follow-up actions and goals (42).

Case Study: mUbuzima (Rwanda)

In Rwanda, decentralizing the health system by focusing on improvements in community-based healthcare and facility-based interventions has been a key part of the government's remarkable efforts to reduce maternal and child mortality. The maternal mortality ratio has been reduced from one of the world's highest in 2005 at 750 deaths per 100,000 live births down to 487 in 2010; the under-5 mortality rate has been reduced by half during the same period. To achieve these results, the Rwanda MOH, in partnership with UNICEF, has deployed an mHealth system—comprising RapidSMS and mUbuzima—to track pregnant women and newborns, promote early detection of life-threatening emergencies, and facilitate reporting on community-level indicators relevant to MDGs 4 and 5.

A cadre of 60,000 volunteer CHWs currently work to strengthen maternal and child health in communities across Rwanda, building awareness on family planning; supplying ORS/zinc to children with diarrhea; distributing contraceptives; promoting ANC visits, facility deliveries, and vaccinations; and tracking and reporting vital events. The Government of Rwanda developed a community health information system to assist CHWs in reporting health information, which is slated for eventual rollout throughout this cadre. mUbuzima offers a mobile mechanism for CHWs to enter and transmit data, offering health officials and supervisors the ability to monitor health services in real time. mUbuzima uses an interactive voice response (IVR) system to help CHWs submit data for a variety of maternal, child, and population health indicators: tuberculosis treatment, case management of sick children, nutrition, and vaccination status. Data submitted monthly can be filtered, displayed, and/or exported according to user preferences. District-level supervisors and MOH officials can log in to a Web dashboard to view CHW performance statistics (in the form of charts and other visual aids, if preferred) and various health indicators.

By the end of 2013, the Government of Rwanda had deployed their system among 15,000 CHWs for maternal and newborn health, and 30,000 CHWs for infant and child health services, covering 15,000 villages overall (43).

MHEALTH INNOVATIONS THAT OVERCOME BARRIERS FOR HEALTH PROVIDERS

The taxonomy of constraints faced by facility- and community-based health providers in low-resource settings is represented in Figure 17.5 as (P). Health providers are tasked with the responsibility of following guidelines to deliver quality health services to beneficiaries, many of whom reside in rural or geographically remote settings. Often, providers receive little to no formal training and lack resources and motivation to perform their duties. We use the example of Sara, a CHW, to illustrate the constraints faced by health providers in low-resource settings, and provide examples of how mHealth innovations are being used in LMICs to overcome those constraints.

Sara is 24 years old, has a high school education, and has worked as a government-salaried health worker for the last 2 years. The health post she staffs with her colleague provides health services to 5,000 households sprawled across a farming community. As a frontline health worker, Sara (who underwent a year-long vocational training for the position) is responsible for providing a full range of family planning, maternal and child health services, and disease prevention counseling and services through home visits and service provision at the health post.

Sara loves her work but often feels as if there is too much for her to keep up with in order to keep their community healthy. 4.2.2 Her colleague is often late to the clinic or absent entirely—when she does come in, she shows little motivation to work, leaving Sara overburdened with clients to treat. 4.3.4 At the same time, Sara knows that some members of her community who are most in need of her attention don't seek it, preferring to seek traditional remedies. 4.4.2 Sara speaks often at community meetings about the importance of ANC and postnatal care (PNC) visits for pregnant women and new mothers and *immunizations for children, but often doesn't have time to follow up with mothers and their babies who miss appointments 4.6.5.*

Sara spends many hours per week walking to the most remote corners of her rural community in order to make home visits, but even after providing counseling at home, she knows that the health post's location makes it difficult for those living further from the community's center to make repeat trips for services like drug refills. 4.5.2 4.5.3 For those who do make the trip, Sara can't guarantee that their facility will have stock of the commodities they need. 4.2.1 Sara is rarely able to tell patients when the clinic will be restocked, something she knows dissuades people from returning. She worries especially for those new mothers awaiting early-infant diagnosis of HIV— they don't always make it back to the health post to get the results, missing a critical window for ensuring that infants with HIV get early access to antiretroviral drugs. 4.5.4

Globally there is a shortage of approximately 2.4 million trained medical professionals and 4 million health workers (10,44). To ameliorate this critical health service gap, many countries have shifted the task of health service provision to CHWs, who are often the only link to the health system for clients residing in rural or remote locations. However, poor communication infrastructures translate into the inability to coordinate care between different providers or facilities, leading to unnecessary referrals or delayed delivery of care. These critical providers become disconnected, working in isolation from the health system they are meant to serve.

Sara is encouraged to see more individuals coming to the health post for the first time, but worries for the more complex cases: her health post is the only easily accessible resource for her community, and the larger, better equipped district health center staffed with doctors and nurses is 20 kilometers away. 4.5.2 Both time and distance make Sara worry about those she refers; Sara has no easy way to reach out for advice or assistance. 4.1.5 Furthermore, difficulty remembering the exact guidelines she was taught in pre-service training on how to diagnose, make decisions on types of treatment, and ensure that her clients are receiving care at the quality that her supervisors and clients expect of her makes Sara uneasy in her daily provision of care 4.3.2 Any formal supervision comes sporadically and infrequently in the form of site visits by district health officers. 4.3.6

Provider Communication Approaches

Text message or voice-based provider-to-client or provider-to-provider communication programs can eliminate communication roadblocks, thereby improving linkages to care, improving counseling and adherence to treatment regimens, and reducing loss to follow-up. For example, clients calling into Village Reach's Chipatala Cha Pa Foni hotline service speak to trained health workers who provide information or, as necessary, refer them to appropriate health facilities (45). Clients can also sign up for a tips and reminders service to receive weekly information on health topics.

In Uganda, a cluster randomized trial to examine the use of mobile technology to support the work of community-based peer health workers providing AIDS care found better task shifting among the health workers and reduced loss to follow-up among patients (46). Additionally, despite no significant differences in health outcomes between patients in the intervention and control groups, peer health workers with mobile phones were able to communicate and seek assistance from clinic staff faster than those without phones (46).

CHAI-Malawi uses SMS-based communication between various cadres of health workers to effectively track patients who miss appointments. This system replaces a paper-based system for communication wherein different cadres of health workers transmitted paper cards with client information to the local CHW, who then located the client lost to follow-up. The use of text messages precludes the need for at least two intermediary health workers in the communication chain, reducing the burden of paperwork. It also reduces the delay in locating the client, thereby supporting faster resumption of health services or critical medication regimens like antiretroviral therapy (ART).

Closed user groups (CUGs) are communication networks whose members can place unlimited calls to each other, at no cost. Eliminating this structural barrier has been the goal Switchboard, a non-governmental organization (NGO) that helps create CUGs of health professionals, to allow them to communicate freely across the urban/rural divide. A survey of 77 physicians from Ghana and 50 physicians from Liberia revealed enhanced physician connectivity, increased frequency of consultation, improved success of diagnosis, increased

speed of referral, and improved patient recovery from the use of a CUG system for communication (47). A social network analysis of a CUG network revealed communication between members even when they were outside of the catchment area, as well as communication with ambulance drivers during emergencies (48).

Decision Support Tools

CHWs face the challenge of delivering health services to substantial populations of beneficiaries in need, with a wide range of health conditions, in the face of limited training and resources, and a frail healthcare infrastructure (49). Decision-support algorithms built into mobile phone applications enable task shifting by aiding the diagnosis and management of diseases in the absence of trained medical providers. Decision-support tools also ensure that providers are appropriately directing only those in need of referral to functioning facilities.

The Electronic Integrated Management of Childhood Illnesses (e-IMCI) decision support system, which guides clinicians step by step through treatment algorithms, was found to increase adherence to IMCI guidelines; 84.7% of investigations required by IMCI were completed by clinicians with the mobile tool compared to 61% otherwise ($p <.01$). In addition, training time per clinician was less than 20 minutes, meaning clinicians can train other clinicians (50).

Another such tool, the Application for Contraceptive Eligibility (ACE), provides guidance to health providers on choosing among 20 different contraceptive methods for their clients, and incorporates knowledge from WHO's *Medical Eligibility Criteria for Contraceptive Use*, and the global handbook for family planning providers (51). The eMocha TB Detect smartphone application assists health workers in the diagnosis of tuberculosis through a screening algorithm based on current WHO guidelines (52,53).

The current system for documenting care and maintaining health records is both tedious and prone to error. 4.1.3 Health records are currently maintained across several topic-specific paper registries, and Sara and her colleague spend the last few days of every month compiling the monthly reports to submit to the district health office. Sara is frustrated at the time she must spend on paperwork, which is time not spent providing services. 4.6.1 Despite submitting reports every month, Sara seldom receives feedback on her performance. 4.3.6

Health providers have poor access to quality information about health of clients, clinical and operational guidelines, as well as functioning of the health system. They face the burden of paper-based reporting, meaning that they must document health service provision activities manually, often duplicating the same information across multiple registers. The drudgery of reporting and completing paperwork often steals time away from service provision. Paper-based data also do not permit continuity in care between visits or when the same client accesses different providers. Tracking services provided requires analysis across multiple documents, which often are not organized by client name. Maintaining lists of clients who are due for services is tedious for similar reasons. Consequently, clients who have missed services or appointments are not identified in a timely fashion, leading to loss to follow-up. Developing aggregate monthly or quarterly reports from paper-based data is error-prone and is often repeated at multiple consecutive levels of supervision, until a compiled report reaches a senior management layer. Lack of appropriate incentives or feedback loops risks engendering poor provider motivation to deliver high-quality care.

Electronic Health Records, Provider Work-Planning, Data Collection and Reporting

Mobile phone–based solutions can streamline the workflow of health providers, allow more efficient data collection, reduce the burden of reporting, support tracking and management of clients, and ensure high quality of service delivery. Specifically, electronic registers of clients, organized by risk status, location, due date, intervention schedules, enable workflow management and facilitate timely provision of services. Moreover, the use of electronic health records and unique identifiers can improve the likelihood that providers are aware of clients' prior health events and treatment, thus improving the quality of care. Alerts and reminders work to maximize the capacity of health providers to be responsive to clients' health service needs.

In Ghana, for instance, health workers use the MOTECH suite to electronically register clients,

capture service delivery information, and look up their medical history (54). Health workers receive alerts on their mobile phones when scheduled cases are missed (54). Health data are also synchronized between phones of multiple health workers, further increasing continuity of care (55). Medical protocols and other job aids are available on the handsets in addition to training modules. The use of electronic reporting templates via mobile clients can enable data uploads to routine information systems or Web-based dashboards that offer real-time data to supervisors.

Financial and Nonfinancial Incentives

Nonfinancial and financial mechanisms can be used via mobile device to reward the provision of timely, appropriate care to clients, positively impacting provider motivation. For example, a financial incentive scheme is built into the Zindagi Mehfooz program in Pakistan (56), where health providers receive compensation each time a child's vaccination card with a radio frequency identification (RFID) tag is scanned at a vaccination center, indicating vaccination provided.

Sensors and Point-of-Care Diagnostics

Health providers in low-resource settings have limited access to diagnostic devices. In many cases, tools may require electricity for operation or simply be too big for carrying on home visits. Sensors and other mobile phone accessories such as accelerometers, mobile phone cameras, and external diagnostic devices can extend the functionality of mobile phones for the provider as well as their clients. Furthermore, they can allow continuous data capture and remote monitoring of vital signs such as blood pressure, heart rate, and respiration rate. Microchips can be used for the diagnosis of diseases (e.g., through a simple reaction of antigens with measurable reactants on the chip surface) or physiological states (e.g., detection of carbon monoxide in breath). Given their small size and portability, sensors linked to mobile phones are viable alternatives to traditional diagnostic devices in LMICs.

There are limited examples for the use of highly sophisticated sensors and other mobile phone accessories in these settings, primarily due to cost constraints, but there is some evidence for simpler applications of mobile phone sensors. In Tanzania, a proof-of-concept study utilizing mobile phone microscopy successfully detected moderate to high parasitic worm infections from fecal samples of individuals living in Pemba (41). As an alternative to traditional light microscopy, the mobile phone microscopy offers potential in cost-efficiency and portability, with the added possibility of linkages to experts who can make a more refined diagnosis and determine whether referral or more tests would be warranted.

Sara is gratified by the warmth and appreciation she receives from her community and loves being a health service provider. She hopes to continue her training as her career progresses, and looks forward to opportunities to go to the health centers for refresher courses and trainings. However, those happen rarely, **4.3.2** *and she doesn't like to leave her health post for long.*

Given the lack of resources and proper training, health workers often feel unable to provide care that positively impacts the health of their clients. Training and in-service refresher content can strengthen providers' ability to provide quality care. The 2012 Dalberg Report acknowledges critical gaps in training of the next generation of CHWs in sub-Saharan Africa and suggests that multimedia applications with digital content can enable more effective training of CHWs at a lower cost compared to traditional methods (44).

Provider Training and Education

Systems such as eMOCHA TB Detect have an education menu that features multimedia content on tuberculosis prevention and care, supporting continuous ongoing medical education. The content is updated regularly and can be accessed via Android smartphones. Use of health content accessible through electronic forms or multimedia can also ensure that health providers are better aligned with local norms. In Dimagi's CommCare ASHA program, audiovisual job aids for maternal and child healthcare are available on the accredited social health activists' (ASHAs') mobile phones. The content is in local languages and in the voice of an elderly woman, in line with local culture that values the wisdom and experience of elders in the community.

Case Study: CommCare ASHA (India)

ASHAs represent an enormous investment by the Government of India and the National Rural Health Mission (NRHM) in the improvement of community health. Since 2005, NRHM has trained over 750,000 ASHAs. These workers are particularly valuable in rural areas, where they may serve as a community's primary healthcare provider. Though trained to be their community's first promoter of maternal and child health, ASHAs face a number of challenges to their job as less-skilled health workers, including high workloads, insufficient training, little support for home visits, and the lack of supervision or feedback on their performance.

Dimagi's CommCare platform provides a supportive tool for these health workers. ASHAs are provided with an inexpensive feature: smartphones running the CommCare software that includes registration forms, checklists, danger sign monitoring, and educational prompts accompanied by audio, visual, and/or video clips. Tracking a woman through pregnancy, an ASHA may use CommCare as follows: during routine surveillance in the community, the ASHA uses her phone to fill in a digital form to register any new pregnancies. She counsels pregnant women to seek antenatal care, and receives decision support by way of the software's audio-visual aids. When a woman comes in for an ANC visit, the ASHA updates her digital form to reflect the services provided. To assist the ASHA with work plan scheduling, the phone can generate a list of women due for ANC visits and can prioritize home visits based on delivery dates. Closer to delivery dates, the ASHA is notified and can return to the woman to counsel her on delivering in a facility; additional audiovisual job aids lend authority to the ASHA's advice. The ASHA registers the birth into the CommCare system; now the ASHA's work plan will include postpartum visits and PNC services to be provided. With these reminders and corresponding updates of the digital form, an ASHA can track a woman through PNC, refer if there are any complications for mother or baby, and keep health records for both mother and baby after each service is provided. Data collection and reporting are continuous: digital form updates are uploaded to a central CommCare server, health records are updated, and the ASHA's digital work plans are downloaded. By 2013, CommCare ASHA had been deployed in three states (Uttar Pradesh, Madhya Pradesh and Maharashtra) and over 500 ASHAs were trained to use the system.

MHEALTH INNOVATIONS THAT OVERCOME BARRIERS FOR CLIENTS

The taxonomy of constraints specific to clients is presented in Figure 17.5 as (C). Clients in LMICs have poor access to health information, are unaware of health services available to them, and often do not have the money or transportation to seek specialized care outside of their communities. We use the example of Yasmeen, a first-time mother-to-be, to illustrate the constraints faced by clients in low-resource settings, and provide examples of how mHealth innovations are being used to overcome those constraints.

Yasmeen is expecting her first baby. She is 18 and lives with her husband and his family in a small, rural community. Her family, like most in her community, are maize farmers. She has just returned from the community's health clinic, where she attended her first ANC visit. Yasmeen has learned that she is 25 weeks pregnant, and was given a package of pills that she was told to take daily for the health of the baby. The health worker gave her an injection—a tetanus vaccination, she was told— along with a dizzying set of instructions on what to eat, planning her delivery, postpartum family planning options, and taking care of herself and her baby in the coming months.

The visit has left her excited but overwhelmed; Yasmeen repeated to herself all the instructions she could remember as she walked home, in order to commit them to memory and share with her husband. Some of them seem contradictory to what she has heard from her in-laws, especially with regard to what she should eat and where she should deliver. 4.4.1 Yasmeen's mother-in-law is planning for a home birth, as is traditional—Yasmeen respects her mother-in-law's opinion immensely but is conflicted and not sure where she should deliver. 4.4.2 Some of the health worker's other advice might raise some difficulties in her home. The health worker warned her about the importance of protecting herself and her unborn child from malaria by using a mosquito net, but Yasmeen hasn't seen her net since her husband's

sister borrowed it 3 months ago. 4.2.3 Yasmeen has been told that as her pregnancy progresses, she should rest when she feels tired, but there is so much work to do around the home and her husband's family expects her to contribute. 4.4.1

Clients in low-resource settings face numerous barriers to care, including poor access to quality health information, delays in receiving care, cultural beliefs and norms leading to stigma of health conditions such as HIV/AIDS, large geographic distances from needed health services, and high direct or indirect costs for accessing or completing treatment. Consequently, there is weak demand for health services and poor adherence to treatment regimens.

Client Education and Behavior Change Communication (BCC)

Evidence is mounting for the effectiveness of using of mobile phone channels such as text messaging, IVR, hotline services, and mobile Web and mobile social media for conveying health information to clients and making it easier for clients to find information themselves. Notably, multiple studies have demonstrated the utility of text messaging as a tool for BCC irrespective of age, minority status, and nationality (57). Text messaging is most commonly used to transmit educational content to beneficiaries regarding health conditions. High subscription rates for mobile phone–based services offering health information to pregnant women, such as the Healthy Pregnancy, Healthy Baby program in Tanzania, suggest high user demand for such services (58).

The Mobile Alliance for Maternal Action (MAMA) South Africa employs five different mobile communication channels to deliver gestational age–specific health information to pregnant women. The channels include text messaging, voice, USSD, mobile Web, and MXit (blogs and social media). In user testing involving 22 pregnant women and mothers subscribing to MAMA, 80% of participants said that they learned new information on pregnancy and child care through the service (41).

Educational multimedia content delivered via mobile devices can empower clients and counter barriers to health-seeking behavior. Results from the evaluation of the Safe Motherhood program in Pakistan show an increase in the number of institutional deliveries, contacts with healthcare providers, and ANC visits among pregnant women in the intervention group who received personalized healthcare messages compared to controls who received standard care (41). In Uganda, the uptake of voluntary testing and counseling increased 40% with the implementation of a quiz by the Text to Change program (59). And a recent pilot evaluation of the Chipatala Cha Pa Foni service in Malawi suggests an increase in the utilization of ANC and PNC services among women in response to calling in to the hotline service (45).

Mobile phone–based strategies have also been used to support family planning initiatives. Examples include CycleTel, a family planning program based on the Standard Days Method that notifies women of days in the month when they are most likely to be fertile (60). Other programs such as the Mobile for Reproductive Health (m4RH) service in Tanzania provide information on contraceptive methods through text messages. Users of m4RH demonstrated increased knowledge on family planning and a change in contraceptive method used (61). In Cambodia, a study investigating the effectiveness of using voice messages to support contraception use in a population with limited literacy is ongoing (62).

Mobile radio has also been used as a channel for communication of health information to the public. The *Galli Galli Sim Sim* project in India delivers information on general health and hygiene to marginalized populations that have access to radiophones. Similarly, in Tanzania, Malaria No More uses radio programming to broadcast promotional messaging related to malaria prevention and insecticide-treated bednet use. Listeners interested in seeking more information can call in to a toll-free number and choose from a menu of voices of their favorite celebrities to hear health messages.

Mobile phones can extend the reach of traditional facilities and provide linkages between clients for empowerment and social support during illness. In a study in South Africa, women were linked with a buddy to help them self-manage their diabetes (63). Despite a negative impact on blood glucose levels, the women exchanged text messages with their buddies on a daily basis and reported higher levels of social support coping at the end of the intervention period (63). Praekelt Foundation's Young Africa Live mobile Web portal offers a medium for young adults to access content on HIV/AIDS and participate in ongoing

discussions about health, with content that constructively counters social stigma and widespread misperceptions (64).

The community health worker scheduled Yasmeen's next ANC check-up for 7 weeks from now, during harvest season. Yasmeen will do her best to remember to go and hopes she can find the time to make the return trip to the clinic **4.6.5***; it will be a busy time for her entire family, and the clinic is at least an hour's walk from home.* **4.5.2** *Returning with her baby to vaccinate, as the CHW advised, will also be time consuming, Yasmeen reflects.* **4.5.3** *Yasmeen has a lot of questions and wishes she had better access to the health worker.* **4.1.5**

A number of factors may contribute to clients not utilizing health services for which they are eligible. First, geographic inaccessibility can serve as a large barrier to accessing care, with clients unable to arrange transportation to the appropriate facility, especially during medical emergencies. Sikder et al. describe the use of mobile phones by families of pregnant women residing in rural Bangladesh, for example, for coordinating transportation in case of obstetric emergencies (65). Additionally, clients may be unaware of services they can access or may forget information provided to them.

Coordination, Referral, and Prevention of Loss to Follow-up

To prevent loss to follow-up, text messages can be used to send reminders and alerts to clients. Studies show that individuals receiving weekly text message reminders are more likely to demonstrate adherence to ART compared to standard practice (66). Two studies in Kenya—one in which participants received text message reminders for ART and were able to talk to their healthcare provider for advice, and another in which participants simply received one-way text message reminders—demonstrated higher adherence and prolonged viral suppression compared to control participants who did not receive any reminders (67–69). Brazilian women receiving text message reminders to take medication through the HIV Alert System (HIVAS) were more adherent to the treatment regimen over a period of 4 months compared to the control group (no reminders) (70). Furthermore, interventions using text messages have been shown to promote smoking cessation (71) and increase healthcare appointment attendance compared to no reminders or postal reminders (72).

Text messages have been used to reduce turnaround time for return of lab results, most notably in the prevention of mother-to-child transmission of HIV in Zambia (73); however, there is limited evidence for the effectiveness of this strategy (72). Programs such as the text message–based Mobile for Reproductive Health (m4RH) in Tanzania and medAfrica include a database of health facilities that can be accessed by beneficiaries.

Validation of Commodities

Counterfeit medications invade marketplaces when there is a shortage of essential medicines, prohibitive prices, or insufficient regulation (74). Counterfeit medicines include those that are manufactured under substandard conditions or which intentionally contain a lower dose of—or frequently, no—active ingredient. A number of applications have been developed to improve clients' ability to protect themselves from counterfeit medicines, targeting markets where this problem is rampant. Sproxil and mPedigree, for example, allow clients to text in a unique "authentication" code affixed to the drug packaging to verify whether the medicines are genuine, at no cost to the client.

Adherence to Treatment Regimens

Text message reminders have also been used to encourage parents to complete timely vaccinations for their infants. Examples include Interactive Research and Development's (IRD's) Zindagi Mehfooz project in Pakistan, the mTikka project in Bangladesh, and PATH's project Optimize in Vietnam. For all three projects, infants are registered at birth and their vaccination status is tracked electronically. In addition, text message reminders are sent to parents of children who are due for upcoming vaccinations. Zindagi Mehfooz employs financial incentives and RFID tags, while the mTikka project uses barcoded bracelets, to uniquely identify infants. mTikka also has a mechanism wherein the vaccine worker can broadcast a text message notification to parents whenever the outreach center is open. This feature can potentially minimize unnecessary travel and time away from employment for parents in the event of outreach center closure or vaccine worker absence.

At a second ANC visit, Yasmeen expresses to the health worker a desire to have her baby in the health facility, but adds that her husband is worried about the expense of maternity services. The health worker refers her to a program offering prepaid cards that Yasmeen and her husband can purchase to pay for discounted maternal services. The card can be topped up via mobile money platforms, meaning that Yasmeen and her husband can gradually set aside money throughout her pregnancy.

Mobile money has been used successfully to incentivize clients to seek healthcare, subsidize their transportation to healthcare facilities, or encourage savings for covering healthcare costs. Provision of financial incentives or vouchers via mobile phones (e.g., mBanking) can mitigate financial barriers or encourage clients to seek and complete appropriate services. For instance, Kenyan hospitals report a 30% increase in the number of women regularly visiting them since they have started accepting Changamka cards (75). Similarly, the number of cases of obstetric fistula treated increased with the introduction of Vodaphone mPESA in Tanzania to cover the transportation and medical costs for surgery in 2011 (76).

Case Study: Zindagi Mehfooz (Pakistan)

In Pakistan, low uptake and delayed immunization of infants and young children result in a large number of vaccine-preventable deaths among children under 5 years of age. In spite of the Government of Pakistan's Expanded Program on Immunization (EPI) prioritizing the immunization of children under 2 years of age, difficulties in accessing these services (clinics operating only for a limited number of hours in the morning, or a perception of poor quality of care) result in many parents not utilizing the services.

IRD's Zindagi Mehfooz system uses client-side SMS reminders and a lottery system with cash prizes to improve age-appropriate immunization coverage. The Zindagi Mehfooz system, in addition to implementing initiatives that seek to improve health system quality (through accurate data collection and health record maintenance) and health worker motivation (incentives based on total children vaccinated), uses this combination of reminder and incentives strategy to encourage parents to make the trip with their child to a vaccination facility multiple times over the course of the first 2 years of their infant's life.

To ensure timeliness of care and adherence to vaccinations, mothers are enrolled into the Zindagi Mehfooz system in their first interaction with the immunization facility: the infant's name, date of birth, vaccine information and parents' information is obtained, as is parental consent to enroll in the SMS reminder program. SMS reminders are sent to mothers 1 day before the next appointment, the day of the appointment, and 2 days after an appointment was missed, if necessary. Mothers bring their infant's vaccination card with them to their baby's appointment. The card is linked to an accompanying tag read using a phone-based RFID system, which allows for the verification of vaccinations and issuance of a lottery. The amount of cash caregivers are eligible for increases with every vaccination their infant receives and for vaccines completed on time, and mothers have a one-in-five chance of winning a lottery voucher. Winnings in the lottery allow caregivers to overcome client-related expenses that may serve as barriers to accessing immunizations for their babies. Additionally, by linking the card to the lottery system (thereby ensuring that caregivers bring their card to every appointment), both caregivers and the EPI system have complete and accurate vaccination records for the infant.

By the end of 2013, the Zindagi Mehfooz system was moving to scale, having registered nearly 17,000 clients by the end of 2103, and adding 1,300 every month. Programs like the Zindagi Mehfooz system could be linked on the client side with additional educational content and health reminders, keeping parents engaged with strategies to promote their child's health and well-being throughout and after the vaccination window.

CONCLUSIONS

There is widespread recognition across development agencies, national governments, the telecommunications sector, and private industry of the *potential* inherent in leveraging information and communications technologies for improvement in public health systems and individual patient outcomes. Despite the proliferation of pilot projects in LMICs, globally few mHealth strategies have scaled to national or regional deployments, and fewer still have been adopted as part of global care standards. Over the past 3 years, there have

been efforts to identify and address obstacles that may be impeding the wider adoption of mHealth strategies (77,78). It is likely that the novelty of the field—characterized by widespread experimentation—along with a lack of a shared vocabulary to describe mHealth innovation, contributed to the initial confusion among potential adopters (22). Additionally, governments—historically the largest providers of health services—are also among the most conservative in adopting health innovations because of financial constraints and a focus on evidence to drive decision-making. These institutions have been faced with a dizzying barrage of mHealth offerings, with few analytic tools or a supporting body of research to distinguish their value or potential for scale.

Currently, most mHealth approaches are narrowly focused solutions aimed at individual health system constraints, operating independently of other information systems. Where there are multiple mHealth deployments in a setting, health workers may be faced with using multiple devices or mHealth solutions on top of an already heavy workload. Many predominant mHealth tools lack consistency in how they function or their user interface, and seldom provide compatibility or linkage with other ICT systems. Non-interoperability and unnecessarily fragmented innovation are frequently cited as barriers to mainstreaming and scaling frontline health worker mHealth solutions. While there may be a growing evidence base for particular mHealth strategies, for broader adoption it will be incumbent upon mHealth solutions to demonstrate interoperability with existing national and regional health information systems, as well as to measure and report on the costs of establishing, maintaining, and institutionalizing these services across health systems.

Governments and large health implementing agencies are beginning to show interest in investing in mHealth solutions, particularly if the coding is flexible and simple to modify, and the generated data are interoperable and complementary to existing ICT investments such as the widely used District Health Information System (DHIS2) and electronic medical record systems like OpenMRS (79,80). However, the current status of most mHealth innovations as narrowly framed solutions, lacking sufficient evidence of improved health intervention coverage and impact, continues to prevent uptake by large health implementers. Insufficient information about the total cost of adoption, as well as the human, technical, and support requirements necessary for scale, render the development of convincing business cases for adoption difficult. Existing systems' dependence on expatriate technical support also impedes country-level ownership, innovation, and customization for growth. Finally, there is widespread consensus that increased consideration of end-user needs and responsive design is required to maximize sustainability. The horizon is looking brighter, however, as countries formulate and adopt national mHealth standards and strategies to help provide the integration layer necessary to facilitate cross-talk and interconnectedness across diverse solutions. Common "backbone" elements such as national unique identifier schema and a central individual health record contribute to an enabling environment that facilitates collaboration. The building of local technical capacity through improved health informatics and telecommunications training generates the human resources needed to foster, adopt, and cultivate local mHealth innovation.

Governments may have less hesitancy about institutionalizing mHealth solutions when there is consolidation of solutions into comprehensive, multifunctional packages that address broader sets of health system constraints; demonstrate integration with other ICT systems and existing work and information flows of their workforce and patient needs; and present obvious health system gains at reduced costs. Already, governments as diverse as Rwanda, Nigeria, Uganda, South Africa, Bangladesh, and the Indian states of Bihar, Gujarat, Andhra Pradesh, and Karnataka have begun to make significant financial and institutional investments into comprehensive mHealth packages that complement existing brick-and-mortar facilities and current eHealth systems.

In the not-too-distant future, a comprehensive mHealth package comprising a diversity of evidence-based approaches to promote existing health interventions may be embraced as a normative standard by donors, countries, technical agencies, and health systems alike. Such a package will likely include deployment of mobile wireless devices to all health providers; closed user groups enabling free communications between providers; electronic enumeration and registration of all eligible clients in the population; unique health identifiers linked to electronic medical records; electronic systems for vital event recording; task management tools for providers that track activities, offer feedback, and provide incentives based on provider performance; systems supporting client-targeted subscriptions of personalized health content available through IVR, text messaging, or mobile applications; and real-time data synced with national health information systems, providing reporting via dashboards.

mHealth in LMICs differs from mHealth implementations in high-resource settings, which have focused primarily on diagnostic tools and sensors to enable real-time data, and consumer-driven apps for empowering and personalizing health monitoring and disease management. In LMICs, mHealth systems are serving not only to catalyze the coverage and quality of health interventions but also to realize specific global health goals that have heretofore languished as pipedreams—to wit: data simplification and harmonization of reporting; population-wide incentive schemes and pay-for-performance mechanisms; task shifting that maintains health service quality; global inclusion facilitated by electronic vital events registration; and continuity of care through the use of electronic medical records. Their realization, along with the substantial benefits likely to result from widespread use of bundled mHealth strategies, will help ensure not only that the Millennium Development Goals are achieved, but also that the post-MDG goals of universal health coverage can become a reality for vulnerable and marginalized populations for whom the benefits of quality health services remain beyond reach.

Three Years Later: A Look into the Future
Kwame

Kwame is at his computer, noting an outbreak of bacterial meningitis in one corner of his district. The incoming data from each of his clinics include statistics on services provided as well as diagnoses, and Kwame calls the health workers at the clinic in question to get details. Kwame pushes out a message to all the health providers in his district alerting them to the outbreak and reminding them of the symptoms and preventative measures they can use to protect their communities. On-demand multimedia refresher training is available through mobile Internet on health workers' smartphones, with quizzes built in to assess their competence. Updated drug inventories show that all of his clinics, except one, appear to be well stocked with necessary antibiotics. He sends a structured message to the central store to check on the status of the supplies being sent in response, knowing that the clinic has already notified the national supply chain system in the previous week's status update. The national health office calls, having also received an alert about the outbreak—Kwame provides them with an update and promises to alert them if he needs any additional resources deployed.

Kwame turns to the district planning for the upcoming year. A higher-than-anticipated number of births in the northern part of the district may require some reshuffling of personnel. He can see that some of his lowest performing health workers operate in this area, and sets up a supervisory visit so he can check in before making any changes—Kwame needs to make sure that these areas will be well equipped to provide the required infant and child services over the next few years. The fact that all clients of reproductive age are entered, and all health events and services provided are registered by health workers using their mobile tablet devices, gives Kwame confidence that the data being reported in real-time and fed up to the national level are reliable and reflective of the actual health situation in his district—a far cry from the previous era when he lacked confidence in the data available to him and consequently faced challenges in responding to needs, planning, and allocating resources. He is able to ride through the community and make sure that all the homes he sees are marked on his tablet's GPS-enabled map, making sure that no families on the outskirts of the area have been missed during the periodic census.

Sara

It is the beginning of another week, and Sara finishes the weekly inventory for her clinic's supply of medicines and equipment, using her phone to send the update to the district health facilities. Antimalarials have gotten a little low, but she knows she can expect more on Thursday, when the health office does commodity disbursements. She consults her registry on her electronic tablet—an integral part of her medical kit—which has been updated to reflect the week's scheduled appointments and home visits. Replacing the multiple paper registries she once had to take with her on visits, the tablet serves as a registry and electronic health record for everyone who has ever received care at their clinics. The electronic registries are dynamic, adding

and withdrawing care recommendations and alerts in accordance with changes in the client's age or status (for example, becoming pregnant, being diagnosed with HIV or tuberculosis). Sara also uses the tablet as a resource during home visits; a variety of video and visual aids provide added information to a client on a wide array of issues, from tuberculosis treatment, sanitation and hygiene, to nutrition, breastfeeding, and maternal and child health. A red notification on the registry alerts Sara to a high-priority pregnancy: the mother, who had high blood pressure in her third trimester, is due this week. Sara will pass by the woman's house during home visits to check on her, and will also check on a woman who missed her second ANC appointment last week.

Sara confers with her colleague, who now shares fully in the responsibilities in the clinic. Sara noticed her colleague's attitude change came about shortly after the implementation of the electronic registries system 2 years ago, which provided all health workers in her district (as well as the district officials) with a dashboard showing performance statistics of each worker, clinic, and the district as a whole. Sara's performance has resulted in her being recognized as an outstanding health worker twice within the last year. These closer ties with the district health facilities are also useful when Sara and her colleague are providing treatment; they have access to a closed network of more skilled health providers at the district and national offices, with whom they can consult on more complex cases. Sara can also track her patient referrals through their treatment at better equipped health centers in the district capital so she can follow up upon their return home. Sara has an hour or so left before the clinic opens and decides to complete the refresher training on postnatal care she had started earlier. A quiz, taken at the end of the module, assures Sara and her superiors that her skills are updated.

Yasmeen

Yasmeen's phone lights up with a reminder of tomorrow's ANC visit—her third. Yasmeen, now 21, is looking forward to meeting the health worker at her new clinic. Not long after Yasmeen's first ANC visit, where she found out she was pregnant for a second time, her husband decided to move the family to the neighboring district, looking for more stable work to support their growing family. Her health records, and those of her 2-year-old daughter, will be accessible at the new clinic, thanks to a national health registry and electronic health record system. Yasmeen has felt *supported throughout the move and her pregnancy, thanks to the personalized text messages she receives as her pregnancy progresses. She also receives messages for her daughter, and is extremely proud of the fact that her daughter will finish her full round of vaccinations in the coming month. Her mother-in-law, Bilkis, also receives messages targeted to her, congratulating her on health checkpoint accomplishments and the role she has played in facilitating a successful pregnancy. Bilkis now feels empowered that she, too, is learning about ways in which to keep her grandchild healthy, and shares messages with her friends in the village. Yasmeen has been extremely appreciative of the interactive child health services, especially during some scary episodes when her daughter was less than a year old. In a week where her daughter had persistent diarrhea, she was able call the child health hotline for advice and received both support and remedies to make sure her baby stayed hydrated while sick. The hotline ultimately recommended she go to the health clinic after a few days with no improvement; the health worker diagnosed an infection and was able to send Yasmeen home with medicine, returning to her home in person a few days later to follow up. Yasmeen is feeling confident and healthy in her second pregnancy and as a mother, and looks forward to the birth of her second child.*

NOTE

1. The rational redistribution of tasks among health workforce teams (10).

REFERENCES

1. World Health Organization, The Partnership for Maternal Newborn and Child Health. The PMNCH 2013 Report: Analysing progress on commitments to the Global Strategy for Women's and Children's Health. Geneva, Switzerland: WHO, 2013.
2. Evans DB, Marten R, Etienne C. Universal health coverage is a development issue. *Lancet* 2012; 380(9845):864–865.
3. Bhutta ZA, Chopra M, Axelson H, Berman P, Boerma T, Bryce J, et al. Countdown to 2015 decade report (2000-10): Taking stock of maternal, newborn, and child survival. *Lancet* 2010; 375(9730):2032–2044.
4. Fraser H, Bailey C, Sinha C, Mehl G, Labrique AB. Call to action on global eHealth evaluation. Consensus statement of the WHO Global eHealth Evaluation Meeting, Bellagio, Italy; 2011.
5. Free C, Phillips G, Watson L, Galli L, Felix L, Edwards P, et al. The effectiveness of mobile-health technologies to improve health care service delivery processes: A systematic review and meta-analysis. *PLoS Medicine* 2013; 10(1):e1001363.
6. World Health Organization. Maternal mortality. Retrieved from http://www.who.int/gho/maternal_health/mortality/maternal/en/
7. Hill K, Thomas K, AbouZahr C, Walker N, Say L, Inoue M, et al. Estimates of maternal mortality worldwide between 1990 and 2005: An assessment of available data. *Lancet* 2007; 370(9595):1311–1319.
8. You D, Bastian P, Wu J, Wardlaw T. *Levels & Trends in Child Mortality: Report 2013.* New York, NY: United Nations Children's Fund, 30 pp. 2013.
9. Measure DHS Demographic and Health Surveys. Unmet need for family planning. 2012. Retrieved from http://www.measuredhs.com/topics/Unmet-Need.cfm
10. World Health Organization. Taking stock: Task shifting to tackle health worker shortages. 2007, pp. 1–12.
11. UN Millennium Project. *Investing in Development: A Practical Plan to Achieve the Millennium Development Goals.* New York: UN; 2005.
12. Telecom Regulatory Authority of India. Highlights on Telecom subscription data as on 31st August 2013. 2013, pp. 1–18. Retrieved from http://pib.nic.in/archieve/others/2013/oct/d2013102503.pdf
13. International Telecommunications Union. World telecommunication/ICT indicators database 2013, Vol. 17. 2013. Retrieved from http://www.itu.int/en/ITU-D/Statistics/Pages/publications/wtid.aspx
14. World Health Organization. Potential and principles for health sector actions to strengthen civil registration and vital statistics systems. Retrieved from http://www.who.int/healthinfo/civil_registration/crvs_meeting_dec2013_discussionpaper.pdf
15. The Partnership for Maternal Newborn and Child Health. *A Global Review of the Key Interventions Related to Reproductive, Maternal, Newborn and Child Health (RMNCH).* Geneva, Switzerland; 2011.
16. World Health Organization. *Packages of Interventions for Family Planing, Safe Abortion Care, Maternal, Newborn and Child Health.* Geneva, Switzerland: WHO; 2010.
17. Bhutta Z, Ahmed T, Black R, Cousens S, Dewey K, Giugliani E, et al. What works? Interventions for maternal and child undernutrition and survival. *Lancet* 2008; 371(9610):417–440.
18. Victora CG. Commentary: LiST: Using epidemiology to guide child survival policymaking and programming. *International Journal of Epidemiology* 2010; 39(Suppl 1):i1–i2.
19. Zurovac D, Otieno G, Kigen S, Mbithi AM, Muturi A, Snow RW, et al. Ownership and use

of mobile phones among health workers, care-givers of sick children and adult patients in Kenya: Cross-sectional national survey. *Global Health* 2013; 9(20).

20. Labrique A. Where there is no "mHealth": Mobile phone ownership and use in rural Bangladesh. mHealth Summit 2012. Washington, DC; 2012. Retrieved from http://www.mhealthsummit.org/sites/default/files/Research - Maternal and Child Health.pdf

21. Mitchell M, Labrique A, Mehl G. *mHealth Logic Model*. Noordhoek, South Africa; 2012. Retrieved from https://www.usaidassist.org/sites/assist/files/marks_mhealth_presentation_core_7may2014.pdf

22. Labrique AB, Vasudevan L, Kochi E, Fabricant R, Mehl G. 12 common applications and a visual framework. *Global Health Science Practice* 2013; 1(2):160–171.

23. World Health Organization. WHO mHealth Technical and Evidence Review Group (mTERG) for reproductive, maternal, newborn and child health. 2013 Retrieved from http://www.who.int/reproductivehealth/topics/mhealth/mterg/en/index.html

24. Mueller D, Lungu D, Acharya A, Palmer N. Constraints to implementing the essential health package in Malawi. *PLoS One* 2011; 6(6).

25. Knippenberg R, Lawn J, Darmstadt G, Begkoyian G, Fogstad H, Walelign N, et al. Systematic scaling up of neonatal care in countries. *Lancet* 2005; 365(9464):1087–1098.

26. Travis P, Bennett S, Haines A, Pang T, Bhutta Z, Hyder A, et al. Overcoming health-systems constraints to achieve the Millennium Development Goals. *Lancet* 2004; 364(9437):900–906.

27. Peters DH, Garg A, Bloom G, Walker DG, Brieger WR, Rahman MH. Poverty and access to health care in developing countries. *Annals of the New York Academy of Science* 2008; 1136:161–171.

28. Christiansen, Clayton M. Grossman JH, Hwang J. *The Innovator's Prescription: A Disruptive Solution for Health Care*. New York: McGraw-Hill; 2009.

29. United Nations Children's Fund. Every child's birth right: Inequities and trends in birth registration. New York; 2013.

30. Health Metrics Network of the World Health Organization. MOVE-IT for the MDGs Africa Initiative. 2012.

31. Uganda Registration Services Bureau. Mobile vital registration system. 2014. Retrieved from: http://www.mobilevrs.co.ug/home.php

32. Center for Health Market Innovations. ChildCount+. 2014. Retrieved from http://healthmarketinnovations.org/program/childcount

33. World Health Organization. Sexual and reproductive health. 2014. Retrieved from http://www.who.int/reproductivehealth/en/

34. Google Play. DRISTHI. 2014. Retrieved from https://play.google.com/store/apps/details?id=org.ei.drishti

35. Barrington J, Wereko-Brobby O, Ward P, Mwafongo W, Kungulwe S. SMS for life: A pilot project to improve anti-malarial drug supply management in rural Tanzania using standard technology. *Malaria Journal*. 2010; 9(1):298.

36. Dimagi. CommTrack: A tool for mobile logistics and supply chain management. 2014. Retrieved from http://www.commtrack.org/home/

37. Dimagi. cStock: Supply chains for community case management. 2014. Retrieved from http://www.commtrack.org/static-resources/docs/case-studies/commtrack-cstock.pdf

38. Rajatonirina S, Heraud J, Randrianasolo L, Orelle A, Razanajatovo NH, Raoelina N, et al. Short message service sentinel surveillance of influenza-like illness in Madagascar, 2008–2012. *World Health* 2012; March:2008–2012.

39. IICD. Combating mother and child malaria mortality with mobiles. 2014. Retrieved from http://www.iicd.org/articles/combating-mother-and-child-malaria-mortality-with-mobiles

40. Yu P, de Courten M, Pan E, Galea G, Pryor J. The development and evaluation of a PDA-based method for public health surveillance data collection in developing countries. *International Journal of Medical Informatics* 2009; 78(8):532–542.

41. Mendoza G, Okoko L, Morgan G, Konopka S. *mHealth Compendium*, Vol 2. Arlington VA; 2013.

42. Dimagi. Active data management—Concept document. Retrieved from: http://bit.ly/dimagi_active_management

43. Ministry of Health Rwanda. mUbuzima. 2014. Retrieved from http://mubuzima.gov.rw/mUbuzima/core/modules/pagelayout/web/showpage.aspx?menukey=1

44. Dalberg Global Development Advisors. Preparing the next generation of community health workers: The power of technology for training. 2012.

45. Mobile Alliance for Maternal Action (MAMA). Chipatala Cha Pa Foni. 2013, pp. 1–9. Retrieved from http://mobilemamaalliance.org/sites/default/files/1772-MAMA-Spotlight-September-v3-JH.pdf

46. Chang LW, Kagaayi J, Arem H, Nakigozi G, Ssempijja V, Serwadda D, et al. Impact of a mHealth intervention for peer health workers on AIDS care in rural Uganda: A mixed methods evaluation of a cluster-randomized trial. *AIDS and Behavior* 2011;15(8):1776–1784.

47. Switchboard. Switchboard: Mobilizing global health. 2014. Retrieved from http://www.switchboard.org/

48. Kaonga NN, Labrique A, Mechael P, Akosah E, Ohemeng-Dapaah S, Baah JS, et al. Mobile phones and social structures: an exploration of a closed user group in rural Ghana. *BMC Medical Informatics and Decision Making* 2013; 13(1):100.

49. Global Health Workforce Alliance. Global experience of community health workers for delivery of health related millennium development goals: A systematic review, country case studies and recommendations for integration into national health systems. 2010.

50. DeRenzi B, Lesh N, Parikh TS, Sims C, Maokola W, Chemba M, et al. e-IMCI: Improving pediatric health care in low-income countries. *Proceedings of the SIGCHI Conference on Human Factors in Computing.* Pages 753–762 (2008) Retrieved from: https://redesign.cs.washington.edu/sites/default/files/hci/papers/tmpbj0qhL.pdf.

51. Knowledge for Health (K4Health). ACE mobile app. 2014. Retrieved from http://www.k4health.org/product/ace-mobile-app

52. Johns Hopkins Center for Clinical Global Health Education. eMOCHA key facts. 2013. Retrieved from http://main.ccghe.net/content/emocha-key-facts

53. The Johns Hopkins Center for Clinical Global Health Education, The Johns Hopkins Center for TB Research. eMocha TB Detect. Retrieved from: http://main.ccghe.net/node/1348

54. Grameen Foundation. MOTECH suite. Retrieved from http://www.motechsuite.org

55. Grameen Foundation. MOTECH suite features. 2014. Retrieved from http://www.motechsuite.org/index.php/features

56. Khan A, Mehl G. mHealth tools: Understanding potential, program integration, and sustainability. Presentation at Saving Lives at Birth, Washington, DC; 2013.

57. Cole-Lewis H, Kershaw T. Text messaging as a tool for behavior change in disease prevention and management. *Epidemiological Review* 2011; 32(1):56–69.

58. Text to Change. Largest scale mHealth project in Africa. 2014. Retrieved from http://projects.texttochange.org/en/project/779/

59. Déglise C, Suggs LS, Odermatt P. Short message service (SMS) applications for disease prevention in developing countries. *Journal of Medical Internet Research* 2012; 14(1):e3.

60. Institute for Reproductive Health, Georgetown University. CycleTel. 2014. Retrieved from http://www.cycletel.org

61. L'Engle KL, Vahdat HL, Ndakidemi E, Lasway C, Zan T. Evaluating feasibility, reach and potential impact of a text message family planning information service in Tanzania. *Contraception* 2013; 87(2):251–256

62. Smith C, Vannak U, Sokhey L, Ngo TD, Gold J, Khut K, et al. MObile Technology for Improved Family Planning Services (MOTIF): Study protocol for a randomised controlled trial. *Trials* 2013; 14:427.

63. Rotheram-Borus MJ, Tomlinson M, Gwegwe M, Comulada WS, Kaufman N, Keim M. Diabetes buddies: Peer support through a mobile phone buddy system. *Diabetes Education* 2012; 38(3):357–365.

64. Praekelt Foundation. Young Africa live. 2014. Retrieved from http://www.praekeltfoundation.org/young-africa-live.html

65. Sikder SS, Labrique AB, Ullah B, Ali H, Rashid M, Mehra S, et al. Accounts of severe acute obstetric complications in rural Bangladesh. *BMC Pregnancy and Childbirth* 2011; 11:76.

66. Horvath T, Azman H, Kennedy GE, Rutherford GW. Mobile phone text messaging to help patients with HIV infection take their antiretroviral medications every day. *Cochrane Database System Review* 2012; (3):CD009756.

67. Pop-Eleches C, Thirumurthy H, Habyarimana JP, Zivin JG, Goldstein MP, de Walque D, et al. Mobile phone technologies improve adherence to antiretroviral treatment in a resource-limited setting: A randomized controlled trial of text message reminders. *AIDS* 2011; 25(6):825–834.

68. Lester RT, Ritvo P, Mills EJ, Kariri A, Karanja S, Chung MH, et al. Effects of a mobile phone short message service on antiretroviral treatment adherence in Kenya (WelTel Kenya1): A randomised trial. *Lancet* 2010; 376(9755):1838–1845.

69. Thirumurthy H, Lester RT. M-health for health behaviour change in resource-limited settings: Applications to HIV care and beyond. *Bulletin of the World Health Organization* 2012; 90:390–392.

70. Da Costa TM, Barbosa BJP, Gomes e Costa DA, Sigulem D, de Fátima Marin H, Filho AC, et al. Results of a randomized controlled trial to assess the effects of a mobile SMS-based intervention on treatment adherence in HIV/AIDS-infected Brazilian women and impressions and satisfaction with respect to incoming messages. *International Journal of Medical Informatics* 2012; 81(4):257–269.

71. Whittaker R, McRobbie H, Bullen C, Borland R, Rodgers A, Gu Y. Mobile phone-based interventions for smoking cessation. *Cochrane Database System Review* 2012; (11): CD006611.

72. Gurol-Urganci I, de Jongh T, Atun R, Car J. Mobile phone messaging reminders for attendance at healthcare appointments (Review). *Cochrane Library* 2013;(12).

73. Seidenberg P, Nicholson S, Schaefer M, Semrau K, Bweupe M, Masese N, et al. Early infant

diagnosis of HIV infection in Zambia through mobile phone texting of blood test results. *Bulletin of the World Health Organization* 2012; 90:348–356.

74. Tremblay M. Medicines counterfeiting is a complex problem: A review of key challenges across the supply chain. *Current Drug Safety* 2013; 8(1):43–55.

75. Center for Health Market Innovations. Changamka Microhealth Limited. 2014. Retrieved from http://healthmarketinnovations.org/program/changamka-microhealth-limited

76. Vodafone foundation. M-Pesa and maternal health. 2011. Retrieved from http://www.vodafone.com/content/dam/vodafone/about/foundation/ccbrt.pdf

77. mHealth Alliance. IWG grants. 2014. Retrieved from http://mhealthalliance.org/our-work/iwg-grants/about-iwg-grants

78. World Health Organization. Use of mobile technology for health. 2014. Retrieved from http://www.who.int/reproductivehealth/topics/mhealth/en/index.html

79. Seebregts C, Mamlin B, Biondich P, Fraser H, Wolfe B, Jazayeri D, et al. The OpenMRS Implementers Network. *International Journal of Medical Informatics* 2009; 78(11):711–20.

80. Braa J, Muquinge H. Building collaborative networks in Africa on health information systems and open source software development—experiences from the HISP/BEANISH network. *IST Africa* 2007; 3. Retrieved from: CiteSeerX: 10.1.1.131.8950

18

Open Architecture and Standards in Mobile Health

JULIA E. HOFFMAN, KELLY M. RAMSEY, AND DEBORAH ESTRIN

INTRODUCTION

In "The Cathedral and the Bazaar" (1) Eric Raymond made the quintessential case for open source software development—the creation of code and processes that are constructed and shared publicly. The analogy made within the central thesis of this essay is easily understood by those outside of software engineering: namely, the teachings and workings of the cathedral are formal, centralized, and tightly held by hierarchical and closed ranks, while the variety and open structure of the bazaar allows for diversity of understanding and, ultimately, a more flexible and self-correcting dissemination of products and processes. The open source model—both well before Raymond's analysis and in the years that have followed—has proven to be a key enabler of rapid collaborative innovation in software (2). However, such a distributed (and, at times, ad-hoc) mode of development also presents many challenges in the healthcare space, where the desire for a coordinated continuum of care can conflict with the freedom to explore new and more effective avenues of healthcare service delivery.

This chapter argues that the health and healthcare challenges of our time are too complex to be approached with closed, siloed approaches, and that the dynamism of the bazaar model can be harnessed to provide the same kind of innovation in behavioral mobile health (mHealth), as it has proven capable of providing in many other domains of information technology. Furthermore, in our view, if a true marketplace for innovative mHealth solutions is to be cultivated, the vendors in such a marketplace must embrace open standards and open architectures to provide the common interfaces and protections that will ensure the safety and liberty of patients.

DEFINING TERMS

In order to best understand—and communicate—the necessity for open architectures in mHealth, it is necessary for behavioral scientists to understand some key terms.

Modularity in psychotherapy and behavioral treatments, as Chorpita, Daleiden, and Weisz conceptualize it (3), is the degree to which a treatment protocol consists of discrete, differentiated, self-contained parts, or "modules." Modules are functionally distinct components (e.g., sessions, activities, or exercises); have a specific purpose (e.g., reducing arousal, countering depressive cognitions, skills training); can be exchanged for equivalent modules without affecting the functioning of the rest of the protocol (e.g., if multiple relaxation modules are available, any can be selected regardless of which relaxation method they use); and can be rearranged and connected interchangeably like building blocks into a variety of prescribed or improvised sequences.

The term has a fully analogous meaning in software design: projects can be decomposed into functional modules in order to optimize implementation and maintenance. The modules can be reused, modified, and reconfigured as needed, to provide similar functionality in different applications. Modularity of software can refer to articulated features and functions (how the software works) or user interface design and user experience.

Designers of new therapeutic treatments or treatment components (i.e., modules) can largely take for granted that they share a similar conceptual language, such as the principles and mechanisms of psychotherapy generally or those of a particular theoretical school of therapy such as cognitive behavioral treatment. The work that they produce can be contributed to a shared knowledge base and can be learned and used by those familiar with other similar tools. These products can be seen as interoperable or as having interoperability: they can communicate and work with each other.

Similarly, in software systems, *interoperability* refers to the extent to which different systems or modules can effectively coordinate and cooperate to provide a more comprehensive solution than either module could individually. Such interoperability usually has at least two main aspects: assuring that systems have mutually comprehensible data, and being able to exchange that data between systems using mutually agreed-upon protocols. Mutual comprehension of data can be achieved by adhering to a common data format. A *data format* is simply a conceptual language and schema that is used to represent accumulated knowledge (e.g., the names of variables and what they each measure), much like the codebook a researcher might create when making a dataset publicly available. Likewise, allowing the exchange of these data between systems or modules requires the use of a common *protocol*—carefully specified rules by which data can be requested and delivered, and by which participants in the exchange can be authenticated. Such a protocol between software components by which one component may share data with another is often called an *API* (application programming interface).

If an industry or community agrees on a common codebook (e.g., a unified format for electronic health records [4]) and a protocol or API to receive or transmit it securely, then that agreement constitutes a *standard*. Such standards are much like the numerous standards that are agreed upon for other tools such as weights and measures, gauges of mechanical components, and the format of calendar dates. While specific definitions of the term vary, an *open standard*, generally, refers to a standard that is produced and maintained by the collaboration of a community (as opposed to being imposed by regulatory mandate or by a few powerful community members) and is available in its entirety to all interested parties either for free or a nominal fee.

Finally, the high-level design of software is referred to as its *architecture*, and a modular computer system that adheres to a set of common standards and which further provides for easy revision

and replacement of its constituent modules by the community can be said to have been designed with an *open architecture*. In a system with an open architecture, the various components of the system—such as an app for the patient to monitor his or her health habits, dashboard software for the provider to review data the patient entered into the app, and a connected sensor to monitor heart rate—are all self-contained parts that serve specific purposes, communicate with each other in mutually agreed-upon ways, and can be swapped out for functionally equivalent parts at will. (A provider might prescribe a different heart rate sensor, for example, or the patient might transition to using a different health monitoring app.)

For reference, the opposite of "open" as it is used here is *siloed*. This refers to architectures, data formats, protocols, and systems that are closed—they are designed to function independently—and do not allow developers or consumers access to generated data, do not allow replacement or customization of individual components except by the original developer, or are defined and controlled by individual (usually private) entities.

THE CURRENT STATE OF MHEALTH: NUMEROUS SINGLE-PURPOSE APPS

As indicated throughout this volume, recent years have seen a massive proliferation of mHealth apps consistent with the increasing ubiquity of app-ready mobile devices. The vast majority of these apps target a single diagnosis, health behavior, and/or treatment regimen. Part of the reason for this is intrinsic to the medium: mobile form factors and usage patterns tend to make narrowly focused, single-purpose apps more popular and thus more successful. In addition, most publicly available apps are produced by independent entrepreneurs and technologists (with the aid of subject matter experts) and aim for broad adoption, which drives them to attempt to solve small, tractable problems that are widely experienced, and have limited potential for adverse events, and which can be addressed independently from other health concerns.

Another less obvious factor driving this trend is that empirical validation of mHealth app efficacy can present many challenges. The empirical literature around behavioral mHealth so far has, understandably, centered around studies of one app at a time: producing a mobile delivery or support app for a psychological treatment is a new, lengthy, and likely expensive endeavor. The justification, development, and initial testing of such an app, consequently, can constitute a useful descriptive paper to inform a community of practice (5,6). Similarly, small-*n* usability trials or case studies demonstrate the feasibility of the innovation (7,8). Larger efficacy studies, which so far have been few, have typically been performed one app at a time, and have taken several different forms: efficacy testing to determine if the mHealth app is better than placebo or control (9,10), augmentation studies to find out if adding the app to standard care improves outcomes (11,12), or efficiency studies to test if the app allows standard care to be performed with more effective use of the provider's time or with less skill or labor (13,14).

Given that each app must be empirically validated as a whole, and that the development and validation of each such app can be costly, it is easy to see why most apps are narrowly focused and try not to introduce multiple different treatments that may add untold additional variables, making research data difficult to interpret. Many of these narrowly focused tools are certainly valuable and are, in fact, aligned with a generally prudent movement toward evidence-based medicine that optimizes care by leveraging solid science.

THE VALUE OF INTEROPERABILITY IN REAL WORLD CLINICAL CARE

It is important to recognize, however, that mHealth apps will increasingly be deployed in *systems* of behavioral healthcare. As more (and more effective) apps become available, as Patrick, Griswold, Raab, and Intille anticipate (15), providers and patients will certainly want to use multiple mHealth apps at once. For example, a patient might use an app to support their smoking cessation therapy, receive reminders and manage cravings, then. once accustomed to the treatment, begin using a diet and exercise tracking app to help manage post-smoking weight gain, while perhaps replacing the stress relief elements of smoking with app-based relaxation exercises. For a patient in intensive psychotherapy, an app to facilitate the provision of a particular protocol (e.g., assignments, readings) could be amplified

by a compatible app for management of self-harm urges, an ecological momentary assessment app to prompt self-care, or an engaging tool such as the Photographic Affect Meter (16) to monitor mood. Patients will also be increasingly likely to come into care while *already* using other apps to support their treatment for other conditions or their maintenance of good health (17).

Behavioral apps, by nature of their technological platform, are prone to be used in this kind of piecewise fashion even when they attempt to combine multiple treatment strategies. Such apps are typically comprised of discrete, purposive components, such as programmed motivational reminders, an anxiety assessment, an audio-guided relaxation exercise, a form to fill in time in bed and hours slept, or a button to make a phone call to a selected emergency contact. In some cases, these components are all used in full in a comprehensive protocol; for example, with a fixed, manualized psychotherapy protocol such as cognitive processing therapy (CPT), the provider and patient might use the various components of a companion app such as CPT Coach (18) thoroughly and in sequence—at least, to the extent that they strictly follow the treatment protocol.

However, more often app features will be mixed and matched by providers and patients to fit the patient's needs. A protocol such as cognitive behavioral therapy (CBT) for insomnia, for example, might be designed with optional components to meet various contingencies. As a result, when using a companion app such as CBT-i Coach (19), a patient might never use a module such as practicing a daily "worry time," or might variously start and stop using such methods as scheduled "winding down" activities before bed to improve calm or "change your perspective" cards to adjust cognitive habits based on collaborative decision-making between provider and patient. A symptom management app such as PTSD Coach (20) (for post-traumatic stress disorder) is intended to be used at will only for those functions the patient finds necessary: one might regularly use only the anger reduction and social isolation tools, for example, and never use the elements targeting anxiety, sleeplessness, or other problems.

These observations suggest that mHealth apps should not be seen as analogs of the implementation of complete treatment plans, but rather as separable treatment *modules*. In fact, the use cases for which behavioral mHealth apps will be applied in the near future—and which these apps will in turn facilitate—are inherently modular. Providers will continue to exercise the flexibility of dropping in components of treatment when they are beneficial to the patient—for example, adding weight loss once a patient has progressed far enough in smoking cessation as to not be overwhelmed by a second regimen—and modifying or removing them as needed. Consequently, the use of apps will mirror this practice: as more app options become available and institutionally sanctioned or even required, providers will prescribe the use of apps as they become beneficial for treatment (e.g., introducing the health insurance plan's sanctioned calorie counting and weighing-in app) and remove them from the regimen as the necessity wanes (e.g., reducing frequency of momentary assessments as the patient improves).

This proper conceptualization of the role of mHealth apps as treatment *modules* (in the full sense of Chorpita, Daleiden, and Weisz's modularity [3]) illuminates the need for these apps to employ common data formats, protocols, and APIs, such that that each app may interoperate with others. Such common protocols are also required to allow sharing of data with providers. A patient's adherence to daily therapy homework, responses to regular assessments, self-tracking of progress indicators, patterns of feature usage, engagement with crisis resources—all of these potential uses of an app generate data that are meaningful to the provider for the purpose of directing and adjusting the course of therapy. Providers will need to be able to leverage this data collection capacity, either for augmenting a course of treatment (e.g., by reaching out to a patient when they lapse or report a high level of distress on a self-assessment) or for making treatment more efficient (e.g., by reviewing adherence and progress indicators before a session begins).

THE CHALLENGES OF INTEROPERABILITY IN REAL-WORLD SCENARIOS

Unfortunately, the level of interoperability among current mHealth solutions and systems is quite poor. As a simple example, consider the tracking of body weight and daily calories consumed—information that people often enter into diet and weight-tracking

apps. A patient receiving care for weight loss might use any number of diet apps to track this information, or might be using a general-purpose tracking app to enter daily or weekly updates. Prior to receiving treatment, a patient might have already been accumulating this information as part of his or her ongoing diet efforts. Rather than be out of contact between visits to the provider, or having the patient come to the care site just to weigh in on a regular basis, a patient and provider might instead want to motivate adherence by authorizing the provider to connect to the patient's tracking app, or to the server where the app stores its data. The provider could ask for just the "weight" and "calories" data that they want to use to inform care and receive the information securely in an understandable format. The provider, then, could readily perform analyses with whatever desktop program they have, such as viewing the weight and calorie entries in a line graph or calculating a correlation, and just as easily record the data in the patient's electronic health record.

Even this straightforward scenario is not yet feasible in the vast majority of cases. The patient's tracking app is in all likelihood storing its data in a unique format, and if it permits other apps to request data at all, it is programmed to do so only with business partners that the app developer has pre-approved (for example, another company who makes an exercise tracking app). Even if the app developer has created and publicized an API (i.e., a protocol that other developers can use to request authorization to transmit and receive data with the app), the developer might impose restrictions on which data are shared or the number of data connections that will be honored for business reasons (21–24). Even if the diet app were to allow all requests in their entirety, such that a patient could authorize their provider to access their data, strong privacy expectations for sensitive health data (e.g., HIPAA rules) would require secure transmission methods with strong authentication of the parties with whom data are shared. The piecewise development of such secure technology on an app-by-app basis can be expensive, and any problems in the design or implementation can lead to patient harm and lawsuits, which disincentivizes vendors from providing the functionality at all.

Simply facilitating patients' "ownership" of their data, for example, by formatting the app's accumulated data in a file that can be downloaded by or sent to the patient, brings additional challenges. Security restrictions for health data often prevent providers from encouraging or cooperating with this approach, or even opening e-mails with clinical information, so providers might not be permitted to receive data directly from their patients. Nor might providers want to drink from the fire hose. Processing an app's (perhaps idiosyncratically formatted) data file to extract only the information they want for informing the current course of care would be a nontrivial burden in terms of both time and technical training. Moreover, having possession of too much patient data could be a liability, or considered as such by the providers' employers or insurers, if it opens providers to later accusations that they could have acted immediately upon receipt of real-time data or diagnosed other conditions had they processed and analyzed all of the data they had received. (Similarly unpalatable to providers would be the organizational mandates or societal expectations that might result: that they, as a liability avoidance strategy, perform comprehensive data mining for symptoms on patient data files that come into their possession.) Providers in behavioral health fields are well trained to erect necessary boundaries to ensure the integrity of the therapeutic work, and a constant influx of data outside of treatment hours is reasonably viewed with some trepidation.

Consequently, without interoperable systems that allow providers to securely acquire patient data, but only the patient data that they need, a patients' data are for all intents and purposes trapped in the app. A patient could, of course, laboriously transcribe the requested information from an app by hand, print it out, and take the paper to the provider, but this would obviate much of the benefit of using the app in the first place.

THE IMPACT OF LIMITED INTEROPERABILITY ON BEHAVIORAL MHEALTH

This lack of interoperability particularly hinders the effectiveness and advancement of behavioral health apps. The same type of data "trap" discussed above applies here as well, but in many ways hampers effective, adaptive treatment far more. A mobile app can be a very effective means of administering a scheduled psychological assessment or EMA to assess symptoms, or apps could be used to support therapy in place of paper handouts, written homework, and audio recordings. But without secure standards for data exchange, all of these data, too, become trapped in individual apps, without any way to inform treatment. For example, CBT for insomnia requires that the provider perform immediate data analysis on patients' daily sleep diaries in order to calculate the prescribed bedtime and wake time, often for several patients at once in a group therapy setting. If patients could use one of the many popular self-tracking apps instead, and these various apps could each send their data to the provider for immediate insertion into the provider's database, more treatment resources could be dedicated to therapy instead of the administrative tasks of collecting and transcribing patient paperwork.

More broadly, when apps are not interoperable, behavioral health providers and app designers cannot rely on being able to access data from other apps performing added or replaced functions. The most beneficial aspects of modularity—the ability to assemble custom protocols from component, outcome-based modules, either as a research question or a field improvisation—are not available. At an app design level, this means that the designer must incorporate every potentially desired feature of therapy into the app, even if alternate tools are available and adaptable from elsewhere. If the therapy involves identifying and tracking progress toward goals, for example, the therapy support app must have its own version of this feature if the patient and provider are to readily use it—even though innumerable specialized goal-tracking apps already exist for this purpose, some of which a patient might already be accustomed to using for other health, professional, or personal reasons. Relaxation exercises or soothing audio, similarly, must be duplicated rather than being potentially referenced from other sources. Any psychological assessments must also be included, even if they are already part of other health apps, and space limitations preclude the incorporation of a large number of alternatives.

As previously discussed, these architectural limitations tilt mHealth app development incentives toward supporting treatment approaches that are already equivalently cohesive and comprehensive: toward producing "one-stop shop" apps designed to complement manualized protocols. While this approach has its advantages—among them, leaning the early focus of development toward supporting established treatments that are applicable to larger populations—it has also tended to incentivize isolated, disorder-specific apps that face similar limitations as disease-oriented treatments (25).

This is not to suggest that cohesive, comprehensive apps are undesirable, or that they are either likely to be or should be abandoned in favor of an array of specialized module apps, micro-apps, or widgets. Designing or modifying a modular therapy consists of assembling and sequencing treatment modules for the therapeutic goal at hand (3,26). When supporting a therapy with an app, a comprehensive app framework or aggregator will in many cases be a far better solution—if not a necessary one—compared to asking a patient to juggle multiple app modules, none of which brings together all of the data from the others in one place. However, the comprehensive apps will need to be able to coordinate with others. To take a practical, non-health-related example, the Pocket Informant productivity app (27) assembles calendar, to-do list, notes, and contacts functions into an integrated system. While it can perform each of those functions internally, the app is able to synchronize with Google Calendar, the Toodledo to-do service/app, and the Evernote note-taking service/app, so that events, tasks, or notes edited in the other apps update in this one and vice-versa. As the field of health apps expand, similarly comprehensive apps will need to be able to do the same.

Another impact of this "all-or-nothing" design approach is that providers, as well as researchers, are severely restricted in their ability to localize treatments for differing local circumstances. Building in language localizations—translations of the app's content for different languages—allows providers to deploy an app for a wider population, but the fundamental limitation of the isolated, siloed app remains: the provider and patient must still take it or leave it as a whole.

Accommodation of more refined localizations, such as those based on region or cultural variation, is most certainly not supported by the mobile device's language settings, and thus is very difficult if not impossible. Language settings are no indication of whether, for example, the mindfulness-based relaxation exercises of a stress relief app are seen as questionable by a specific religious community or skirt a locality's blasphemy laws. A provider in those circumstances is left

with no option except to eschew the app entirely. Similarly, a provider may be stuck with therapy education or examples that are so outside the experience of a community as to be ridiculous—for example, in an area recovering from recent disaster, or in an impoverished neighborhood.

These app "silos" also have implications for operationalizing deployment of apps in behavioral health settings. Learning a new form of therapy, and integrating it into practice, is a recurring difficulty for providers all by itself (26). It places an undue burden on providers if, in order to integrate apps into therapy, they must learn how each app conglomerates or separates functions, and how each collects and reports data. Adding another layer of complexity on top of that at the office level—having to learn a new specialized, proprietary data dashboard interface for each therapy support app one is considering using—would be as unreasonable as attempting to integrate multiple formats of laboratory results or patient records. Such an arrangement would also likely be infeasible in a bureaucratic healthcare workplace that would have to attach these multiple data interfaces onto its existing systems, under what are likely to be heavy security restrictions or organizational inertia. This arrangement is not scalable: what is feasible at a very small scale becomes unworkable in a large implementation.

IMPACTS OF LIMITED MODULARITY ON BEHAVIORAL MHEALTH RESEARCH

One of the most profound problems with the current lack of interoperability is the unacceptable limits it places on mHealth research, and, by extension, future development of optimally effective mHealth systems. As mentioned previously, just as providers will find it not just useful but necessary to analyze patient data from mHealth apps, researchers studying the use of apps to complement behavioral health treatments will need to be able to analyze these data in order to perform evaluations of protocols that incorporate apps. At the simplest level, researchers are already studying apps one at a time, as stand-alone stop-gap treatments (9,10), augmentations to improve the outcomes of care (11,12), or aids to efficiency that could reduce the time or skill needed to attain the same outcomes (13,14). Blunt comparisons can currently be tested without requiring data from the app; for example, a treatment-plus-app condition or a brief-treatment-with-app condition can be compared to a treatment-as-usual condition.

Anything more refined, though, requires that the researcher be able to view the patient's interactions with the app. Like providers, researchers will want to view assessment responses over time to track symptom progression. Researchers will want to quantify the with-app/without-app distinction, so they will need to know not just if but how much a patient used the app, or when, or at which locations. As research progresses, they will also want these usage data broken down by app feature, such as SMS/momentary intervention, self-management exercise, or behavior tracking, in order to better understand dose and to identify the mechanisms and empirically supported principles (28) driving the outcomes that come with use of the app, as well as to design and compare modular app-complemented protocols that prescribe different combinations of mechanisms in different sequences (26). Studies will eventually progress to more complex treatment scenarios involving more than one app (for example, treatment for PTSD with sleep difficulties, incorporating a PTSD symptom management app and a sleep hygiene treatment + app), requiring either that the apps be able to retrieve data from each other or that data from the same participant across multiple apps be identifiable as such to the research team. On a wider scale, large-n research studies will be increasingly desirable that aggregate anonymized data from large numbers of patients, as Estrin and Sim envisiage (29), or that aggregate anonymized treatment data from large numbers of providers to compile databases of what was encountered, what was tried, and what worked, as Kazdin imagines (30).

Furthermore, mHealth apps can be used to overcome the standard challenges of self-report data in both clinical and research scenarios. *Passive sensing*—the identification of activity, biomarkers related to behavioral health, or other cues without the user taking specific action—can be measured and analyzed in order to add a richness of data that was never before possible. For example, consider the value of measuring a depressed patient's hours spent in vs. out of her house, or her daily geodiameter (distance traveled from home). Not only

is a new type of data available for analysis, but it is without additional patient burden, and suffers none of the oft-cited challenges of self-report.

While all of these kinds of data and more can be collected within an app with relative ease, currently getting the data off of a treatment support app into the researcher's hands presents difficult logistical and policy challenges. At best, currently, a fleshed-out commercial behavior-tracking app *might* permit *selected* commercial partners to retrieve and send *some* kinds of data at its discretion. In the example above, workouts or calories tracked with one fitness app could be transmitted to another fitness app—for as long as the business relationship between the two ventures persists (31,32). Patients cannot yet expect to be able to share their data with designated recipients or export their data at will, the way users usually can with their online calendars or website bookmarks. This is far cry from the kind of access researchers would need to collect data from study participants, especially when added data security is mandated by law or organization policy in order to protect sensitive patient information. HIPAA-compliant solutions for the secure transmission of health data from U.S. apps, as described above, are only in the prototype stage (29,33). While lack of agreed-upon data standards forces these solutions to remain bespoke projects that must be built anew for each study, and data from popular commercial mHealth apps remain locked away behind business strategies and proprietary data stovepipes, the pace of research to evaluate and improve apps for behavioral mHealth will be very slow.

THE VALUE OF OPENNESS IN MHEALTH STANDARDS AND ARCHITECTURES

All of this points toward the need for robust standards governing interoperability between mHealth apps and systems. Indeed, the problems cited above could be plucked from software engineering textbook case studies on the benefits of modular architecture, common data formats and protocols, and standards compliance. But why must these standards and architectures be "open"? These problems are not unanticipated by the mHealth industry; various proprietary mHealth data exchange systems are being developed, such as Aetna's CarePass or Microsoft's HealthVault, and some of these are starting to gain adoption. What is wrong with settling on a proprietary standard, if it seems to solve the problem?

Here, we must return to Raymond (1), and his analogy of the cathedral and the bazaar. His argument's central thesis is sometimes stated as, "given enough eyeballs, all bugs are shallow"— that is, the democratic nature of the bazaar model leads to a higher quality product, because a much larger group of contributors are free to inspect and improve the code. This property of the bazaar model is particularly useful when the technology being developed is the shared foundation of multiple other projects and products, because those who make use of the product can take their experience with using it and bring that experience to bear in improving and extending the foundations for the benefit of all other users. Raymond's frame of reference for his argument was the development process of Linux, an open-source operating system that in the time since has come to dominate as the operating system of choice for Internet servers, as well as being used as the foundation of the Android mobile operating system. Linux was just such a shared foundational technology, and its success has in large part been due to that fact that is freely available, and to this ability by its various users to be able to inspect and contribute back to the foundation. Linux's development model and place in the information technology ecosystem make it a sort of public trust resource for the entire industry—owned by everyone, controlled by collaboration, and not subject to the whims or profit motives of any one actor. Today, Linux is just one example from a deep bench of such success stories: from HTTP to HTML, from MySQL to the Apache Web server, today's Internet (and Internet businesses) are built atop a vast number of free and open architectures and standards. In fact, it is commonly held that the prevalence and flexibility of such readily available foundational technology has been and remains one of the most crucial enablers of the Internet as we know it today. No single entity, had it been in control of these various pieces of technology, would have been able to deal with the scale of demand for different use cases, nor would these standards have achieved such wide adoption (and the interoperability benefits that adoption has yielded) if they had been closed and there were profit incentives to produce a competing "standard."

As a shared foundation for the representation and exchange of something as existentially vital and sensitive as healthcare information, an architecture and set of standards for mHealth should also be considered a public trust resource. Only an open architecture based on open standards— especially if most or all of the constituent foundational software components are free—seems capable of gaining the ubiquitous adoption that will guarantee the interoperability that is so desperately needed, while allowing the explosive, bazaar-like innovation in mHealth to continue without being centrally controlled (and undoubtedly slowed and manipulated) by individual actors with unknown motives.

While behavioral health practitioners and researchers may be expert in the *content* of treatments and assessments, they rarely attend to how to translate the "nonspecific" factors of patient engagement onto a mobile platform. Beautiful design and gaming mechanics ("gamificiation") are expected by app users, and no exceptions are made for mHealth apps, in spite of the limited focus and expertise subject matter experts tend to allot to this domain. In an open ecosystem, design elements and game mechanics can be evaluated, fine-tuned, reused, and personalized through the use of APIs (e.g., with Pollak's Wellcoin [34]).

The most important reason for our call for openness is simply that it is in the best interest of patients. The ownership by a single (usually private) entity of any type of computing *platform*—that is, a foundational technology (such as an operating system like Linux or a protocol like TCP/IP) that enables an ecosystem of other, higher level components and defines the standards and architectures by which interoperability between those components may occur—gives that entity long-lasting influence over the ecosystem, which is not necessarily (and in practice, rarely) aligned with the interests of the ecosystem and those it serves. Once a platform achieves dominance, that dominance is self-perpetuating—because so much investment has been made in building on the provided foundation, moving to another foundation can be prohibitively expensive or impossible. This is known as platform "lock-in," and it can make it exceedingly difficult or completely infeasible for a new entrant to compete against an entrenched incumbent. This is bad enough when the result is slower, less vigorous innovation and a lack of user choice (e.g., I may need to choose this mHealth app over that one, not based on merit but because this one is compatible with my insurer's mHealth data exchange architecture and the other is not). But when it comes to an infrastructure for mHealth interoperability, in the worst case such lock-in could apply not simply to software compatibility but also to the patient's own health data.

Consider a scenario where an Aetna patient's mHealth data can be shared freely between apps and providers using Aetna's CarePass architecture, and the patient's providers are able to analyze a rich, accumulated store of historical health data to inform each intervention. Imagine then, that the patient wants (or is required) to change insurance providers. Unless Aetna has decided to provide robust export facilities (which is not aligned with their own profit motives), and the patient's new insurer is able to import that proprietary data format, the patient may be forced to abandon the rich mHealth data they have accumulated and start over with some new system (or, worse, be left with no path for ongoing mHealth interoperability at all). Patients should not be placed in a position where they forced to choose between having the right provider and having the right data.

Scenarios like this make it clear that the arguments for an open architecture for mHealth are not simply technological, but ethical as well. We strive for an mHealth industry that serves patients most effectively and where solutions compete on their merits (rather than on secondary factors irrelevant to outcomes). Designing the foundational components required for mHealth interoperability around an open architecture is quite simply the best way the software industry has found to bring this about.

DEFINING SUCCESS IN OPEN MHEALTH

What would a successful open mHealth architecture look like? The technical details of such an architecture are well outside the scope of this chapter, but perhaps such an architecture is most easily specified by describing the healthy mHealth ecosystem that could result.

Suppose that the various apps and clinical dashboard programs were thoroughly interoperable and compliant with any health data security policies their users might encounter. Developers would not have to invest in designing their own unique data transmission systems; they could just incorporate the thoroughly field-tested, agreed-upon standard. Moreover, incorporating the standards would be not just optional but expected, due to some combination of efficiency, industry consensus, user demand, or other factors that tend to drive standardization of methods (35). This would ultimately impact not only the value of the mHealth apps to patients but also the rapid dissemination and implementation of these in self-management and clinical practice.

These same benefits would manifest for subject matter experts and app designers when exploring more options for customized therapy and integrated health approaches beyond what is built into one app alone. A provider, for example, might want to be able to reinforce an anxiety treatment with having the patient keep a typed journal or make audio recordings; a treatment support app that can pull tagged notes from a note-taking app or link to recordings from a separate audio app would be more useful than an app that either has no such options (perhaps due to their absence in the source protocol) or that has its own, bare-bones version of these features that are unlikely to match the feature sets of specialized apps. Similarly, a provider might want to integrate a panic button or crisis safety plan into treatment for patients who are in unusually dangerous situations; this would be greatly facilitated if the therapy support app can communicate data back and forth with a safety plan app.

Modular mHealth apps that can pull alternate versions of content—either from another app or a server—would similarly be more useful to providers in the field. A provider prescribing a support app might need to substitute the civilian version of a validated assessment with the military version, for example, or might need to have patients use a particular version or frequency of an assessment in order to conform with their institution's preferred practices. Rather than wait for an app's designer to accommodate all possible use scenarios (which may very well never occur, resources being finite), a provider equipped with interoperable apps might simply have the treatment app retrieve an alternate assessment version from a library app or server, and in turn also be able to rely on these new response data being no less interpretable to a display dashboard or complementary mHealth app. Similarly, a provider might want to swap educational material or therapy homework for those from a different version of a manual, or from a specialized version developed by a particular community of practice, or just to a slightly different permutation that was used in a published study or by the institution's practices, so that treatment is thoroughly comparable to past results.

If providers are able to have apps pull in alternate versions of content from other apps or servers, or replace an app's modules with those more suitable to local restrictions and preferences, then possibilities greatly open up. A provider serving an observant religious community might replace an app's relaxation module with a set of appropriate scriptural meditations, or might simply have that portion of the app connect to a daily prayer app that the patient is already using. A provider with poor patients might want to replace a socialization skills module with one that does not reference out-of-touch examples, such as taking a Pilates class or planning a vacation, that would chip at the therapeutic alliance.

Likewise, implementation challenges associated with integrating heterogeneous apps into practice become easier to deal with. An app would merely need to meet the prevailing mHealth data transmission standards in order to be compatible with the provider's computer system. Conversely, the provider's computer system would just need to meet those standards in order to be compatible with whatever app or apps the patient is using. As a result, the provider would not have to install and learn new software suites in order to review patients' health app data at any scale, from monthly assessments to multiple daily coping and homework activities, nor would the provider's institution have to approve and maintain these new suites; they could continue to use the standards-compliant ones they already have. Rollouts for app-supported therapy protocols would then be better able to focus just on the already challenging tasks of implementing the therapy into the provider's work practices.

At the provider learning level, treatment support apps will be more readily integrated into care as they solidify around sets of functionally equivalent modules. What do the pieces of apps do, and what do they do with the data? With a psychological assessment or EMA, this is familiar and comparatively straightforward: the patient completes a survey, the results are totaled or otherwise

transformed, and the results are translated by the provider into idiosyncratic, clinically significant indicators. On the other hand, a momentary intervention (36) is conceptually less self-evident because it can have different technological implementations—from automatically generated SMS messages from a server (37–39), to regular reminders from within the app (9,40,41), to various kinds of sensor-triggered notifications made viable by university labs (42) and commercial enterprises such as Ginger.io (43,44)—and variants depending on what the intended outcome is. If apps—and their designers—make it easier for providers to look past the distracting technical specifics of *how* (which, like devices, will become obsolete anyway as time passes) and focus on the treatment *mechanism* a module is implementing, providers will in turn find it much easier to integrate mHealth apps into their data-processing systems and their institutions of care.

A well-designed provider dashboard will identify and summarize data from the standardized component modules of an app that supports a therapy protocol. For example, a manual or improvised protocol might consist of a weekly assessment module to monitor symptoms; a twice-daily momentary intervention module to motivate adherence; cognitive homework exercises; a daily tracking module for the patient to check off, and be accountable for, having done the homework exercises; and at-will use of calming, distraction, and habituation exercise modules. The provider will be able to rely on all assessment data being presented, analyzed, and, if desired, copied to the patient's medical record in the same, standardized way; similarly tracking of adherence to exercises, activations of "get crisis support now" modules, stress levels from momentary assessments, and so on. New therapy protocols and their supporting mHealth apps, to the extent that they consist of recognizable component modules, will be easy to integrate into this system, both conceptually and pragmatically.

Open architectures allow for a *learning health-care system* in which all actors in healthcare, from patients, to providers, to the system administrators, can improve over time using the wealth of nearly real-time data collected from mHealth assessments and interventions. Analytics from usage can inform rapid iteration and performance improvement across the system. Whether the goal is more successful personalized medicine that takes into account idiosyncratic reactions to interventions or decreased healthcare utilization to control costs, all can benefit from the transparent and continuous flow and interpretation of data.

Finally, the pace of research and empirical validation of mHealth approaches in an interoperable, open world will be dramatically faster. Researchers will be able to rely on study participants being able to simply opt in to secure data collection with the apps they are using, and will not be dependent on the business strategy or partnerships of common commercial apps in order to collect research data from participants who are using them. Various elements of usability and feasibility can become accepted so that researchers can set their sights on the more ambitious goals of efficacy and effectiveness testing, or the study of dissemination and implementation. The complexity of large studies can flourish as the typical randomized, controlled designs used in behavioral science can be replaced with the diverse and dynamic A-B testing enabled by sophisticated mobile technology and/or a series of structured n of 1 studies.

CHALLENGES ASSOCIATED WITH OPEN ARCHITECTURES

It should be noted that engaging an open approach is not a panacea. Challenges are to be expected in the development, promotion, and sustainment of open architectures (2). Adequate participation—both in number and quality of contributors—can determine the success or failure of an open endeavor. A critical mass of viable resulting products is needed that will ensure that the underlying structures are worth maintaining. Commercial interests and those who require branded options may have limited tolerance for contributing development resources to products that they will not ultimately own. Intricate security issues, which are generally facilitated by openness, can slip through due to the diversity of contributors to the code base or assumptions that do not hold up when exposed for all to see.

Beyond these technical issues, researchers and developers of behavioral interventions may find that their requirements are so specific that working to fit in or contribute to a larger system is hardly worth the effort. And furthermore, those with specific populations to treat or healthcare delivery systems with which to integrate may find that open architectures provide a one-size-fits-all approach that causes usability to suffer for patients, providers, or researchers. Ultimately, if open architectures are to be successful in this domain, they must be compelling enough for software developers to participate in and flexible enough to allow for creation of consumer-usable products that do not require technical expertise to navigate.

CONCLUSIONS

Technological innovations, including but not limited to mobile apps, have the potential to disrupt and enhance behavioral health and healthcare. As these novel products and processes emerge, the case for open standards and open architecture requires immediate and critical attention in order to optimize products, maximize safety and security, and integrate products meaningfully into existing models of care. Recommendations for behavioral health subject matter experts, healthcare innovators, and policymakers follow.

1. *Use—or develop with colleagues—open data and exchange formats that can be used to represent the same information to multiple parties.* Ensure application programming interfaces are created to allow cross-updating, data portability, and protection from obsolescence. Proprietary data formats dramatically limit the population that can be reached and the range of treatments that such information may inform. Having a wealth of information available about a patient is only useful if it can be understood by the system currently guiding interventions at any given time.

2. *Share data via protocols and interfaces that are secure, common, and transparent.* Any notion that patients are best protected by closed systems is misguided, since all this does is hide all of the inevitable bugs and weaknesses until they can be exploited. This is known as "security by obscurity," and it is no true security at all. Secure systems are built by establishing clear chains of trust and keeping the pieces that need to remain secret for security to be maintained as small as possible.

3. *Don't try to provide all-in-one solutions; build within your own domain of expertise and look to integrate or partner*

with existing solutions that are good at what they do. Open standards allow straightforward integration, which has financial, efficiency, and quality benefits for developers, providers, and consumers. This guidance is intended to apply isomorphically: whole programs can be integrated, as can specific elements of them. This can happen on the front end, where the integrated elements are visible to users, or on the back end, where disparate data sources can be combined post-hoc.

4. *Strive for an mHealth meritocracy.* For precisely the same reason that open architectures create an excellent foundation for innovation, they threaten any dominance of a category by suboptimal existing solutions (see: the current state of the healthcare industry). In the level playing field that open systems provide, the best solutions can compete and win against established systems that don't best serve the needs of patients, whereas closed systems usually make this kind of competition a foregone conclusion in favor of the status quo.

5. *Don't be afraid to climb the value chain.* Open architectures naturally lead to the commoditization of lower layers of technology, which opens new opportunities to innovate in higher level (and higher value) services. In 10 years, no one should want to be competing merely on the grounds that they provide the ability to securely share basic healthcare information with other solutions—that should be a given, and instead, the competition should be about who can best use those common facilities to optimize patient self- or supported care.

6. *Embrace the medium and learn what you need to use it effectively.* Many subject matter experts invested in developing novel mHealth tools purposely divorce themselves from technical details, either from fear that the decisions will be too complex to understand or that the technical team members will find the discussions intrusive. Both of these fears are unfounded. Consider that the true

value of a transdisciplinary team is only available when silos are broken down, not when work is divided up along strict lines. This reciprocally implies that health jargon should also be eliminated or explained to technical team members.

7. *Beginning with early designs, place value on interoperability over brand distinctiveness or platform "lock-in."* We recognize that this is not the path of least resistance. This is serious, collaborative mHealth work with the goal of building community capacity for everyone, not a gold rush to churn out cheap, minimal isolated apps or HTML5 Web apps that lack the sophistication to meaningfully integrate with others and are likely to be abandoned as quickly as they are produced.

8. *Provide unrestricted access to users' data for users or authenticated others.* Facilitate users' exporting all of their data into another app/protocol at will and, if possible, importing all of their data from another app, either directly or via an intermediary system such as a standardized electronic medical record. Users' needs will change throughout their lives, so they will be regularly switching apps regardless, and as mHealth becomes routine will simply expect as a matter of course that their health data will be compatible with not only existing alternatives but also with future systems not yet conceived.

9. *Develop or participate in communities and/or nonprofits that advance these technical projects and ecosystems.* Companies that are erecting branded walls around their moldering demonstration gardens already have numerous incentives and institutions for doing so—and when they ultimately deliquesce will leave their users with little or no provision for escape. Building a more sustainable, durable, forward-looking system will require its own incentives and institutions to overcome this imbalance as well as cultivate opportunities for investment and public–private partnerships. Open

mHealth (45) is one such nonprofit, which is "building an open architecture for improved, integrated health," and others are emerging as the need for standards comes further into focus. These organizations offer valuable consultation and resources for those seeking to build open products.

10. *Never lose sight of what real patients—real people—need, have, and want.* Humans seeking better health are complex entities who exist within an ever-changing context and are poorly served by single-purpose solutions made with the resource constraints of any individual team. The value of broadening teamwork and creating a fair and open playing field is no different in mHealth technology than it is in any other domain: in order to move toward resolution of the most complex health and healthcare challenges of our time, we must find ways to stand on the shoulders of giants. As creators of mHealth technologies we must learn to grasp our responsibility to avail our own shoulders for the standing.

REFERENCES

1. Raymond ES. *The Cathedral and the Bazaar.* Sebastopol, CA: O'Reilly; 1999, pp. 19–64.
2. Weber S. *The Success of Open Source.* Vol. 368. Cambridge, MA: Harvard University Press, 2004.
3. Chorpita BF, Daleiden EL, Weisz JR. Modularity in the design and application of therapeutic interventions. *Applied and Preventive Psychology* 2005; 11(3):141–156.
4. Hammond WE. The making and adoption of health data standards. *Health Affairs* 2005; 24(5):1205–1213.
5. Newman MG, Kenardy J. Comparison of palmtop-computer-assisted brief cognitive-behavioral treatment for panic disorder. *Journal of Consulting and Clinical Psychology* 1996; 65(1):178–183.
6. Przeworski A, Newman MG. Palmtop computer-assisted group therapy for social phobia. *Journal of Clinical Psychology* 2004; 60(2):179–188.
7. Rizvi SL, Dimeff LA, Skutch JM, Carroll D, Linehan MM. A pilot study of the DBT Coach: An interactive mobile phone application for individuals with borderline personality disorder and substance use disorder. *Behavior Therapy* 2011; 42:589–600.
8. Buchanan LM, Khazanchi D. A PDA intervention to sustain smoking cessation in clients with socioeconomic vulnerability. *Western Journal of Nursing Research* 2010; 32(3):281–304.
9. Oerlemans S, van Cranenburgh O, Herremans PJ, Spreeuwenberg P, van Dulmen S. Intervening on cognitions and behavior in irritable bowel syndrome: A feasibility trial using PDAs. *Journal of Psychosomatic Research* 2011; 70(3):267–277.
10. Atienza AA, King AC, Oliveira BM, Ahn DK, Gardner CD. Using hand-held computer technologies to improve dietary intake. *American Journal of Preventative Medicine* 2008; 34(6):514–518.
11. Gorini A, Pallavicini F, Algeri D, Repetto C, Gaggioli A, Riva G. Virtual reality in the treatment of generalized anxiety disorders. *Studies in Health Technology and Informatics* 2010; 154:39–43.
12. Askins MA, Sahler OJ, Sherman SA, Fairclough DL, Butler RW, Katz ER, et al. Report from a multi-institutional randomized clinical trial examining computer-assisted problem-solving skills training for English- and Spanish-speaking mothers of children with newly diagnosed cancer. *Journal of Pediatric Psychology* 2009; 34(5):551–563.
13. Kenardy JA, Dow MGT, Johnston DW, Newman MG. A comparison of delivery methods of cognitive-behavioral therapy for panic disorder: An international multicenter trial. *Journal of Consulting and Clinical Psychology* 2003; 71(6):1068–1075.
14. Gruber K, Moran PJ, Roth WT, Taylor CB. Computer-assisted cognitive behavioral group therapy for social phobia. *Behavior Therapy* 2001; 32(1):155–165.
15. Patrick K, Griswold WG, Raab F, Intille SS. Health and the mobile phone. *American Journal of Preventive Medicine* 2008; 35(2):177–181.
16. Pollack JP, Adams P, Gay G. PAM: A photographic affect meter for frequent, in situ measurement of affect. In Tan D, Fitzpatrick G, Gutwin C, Begole B, Kelllogg WA (eds.), *Proceedings of the SIGCHI Conference on Human Factors in Computing Systems,* 2011 May 7–May 12; Vancouver, BC. New York: Association for Computing Machinery; 2011, pp. 725–734.
17. Fox S, Duggan M. Tracking for health. Washington, DC: Pew Internet & American Life Project; 2013 (Jan. 28).
18. Hoffman JE, Kuhn E, Chard K, Resick P, Greene C, Weingardt K, Ruzek, JI. CPT Coach [Mobile application software]. Version 1.0. Menlo Park, CA: VA National Center for PTSD; 2013. Retrieved from http://myvaapps.com
19. Hoffman JE, Taylor K, Manber R, Trockel M, Gehrman P, Woodward S, et al. CBT-i Coach [Mobile application software]. Version 1.0. Menlo Park, CA: VA National Center for PTSD; 2013.

20. Hoffman JE, Wald LJ, Kuhn E, Greene C, Ruzek JI, Weingardt K. PTSD Coach [Mobile application software]. Version 1.0. Menlo Park, CA: VA National Center for PTSD; 2013.

21. Warren C. Twitter's API update cuts off oxygen to third-party clients. New York, NY; 2012 (Aug. 16). Retrieved from http://mashable.com/2012/08/16/twitter-api-big-changes/

22. Tsotsis A. No API for you: Twitter shuts off "find friends" feature for Instagram. New York, NY; 2012 (July 26). Retrieved from http://techcrunch.com/2012/07/26/no-api-for-you-twitter-shuts-off-find-friends-feature-for-instagram/

23. Mlot S. Twitter API restrictions cut off Tumblr access. New York, NY; 2012 (Aug 23). Retrieved from http://www.pcmag.com/article2/0,2817,2408853,00.asp

24. Dash A. Facebook is gaslighting the Web. We can fix it. New York, NY; 2011 (Nov 21). Retrieved from: http://dashes.com/anil/2011/11/facebook-is-gaslighting-the-web.html

25. De Maeseneer J, Boeckxstaens P. Care for non-communicable diseases (NCDs): Time for a paradigm-shift. *World Hospitals and Health Services* 2011; 47(4):30–33.

26. Chorpita BF, Daleiden EL, Weisz JR. Identifying and selecting the common elements of evidence based interventions: A distillation and matching model. *Mental Health Services Research* 2005; 7(1):5–20.

27. Web Information Solutions Inc. Pocket Informant. Web Information Solutions Inc.; 2012.

28. Rosen GM, Davison GC. Psychology should list empirically supported principles of change (ESPs) and not credential trademarked therapies or other treatment packages. *Behavior Modification* 2003; 27(3):300–312.

29. Estrin D, Sim I. Open mHealth architecture: An engine for health care innovation. *Science* 2010; 330(6005):759–760.

30. Kazdin AE. Evidence-based treatment and practice: New opportunities to bridge clinical research and practice, enhance the knowledge base, and improve patient care. *American Psychologist* 2008; 63(3):146–159.

31. Ha A. MyFitnessPal launches API to sync its 30m users with other fitness apps and devices. New York, NY; 2012 (Oct 16). Retrieved from http://techcrunch.com/2012/10/16/myfitnesspal-api/

32. D'Orazio D. Jawbone launches an ecosystem for Up, lets other apps tap into your fitness data. New York, NY; 2013 (April 30). Retrieved from http://www.theverge.com/2013/4/30/4283626/jawbone-bodymedia-acquisition-up-platform-api-fitness-data-share

33. Chen C, Haddad D, Selsky J, Hoffman JE, Kravitz RL, Estrin DE, et al. Making sense of mobile health data: An open architecture to improve individual-and population-level health. *Journal of Medical Internet Research* 2012; 14(4):e112.

34. Laffel G. Track your healthy activities on Wellcoin. Newton, MA; 2013 (Feb 9). Retrieved from http://wellcoin.tumblr.com/post/42675544744/track-your-healthy-activities-on-wellcoin

35. West J. The economic realities of open standards: Black, white and many shades of gray. In *Standards and Public Policy*. Cambridge, UK: Cambridge University Press; 2007, pp. 87–122.

36. Heron KE, Smyth JM. Ecological momentary interventions: Incorporating mobile technology into psychosocial and health behavior treatments. *British Journal of Health Psychology* 2010; 15(1):1–39.

37. Agyapong VI, Ahern S, McLoughlin DM, Farren CK. Supportive text messaging for depression and comorbid alcohol use disorder: Single-blind randomised trial. *Journal of Affective Disorders* 2012; 141(2-3):168–176.

38. Naughton F, Prevost AT, Gilbert H, Sutton S. Randomized controlled trial evaluation of a tailored leaflet and SMS text message self-help intervention for pregnant smokers (MiQuit). *Nicotine & Tobacco Research* 2012; 14(5):569–577.

39. Free C, Knight R, Robertson S, Whittaker R, Edwards P, Zhou W, et al. Smoking cessation support delivered via mobile phone text messaging (txt2stop): A single-blind, randomised trial. *Lancet* 2011; 378(9785):49–55.

40. Sorbi MJ, Mak SB, Houtveen JH, Kleiboer AM, van Doornen LJ. Mobile web-based monitoring and coaching: Feasibility in chronic migraine. *Journal of Medical Internet Research* 2007; 9(5):e38.

41. Burns MN, Begale M, Duffecy J, Gergle D, Karr CJ, Giangrande E, et al. Harnessing context sensing to develop a mobile intervention for depression. *Journal of Medical Internet Research* 2011; 13(3):e55.

42. Massachusets Institute of Technology Media Lab. Affective computing. Retrieved from http://affect.media.mit.edu/index.php

43. Ginger.io. http://www.ginger.io

44. Hodson H. Ditch the pedometer–an AI in your smartphone knows better. *New Scientist* 2013; 220(2941):23.

45. Open mHealth. http://www.openmhealth.org

SECTION V

Public Health and
Policy Implications

19

Using Technology to Integrate Behavioral Health into Primary Care

LOLA AWOYINKA, DAVID H. GUSTAFSON, AND ROBERTA JOHNSON

THE IMPORTANCE OF INTEGRATING BEHAVIORAL HEALTH AND PRIMARY CARE

INTRODUCTION

Decades of increasing specialization and fragmentation in healthcare have produced an increasingly persistent call for the integration of care. The goal is for providers to care for the whole patient rather than just aspects of the patient's health—for example, one provider treating a patient's diabetes while another treats her depression. Integrated care typically refers to teamwork between primary care and behavioral health providers with a unified patient care plan; it often connotes close organizational integration, perhaps involving social and other services (1,2), though the degree of integration may vary. Traditional models of integration often assume that the various services are delivered in the same physical space, although this doesn't have to be the case. Primary care has sometimes been integrated into behavioral health, but the reverse is normally the case—behavioral health is typically integrated into primary care—and this is the type of integration discussed in this chapter. Although research on integrating care is still developing, evidence has begun to show that it can improve the quality of patient care, patient satisfaction, clinician job satisfaction, and other outcomes (3–8).

The co-occurrence of chronic physical conditions and behavioral health problems accounts in part for the call for integration. By one estimate, 68% of adults with behavioral health problems also have one or more chronic physical illnesses (9). Further, patients with behavioral health problems have high rates of risk factors that exacerbate chronic conditions, such as poor nutrition, physical inactivity, and smoking (10). Similarly, those with chronic physical conditions often have behavioral health problems. For example, up to one-third of patients with a serious medical condition experience depression (11). Consider again the patient with diabetes and depression. Her depression may contribute to her not regularly checking her blood sugar, but depression might not be a priority for her primary care physician, and the role of depression in managing diabetes may not come to the attention of the behavioral health specialist. When patients are treated in two different systems, practitioners in each system are likely to focus on the problem each system is comfortable dealing with. An integrated view of the patient's situation can lead to more effective diagnosis and treatment. In fact, technologies exist that are designed to take two or more conditions into account to develop a plan for prevention among patients at risk and, for patients suffering from the conditions, a plan for treatment and recovery (12).

The federal Agency for Healthcare Research and Quality (13), the Institute of Medicine (14), and the Substance Abuse and Mental Health Services Administration (15,16) have all advocated for the integration of physical and behavioral healthcare. The Affordable Care Act and its promotion of the patient-centered medical home (PCMH) care model and accountable care organizations have expanded the conversation about integration as a way to coordinate care and reduce costs. The PCMH model is intended to coordinate care for people with multiple chronic conditions. The model attempts to provide direction about how to bundle care and how better to pay for coordinated services (17). Though PCMHs remain a work in progress, the Affordable Care

Act has clearly made behavioral health important. In order to qualify as a PCMH, a health team must include behavioral health providers (18). Accountable care organizations—HMOs that have agreements with the federal government by which they share with the government the cost savings of improved care and improved outcomes—are interested in integration in part because of the expected savings.

The integration of physical and behavioral health requires changes both for organizations and for individuals in the systems—patients, their family members, and providers—and technology can support change at both levels. In fact, technology is essential to surmounting some of the obstacles to integration because while integration makes clinical, financial, and common sense, it also makes care more complex, and technology can provide the communication, information, decision support, prediction models, and other tools essential to successful integration.

USING TECHNOLOGY TO SUPPORT ORGANIZATIONAL CHANGE
Organizational Challenges to Integration

Many challenges exist at the organizational level to integrating behavioral health into primary care (19), and many of them arise in other industries undergoing organizational changes. For example, the integration of behavioral health into primary care requires the merging of two fields with substantially different cultures. This is usually the case when companies combine, and the literature shows that culture clashes are a primary cause of merger failures (20). Primary care is often driven by productivity incentives that can limit patient visits to 20 minutes or less, while behavioral health operates on the belief that more face time with the patient is essential. In general, primary care systems measure productivity more strictly and report outcomes more consistently than behavioral health. Physical health record systems have well-structured data to be collected on many conditions; behavioral health systems often lack electronic health records entirely and agreement is still being developed on which indicators to capture (21).

Making Patient Information Available to All Providers

Although some of the challenges to integration result from technology (e.g., different screening, records, and monitoring systems), technology also solves many of the problems created by the existence of two systems. Perhaps most importantly, a uniform set of technologies across behavioral health and primary care can consistently provide patient information to all providers—an essential element in addressing a patient's multiple, interdependent conditions. Currently, primary care has data on some aspects of a patient's health while behavioral health has data on other aspects of the same patient's health. Without a common set of accessible information, care is virtually guaranteed to be suboptimal. Integrated electronic health records will allow each member of a patient's care team to see the full picture of the patient. Although many studies demonstrate the importance of record systems and give guidance about implementing electronic records (22), we found no studies about integrating behavioral and physical health record systems. An integrated health record, combined with other telehealth tools, can also relieve the need for care groups to be located in the same physical place. In fact, having staff located in different places could have advantages, such as providing a wider base of clinicians, though we have not been able to find research addressing this subject.

Improving Transitions and Handoffs

Technology can also improve transitions and handoffs between care groups. Patients with several behavioral and physical health conditions often require multiple laboratory investigations and coordinated visits to various specialists. To make these processes run well, scheduling, communication, and resource allocation all need to operate smoothly. One delay or missed appointment could force substantial changes in plans, creating unused capacity and delayed or inhibited recovery. Technology can be used to map out registration processes, appointment scheduling, and treatment plans and to display and monitor progress. For instance, Marrie et al. (23) conducted a cluster-randomized trial in 19 Canadian hospitals (1,743 patients) to test whether the critical path method (CPM) (24) could improve the efficiency (bed days per patient managed, or BDPM) of treating community-acquired pneumonia without compromising patient well-being (from the Short Form 36 Physical Component Survey [SF-36 PCS], which measures health-related quality of life). Using the CPM, practitioners name the necessary steps to reach a desired outcome in a timely manner and indicate the temporal relationships of the steps (A must precede B). CPM is supported by various computer programs that create a picture of various work flows and identify which flow of work will take the most time to complete, thus identifying the set of activities that can least afford to be late if the work is to be completed on time. In the Canadian study, CPM produced a 26% reduction in BDPM with no change in well-being and required fewer days of intravenous (IV) therapy. While this was not a study of primary care or behavioral health, it provides evidence of the potential of this technology in integrated primary care.

Handoffs between providers are enhanced by providing convenient ways to share information with staff and colleagues in other parts of an organization or between organizations struggling with similar issues (25). Research has shown that feedback to and from clinicians during a referral is fraught with problems, as are communications between the patient, family members, and clinicians (26). Distance communication to subspecialists could be eased with video counseling and related functionality. Feedback to patients and primary providers can be enhanced; patient data can be more easily shared between providers. Communication services are particularly important for integrated systems addressing the whole patient, though the best way(s) to provide these services is open to conjecture. The effect of "provider-to-provider communication within the electronic domain is not well understood (27)." Can we rely on the clinical team to do that well? This issue has been present for decades and little progress has been made. Are there ways in which the patient and family can play a more central role in communicating key information about referrals and handoffs? Can patients and families be trained to play that role effectively and can technology support that effort? These and many other questions remain, and further research is needed to develop answers.

Training

Integrated primary care systems will require that patients, families, and providers take on unfamiliar roles and relationships. Support systems (such as dashboards, location and status monitors, and decision support systems) can help reduce the difficulty of such adaptations, but there will be new roles to learn and cultural shifts occurring that can be difficult to address. Given that staff issues and culture clashes are primary causes of merger failures, it can be particularly important to prepare staff for what to expect. Simulations can be used for role-playing in the new environment. Shapiro et al. (28) used a crossover, prospective, blinded, and controlled observational study to evaluate the effect on team behavior of a simulation-based training program designed to improve teamwork skills in the ED and found a trend ($p = .07$) toward improved team behavior compared to a control group. While simulations can be effective in such circumstances, research is needed to assess impact on cultural adjustments during integration.

Patients with multiple chronic conditions are likely to face new situations as they are referred to specialists or new types of care. It is so difficult for a patient to move (for instance) from residential care to a halfway house or intensive outpatient care that this transition often fails (29). The challenge is multiplied in an integrated setting where patients with multiple chronic conditions are often referred to several specialists. Videography may be able to help patients virtually walk through the experience they will face (e.g., introduce them to staff they are likely to meet; see the facility; meet other patients; get hints on how to make the most of the experience). At this time, though, this idea remains speculative. Research is needed to empirically examine its potential.

Providing More Data

Dealing with multiple chronic conditions is a very complex process involving more information than any single human being can process at once. Technology can make things better or worse by giving clinicians and researchers more data than they have ever had access to before. For example, technology can collect data through sensors, such as those found on smartphones—for example, cameras to measure pupillary dilation, GPS to document location, voice recorders to measure voice intonation, proximity sensors, compass, gyroscopes, ambient light and back-illuminated sensors (30), and accelerometers to measure tremors and gait (31). Sensors external to smartphones can measure blood pressure, blood sugar level, and blood alcohol levels as well as exercise, nutrition, and sleep (32). Survey data can be requested via e-mail, ecological momentary ssessments (EMAs, which are real-time reports by the patient about aspects of his or her health), SMS messaging (text messaging), or interactive voice response (IVR) collection methods. These can be administered as often as necessary and the information can then be used to determine any changes in health or plans for care. Alerts can also be established, notifying providers of any notable changes in patient health. These methods have been shown to be as valid as face-to-face interviews and questionnaires and in some cases more valid (33).

Using EMAs (34), the patient might report on his or her mood, physical symptoms, drug use, relationships, and other factors. EMAs can be very brief (one question collected once a day) or more extensive, and can lead to ecological momentary interventions (which could be, for example, suggestions, problem-solving tips, or other types of information programmed to be delivered in the moment to the patient in response to a problem revealed by the EMA). Having observed extensive compliance with EMAs delivered six times a day with questions that took almost 2 minutes to complete, we are excited about their potential. However, the study in which we observed the effects of EMAs involved handsomely paying people who had been recently discharged from drug-related imprisonment. We don't yet fully understand what is practical to push via EMAs.

Providers can also explore the use of sensor technology to monitor patients in real time. Sensors (e.g., ones that measure gait or driving performance) may influence care in an integrated system. A person's driving or gait can be a sensitive indicator of health status. For instance, driving performance is strongly associated with sleep apnea. And of course, driving performance strongly relates to a patient's use of alcohol and other drugs. Sensors that measure these conditions can send early warnings that can be pursued by automated and manual interventions from the primary care clinic (35). Although it may take time for healthcare to use environmental information

and measures such as driving performance or changes in gait to alone identify what a problem is, early evidence suggests that such information may eventually be able to be used to identify a problem (31). Meanwhile, such information can *indicate* a problem. In an integrated clinic, these warnings can initiate a wide-ranging analysis of problems, an analysis that would be more limited if the warning came to just a behavioral health provider or just a primary care clinician.

Nothing is perfect, and every data collection system has disadvantages. Using GPS systems to monitor location works well if signal strength is strong and if a high-risk location can be differentiated from other activities in the same area. Other sensors work well if they are properly charged, or if the environment has the proper light or background sound. Each data collection system must be thoroughly tested so that its limits and benefits are understood before wide implementation. Without some way to process all this information, its complexity can overwhelm the human mind.

Tools for Making Use of Additional Data

Technology can provide the tools to make use of voluminous data, which must often be combined to reach conclusions on how the patient is progressing (36). These measurement tools become particularly important when the patient is dealing with several health problems, because the data may help identify an unsuspected cause of a symptom or help validate an interpretation. Information and communication technologies are natural mechanisms for building and analyzing large data sets. Keystrokes can be examined to understand how synchronous and asynchronous communication devices are being used (37,38). Sensors can provide continuous streams of information on how patients are doing and how they respond to interventions. Ecological momentary assessments can collect large amounts of data on how patients are doing.

All these data can be subjected to analyses through systems for machine learning (39), sequential decision support (40), and predictive modeling (41). For instance, asynchronous communications could be analyzed to identify worrisome words that may predict relapse or harmful behavior. Decision support modules can help primary care providers in an integrated system better determine when to seek the assistance of behavioral health or other specialists. Technology can help plan a sequence of steps depending on how a patient responds earlier in the sequence; predict the likelihood of risky events, such as relapse; and help tailor interventions to specific needs, taking the whole patient into account. These technologies and the enormous amount of data they can process in an integrated system offer great potential to tailor interventions based on a broad knowledge of patient conditions as well as the environment in which the patient functions.

Using Dashboards

The wealth of new information available from technology can also be used—and made sense of—by dashboards of different types. Dashboards have been a central tool for progress monitoring in many fields, one that strongly relates to data visualization (42). Healthcare dashboards have been used for patient and population management. Their purpose is to provide at-a-glance information about key performance indicators. Typically they show (in easy-to-digest pictures) summaries, trends, and alerts. Dashboards can track changes in patient status over time and alert providers, family, and patients to significant changes. Data analysis packages can be tied to dashboards that track both individual and collective patient trends over time and allow a quick analysis or a deeper study. While dashboards have been extensively used, only a few studies have evaluated the impact of dashboards. In theory at least, dashboards should enable healthcare providers, patients, and families to be aware of and act on important changes in health status and behaviors at both the patient and population levels. Koopman et al. (43) found that dashboards enabled physicians to find information in the medical record more quickly. Hunt et al. (44) found that diabetes control improved when a multifeatured health information technology (including dashboards) was implemented.

This raises two important issues: 1) Is there a special role for dashboards in an integrated system? 2) What research questions do dashboards raise? Integrated primary care systems deal with multiple chronic conditions. Parthasarathy, Mertens, Moore, and Weisner (45) and Weisner, Mertens, Parthasarathy, Moore, and Lu (46) found that integrated care was helpful for substance use disorder patients with multiple chronic conditions. It is reasonable to assume that the more complex a patient's health is, the more difficult it will be to monitor and manage the conditions, not only from the provider's perspective but from the patient and family's perspective as well. Bharosa, Janssen, Meijer, and Brave (47) empirically evaluated alternative design configurations for dashboards. Continued work is needed on how best to display information in dashboards so it is easily understood by all concerned, and research is needed into the impact of dashboards on outcomes in integrated clinics.

Improving Population Health

Finally, technologies can make available the tools needed to manipulate data in ways that serve population health. For example, how do diabetics without depression differ from diabetics with depression in adherence to treatment? How do asthmatic patients differ in asthma control if they abuse alcohol? What demographic characteristics are associated with failure and success of a particular intervention? These questions are nearly impossible to answer in a non-integrated system, but are available in a system with an integrated health record with an easy-to-use registry (a list of names of patients grouped by specific shared characteristics). Technologies such as advanced registries allow users to see interactions between various diseases, such as the relationship between addiction, depression, and obesity. Knowledge of all conditions can redefine which conditions to focus on and how to do so. For instance, knowing that 30% of people being treated for chronic pain are also addicted to pain-killers and 40% of those have an anxiety disorder may lead to important policy initiatives, such as having the patient review prevention material before receiving a prescription for opioids. Well-designed registries also allow clinicians to conduct their own research and quality improvement on the spot with their own population or with a larger patient set. For instance, clinicians can examine the progress of the population as a whole and pull out the patients who are progressing differently.

Registries can routinely collect, receive, and store data, such as health status and adherence to treatment plans (e.g., treatment session attendance; self-reported medication adherence) for substance use disorders and selected co-occurring illnesses (e.g., diabetes, hypertension, depression, and chronic pain). Registries can store, integrate, and share data collected by the primary care site and referral agencies, such as HIV specialists and addiction treatment specialists, even if data come from different record systems. Well-designed registries allow staff to easily and quickly aggregate, display, and examine information about patients in several ways, for example, by patient type, provider, health problem(s), appointment dates, level of treatment adherence (e.g., time since a medical appointment), source of care, and behavioral adherence, over time and within a certain period.

Primary care providers, behavioral health specialists, patients, and families can access these data any time they wish and access a summary of the data before appointments. Staff can be also notified if an indicator exceeds a predefined threshold so they can intervene (e.g., by offering relaxation recordings if a person has high anxiety) and send reminders to patients, family, and staff of appointments, medication schedules, and so on. Registries can also store key actions taken by clinicians or referral agencies and automatically share that information between providers according to instructions from patients, family, and staff. Data visualization (48) technologies will allow registries to display results of analyses in ways that will make them easy to understand. While data visualization is finally being recognized for its importance, we have a long way to go before we understand which techniques work best for which audiences. The power of computers to display data in many different ways can lead to confusion rather than simplification.

Tools for Managing Integration Assessment and Planning

Integrating behavioral health into primary care is similar to a merger of related but not competing organizations, and tools used in other industries can be adapted to benefit the integration process. As in any merger, is important to conduct due diligence before deciding to go ahead. Examining the potential to improve care is the central question of such analyses, but other issues include 1) assessing the potential to reduce total costs by combining operations and workforces, and 2) assessing the potential to more effectively use resources by treating whole patients. Computer-based protocols for such assessments exist and can be adapted to the integration of behavioral health into primary care

(49). Computer simulation can help the parties understand the risks and benefits of integration, including space demands (e.g., a change in number of examining rooms), staffing (e.g., the number of counselors needed to meet demand), and bottlenecks in work flow. Simulation can also be used to conduct sensitivity analyses. For instance, a range of demand estimates can be entered into a simulation system to see how variations can affect resource requirements. A simulation can also be used to estimate the effects of different care strategies on resources, for example, if video counseling were to complement face-to-face counseling, or if chat rooms were to be used between clinic visits. While all of these analyses would help in a freestanding treatment agency, they are even more important when conducted in the context of integration (50). Finally, simulation can be used to estimate the impact of integration and new technologies on treatment measures such as time to treatment, dropout rates, and attendance at both behavioral interventions and treatments for physical problems (e.g., chronic care visits). For instance, evidence shows that computer-based chat rooms can increase attendance at group psychotherapy sessions (51). Simulations can use these data to estimate the impact of a new technology on outcomes and resource requirements.

Project Management Systems

When two systems are merged, the process for doing so needs to be carefully thought through and plans carefully followed for the integration to take place on time and within budget. Patients need to be cared for and families need to be properly involved during the integration process. The longer the process takes and the more rework is involved, the more likely it is that staff, patient, and family satisfaction will deteriorate. In an environment in which both primary care and behavioral health staff may resist change, implementation needs to go smoothly. A number of project management tools, many of them computerized, can be used to improve planning and implementation. For example, PERT (Project Evaluation and Review Technique) charts identify the tasks necessary to reach a goal, the sequence of the tasks, and the shortest and longest times required to complete each task. PERT charts are often used with the critical path method mentioned earlier (24). PERT charts and CPM can be used to identify bottlenecks that need special attention to keep implementation on track. Dashboards can track the integration to help management quickly identify activities and other system outcome measures that are off schedule. Gantt charts use bars to show the tasks necessary to reach a goal as well as other information, such as the length of time required by each task, start and finish dates, and who will perform the tasks. Gantt charts can provide timelines and staff assignments. Computer-based project management tools are available for these and many other tasks involved in integrating programs, such as facility planning, financial forecasting, work specifications, space management, new construction and renovation, maintenance, operations management, telecommunications integration, and security. To our knowledge, no demonstrations or evaluations have examined the impact of such systems in the integration process, but their application in other fields is well documented (52). Studies of their application to integration would be helpful.

Data Collection

Research (53) has shown that human issues—such as poor management, the clash of cultures or egos, and the inability to manage change—are the primary reason for merger failures. These are issues that fester over time and must be addressed very quickly. An article by Walker and Price (54) identifies problems that may need to be addressed in an integration, such as a poor understanding of what the integration is intended to do or how it will do it; unclear impact on staff; how will talent be integrated; and how cultures will change. A key message from this literature seems to be that staff and customer attitudes need to be carefully monitored. It is important to collect, analyze, and act on satisfaction and experience data before, during, and after integration. Technology can be effective in collecting such data, assuming the data can be collected in a way that is (and is perceived to be) risk-free for respondents. EMAs, Twitter, more extensive surveys, and even sensors have potential value here. But a key is that the data must be analyzed and used quickly. Very often satisfaction data are not acted upon. This cannot be the case with a goal as fragile as integration. To increase the chance that data are used, analyses must be presented in an easy-to-use and understandable way (data visualization) and communicated on a management-by-exception basis (sharing only the information that leaders need).

Communication Systems

Integration of systems can create enormous uncertainty related to future roles, responsibilities, and culture. People don't know if they will keep their jobs, who they will report to, and what expectations will change. The whole issue of "what does it take to get ahead around here" may change. To reduce this uncertainty, it is important that regular and honest communication take place. In its absence, the rumor mill takes over. Communication systems can be used to engage broad populations in setting integration priorities; developing and communicating the vision; engaging patients, families, and staff in designing the integration plan; redefining a business model by better understanding opportunities for growth; and sharing progress on integration. While face-to-face communication is critically important under these circumstances, providing opportunities for anonymous communications can give those involved a way to share their concerns without fear of retribution.

Employees will be particularly affected by integration. Patients and families will be, too. It is probably inevitable that some patients from both primary care and behavioral health clinics will leave as integration proceeds. For instance, a different clientele may appear in the waiting room. Those with behavioral health problems may be embarrassed by their health problems. Others may be intimidated or afraid. Careful planning is required to ensure that the merger is seen as improving service. But unless changes are marketed properly, patients and families may not aware of the improvements. Hence it is also essential to communicate to patients how services have improved. It is important to embrace, not hide, the integration.

Technology can play a critical role in communication. We know that a large proportion of minorities as well as Caucasians use mobile phones and thus can receive communications from the primary care clinic to inform them of changes, remind them of appointments, follow up on status, and link patients together between appointments.

From a corporate perspective, the merits of integration must be sold to influential people in the community. Computers can be combined with social network analyses (55) to plan appropriate information campaigns. Twitter can be an effective way for concerns to be raised and an effective way for management to track the reaction of the community and the organization to integration (56). Twitter chat can be a way to focus conversations in a specific time frame and engage a very large number of people at one time. Computerized Delphi processes offer an effective way to anonymously engage a moderately large group of people in identifying options, setting priorities, and giving feedback (57,58). Data visualization tools also provide important ways to present data so they are easy to understand, which is essential to effective communication. One particularly important application is to keep interested parties regularly updated on the progress of integration. Another is to quickly identify when progress is deviating from the plan and understand the source of that deviance.

USING TECHNOLOGY TO SUPPORT PATIENTS, THEIR FAMILIES, AND CLINICIANS
Serving Patients and Their Families

Just as technology can support organizations in making the changes required by integration, technology can support individuals in the integrated system. Our discussion of technology supporting individuals rests on the assumption that patient disease is a rare thing. Except for isolated individuals with no close family or friends, patients are part of a social circle, and serious illness affects the entire social network, not just the patient. A patient's recovery depends on the network as well the patient. A person dealing with depression can have a negative effect on his or her network; so can someone dealing with heart failure. One of the authors had a heart attack, followed eventually by a heart transplant. He was not the one to listen to the discharge nurse's instructions; he slept. He did not buy or cook food, monitor his medications, or report on his progress. In the hospital, he did not choose whether to continue treatment or monitor his medications to prevent errors or arrange to get to cardiac rehab on time. When the acute phase of recovery ended, he did not have post-traumatic stress disorder (PTSD); his wife did. Hence we address the role of technology in integrated care by focusing on the family as well as the patient.

Screening, Diagnosis, and Treatment Planning
Different Treatment Cultures and the Need for Combinations

Primary care and behavioral health have operated on different assumptions about the role of medications and cognitive therapies in treatment. Primary care uses medications extensively to prevent and treat disease. Mental illnesses are often treated with multiple medications that may or may not be combined with cognitive therapy. Behavioral health clinicians mainly have focused on cognitive aspects of treatment, although medication-assisted therapy is gaining ground in treating behavioral health conditions.

Combinations of therapies often work best for chronic conditions or multiple concurrent illnesses. In HIV and hypertension, cocktails of medications have proven more effective than a single drug. Optimal treatment for metabolic syndrome consists of medications, exercise, improved nutrition, and cognitive restructuring. An integrated system provides the opportunity to optimize the combinations of interventions, and technology may help us understand appropriate combinations for different combinations of conditions. Many other fields face this issue daily and use technologies to accomplish these goals. For instance, makers of hot dogs use mathematical models to optimize the combinations of ingredients (without changing taste) based on daily shifts in cost and availability to maintain the cost and quality of their product. We are not suggesting that making a hot dog is as complex as dealing with depression, but more research is needed into finding optimal combinations of interventions, given the enormous amount of evidence about individual interventions, especially as healthcare increasingly addresses combinations of physical and behavioral conditions (59).

Problem knowledge couplers (PKCs) offer insights into ways in which technology may be able to improve screening, diagnosis, and treatment planning in the face of an overwhelming evidence base. To develop PKCs, medical librarians identify evidence-based practices (EBPs) related to patient problems (not diagnoses). For example, EBPs would be identified for patients who have a runny nose; another set of EBPs would be identified for patients who have an earache. The set of

EBPs delivered by the PKC for a patient who complains of *both* a runny nose and an earache would be smaller than the sets of EBPs for runny nose and earache combined. PKCs were implemented in defense department settings. While PKCs are conceptually appealing, a randomized trial (60) did not find significant results, leading the evaluators to question the approach. In an integrated system, such an approach could help clinicians develop alternative explanations for their observations and offer several evidence-based interventions rather than rapidly focusing on one cause (e.g., depression). Although research in this area is in its early stages, further trials are now underway.

Using Technology for Screening

In an integrated system, screening needs to be more inclusive than it has been in independent primary care and behavioral health. Particular symptoms can have many causes, and many steps may be required to address the causes. In an ideal world, clinicians would be able to remember all possible signs and all possible actions. But this is an impossible challenge made even harder in an integrated system. Screening technologies offer one way to help meet the challenge. Although we are not aware of evaluations of technologies specifically designed for integrated clinics, technology has been developed to help screen for problems such as depression (61) and addiction (19). In theory, clinic staff could ask patients to complete online evaluations before office visits. Practitioners could also incorporate screening at clinic check-in using tablets or kiosks prepared for this purpose. Algorithms could be used to alert the clinician about patient results that meet defined criteria and require follow-up. Results could then be embedded into patient health records. This type of system allows for universal screening in primary care clinics, increasing the likelihood of connecting those in need of behavioral healthcare with the necessary resources, whether in-house or through referral. Several evaluations have been conducted of computerized screening for behavioral health in a primary care setting. Apkon et al. (60) evaluated a computerized psychosocial assessment that generated a report for the primary care provider, including patient-specific treatment recommendations. This randomized trial of 762 individuals who scored ≥12 on the Clinical Interview

Schedule Revised found significant improvements in quality of care (compared to the control group) at 6 weeks but not at 6 months. While the Apkon evaluation addressed behavioral health problems, it did not examine patients who had multiple diagnoses, one of which was a behavioral health condition.

How will such systems address the interactions of multiple chronic conditions to be addressed in an integrated system? Models could be developed that combine indicators from several different conditions into a more precise monitoring and alert tool. For instance, it may be that small changes in a patient's level of depression and pain may predict alcohol relapse more strongly than a single indicator, such as cravings. If so, these indicators could be used in a model upon which more targeted treatment plans can be constructed. Research is needed to develop and evaluate such models.

Treatment and Monitoring

The potential of technology to improve treatment has received extensive study. Pearson et al.'s review (62) found mixed results, but one clear point emerged: the need for interventions to improve safety and monitor care. One of our randomized trials evaluating an eHealth system designed for family caregivers of lung cancer patients (63) demonstrated such an effect. When the eHealth system sent an alert to the clinical team that a patient's symptom exceeded a threshold set by the team, the problem was resolved more quickly and symptom distress was reduced (64). In a secondary analysis, even length of survival appeared to improve. In integrated care, monitoring will become more complex. Added complexity increases the need to focus on the issues that matter. Technology may be able to help reduce that complexity.

Growing evidence suggests that psychological interventions may speed recovery from physical problems (65), and cognitive behavior therapy (CBT) is a particularly promising tool. But delivering CBT is time-consuming—and therefore not an easy fit in primary care. A number of online versions of CBT have been developed. Two that have been extensively studied with positive results were developed by Marsch et al. (66) and Carroll et al. (67). Both of these systems could effectively play the role of a clinician extender.

Chronic Disease Self-Management

Patients in active treatment receive consistent attention that goes away when they progress to the maintenance phase of treatment, sometimes called continuing care or relapse prevention. During the maintenance phase, patients often have a self-management plan to follow. Led by the pioneering work of Kate Lorig (68), a number of interventions have emerged, including her Internet-based version of the chronic disease self-management program she developed (69). While these programs have had mixed reviews (70), they point to the importance of self-management programs in treating chronic diseases. These programs have generally focused on one disease at a time (71). Gellis et al. (72) conducted a randomized trial to evaluate a telehealth system designed for patients with heart failure or COPD that monitored key indicators and transmitted the results to a nurse who could then initiate contacts with patients if the data justified it. They found significant effects on quality-of-life indicators and emergency department (ED) visits, with a promising trend in hospital days, though still with just one disease. In contrast, Darkins et al. (73) used a telehealth system of data collection and monitoring to help veterans, some with multiple chronic conditions. They found 26% reduction in bed days of care. Systems to address combinations of diseases are needed, as are research studies to evaluate them.

Telehealth and Mobile Health

Telehealth (remote communication designed to improve health) and mHealth (mobile health) platforms are becoming catalysts to improving care. Patients appreciate the easy access to diagnosis and treatment provided by remote and electronic platforms and often feel less stigmatized than in on-site systems of care. Providers get instantaneous, real-time information and communication, allowing them to intervene rapidly. Efficiency and effectiveness improve. Moreover, the patient can access at any time health information, training, and support offered through the clinic via tablets and smartphones. Mobile phones can now be docked to something that looks like a laptop to offer a big screen and keyboard, making it easier for older adults and people with disabilities to have large-screen visibility and phone capability in one unit (74). Telehealth can also play a huge

role in self-management. Among patients with multiple chronic conditions, behavior changes associated with effective self-management often benefit both physical and behavioral problems. For instance Wijsman et al. (75) conducted a 3-month randomized trial with 235 inactive older adults of a Web-based intervention designed to increase physical activity. They found that the intervention was effective in increasing daily physical activity and improving metabolic health. When behavioral health is integrated into primary care, this type of Web-based behavioral intervention could be added to the treatment of many physical health problems. For instance, although heart disease can be addressed with medications, a more beneficial treatment plan also addressed a patient's nutrition, exercise, and stress.

Reminder Systems

Reminders are a key part of chronic disease self-management. Patients and their family members need to be reminded of their behavioral responsibilities (medication adherence, appointments, exercises, sleep, and so on) to help ensure that complex treatment plans (which are likely when treating several conditions rather than one) are carried out as planned. Clinicians need to be alerted if a patient begins to deteriorate, especially because deterioration is more likely to be prevented if action is taken quickly (63). Such systems can also remind clinicians to take specific steps to prevent errors. Reminders and alerts are particularly important when a patient's health warrants collecting, analyzing, and reporting data on multiple systems to multiple providers. Moreover, adding behavioral health professionals to a clinic's staff will increase the focus on behavior change and, as a result, on reminder systems.

THE FUTURE OF USING TECHNOLOGY TO INTEGRATE BEHAVIORAL HEALTH AND PRIMARY CARE

Integrating behavioral health into primary care will pose difficulties. While both systems will be changed as a result of integration, the culture, expectations, and operations of traditional behavioral health will be changed more substantially because behavioral health organizations usually will be smaller than the primary care organizations into which they will be integrated.

The pressure will be on behavior health professionals to adapt. Data that may have been collected manually in a behavioral health organization will be electronically collected in real time at the integrated organization, and stored and analyzed. Security restrictions will change to allow different healthcare providers access to information that until now has been restricted. Clinician face time with patients will be dramatically reduced. The goals and philosophy of care in traditional behavioral health will shift to a medical model that addresses multiple conditions at once. The timing of interventions will change, with a growing focus on prevention and early identification. Personnel will change to include staff who understand addiction as just one more chronic condition and treat it that way. Payment models will be more outcome oriented and focus on bundled payments. Telehealth and mobile health will reduce the problem of distance and access that exist with mainly on-site care. Treatment plans should consider the needs of the whole patient with possibly several health conditions. Productivity measurement will become important, with increasing pressure to do more with less. Many of these essential transformations will require extensive use of technology both for bringing about the systems and procedural changes needed and for the direct support of patients and families.

With policy shifts encouraging change and integrated models of care are increasing in popularity, efforts continue to make care more affordable and efficient. Specific mechanisms required to make an integrated care model work are still being evaluated. The options for using technology in integration are open-ended and can easily be adjusted based on the needs, goals, and resources of the clinic seeking to integrate behavioral health and primary care. This is perhaps one of the greatest benefits of technology—its capacity to be scaled up or down to address the needs of a given situation.

The core of integrated care is to move from a program-centric paradigm, in which the program prescribes the same thing over and over again, to a paradigm in which care is blended and adapted to the whole patient and the patient's family. Behavioral health has been criticized for using a one-size-fits-all approach to treatment. Technology will allow a primary care practice to efficiently and productively integrate a more tailored behavioral health approach into its normal operations. For instance, reminder systems can alert a primary care clinician to an anniversary (e.g., the death of a spouse) that has in the past triggered binge drinking. Rather than adding work to an already overburdened staff, additional use of technology can reduce staff burden. The same technology that alerts the clinician can also initiate an intervention with the patient and family, such as sending tips on how to cope with sad memories. But such capabilities will require extensive systems development and, in the short run, time from staff to be part of that development.

Because integrating behavioral health into primary care will be challenging, requiring the melding of different cultures and subsystems (health records, privacy practices, payment systems, and so on), it may be tempting to maintain separate operations. But doing this will dramatically reduce the benefits of integration. Substantial evidence from other fields suggests that technology can aid in integrating and cost-effectively operating an integrated system.

Although the essence of what has worked in other fields may pertain to integrating behavioral health into primary care, specifics must be worked out. Little research has been done on technologies for integrated systems, in part because of the added complexity of the issues and the greater sophistication of technologies capable of making a difference. Although the use of technology in integrated systems has been receiving more attention recently, research is still needed to find the best ways to use technological advances in social marketing (which can individualize behavior change campaigns to address both health problems and culture shifts at the organizational level [76]) in supply chain management, program planning, and monitoring resources. A study by McKinsey and Company (77) reported on the increasing adoption of social technology for organizational purposes, such as scanning the environment, finding new ideas, managing projects, developing strategic plans, allocating resources, and so on. They found that social networking, blogs, video sharing, RSS (Rich Site Summaries), Wikis, podcasts, and micro-blogging are becoming important means by which organizations can better understand their environment and gain ideas for future development. This is particularly important in the integration of behavioral health into primary care, because this is a relatively new endeavor. We don't yet know how to do this well. Social marketing mechanisms may help us keep a pulse on what is happening and suggest how we can improve integration efforts. Creative ways also need to be developed to engage simulation, big data, and machine learning to guide integration. We have our work to do.

REFERENCES

1. Blount A. Integrated primary care: Organizing the evidence. *Families, Systems and Health* 2003; 21(2):121–133.

2. Blount A, Schoenbaum M, Kathol R, Rollman BL, Thomas M, O'Donohue W, Peek CJ. The economics of behavioral health services in medical settings: A summary of the evidence. *Professional Psychology: Research and Practice* 2007; 38(3):290–297.

3. Strosahl K. The integration of primary care and behavioral health: Type II changes in the era of managed care. In Cummings N, O'Donohue W, Hayes SC, Follette V (eds.), *Integrated Behavioral Healthcare: Positioning Mental Health Practice with Medical/Surgical Practice* (pp. 45–69). San Diego, CA: Academic Press; 2001.

4. Unützer J, Katon W, Callahan CM, Williams Jr JW, Hunkeler E, Harpole L, et al. Collaborative care management of late-life depression in the primary care setting. *Journal of the American Medical Association* 2002; 288(22):2836–2845.

5. Asarnow JR, Jaycox LH, Duan N, LaBorde AP, Rea MM, Murray P, et al. Effectiveness of a quality improvement intervention for adolescent depression in primary care clinics. *Journal of the American Medical Association* 2005; 293(3):311–319.

6. Partners in Health: Primary Care/County Mental Health Collaboration, Toolkit First Edition (Oct 2009). Integrated Behavioral Health Project (IBHP). Retrieved from http://www.ibhp.org/uploads/file/IBHP%20Collaborative%20Tool%20Kit%20final.pdf

7. Gilbody S, Bower P, Whitty P. Costs and consequences of enhanced primary care for depression: Systematic review of randomised economic evaluations. *British Journal of Psychiatry* 2006; 189(4):297–308.

8. Mauksch LB, Tucker SM, Katon WJ, Russo J, Cameron J, Walker E, Spitzer R. Mental illness, functional impairment, and patient preferences for collaborative care in an uninsured, primary care population. *Journal of Family Practice* 2001; 50(1):41–50.

9. Substance Abuse and Mental Health Services Administration (SAMHSA). Primary and Behavioral Health Care Integration (PBHCI) grant program. Retrieved from http://www.integration.samhsa.gov/about-us/pbhci

10. Davidson S, Judd F, Jolley D, Hocking B, Thompson S, Hyland B. Cardiovascular risk factors for people with mental illness. *Australian and New Zealand Journal of Psychiatry* 2001; 35(2):196–202.

11. National Alliance on Mental Illness (NAMI) (2009). Depression and chronic illness fact sheet. Retrieved from http://www.nami.org/Template.cfm?Section=Depression&Template=/ContentManagement/ContentDisplay.cfm&ContentID=88875

12. Kaplan B. Evaluating informatics applications—some alternative approaches: Theory, social interactionism, and call for methodological pluralism. *International Journal of Medical Informatics* 2001; 64(1):39–56.

13. Agency for Healthcare Research and Quality (AHRQ). Experts call for integrating mental health into primary care. Research Activities, January 2012, No. 377, U.S. Department of Health & Human Services. Retrieved from http://www.ahrq.gov/news/newsletters/research-activities/jan12/0112RA1.html

14. Institute of Medicine. *Improving the Quality of Health Care for Mental and Substance-Use Conditions: Quality Chasm Series.* Washington, DC: National Academies Press; 2006. Retrieved from http://www.iom.edu/Reports/2005/Improving-the-Quality-of-Health-Care-for-Mental-and-Substance-Use-Conditions-Quality-Chasm-Series.aspx

15. Croghan TW, Brown JD. *Integrating Mental Health Treatment into the Patient-Centered Medical Home.* Rockville, MD: Agency for Healthcare Research and Quality; 2010. Retrieved from http://www.pcpcc.org/

16. Butler M, Kane RL, McAlpine D, et al. Integration of mental health/substance abuse and primary care. Evidence Report/Technology Assessments No. 173. Rockville, MD: Agency for Healthcare Research and Quality; 2008. Retrieved from http://www.ncbi.nlm.nih.gov/books/NBK38632/

17. Health Homes. Affordable Care Act, Public Laws 111-148 & 111-152, §2703. Retrieved from http://www.medicaid.gov/Medicaid-CHIP-Program-Information/By-Topics/Long-Term-Services-and-Support/Integrating-Care/Health-Homes/Health-Homes.html

18. Substance Abuse and Mental Health Services Administration (SAMHSA). 100

Strong:Integrationcontinuestogrow.Retrievedfrom http://www.integration.samhsa.gov/about-us/ esolutions-newsletter/september-2013-esolutions #quick

19. Cunningham JA, Kypri K, McCambridge J. The use of emerging technologies in alcohol treatment. *Alcohol Research & Health* 2011; 33(4), 320.

20. Jacobsen D. 6 big mergers that were killed by culture (and how to stop it from killing yours) [Web log post]; 2012 (September 26). Retrieved from http://www.globoforce.com/gfblog/201 2/6-big-mergers-that-were-killed-by-culture/

21. Nutting PA, Miller WL, Crabtree BF, Jaen CR, Stewart EE, Stange KC. Initial lessons from the first national demonstration project on practice transformation to a patient-centered medical home. *Annals of Family Medicine* 2009; 7(3):254–260.

22. Lærum H, Ellingsen G, Faxvaag A. Doctors' use of electronic medical records systems in hospitals: Cross sectional survey. *British Medical Journal* 2001; 323(7325):1344–1348.

23. Marrie TJ, Lau CY, Wheeler SL, Wong CJ, Vandervoort MK, Feagan BG. A controlled trial of a critical pathway for treatment of community-acquired pneumonia. *Journal of the American Medical Association* 2000; 283(6):749–755.

24. Critical Path Method (CPM). A quick introduction to CPM (training video); 2012 (July 1). Retrieved from http://www.youtube.com/ watch?v=SF53ZZsP4ik

25. Gustafson DH, Resar R, Johnson K, Daigle JG. Don't fumble the treatment handoff. *Addiction Professional* 2008; 6(5), 30–33.

26. Arora NK, Gustafson DH. Perceived helpfulness of physicians' communication behavior and breast cancer patients' level of trust over time. *Journal of General Internal Medicine* 2009; 24(2):252–255.

27. Walsh C, Siegler EL, Cheston E, O'Donnell H, Collins S, Stein D, et al. Provider-to-provider electronic communication in the era of meaningful use: A review of the evidence. *Journal of Hospital Medicine* 2013; 8(10):589–597.

28. Shapiro MJ, Morey JC, Small SD, Langford V, Kaylor CJ, Jagminas L, et al. Simulation based teamwork training for emergency department staff: Does it improve clinical team performance when added to an existing didactic teamwork curriculum? *Quality and Safety in Health Care* 2004; 13(6):417–421.

29. Carter RE, Haynes LF, Back SE, Herrin AE, Brady KT, Leimberger JD, et al. Improving the transition from residential to outpatient addiction treatment: Gender differences in response to supportive telephone calls. *American Journal of Drug and Alcohol Abuse* 2008; 34(1):47–59.

30. Asad-Uj-Jaman. Sensors in smartphones. 2011 (Dec.). Retrieved from http://mobiledeviceinsight. com/2011/12/sensors-in-smartphones/

31. Michalak J, Troje NF, Fischer J, Vollmar P, Heidenreich T, Schulte D. Embodiment of sadness and depression—Gait patterns associated with dysphoric mood. *Psychosomatic Medicine* 2009; 71(5), 580–587.

32. Tsubouchi K, Kawajiri R, Shimosaka M. Working-relationship detection from fitbit sensor data. In *Proceedings of the 2013 ACM International Joint Conference on Pervasive and Ubiquitous Computing* (UbiComp '13) (pp. 115–118). New York: ACM; 2013.

33. Lieberman G, Naylor MR. Interactive voice response technology for symptom monitoring and as an adjunct to the treatment of chronic pain. *Translational Behavioral Medicine* 2012; 2(1):93–101.

34. Shiffman S, Stone AA, Hufford MR. Ecological momentary assessment. *Annual Review of Clinical Psychology* 2008; 4:1–32.

35. Schultheis MT, Garay E, DeLuca J. The influence of cognitive impairment on driving performance in multiple sclerosis. *Neurology* 2001; 56(8):1089–1094.

36. Beach A, Gartrell M, Xing X, Han R, Lv Q, Mishra S, Seada K. Fusing mobile, sensor, and social data to fully enable context-aware computing. In *Proceedings of the Eleventh Workshop on Mobile Computing Systems & Applications* (pp. 60–65). New York: ACM; 2010.

37. Namkoong K, McLaughlin B, Yoo W, Hull S, Shah D, Kim S, et al. The effects of expression: How providing emotional support online improves cancer patients coping strategies. *Journal of the National Cancer Institute Monograph* 2013; (47):169–174.

38. Yoo W, Namkoong K, Choi M, Shah DV, Tsang S, Hong Y, et al. Giving and receiving emotional support online: Communication competence as a moderator of psychosocial benefits for women with breast cancer. *Computers in Human Behavior* 2014; 30:13–22.

39. Mannini A, Sabatini AM. Machine learning methods for classifying human physical activity from on-body accelerometers. *Sensors* 2010; 10(2):1154–1175.

40. Murphy SA, Bingham D. Screening experiments for developing dynamic treatment regimes. *Journal of the American Statistical Association* 2009; 104(485), 391–408.

41. Gustafson DH, Sainfort F, Eichler M, Adams L, Bisognano M, Steudel H. Developing and testing a model to predict outcomes of organizational change. *Health Services Research* 2003; 38(2):751–776.

42. Clarke S. Your business dashboard: Knowing when to change the oil. *Journal of Corporate Accounting & Finance* 2005; 16(2):51–54.

43. Koopman RJ, Kochendorfer KM, Moore JL, Mehr DR, Wakefield DS, Yadamsuren B, et al. A diabetes dashboard and physician efficiency and accuracy in accessing data needed for high-quality diabetes care. *Annals of Family Medicine* 2011; 9(5):398–405.

44. Hunt JS, Siemienczuk J, Gillanders W, LeBlanc BH, Rozenfeld Y, Bonin K, Pape G. The impact of a physician-directed health information technology system on diabetes outcomes in primary care: A pre-and post-implementation study. *Informatics in Primary Care* 2009; 17(3):165–174.

45. Parthasarathy S, Mertens J, Moore C, Weisner C. (2003). Utilization and cost impact of integrating substance abuse treatment and primary care. *Medical Care* 2003; 41(3):357–367.

46. Weisner C, Mertens J, Parthasarathy S, Moore C, Lu Y. (2001). Integrating primary medical care with addiction treatment. *Journal of the American Medical Association* 2001; 286(14):1715–1723.

47. Bharosa N, Janssen M, Meijer S, Brave F. Designing and evaluating dashboards for multi-agency crisis preparation: A living lab. In *Electronic Government* (pp. 180–191). Berlin, Heidelberg: Springer; 2010.

48. Tufte ER. *The Visual Display of Quantitative Information* (2nd ed.). Cheshire, CT: Graphics Press; 2001.

49. Boyle R, Solberg L, Fiore M. Use of electronic health records to support smoking cessation. *Cochrane Database of Systematic Reviews* 2011; Issue 12.

50. Nevo A, Whinston MD. Taking the dogma out of econometrics: Structural modeling and credible inference. *Journal of Economic Perspectives* 2010; 24(2):69–81.

51. Gustafson D, McTavish F, Schubert C, Johnson RA. The effect of a computer-based intervention on adult children of alcoholics. *Journal of Addiction Medicine* 2012; 6(1):24–28.

52. Kerzner HR. *Project Management: A Systems Approach to Planning, Scheduling, and Controlling* (11th ed.). Hoboken, NJ: John Wiley and Sons; 2013.

53. Weber RA, Camerer CF. Cultural conflict and merger failure: An experimental approach. *Management Science* 2003; 49(4):400–415.

54. Walker JW, Price KF. Why do mergers go right? *Human Resource Planning* 2000; 23(2):6–8.

55. Scott JG, Carrington PJ. (eds.) *The SAGE Handbook of Social Network Analysis*. Thousand Oaks, CA: Sage Publications; 2011.

56. Attaran M. Exploring the relationship between information technology and business process reengineering. *Information & Management* 2004; 41(5):585–596.

57. Turoff M, Hiltz S. Computer based Delphi processes. In Adler M, Ziglio E, (eds.), *Gazing into the Oracle*. (pp. 56–88). London: Jessica Kingsley Publishers; 1995.

58. Monguet J, Ferruzca M, Gutiérrez A, Alatriste Y, Martínez C, Cordoba C, et al. Vector consensus: Decision making for collaborative innovation communities. In *ENTERprise Information Systems* (pp. 218–227). Berlin, Heidelberg: Springer; 2010.

59. Brandeau ML, Sainfort F, Pierskalla WP (eds.). *Operations Research and Health Care: A Handbook of Methods and Applications* (Vol. 70). Norwell, MA: Kluwer Academic Publishers, Springer; 2004.

60. Apkon M, Mattera JA, Lin Z, Herrin J, Bradley EH, Carbone M, et al. A randomized outpatient trial of a decision-support information technology tool. *Archives of Internal Medicine* 2005; 165(20):2388–2394.

61. Davis M, Balasubramanian BA, Waller E, Miller BF, Green LA, Cohen DJ. Integrating behavioral and physical health care in the real world: Early lessons from advancing care together. *Journal of the American Board of Family Medicine* 2013; 26(5):588–602.

62. Pearson SA, Moxey A, Robertson J, Hains I, Williamson M, Reeve J, Newby D. Do computerised clinical decision support systems for prescribing change practice? A systematic review of the literature (1990-2007). *BMC Health Services Research* 2009; 9(1), 154.

63. Chih MY, Dubenski LL, Hawkins RP, Brown RL, Dinauer SK, Cleary JF, Gustafson DH. Communicating advanced cancer patients' symptoms via the Internet: A pooled analysis of two randomized trials examining caregiver preparedness, physical burden, and negative mood. *Palliative Medicine* 2012; 27(6):533–543.

64. Gustafson DH, DuBenske LL, Namkoong K, Hawkins R, Chih MY, Atwood AK, et al. An eHealth system supporting palliative care for patients with non-small cell lung cancer: A randomized trial. *Cancer* 2013; 119(9):1744–1751.

65. Mumford E, Schlesinger HJ, Glass GV. The effect of psychological intervention on recovery from surgery and heart attacks: An analysis of the literature. *American Journal of Public Health* 1982; 72(2):141–151.

66. Marsch LA, Bickel WK, Badger GJ, Stothart ME, Quesnel KJ, Stanger C, Brooklyn J. Comparison of pharmacological treatments for opioid-dependent adolescents: A randomized controlled trial. *Archives of General Psychiatry* 2005; 62(10):1157–1164.

67. Kiluk BD, Sugarman DE, Nich C, Gibbons CJ, Martino S, Rounsaville BJ, Carroll KM. A methodological analysis of randomized clinical trials of computer-assisted therapies for psychiatric

disorders: Toward improved standards for an emerging field. *American Journal of Psychiatry* 2011; 168(8):790–799.

68. Bodenheimer T, Lorig K, Holman H, Grumbach K. Patient self-management of chronic disease in primary care. *Journal of the American Medical Association* 2002; 288(19):2469–2475.

69. Lorig KR, Ritter PL, Laurent DD, Plant K. The Internet-based arthritis self-management program: A one-year randomized trial for patients with arthritis or fibromyalgia. *Arthritis Care & Research* 2008; 59(7):1009–1017.

70. Elzen H, Slaets JP, Snijders TA, Steverink N. Evaluation of the chronic disease self-management program (CDSMP) among chronically ill older people in the Netherlands. *Social Science & Medicine* 2007; 64(9):1832–1841.

71. De San Miguel K, Smith J, Lewin G. Telehealth remote monitoring for community-dwelling older adults with chronic obstructive pulmonary disease. *Telemedicine and e-Health* 2013; 19(9):652–657.

72. Gellis ZD, Kenaley B, McGinty J, Bardelli E, Davitt J, Ten Have T. Outcomes of a telehealth intervention for homebound older adults with heart or chronic respiratory failure: a randomized controlled trial. *Gerontologist* 2012; 52(4):541–552.

73. Darkins A, Ryan P, Kobb R, Foster L, Edmonson E, Wakefield B, Lancaster AE. (2008). Care coordination/home telehealth: The systematic implementation of health informatics, home telehealth, and disease management to support the care of veteran patients with chronic conditions. *Telemedicine and e-Health* 2008; 14(10):1118–1126.

74. Gustafson DH, Boyle MG, Shaw BR, Isham A, McTavish F, Richards S, et al. An e-Health solution for people with alcohol problems. *Alcohol Research & Health* 2011; 33(4):327–337.

75. Wijsman CA, Westendorp RG, Verhagen EA, Catt M, Slagboom PE, de Craen AJ, et al. (2013). Effects of a Web-based intervention on physical activity and metabolism in older adults: Randomized controlled trial. *Journal of Medical Internet Research* 15(11):e233.

76. Cugelman B, Thelwall M, Dawes P. Online interventions for social marketing health behavior change campaigns: A meta-analysis of psychological architectures and adherence factors. *Journal of Medical Internet Research* 2011; 13(1):e17.

77. Bughin J, Byers AH, Chui M. How social technologies are extending the organization. 2011 (November). Retrieved from http://www.mckinsey.com/insights/high_tech_telecoms_internet/how_social_technologies_are_extending_the_organization

20

The Potential of Technology Solutions for Behavioral Healthcare Disparities

MICHAEL CHRISTOPHER GIBBONS

DISPARITIES DEFINITIONS AND DETERMINANTS

Unfortunately, a large and growing base of scientific evidence indicates that healthcare disparities are an undeniable reality (1). In the literature the term *health disparities* is often used synonymously with healthcare disparities. As the names imply, it is at least theoretically possible to separate health disparities from healthcare disparities. Proponents of this distinction insist that the major difference between the two groups of disparities is that health disparities are primarily caused by broad family, social, environmental, and societal factors, or the so-called social determinants of health (2–7). In contrast, healthcare disparities are primarily associated with factors pertaining to the healthcare system and the provision (or lack of provision) of healthcare services (1). While this distinction is logical and at times useful, as the discussion in the remainder of this chapter will show, it is also of diminishing significance.

To illustrate the lack of meaningful distinction in terms of causes of health and healthcare disparities, consider that the societal burden of disparities in the United States can be seen in the more than 35-year discrepancy in longevity between the longest living and shortest living groups (8,9). The economic burden of disparities has been estimated to be approximately $1.24 trillion between 2003 and 2006 alone (10). These disparities arise from the healthcare system, and from biological, environmental, and social factors that affect individuals across their lifespan (11). In the United States, significant differences in social determinants exist along racial and ethnic lines and contribute to poorer health status seen across these populations. These social determinants are also associated with disparities in access to healthcare services, the quality of healthcare services provided, and the health outcomes achieved by these populations.

To fully comprehend the complexity of the factors associated with health or healthcare disparities, it is also important to consider determinants that operate at the level of healthcare systems and in the broader society. For example, the predominant diseases that afflict our society today are chronic diseases such as cancer, cardiovascular disease, and diabetes mellitus. Today, chronic diseases are among the most common health problems in the United States. In 2005, almost 50% of adults (133 million) had at least one chronic illness (12). Behavioral health problems such as excessive alcohol consumption are the third leading preventable cause of death in the United States (13), while mood disorders such as major depression affect over 20 million people and are the leading cause of disability among adults aged 15–44 (14). By definition, these diseases afflict individuals for years and often decades. Yet our healthcare system is still largely oriented toward treating acute episodic illnesses, like those that predominated when our healthcare system was being formed. It also struggles to provide high-quality care to most patients. As such, certain groups of patients are less able to successfully surmount the many challenges associated with the system to maximally benefit from the system. The resulting disparities are often seen along race and ethnicity lines (15,16). Indeed, healthcare quality and healthcare disparities are related to each other. Efforts to eliminate disparities and efforts to improve the quality of care provided in our healthcare system are two inseparable components of high-quality healthcare for all citizens (17).

Another societal influence contributing to the existence of disparities is the significant change in demographics occurring in our society. Within the United States, soon approximately 30% of the population (70+ million) will be over the age of 65 and 20% will be over the age of 85 (18). This presents challenges because in addition to being at much higher risk for having a chronic disease, seniors often have from two to five concurrent chronic illnesses (19). As such, seniors have more complex chronic disease–related needs, and they also have these needs for many more years than did those living generations ago. Among seniors, those with chronic diseases who are also of immigrant and/or racial and ethnic minority backgrounds are often at greatest risk for health or healthcare disparities (1,18).

Thus, both health and healthcare disparities are associated with biological, behavioral, social, environmental, and societal factors that cannot be disentangled. To artificially separate determinants for analytic or methodological reasons denies the reality of their coexistence and interdependence.

PROGRESS IN REDUCING DISPARITIES

For the tenth year in a row, the Agency for Healthcare Research and Quality (AHRQ) has produced the *National Healthcare Quality Report* (NHQR) and the *National Healthcare Disparities Report* (NHDR). These reports measure trends in effectiveness of care, patient safety, timeliness of care, patient centeredness, and efficiency of care. New in 2013 are chapters on care coordination and health system infrastructure (20). The *National Healthcare Quality Report* tracks the healthcare system through quality measures, such as the percentage of heart attack patients who received recommended care when they reached the hospital, or the percentage of children who received recommended vaccinations (20). The *National Healthcare Disparities Report* summarizes healthcare quality and access among various racial, ethnic, and income groups and other priority populations, such as residents of rural areas and people with disabilities (20). A review of the findings of these reports over the last decade indicated that while healthcare quality has improved slightly, there has been no systematic and sustained reduction in healthcare disparities (20).

Interestingly, the domestic and international experience, which has focused on the social determinants of health, has not fared much better. In the United Kingdom, government-level national policies meant to address the social determinants of health inequalities have had little impact over a 20-year period (21,22). Despite the best of intentions and a great deal of hard work, the evidence indicates that neither a medical approach nor a social determinant approach to the elimination of healthcare disparities has been successful at a national level. Thus the global experience in large-scale disparities reduction interventions suggests that, in the future, approaches integrating both medical and social determinants approaches may be needed to enhance our understanding of behavioral healthcare disparities and improve efforts to reduce disparities.

CHALLENGES TO UNDERSTANDING AND ADDRESSING DISPARITIES
Definitional Imprecision and Duplicity

The first challenge to address disparities concerns the terminology and definitions used in the field. As noted earlier, several terms have been used synonymously when talking about disparities. For example, healthcare disparities have been defined as "differences in the quality of healthcare that are not due to access-related factors or clinical needs, preferences, and appropriateness of intervention" by the Institute of Medicine, in their classic report entitled *Unequal Treatment* (1). *Healthcare* disparities have also been defined as "any differences among populations that are statistically significant and differ from the reference group by at least 10%" (23). *Health* disparities have been defined as differences in health outcomes and their determinants between segments of the population, as defined by social, demographic, environmental, and geographic attributes (24). A similar term, *health inequalities*, signifies summary measures of population health that are associated with individual- or group-specific attributes (e.g., income, education, or race/ethnicity) (25). A third term, *health inequities*, has been defined as health inequalities that are modifiable, associated with social disadvantage, and considered ethically unfair (26).

A central component of all the definitions is the notion of population-level differences. However, even the definition of population can be problematic, because while the idea of population is central to many disciplines and fields of study, it is rarely defined, except in abstract statistical terms (27). To complicate matters further, the terms *inequality* and *inequity* have been introduced in the disparities literature and have often been used synonymously with the term *disparities*. The latter terms were introduced to instantiate the connotation of injustice, social privilege, or unfairness into the emerging definition of disparities (28). These terminology differences underlie differing disciplinary orientations and perspectives and inevitably lead to confusion. This inhibits the transdisciplinary investigation and collaboration that are needed to comprehensively understand how disparities happen and to craft effective disparities solutions. As will emerge from discussion in the remainder of this chapter, a technology-based approach to disparities research helps to overcome these challenges, by providing a framework and orientation using discipline-independent nomenclature. As such, differing disciplinary perspectives may be incorporated in a way that facilitates insights not possible within the context of any one scientific field of study.

Poor Understanding of Links between Biology, Behavior, and Environment

Another challenge found in much of the disparities literature relates to a relatively poor understanding of the links between molecular biology, physiology, behavior, and environmental factors. Bench scientists often do not account for social and behavioral factors that may impact the development of health disparities (29,30). While sociobehavioral scientists generally acknowledge that links exist, the exact nature of the links remains obscure and imprecise, especially when describing cellular and molecular connections to behavior or environmental factors (21,31–33). The one exception is found in the articulation of stress (neuroimmunological) mechanisms, which many social scientists suggest is the pathway underlying all connections between the biological and socioenvironmental worlds (31,33,34).

Categorical Conceptions of Disparities Determinants

A third challenge to fully understanding and addressing disparities relates to what might be called disciplinary perspectivism. On the one hand, scientists and investigators trained in the clinical and bench sciences generally consider discreet, quantitative exposures (viral, bacterial, toxicological, psychological, etc.) as the etiological agents of disease. Historically, these exposures were studied in isolation from the broader sociobehavioral contexts in which they exist. On the other hand, social scientists often consider more qualitative social factors like poverty, socioeconomic status (SES), and racial segregation as the key drivers of health (27,31). They often assert that other, more quantitative exposures are factors that alter the nature of the association between the social factor and a given health outcome (35). They also draw a distinction between so-called proximal social factors, which are the settings in which people live (family, work, school, and neighborhood), and distal social factors, which are the pervasive forces in society (culture, SES, and race relations) (35).

Unfortunately, rather than spurring efforts to come together, disciplinary elitism has led to academic "debate" regarding the causes of disparities vs. the causes of the causes, or the "fundamental" causes of disparities (36). The inevitable implication of these positions is that some determinants (and their corresponding experts and fields of study) are more valid or important to our understanding of disparities than others.

Transdisciplinary Disparities Investigation

The final challenge relates to the significant inertia needed to overcome unidisciplinary, single-level, non-systems-oriented approaches to disparities investigation. In reality, important determinants or hypothesized causes of disparities have been identified at many levels of analysis (molecular biology, behavioral sciences, environmental sciences and population science), and all within complex interrelated systems (11,37). As such, disentangling the myriad determinants and connections between these determinants over the lifespan and understanding how these determinants cause disparities will require insight and expertise from multiple scientific perspectives (11). Likewise, interventions—be they individual, clinical, community, or population based—that operate at only one level or system are likely to have only limited ability to improve a given disparity because they inevitably are dealing only with one level of determinants in a multilevel, integrated system. In some ways it is like trying to build an automobile or understand how they are built by only studying the tires, body, axle, or muffler. Important? Yes. Necessary? Yes, but not sufficient to comprehensively understand automobiles or adequately prepare the investigator or practitioner to make better cars.

ACHIEVING THE GOAL: THE ROLE OF TECHNOLOGY
Improving our Understanding of Disparities Pathogenesis

There are two basic ways in which technology can potentially help us achieve the goal of reducing disparities. First, technology may help us enhance our understanding of how or why disparities occur (disparities pathogenesis). Second, technology can potentially help reduce disparities by improving disparities interventions.

In terms of understanding how disparities happen in a population, most conceptual models of population health were derived from either the sociobehavioral sciences or the biomolecular sciences. Those models from the sociobehavioral sciences generally lack detailed physiological and molecular mechanisms of action, whereas those from the biomolecular sciences largely do not seriously consider the vast majority of socioenvironmental determinants (11). Systems scientists have attempted to overcome this problem by regarding health within the context of a broad set of interrelated phenomena. The challenging reality is that even systems themselves exist at multiple levels. These include molecular systems, biological systems, family or neighborhood systems, environmental systems, political systems, and societal systems, to name a few. In reality, all of these systems coexist, and substantial scientific evidence suggests that these systems impact one another in complicated ways to produce health outcomes in individuals and populations (11). The reality is that we do ourselves no favors by ignoring some systems and focusing on others. Nor do we help the cause by spending time arguing over which systems are most important, as if any one system

would be important at all times over the lifespan. Until we have a more sophisticated understanding that is comprehensive, integrative, and systems oriented, there may be little hope of developing effective interventions, because we will continue to rely on our partial or limited understanding of how disparities truly happen.

Certainly, achieving this goal will be incredibly challenging; however, some scientists are taking important first steps toward creating a technology that will aid us in dealing adequately with the exploding complexity of today's world and successfully addressing interlocking problems such as disease, poverty, and stress (38). In 2007, IBM scientists began a project to build an intelligent computer system that could deeply analyze any and all kinds of data at once. The prototype system, dubbed "Watson," is a computer system that recognizes concepts by decomposing expressions of an idea and then combining the results with available contextual information. Watson can recompose the elements in various ways, each of which can be tested to imagine new concepts. These combinations can then be used to drive new discovery and insight, helping us to find answers to questions and to realize the questions that were never even asked. Technologies like Watson may in the future be used to solve problems that fit certain common patterns, such as understanding why certain diseases have common characteristics or which populations will develop certain diseases. In so doing, Watson can be asked questions that yield answers, or it can also be used to discover new insights and realize concepts that were not previously recognized (39).

Analysis and interpretation of the many factors existing within and across systems in a population that cause disparities will require advanced computing power, like Watson, that goes far beyond the capacity of a desktop computer. Similarly, understanding the relationships between these factors over time will require the development of novel analytic methodologies that go beyond the capacities of those currently available. Once again, this will require advanced computing power and computer-based methods like machine learning, data mining, and perhaps other methods yet to be developed.

From a theoretical and conceptual perspective, the term *populomics* has been suggested to embody a scientific perspective that embraces the challenge of integrative analysis of complex and disparate multilevel data, and to articulate a general conceptual approach and goal (40). The term *populomics* is derived from the synthesis of population sciences, medicine, and informatics. It is defined as the discipline that employs a population level, transdisciplinary, integrative approach to disease and risk characterization, interdiction, and mitigation. At the core of a populomics orientation is an enhanced reliance on advanced computing methods to enable the characterization of the interplay of sociobehavioral pathways and biophysiological and molecular mechanisms that work across levels of existence, to impact the health of populations (40,41). Populomics is novel in that it specifically focuses on the integration of medical, social, and population sciences and the relationships between determinants across these domains to explain health outcomes among populations. A populomics orientation can lead to understanding and insights as well as analytic methodologies that are superior to contemporary approaches based on probabilistic statistics, race, socioeconomic status, educational status, or genetic mutations.

A populomics-based approach to disparities research may facilitate the analysis and interpretation of population-level data to enable the development of community-wide risk profiles based on clinical and socioenvironmental data. This population-level risk characterization could potentially go beyond the limitations of current analyses (surveillance, monitoring, cross-sectional, or even cohort analyses). In addition, these risk profiles, when linked to the underlying molecular genetic mechanisms, may enable the development of population-wide disparities signatures or profiles (groups of determinants or causative factors that predictably coexist among given populations exhibiting a defined health or healthcare disparity). These disparities profiles may in fact be a far more accurate and precise way to characterize the causes of disparities than current single-level, single-disciplinary determinants such as genetics, behavior, poverty, or race, or even better than broader social determinants of health. Once these disparities profiles are known, it should then be possible to evaluate the existence of the determinants in question among non-disparities populations. If found, they could provide strong evidence suggesting the possibility of the development of future disparities in that population,

should current conditions and determinants remain unaltered. This would essentially equate to population-level disparities-predictive analytics, which is currently not possible to do. In addition, primary prevention of disparities (preventing disparities from occurring in the first place) may also be possible in that interventions could be put in place to prevent the future occurrence of a given disparity before the disparity even exists. Again, currently, this level of disparities research is simply not possible and remains the stuff of imagination, unless the disparities sciences embrace the full potential that advanced computer-based analytic research approaches have to offer.

In summary, considering the number of potential factors existing at the cellular, individual, population, and environmental levels that may be important in the genesis of disease or behavioral healthcare disparities (11,42), advanced computing technologies may offer hope of harnessing this vast array of information and using it to understand disease or disparities as they exist in populations. New computer-based, Internet-based, and Internet-enabled electronic health (eHealth) solutions can enable the real-time integrative utilization of petabyte amounts of behavioral, biological, and community-level information in ways not previously possible (41). As outlined above, integrative behavioral algorithms and decision support tools for scientists and clinicians, like IBM's Watson, could facilitate the analysis and interpretation of population- and individual-level data and go beyond current possibilities and overcome existing limitations (41).

Improving Disparities Interventions

In addition to being an analytic and decision support tool for scientists, providers, and practitioners, technology can also be an important interventional agent for both clinicians and patients. Technology may play a significant role in the development of effective disparities solutions. Because there already exists a significant literature, and much public discourse, that focuses on the role of technology-based clinical interventional tools (43–54), these technologies will not be reviewed here. Rather, the remainder of this chapter will focus on patient- and consumer-oriented tools that have received comparatively little scientific attention. In some ways, these technologies may offer much more promise than the clinical tools in helping us reach the goal of eliminating disparities and enhancing health for all. This is because the healthcare system provides only episodic support, primarily in the later years of life, to patients managing chronic diseases. The current system also offers little to family caregivers who provide the bulk of the care patients receive. In addition, the current healthcare system has little ability to monitor or otherwise interact "on demand" with community-dwelling patients proactively and in real time. Because most individuals spend relatively little time in the healthcare system over the course of their lifetime, how effectively can the system reduce and eliminate disparities (health or healthcare)?

Information technologies that function as interventional tools and/or decision aids primarily for patients, clients, family members, and caregivers, with or without the direct involvement of their formal clinical providers, are collectively termed consumer health technologies or consumer health informatics. Specifically, they are defined as any electronic tool, technology, or system that (a) is primarily designed to interact with individuals who seek or use healthcare information for nonprofessional work, (b) interacts directly with the consumer who provides personal health information to the system and receives personalized health information from the electronic tool, and (c) is one in which the data, information, recommendations, or other benefits provided to the consumer may be used with a healthcare professional but is not dependent on a healthcare professional (55).

Early examples of these types of tools include websites providing self-care information, online health risk calculators, personal health records (PHRs), and online support groups. Today, however, the numbers, growth, and types of these tools are staggering. They include online support groups like Nike+, Patients Like Me, Cure Together, and Second Life. Cell phone applications (apps) being designed for smartphone and non-smartphones, as well as other mobile health (mHealth) tools, form another genre of these tools. It has been reported that over 1 million apps are available across Android, Google, and Apple app stores (56), with 40,000 health apps being available on the iTunes store alone (57)!

Health interventions delivered or used primarily via gaming devices (health gaming) are another emerging genre of consumer health technology found in this domain (58,59). Finally, sensor-based technologies and wearable technologies that are able to automatically detect a number of physical, psychological, or environmental factors and wirelessly relay this information to a provider, consumer, website, smartphone, electronic health record or personal health record are becoming increasingly available. Examples include Fitbit® (www.fitbit.com), which is a wristband-like activity tracker able to track steps, distance, stairs climbed, calories burned, and active minutes; monitor sleep; and wake users with a silent alarm. Propellar Health® (www.propellarhealth.com) is another example of this type of health tool. Propellar Health is a sensor that tracks asthma medication use and records the time and place of use. It is attached to the top of an asthma inhaler. It wirelessly syncs with a smartphone via Bluetooth technology to input the data into the Propeller mobile app, which allows the user to view the data and gives the user personalized feedback and education on ways to improve his or her asthma control.

In a systematic review of the impact of these consumer health applications, eight studies were identified and evaluated for the evidence of impact on intermediate mental health outcomes and mental health–oriented clinical outcomes (60). Intermediate outcomes of interest included work and social adjustment, perceived stress, self-rated self-management, sleep quality, mental energy, and concentration. Seven of the eight studies found evidence of positive effect on one or more intermediate outcomes. In addition, seven studies showed evidence of significant impact on one or more clinical outcomes related to mental health. No study found any evidence of harm attributable to the consumer technology (60). Thus there is increasing interest in evaluating the potential of these technologies in reaching consumers at a low cost and in obviating the need for some activities currently performed by humans. The data additionally suggest that these technologies may enhance the effectiveness of current non-technological interventions. Finally, individual tailoring, personalization, and behavioral consumer feedback were critical elements found among those electronic tools demonstrating positive impact (60).

TECHNOLOGY DISPARITIES

Over the last decade, many of the gaps in technology access and usage that have been reported have narrowed significantly. However, significant gaps remain and suggest both challenges and opportunities for using technology to reduce behavioral healthcare disparities. For example, in 1995, approximately 10% of adults in the United States were going online. In 2013 almost 80% of adults and 95% of teens did so (61). Among African Americans Internet use has more than doubled, from 35% to 71%. Among Hispanics the rate has increased from 40% to 68% over the same time period (61). Similarly, among individuals earning less than $30,000 per year, Internet utilization has gone from 28% to 62%, while also increasing from 16% to 43% and 33% to 71% among those who have less than a high school diploma or are high school graduates, respectively (61). In terms of broadband access at home, only 62% of African Americans have such access as compared to 74% of whites (62).

Overall, 85% of U.S. adults own a cell phone, with 53% being smartphone owners (63). In addition, 31% of cell phone owners say they use their phone to look for health or medical information online. Younger adults, minorities, and those in particular need of health information are most likely to use their phones to obtain health information (63). African Americans are twice as likely as whites to use their phones as the primary method of getting online (38% vs. 17%), and they are more likely to own a mobile device and use a wider array of functions on these devices than whites (61). Finally, there is mixed evidence regarding the use of social media by race. Some reports suggest significantly higher utilization of social media by minorities, and other reports suggest uniformly high rates of social media across racial subgroups (64,65).

As these data indicate, gaps in technology access and utilization remain despite significant narrowing of such gaps over time. In addition, minorities appear to preferentially use mobile technologies to a greater degree than non-minorities. Given this reality, technology may enable the delivery of behavioral interventions to historically underserved populations. If, however, the benefits of using technologies in this way are not realized among these populations, disparities may not be reduced and, in some cases, may even

increase. There are several reasons why this could occur. Emerging evidence suggests that while technology access and utilization are necessary in order to produce benefit, access and utilization alone cannot guarantee beneficial impact (66–70). Factors related to the design of the tools, the environment in which the tools are being used, and the users themselves can significantly impact the safe, effective, satisfactory, and error-free utilization of a device and therefore also affect the likelihood of the user experiencing health benefits attributable to the use of the device.

The Institute of Medicine has called for the development and deployment of culturally appropriate healthcare services to mitigate disparities (1). The role of culture on healthcare processes and outcomes is both complex and undeniable. Culture has been shown to affect how individuals think about the causes of disease, choices regarding the use of life-sustaining technology, provider–patient interaction, and the role of family and others in the caregiving process (71). To date, most of the work that has been done seeking to address the role of culture in health and disparities has focused primarily on the role of cross-cultural competency, sensitivity, and awareness among providers and healthcare institutions, and on the need for cultural tailoring of healthcare processes and public health interventions (72–74). In addition, however, information and computer scientists have suggested that technology-based health tools are embedded with "hidden cultural assumptions." For example, a European developer may assume that all users of the emerging technology will seek to engage a doctor or nurse when the individual is experiencing a perceived heart attack or stroke, as the developer would do. However, well-documented levels of mistrust among certain racial and ethnic groups may cause members of that group to consult medical professionals only after discussing their concerns with trusted members of their community. In this case, a technology that helps a consumer recognize symptoms of a stroke and immediately contact a healthcare professional might not be trusted, valued, or used in the way the developer intends. In addition, while technology designers often believe their creations to be culturally neutral, health technology often embodies cultural assumptions that may not always be appropriate for the intended user (71). Continuing with our previous example then, developing a technology relying on the assumption that all patients need the best scientific evidence to make choices regarding their health might lead a developer to design a technology that highlights the availability of the scientific literature but provides no functionality for social support or peer interaction. While logical, this assumption could prove problematic for users from racial and ethnic minority populations. In turn, the efficacy of the tool may be limited among certain users. Thus consumer health technologies could, in part or in whole, render these tools ineffective or less valuable and preclude the realization of any health benefit, even if the target population has adequate access to the technology. Further, if the technology is used widely, but the underlying developmental assumptions are appropriate for only one group of intended users, the benefits attributable to the use of the technology could differentially accrue to one population and actually increase disparities between the two populations (71).

POTENTIAL IMPACT OF NEW TECHNOLOGY-BASED TOOLS

The preceding discussion briefly outlined the basis for the growing optimism regarding the potential of technology-based approaches to help improve behavioral health outcomes and address behavioral healthcare disparities. For consumers, caregivers, and family members, emerging tools could help enable or enhance patients' desire to document the illness experience, facilitate the reporting of this information to their clinicians, and provide real-time consumer decision support regarding the many questions that arise in the course of care-giving for patients with behavioral health issues. Technology-based approaches could prove valuable for patient and caregiver training and/or patient education. This could occur in the pre-hospital discharge context or on demand from home as needed. In turn, consumer health technologies may, in certain patients, enable the users to receive needed social support, thus enhancing patient satisfaction with care and with trust in the healthcare system while also helping to improve the quality and cultural appropriateness of clinical interventions.

It is possible to also understand the potential benefits of technology-based approaches

from a health systems perspective. From this perspective health technology benefits could accrue across the entire health and care continuum (screening, diagnosis, treatment, monitoring, survivorship). In the future, technology may even enable the development of enhanced prevention and wellness interventions, as well as better screening, diagnostic, and therapeutic interventions that can reach people even when they are not in the hospital, clinic, or office setting during normal business hours. In addition, these interventions potentially could support and enhance self-care and disease self-management where appropriate, improve shared decision-making, enhance patient engagement, and promote adherence.

Finally, the benefits of technology-based approaches, even consumer health technologies, will likely also impact clinical providers. They will inevitably impact information sharing at the point of care and in so doing spur greater patient-centered collaborative care. For example, some experts have highlighted the need for providers to know and understand important nonclinical information that occurs in the lives of their patients. These have been collectively termed observations of daily living (ODLs) and have in some cases been found to be of benefit to clinicians (75,76). Consumer health technologies could provide a mechanism to track, summarize, and efficiently communicate important ODLs that are currently largely unknown to the healthcare system but occurring in the lives of disparities populations and could prove critical in overcoming these challenges. Finally, technology-based approaches could significantly improve our understanding of the genesis, development, and natural history of disparities.

CONCLUSIONS

In conclusion, significant scientific evidence attests to the fact that healthcare disparities exist; they are intractable and associated with increased healthcare costs, premature morbidity, and excess mortality. Increasing demand and adoption of digital and information technologies by providers and patients will likely affect behavioral healthcare disparities. The impact of information technologies on behavioral healthcare disparities is almost certainly going to be multifaceted, nuanced, and, in some cases, indirect, yet cumulatively significant. Disparities could be reduced if technology use and benefits are equitably distributed across user populations. Alternatively, disparities could worsen if some patients are not able to benefit from use of such technologies.

Despite these challenges, there is real potential to make a significant impact toward the goal of enhancing our understanding of behavioral healthcare disparities pathogenesis through technology. This understanding will lead to improved clinical effectiveness of disparities interventions and health outcomes, and ultimately eliminate health and healthcare disparities from our society.

REFERENCES

1. Committee on Understanding and Eliminating Racial and Ethnic Disparities in Health Care. *Unequal Treatment; Confronting Racial and Ethnic Disparities in Health Care.* Washington DC, National Academies Press; 2002.

2. Wilkinson RG. Socioeconomic determinants of health. Health inequalities: relative or absolute material standards? *British Journal of Medicine* 1997; 314(7080):591–595.

3. Marmot MG. Does stress cause heart attacks? *Postgraduate Medical Journal* 1986; 62(729):683–686.

4. Wilkinson RG, Pickett KE. Income inequality and socioeconomic gradients in mortality. *American Journal of Public Health* 2008; 98(4):699–704.

5. Wilkinson RG. "Variations" in health. *British Journal of Medicine* 1995; 311(7014):1177–1178.

6. Wilkinson RG. Inequalities and health. *Lancet* 1994; 343(8896):538.

7. Pickett KE, Wilkinson RG. Greater equality and better health. *British Journal of Medicine* 2009; 339:b4320.

8. Murray CJ, Kulkarni SC, Michaud C, Tomijima N, Bulzacchelli MT, Iandiorio TJ, et al. Eight Americas: Investigating mortality disparities across races, counties, and race-counties in the United States. *PLoS Medicine* 2006; 3(9):e260.

9. Murray CJ, Kulkarni S, Ezzati M. Eight Americas: New perspectives on U.S. health disparities. *American Journal of Preventive Medicine* 2005; 29(5 Suppl 1):4–10.

10. LaVeist T, Gaskin D, Richard P. The economic burden of health inequalities in the United States. Washington, DC: The Joint Center for Political and Economic Studies; 2009.

11. Gibbons MC, Brock M, Alberg AJ, Glass T, LaVeist TA, Baylin S, et al. The sociobiologic integrative model (SBIM): Enhancing the integration of sociobehavioral, environmental, and biomolecular knowledge in urban health and disparities research. *Journal of Urban Health* 2007; 84(2):198–211.

12. Wu SY, Green A. Projection of chronic illness prevalence and cost inflation. Santa Monica, CA, RAND Corp.; 2000.

13. Mokdad AH, Marks JS, Stroup DF, Gerberding JL. Actual causes of death in the United States, 2000. *Journal of the American Medical Association* 2004; 291(10):1238–1245.

14. World Health Organization. The global burden of disease: 2004 update, Table A2: Burden of disease in DALYs by cause, sex and income group in WHO regions, estimates for 2004. Retreived from http://www.who.int/healthinfo/global_burden_disease/GBD_report_2004update_AnnexA.pdf

15. Committee on Quality of Health Care in America. *Crossing the Quality Chasm.* Washington DC: National Academy Press; 2001.

16. Gibbons MC. Emerging e-Health response to contemporary healthcare realities. In Wickramasinghe N, Geisler E (eds.). *Encyclopedia of Healthcare Information Systems.* Hershey, NY: Illinois Institute of Technology; 2013.

17. Fiscella K, Franks P, Gold MR, Clancy CM. Inequality in quality: Addressing socioeconomic, racial, and ethnic disparities in health care. *Journal of the American Medical Association* 2000; 283(19):2579–2584.

18. Shrestha L. The Changing Demographic Profile of the United States. RL32701. 2006. Washington, DC: Congressional Research Service—The Library of Congress.

19. Changing Demographics: Implications for Physicians, Nurses, and Other Health Workers. Washington, DC; U.S. DHHS, Health Resources and Services Administration, Bureau of Health Professions; 2003.

20. Agency for Healthcare Research and Quality. The National Healthcare Disparities Reporrt 2012. Washington, DC; Government Printing Office; 2013.

21. Acheson D. Independent Inquiry into Inequalities in Health Report. London: Stationery Office; 1998

22. Black D. Inequalities in Health: Report of a Working Group. London: Department of Health and Social Security; 1980.

23. The Agency for Healthcare Research and Quality. The National Healthcare Disparities Report 2009. Washington DC: AHRQ, 2010.

24. Carter-Pokras O, Baquet C. What is a "health disparity"? *Public Health Report* 2002; 117(5):426–434.

25. Asada Y. A summary measure of health inequalities for a pay-for-population health performance system. *Prevention of Chronic Disease* 2010; 7(4):A72.

26. Braveman P, Gruskin S. Defining equity in health. *Journal of Epidemiology and Community Health* 2003; 57(4):254–258.

27. Krieger N. Who and what is a "population"? Historical debates, current controversies, and implications for understanding "population health" and rectifying health inequities. *Milbank Quarterly* 2012; 90(4):634–681.

28. Braveman P, Krieger N, Lynch J. Health inequalities and social inequalities in health. *Bulletin of the World Health Organization* 2000; 78(2):232–234.

29. Burger R, Gimelfarb A. Genetic variation maintained in multilocus models of additive quantitative traits under stabilizing selection. *Genetics* 1999; 152(2):807–820.

30. Sharma AM. The thrifty-genotype hypothesis and its implications for the study of complex genetic disorders in man. *Journal of Molecular Medicine (Berlin)* 1998; 76(8):568–571.

31. Adler NE, Rehkopf DH. U.S. disparities in health: Descriptions, causes, and mechanisms. *Annual Review of Public Health* 2008; 29:235–252.

32. Capitman J, Bhalotra SM, Calderon-Rosado V, Gibbons MC. Cancer prevention and treatment demonstration for racial and ethnic minorities; Evidence report and evidence-based reccomendations. 1500-00-0031. 2003. Washington DC: Department of Health and Human Services Government Printing Office; 2003

33. Macintyre S. The Black Report and beyond: What are the issues? *Social Science Medicine* 1997; 44(6):723–745.

34. Lupie SJ, King S, Meaney MJ, McEwen BS. Can poverty get under your skin? Basal cortisol levels and cognitive function in children from low and high socioeconomic status. *Developmental Psychopathology* 2001; 13(3):653–676.

35. Amick BC, Levine S, Tarlov AR, Walsh DC. *Society and Health.* New York: Oxford University Press; 1995.

36. Wilson AE. "Fundamental causes" of health disparities; A comparative analysis of Canada and the United States. *International Sociology* 2009; 24(1):93–113.

37. Abrams DB. Applying transdisciplinary research strategies to understanding and eliminating health disparities. *Health Education Behavior* 2006; 33(4):515–531.

38. Kelly J, Hamm S. *Smart Machines IBM'S Watson and the Era of Cognative Computing.* New York: Columbia University Press; 2013.

39. High R. The era of cognitive systems: An inside look at IBM Watson and how it works. REDP-4955-00. IBM Corporation; 2012.

40. Gibbons MC. Populomics. *Studies in Health Technology Information* 2008; 137:265–268.

41. Gibbons MC. A historical overview of health disparities and the potential of eHealth solutions. *Journal of Medical Internet Research* 2005; 7(5):e50.

42. National Research Council. *New Horizons in Health: An Integrative Approach.* Singer B, Ryff C (eds.). Washington, DC: National Academy Press; 2001.

43. Hoyt RE, Bailey N, Yoshihashi AK. *Health Informatics: Practical Guide for Healthcare and Information Technology Professionals* (5th ed.). Lulu Publishers; 2012.

44. Ajami S, Rajabzadeh A. Radio frequency identification (RFID) technology and patient safety. *Journal of Research and Medical Science* 2013; 18(9):809–813.

45. Ajami S, Arab-Chadegani R. Barriers to implement electronic health records (EHRs). *Material Sociomedicine* 2013; 25(3):213–215.

46. Gillum RF. From papyrus to the electronic tablet: A brief history of the clinical medical record with lessons for the digital age. *American Journal of Medicine* 2013; 126(10):853–857.

47. Lally JF. Telemedicine: winners and losers. *Delaware Medical Journal* 2013; 85(8):245–246.

48. Logan AG. Transforming hypertension management using mobile health technology for telemonitoring and self-care support. *Canadian Journal of Cardiology* 2013; 29(5):579–585.

49. Morales-Vidal S, Ruland S. Telemedicine in stroke care and rehabilitation. *Topics in Stroke Rehabilitation* 2013; 20(2):101–107.

50. Stellefson M, Chaney B, Barry AE, Chavarria E, Tennant B, Walsh-Childers K, et al. Web 2.0 chronic disease self-management for older adults: A systematic review. *Journal of Medical Internet Research* 2013; 15(2):e35.

51. Rubin MN, Wellik KE, Channer DD, Demaerschalk BM. A systematic review of telestroke. *Postgraduate Medicine* 2013; 125(1):45–50.

52. Maat B, Bollen CW, van Vught AJ, Egberts TC, Rademaker CM. Impact of computerized physician order entry (CPOE) on PICU prescribing errors. *Intensive Care Medicine* 2014; 0(3):458–459.

53. Armada ER, Villamanan E, Lopez-de-Sa E, Rosillo S, Rey-Blas JR, Testillano ML, et al. Computerized physician order entry in the cardiac intensive care unit: Effects on prescription errors and workflow conditions. *Journal of Critical Care* 2014; 29(2):188–193.

54. Al Rowibah FA, Younis MZ, Parkash J. The impact of computerized physician order entry on medication errors and adverse drug events. *Journal of Health Care Finance* 2013; 40(1):93–102.

55. Gibbons MC, Wilson RF, Samal L, Lehman CU, Dickersin K, Lehmann HP, et al. Impact of consumer health informatics applications. *Evididence Report Technology Assessment* 2009;188:1–546.

56. Freierman S. One million apps and counting at a fast pace. *New York Times*, December 11, 2011.

57. Aitken M, Gauntlet C. *Patient Apps for Improved Healthcare: From Novelty to Mainstream* (pp. 1–65). Parsippany, NJ: IMS Institute for Healthcare Informatics; 2013.

58. Lamboglia CM, da Silva VT, Vasconcelos Filho JE, Pinheiro MH, Munguba MC, Silva Junior FV, et al. Exergaming as a strategic tool in the fight against childhood obesity: A systematic review. *Journal of Obesity* 2013; 2013:438364.

59. Studenski S, Perera S, Hile E, Keller V, Spadola-Bogard J, Garcia J. Interactive video dance games for healthy older adults. *Journal of Nutrition, Health & Aging* 2010; 14(10):850–852.

60. Gibbons MC, Wilson RF, Samal L, Lehmann CU, Dickersin K, Lehmann HP, et al. Consumer health informatics: Results of a systematic evidence review and evidence based recommendations. *Translational Behavior Medicine* 2011; 1(1):72–82.

61. Zickuhr K, Smith A. Digital differences. Washington DC: Pew Internet and American Life Project, Pew Charitable Trusts; 2012.

62. Smith A. African Americans and technology use. Pew Internet and American Life Project. 2014. Retrieved from http://pewinternet. org/Reports/2014/African-American-Tech-Use/ Detailed-Demographic-Tables/ Internet-mobile-and-social-networking-adoption.aspx

63. Fox S, Duggan M. Mobile health 2012 (pp. 1–29). Pew Charitable Trusts; 2012.

64. Gibbons MC, Fleisher L, Slamon RE, Bass S, Kandadai V, Beck JR. Exploring the potential of Web 2.0 to address health disparities. *Journal of Health Communication* 2011; 16(Suppl 1):77–89.

65. Korzenny F, Vann L. Tapping into their connections: The multicultural world of social media marketing. Tallahassee, FL: Florida State University Center for Hispanic Marketing Communication; 2009.

66. Yamin CK, Emani S, Williams DH, Lipsitz SR, Karson AS, Wald JS, et al. The digital divide in adoption and use of a personal health record. *Archives of Internal Medicine* 2011; 171(6):568–574.

67. Roblin DW, Houston TK, Allison JJ, Joski PJ, Becker ER. Disparities in use of a personal health record in a managed care organization. *Journal of the American Medical Informatics Association* 2009; 16(5):683–689.

68. Hing E, Burt CW. Are there patient disparities when electronic health records are adopted? *Journal of Health Care for the Poor and Underserved* 2009; 20(2):473–488.

69. Sarkar U, Karter AJ, Liu JY, Adler NE, Nguyen R, Lopez A, et al. Social disparities in internet patient portal use in diabetes: Evidence that the digital divide extends beyond access. *Journal of the American Medical Informatics Association* 2011; 18(3):318–321.

70. Sarkar U, Karter AJ, Liu JY, Adler NE, Nguyen R, Lopez A, et al. The literacy divide: Health literacy and the use of an Internet-based patient portal in an integrated health system-results from the diabetes study of northern California (DISTANCE). *Journal of Health Communication* 2010; 15(Suppl 2):183–196.

71. Valdez RS, Gibbons MC, Siegel ER, Kukafka R, Brennan PF. Designing consumer health IT to enhance usability among different racial and ethnic groups within the United States. *Health and Technology* 2012;2(4):225–233.

72. Hobgood C, Sawning S, Bowen J, Savage K. Teaching culturally appropriate care: a review of educational models and methods. *Academy of Emergency Medicine* 2006; 13(12):1288–1295.

73. Juckett G. Cross-cultural medicine. *American Family Physician* 2005; 72(11):2267–2274.

74. Brach C, Fraser I. Can cultural competency reduce racial and ethnic health disparities? A review and conceptual model. *Medical Care Research and Review* 2000; 57(Suppl 1):181–217.

75. Backonja U, Kim K, Casper GR, Patton T, Ramly E, Brennan PF. Observations of daily living: putting the "personal" in personal health records. *Nursing Informatics* 2012; 2012:6.

76. Brennan PF, Downs S, Casper G. Project HealthDesign: Rethinking the power and potential of personal health records. *Journal of Biomedical Informatics* 2010; 43(5 Suppl):S3–S5.

21

Behavioral Health Information Technology Adoption in the Context of a Changing Healthcare Landscape

WENDY J. NILSEN AND MISHA PAVEL

BRAVE NEW WORLD

By all accounts, technology has profoundly changed the human experience. In a century, the world has been transformed from a place in which real-time interactions were face to face to one in which information technology, such as computers and cellular phones, make immediate, virtual communication the norm, regardless of where each party happens to be. Despite the pace of these developments, healthcare has been late to adopt technology in the support and provision of care. Changes in U.S policy over the last 5 years represent an attempt to shift the emphasis, however. While technology has been creeping into healthcare since the widespread diffusion of computers, the Health Information Technology for Economic and Clinical Health (HITECH) initiative (www.healthit.hhs.gov) in 2009 began the systematic adoption of technology into healthcare. This initiative set up standards for electronic health records (EHRs) and put in place $2 billion in incentives to support healthcare agencies in the meaningful use of EHRs. According to David Blumenthal, Director of the Office of the National Coordinator of Health Information Technology (ONC) at the time, the "HITECH Act's programs strive to create an electronic circulatory system for health information that nourishes the practice of medicine, research, and public health, making healthcare professionals better at what they do and the American people healthier" (1). The lofty goals of the HITECH initiative are to improve care coordination, quality, efficiency, and patient safety; reduce health disparities; promote public and population health; engage patients and families; and ensure privacy and security (http://aspe.hhs.gov/daltcp/reports/2013/ehrpi.shtml#figure1). Presumably, meaningful use of EHR data will change practice standards and patterns to enhance healthcare at the level of the patient, as well as the population.

In 2008, only 13% of physicians had access to an EHR. In 2011, the number was estimated to be 57%. In behavioral health (i.e., substance use and mental health), the rate of EHR adoption is lower than that in general healthcare (2). Reasons for this discrepancy are unclear but seem to include the fact that behavioral health clinics are more likely to be small or solo practices and are not connected to a larger health system (which are incentivized for the use of EHRs [3]). Further, behavioral health clinics report designating a much smaller percentage of revenue to HIT development than general health clinics (1.8 vs. 3.5%), as well as assigning a third of the staff to HIT issues compared to the portion assigned in other healthcare settings (3). Combined, these data suggest that behavioral health clinics are not investing in the complex electronic record systems that are thought to facilitate care. In addition, the electronic exchange of data associated with EHRs is complicated by 42 Code of Federal Regulations (CFR) Part II, which mandates the confidentiality of alcohol and drug abuse patient records.

Unfortunately, the uptake of information technology in healthcare in general, and behavioral health in particular, has not been as fast as predicted (1,3). The reasons for this are myriad, but generally focus on the lack of empirical support for information technologies (4,5) and the technological challenges to security and privacy, especially as addressed by the Health Insurance Portability and Accountability Act of 1996 (HIPAA, http://www.hhs.gov/ocr/privacy/hipaa/understanding/index.html).

Although these issues are important, it is also crucial to compare the challenges of technology adoption in healthcare to other industries. For example, banking has been radically transformed in the past decade. In the past, many daily interactions took place face to face: consumers had to go to the bank to access money or loans or access information about their account. Electronic transactions involved checks, credit cards, or wire transfers, the latter of which generally required a visit to a bank. This banking world, which is flush with personal and financial information, traditionally relied on face-to-face interactions to verify information. This all changed as technology made it possible for these transactions to be handled remotely and in a secure fashion. In a very short period of time, modern banking has been transformed into an industry in which most transactions no longer require in-person transactions. Deposits are managed with cell phone cameras, and withdrawals are made at 24-hour automatic tellers. These changes are possible not only because of changes in technology that provide a platform for interaction but also because the regulatory and business agendas were aligned to enhance adoption. The banking industry convinced consumers that the lack of human interaction was to their benefit (e.g., convenience and timing), while allowing for significant reductions in staffing and building space. Regulators (e.g., the Federal Deposit and Insurance Corp.), when convinced of the relative safety of remote transactions, developed policies that enhanced the use of technology to facilitate online and remote finance. This confluence of value for both the consumer and industry has led to the success of remote banking services.

When this history of remote banking is compared to the adoption of HIT, some obvious similarities and differences are apparent. First, both healthcare and finance deal in very sensitive information. Privacy and security are essential to success in either area. Consumers will leave a system in which their important personal information is not secure or private. Although some may argue that personal health information is more sensitive than financial data, no one would dispute that financial information must be secure and private. Therefore, it is not the type of information per se that is inhibiting HIT adoption. There is and should be more caution in using HIT because of safety in a health context, although much of the technology in current use, such as EHRs, have not been evaluated for efficacy (6).

There are clear regulatory differences between the healthcare and financial industry that affect adoption of technology. In finance, the regulatory framework for remote banking was developed to support an electronic approach. That same type of framework is currently under development for health. For instance, the mobile health (mHealth) guidance on the regulation of mobile apps from the Food and Drug Administration was released in September 2013 (http://www.fda.gov/downloads/MedicalDevices/.../UCM263366.pdf). In addition, the Office of the National Coordinator of Health Information Technology (ONC) has been continuously drafting guidance for healthcare agencies on managing their HIT since the HITECH act. Also, in 2012, an update was made to the Health insurance Portability and Accountability Act of 1996 regulations (HIPAA, http://www.hhs.gov/ocr/privacy) to address remote transmissions. Thus, the regulatory framework for HIT, unlike remote banking, has been developing slowly and has not kept pace with the rapid growth of technology. That said, these recent changes in the HIT regulatory arena and the healthcare landscape have created an environment in which HIT in behavioral health and healthcare in general may begin to flourish.

THE AFFORDABLE CARE ACT AND HIT

The Affordable Care Act (ACA) of 2008 was developed as a way to address the rising costs of healthcare. New policy was needed to address the spiraling costs of healthcare in the United States, paired with poor health outcomes. The United States pays more per capita for healthcare than any other developed country, but also has the poorest health outcomes per dollar spent among Western countries (7). The ACA addresses both of these issues by reducing cost and improving health through enhancing the quality of care.

At its most basic level, the goal of the ACA is to ensure that all Americans have health insurance. The legislation addresses two factors that affect health and the cost of healthcare: 1) people without insurance, as well as those who are underinsured (e.g., catastrophic coverage only), are less likely to get timely and preventive healthcare services, which leads to poorer health outcomes in the long term, and 2) because hospitals cannot refuse emergency care to people in need and the costs are not fully reimbursed (if at all), the cost of these acute care services are born by healthcare industries and passed on to consumers as increased costs to those who have insurance. Thus, insuring everyone would allow people to get care before they were very sick, thereby potentially avoiding expensive acute care services.

The difference is not only one of cost, but also the focus of care. Primary care provides services to treat immediate illness, but also offers preventive services, while emergency care is focused on acute solutions and not prevention. Indeed, a major focus of the ACA is on prevention. Health insurance is now required to include preventive services. A strong preventive approach should result in people avoiding or delaying new disease onset or ensuring that those who have illnesses do not deteriorate. This preventive focus also includes screening for diseases before they become problematic.

In the ACA model, the focus on prevention means that diseases are either prevented or morbidities for existing illness are reduced, resulting in a healthier population. Also, because the young and healthy are insured as well as those who have already developed a disease, the young should be healthier as they age, and the costs of care would be spread across an entire population, reducing the cost of health insurance.

The other main focus of the ACA is on integration of care. For example, the ACA has provided support for the integration of care and the development of medical teams. Dubbed the primary care "medical home," this model designates that all healthcare services should be coordinated by the person's primary care medical team. This team is designed to reduce duplication of services and to reduce reliance on specialty care. The medical home team can make sure patients are getting the services they need in a timely fashion without duplicating costly tests or procedures. The medical care model has also been expanded into accountable care organizations (ACOs), which are larger organizations that provide unified systems of care. Both systems are designed to better integrate and coordinate care.

The medical home approach also addresses another area of the ACA, which is patient-centered care. Instead of being passive recipients of treatment proscribed by physicians, patients now become partners in a dialogue with their healthcare providers. Recognizing that relationships between providers and patients are a key factor in the therapeutic relationship (8), the ACA includes provisions that allow healthcare to become more patient centered, focusing on the best care options for a person based on their goals, beliefs, and preferences. Patient-centered care includes shared decision-making, in which the patient and provider explore treatment options and decide on the plan together (9). The ACA also includes the development of the Patient-Centered Outcomes Research Institute (PCORI; http://www.pcori.org/) to support the patient-centered model of healthcare and provide needed research on comparative effectiveness that will support better joint decisions.

In addition to restructuring healthcare services, the ACA has also begun to institute financial reform, including recent demonstration projects for payment reform by the Center for Medicaid and Medicare Services (CMS). As one of the country's largest healthcare insurers, CMS is working with ACOs throughout the country to explore new ways to pay for healthcare. In the past, payment was based on a fee-for-service model in which providers were paid by the procedure or visit, regardless of the outcome. Current work focuses on a bundled payment approach in which organizations are paid a set rate for a problem and, if they can treat it successfully for less than the cost estimated, they share in the surplus. This model gives them incentives to reduce costly and less efficacious treatments and to be innovative in their provision of care. Also, because evidenced-based treatments should be the most effective, the bundled payment approach supports better use of the science in treatment decisions.

The ACA also requires new insurance coverage to include treatment for mental health and substance use disorders, as well as to extend parity for substance use disorders and mental health treatment. Table 21.1 highlights the expected increases in

TABLE 21.1. INCREASES IN INSURED AMERICANS AND THOSE WHO GAIN
BEHAVIORAL HEALTH INSURANCE, OR SUBSTANCE USE DISORDER AND
MENTAL ILLNESS BENEFITS WITH PARITY TO GENERAL HEALTHCARE

	Individuals who will gain mental health, substance use disorder, or both benefits under the Affordable Care Act, including federal parity protections	Individuals with existing mental health and substance use disorder benefits who will benefit from federal parity protections	Total individuals who **will** benefit from federal parity protections as a result of the Affordable Care Act
Individuals currently with insurance plans	5.1 million	30.4 million	35.5 million
Individuals currently uninsured	27 million	n/a	27 million
Total	**32.1 million**	**30.4 million**	**62.5 million**

Adapted from http://aspe.hhs.gov/health/reports/2013/mental/rb_mental.cfm.

insured individuals with the ACA, as well as the numbers who will gain parity for mental health and substance abuse treatment. These newly insured individuals will be able to get care for their behavioral health needs and, ideally, see a positive health spiral.

The efforts to reduce cost through prevention and integration of service, as well as increasing insurance coverage for behavioral health, have created a perfect storm for substance abuse and mental health treatment in the 21st century. This is because medical teams will screen patients for common problems, including mental health and substance use. Because patients have insurance that includes behavioral health, patients can then be treated before their problems develop into disorders that disrupt their lives. Further, because care is integrated and outcomes rather than services are incentivized, the whole team is involved in ensuring that the patient is improving and that normal functioning is restored. In the past, specialty care like behavioral health was provided outside of the general system of care; primary care clinicians might never have known that a patient was seeking treatment for mental health or substance use. The ACA creates a system in which the entire team, including the patient, is accountable for care. For behavioral health, this means that timely screening and care are facilitated and that mental health and substance use treatment are members of the medical team. It also means that

substance and mental health issues, which commonly co-occur with other health problems, will now be seen as an essential part of helping a patient to get healthy.

CHALLENGES FOR HIT ADOPTION IN BEHAVIORAL HEALTH
Ineligible Providers

Despite the potential for the ACA and HIT to positively affect behavioral health, adoption of technology in these areas has not advanced as quickly as in general healthcare (1,8). Recent work commissioned by the Secretary of the Department of Health and Human Services found in a 2012 study of HIT that 21% of community behavioral health organizations have EHRs at all of their sites, while 65% of respondents reported having adopted some form of an EHR at least at some of their sites. Importantly, only 2% of responding community behavioral health organizations reported adopting technology that could meet the base requirements of the HITECH's standards for the EHR Incentive Program for general healthcare (3). Reasons for the low rate of adoption are complex, but the identification of behavioral health as ineligible providers for EHR incentives, the status of behavioral health as primarily a specialty care service, the privacy and security concerns in substance abuse and mental health treatment, and the lack of evidence-based work in HIT for behavioral health all play a role. Each one of these topics is addressed below.

When the HITECH Act was developed, behavioral health practitioners were deemed ineligible providers (i.e., behavioral health providers are not eligible for the EHR adoption incentives developed in the HITEC Act). Ineligible providers were those outside of the general healthcare system, such as behavioral health, long-term care, and residential facilities, who provide a range of services and who would face undue burdens setting up an EHR. Further, the needs of many of the ineligible providers were not well accommodated within commercially available EHR systems. Although behavioral health was not pushed to adopt an EHR, it also did not qualify for incentives associated with meaningful use of EHRs. It is important to note that this does not mean that behavioral health would not benefit from these incentives or that information exchange would not enhance coordination and benefit the populations served by the ineligible providers. In fact, behavioral health providers' use of EHRs within hospitals or general healthcare settings was encouraged (3). Significant efforts through the Substance Abuse and Mental Health Services Administration (SAMHSA) and the National Council for Community Behavioral Healthcare have identified opportunities to advance data exchange on behalf of behavioral health providers, and new standards have been developed. In 2012, SAMHSA directed $23 million toward development of a HIT infrastructure and the use of technology by behavioral health providers.

This work is currently being piloted for electronic exchange of health information that is subject to the increased privacy protections of 42 CFR Part II. As noted earlier, behavioral health offers some special challenges for HIT because of the strictures of this legislation. These regulations limit the exchange of behavioral health data in addition to the requirements of HIPAA. Although this protection is in support of patients, the lack of customizable privacy settings to electronically exchange data creates disincentives for providers to work within an EHR system (3). Recent research undertaken by the Secretary of Health and Human Services about HIT adoption in ineligible providers, such as behavioral health, suggests ways to incentivize growth in this area and to reduce some of the financial and technical burdens

(3). It is unclear now whether these findings will drive new policy.

Specialty Care

Behavioral health is traditionally a specialty care service and not integrated into the larger healthcare system. This lack of integration results in a limited push to share information and integrate and coordinate care. Further, research suggests that mental health providers are less comfortable with technology, in general, than other healthcare practitioners. Thus, the value of technology in the view of providers may be limited and may not justify the cost and potential risk associated with HIT adoption (3). Further, if providers do not value the technology, they may assume that patients are also not interested in utilizing these tools. With a limited research base for HIT in behavioral health (10), the value of technology for the support and provision of practice and treatment may not be clear.

Privacy and Security

Privacy and security are also frequently cited as reasons for behavioral health non-adoption of HIT, as well as for not integrating with primary care and other specialties. As noted earlier, the bar for confidentiality is higher in substance abuse practice than in other areas of healthcare. Thus, providers are duly concerned that, by utilizing technology, they put themselves and their patients at risk. Similar to the world of finance, behavioral health will need to operate within standards that reduce these risks and not only support the use of technology to improve health outcomes but also appropriately protect patient information. While security and privacy will likely always be an issue in a technological world, these are areas of dynamic research growth, and, solutions to these issues are currently being tested and implemented.

Evidence

The full promise of technology has not yet been demonstrated empirically (4,5,11). Thus, we do not have the research findings available currently to demonstrate that HIT is advantageous. In fact, in the general area of IT, there is a well-known paradox showing that growth in computing capabilities was not initially coupled with increased productivity (11). Instead, they require a retooling of the system to realize the value of the technologies. Healthcare in general, and behavioral health in particular, are likely a case where we will need to invest in rethinking and creating user-centered systems—that is, not just make paper materials electronic or code in-person activities into code. Instead, we will need to develop systems that address challenges that healthcare systems, providers, and patients face and develop technological solutions to address the challenges.

Despite these challenges, the empirical literature for behavioral health HIT is growing rapidly, some of which is described within this book. That said, even when we know that an HIT technology is efficacious for improving health in one domain, we do not yet have the effectiveness or comparative data to show when, where, or with whom HIT works best. Future research will need to focus on conventional research to assess efficacy (e.g., randomized control trials). It will also need to include more fundamental research on how patients interact with their technology, how they best understand and utilize data, and how we can best monitor health without raising privacy concerns or creating burden.

These challenges to the adoption of HIT in behavioral health are vexing. Current efforts are underway and will soon begin addressing some of the challenges highlighted here. For instance, SAMHSA's work to develop a behavioral health EHR system may make adoption in smaller clinics feasible. In the privacy and research areas, studies are underway to provide an evidence base for enabling secure and effective use of HIT in behavioral health.

FUTURE DIRECTIONS: USING TECHNOLOGIES TO INFORM POLICIES TO PROMOTE BEHAVIORAL HEALTH

Setting policy is one of the most important societal decisions. It should be, as much as possible, based on our best evidence. In order to optimize outcomes, the policy-setting process should be based on the likely outcomes resulting from alternative policy adoption. Thus, when evaluating various alternatives, it would be helpful to know which combination has the best chance of achieving desired outcomes while keeping costs in check and minimizing undesirable consequences. Optimally, the evidence-based approach requires

quantification of many of the concepts that until now have been the domain of subjective or indirect assessment. New methods of evaluation have already begun to influence data gathering, including the use of technologies for unobtrusive monitoring (12), data collection from new types of sensors, sources based on localization and environmental context (13), and sophisticated algorithms and modeling for inference and prediction. New methods based on *big data* and their utilization are likely to revamp the healthcare delivery landscape and will require transformative change in the way that policies are determined and implemented.

Evidence-based policy brings with it both advantages and challenges. Because of technology-based data collection, one important advantage is that the future policymakers will be able to get relatively rapid feedback regarding the effects of their policies. Moreover, algorithms and computational models based on the collected data to forecast plausible scenarios will help inform policymakers anticipate the effects of their decisions. Effective data gathering should allow one to assess a variety of policy interventions, such as traveling restrictions during epidemics (14) and the labeling of products (e.g., cigarette packages [15]), in near real time instead of waiting years to indirectly assess the data. The development of these computational models and corresponding algorithms that will enable these evaluations will require a fundamental scientific basis to enhance their accuracy. An example of this approach is the use of many of the consumer monitors for assessing behavior. Although they provide information to consumers, research is required to find out whether they are reliable, valid, or useful. Thus, if a bike lane is being added in a community to enhance physical activity and policymakers want to use data from consumer physical activity monitors, for example, accelerometer-based monitors, to quantify outcomes, they will need to know whether the data being collected track cycling activity. It may be that accelerometers are sufficiently accurate for walking and running, but do not adequately capture cycling. Rapid advances in technology will also require responses on the part of various policy-setting governmental organizations, such as the ONC and the Food and Drug Administration, to ensure that data collection is not only valid but also used appropriately in a health context. All of this will require quantification of a variety of aspects of human behavior and development of the scientific basis for informing policy-making decisions. These issues are addressed in more detail next.

Monitoring

As noted earlier, sensor technologies, especially mHealth technologies, now permit researchers and healthcare workers to unobtrusively capture aspects of individuals' health states, vital signs, and aspects of behaviors. Without much additional work, mHealth technologies based on current smartphone technology can enable frequent and/or continuous sampling of a variety of behavior-related data, such as location tracking (GPS), accelerometry (estimating energy expenditure), speech recognition (health state derived from speech signal and patterns), and other physical interactions with the devices (see reference 12 for additional possibilities). These data, combined with appropriate inference algorithms, can potentially deliver new behavioral metrics and support the development of behavioral phenotypes. As such, these data may enable researchers to connect the vast genomic data to their health, clinical, and behavioral consequences. In behavioral healthcare practice, these data will provide a baseline for each individual and, as such, provide insights into the evolution of health states over time, detecting early changes due to onset of disease and estimating the slow decline in various physical and cognitive capabilities resulting from aging. Frequent sampling of a variety of variables can also provide information about the variability in the behavioral metrics that has not been possible to date (16).

Real-Time Assessment and Intervention

There is also experimental evidence indicating that asking individuals about their states and activities close in time to the occurrence of the events of interest is significantly more accurate than posing the same questions later (17–19). This relatively recent paradigm is termed ecological momentary assessment (EMA [18]) and is clearly easier to implement within the mHealth technology than with other more traditional communication technologies such as wired telephony. In fact, mHealth can be far more effective because it may be possible to use sensing and interpretation of the individual's context to make the assessment at the most appropriate times. In a similar way, ecological momentary intervention (EMI) can be made most effective if the time of the intervention is appropriately synchronized with the events that require behavioral modification. It would be reasonable to conjecture that using technology to intervene at the very moment an individual is likely to reach for a substance, in conjunction with motivational interviewing, is likely to be much more effective than motivational interviewing alone. The event-based sampling and interventions in mHealth are relatively recent advances and will require further scientific and engineering development to enable model-based optimization. By the same token, policies concerning the data collected via EMA and intervention will require the development of the scientific foundations for these approaches.

Social Networks Enhanced by Social Media

Another transformative consequence of changes in information technologies and their implementation is the creation and support of active social networks that are accessible anywhere, any time, and by anyone. The ability to connect and communicate in this manner provides the capability of rapid distribution of information, warnings, and feedback. These capabilities also provide the opportunity for real-time intervention in the form of social support and virtual competitive scenarios. In behavioral health, this can mean that patients and providers receive information when it is most needed. Although this has great potential benefit, the science of how to best use information, and when, is needed to help develop appropriate policies.

At the same time, these technologies can be used to distribute misinformation and spread rapidly a variety of rumors. Online social networks, without careful design, and by their nature can present challenges with respect to privacy and security for patients and their families. Estimation and prediction of the possible implications of these systems need to be addressed scientifically and by implementation of new policies. This is not a trivial task. Early understanding of potential policy issues will be critical in reducing risk, such as bullying, spreading rumors, and social controls.

Gaming

Concurrently with the development of IT, we have experienced an exponential explosion in gaming. Numerous types of games exist, in various formats and on various platforms, which were made possible by advances in game technology and design. Although most efforts in game development, implementation, and distribution have been focused on entertainment, there significant efforts have been made to apply gaming in education, health assessment, and patient empowerment and rehabilitation (20,21). The games in the latter category have been referred to as "serious" games or games for impact and are currently the subject of intensive research and development.

Although there is no unanimous agreement regarding the effectiveness of serious computer games and gaming for healthcare and education, there is no question that the population of players of these games is significant and that game playing now penetrates all age groups, including elders. Computer games thus have the potential to contribute in an important way to the continuous, unobtrusive assessment and remediation of a variety of functions, both cognitive and physical. There is agreement that players improve in playing the games, but the question of whether these improvements generalize to other activities has not yet been answered (22). A plausible hypothesis is that one of the reasons for the inconsistent results is the lack of a sufficiently rigorous theoretical understanding of how to map game performance to the underlying cognitive and sensory-motor processes. As a result, the games under investigation thus far may not exercise the appropriate underlying processes and set of skills. Research is needed to develop more rigorous designs and analytic frameworks for evaluating computer games for reporting health outcomes. If successful, gaming may become an important therapeutic component and could become a readily scalable intervention.

Big Data and Computational Modeling

As noted earlier, one feature of health technology is the potential for frequent or continuous monitoring of a variety of behavioral, physiological, and environmental variables. This monitoring is beginning to generate unprecedented amounts of data. In this respect, HIT parallels the developments of data gathering in other areas, resulting in a similar explosion of available data from a variety of sources including physical sensors, genomic data, earth observation systems, EHRs, users browsing the Web, and so on. This exponential increase in the available data is challenging our ability to analyze them with the current approaches and algorithms and has stimulated the development of a new area called "big data." *Big data* is a term used to describe the challenges of storing, transferring, and analyzing large, complex datasets (23). One of the key promises of big data is that the data mining of large data sets, without any prior hypotheses, will enable discoveries of relationships among the many observed and measured variables (24). Although this may be a successful approach in a small number of cases, in most situations it is necessary to have an explicit starting hypothesis that governs the choice of features and variables to be used in the data mining analysis or to use data mining as an exploratory science tool for extracting possible hypotheses (25). The extracted relationships should be formally evaluated and, if possible, tested experimentally. It is important to note that the data-mining framework for finding new relationships, including the choice of the variables, features, and data-mining algorithms, constitutes a data-driven computational model of the underlying processes. A careful analysis of the results is also necessary in order to avoid erroneous conclusions resulting from spurious correlations caused by latent variables (25).

Personalized Treatment Based on the Full Factors Affecting Behavioral Health

One of the goals of the HIT is to enable person-centered, "precision" care by tailoring diagnostics, therapeutics, as well as proactive care to the characteristics of each individual, even prior to them getting sick. Achieving this goal requires relatively complete personal background data and information. Ideally, this background information could be compiled in the form of a computational model. The model could be used to estimate the person's response to a therapeutic intervention. This could be seen as analogous to X-ray or MRI images from the target individual that a surgeon would use to plan surgery; the surgeon would not use an image averaged over a set of patients. This information can be thought of as an extension of the EHR and, as such, it is sensitive and would require careful considerations with respect to privacy and security. It also requires careful scientific validation so that intervention planning can move from assessment and treatment based on averages to a health plan that is developed and tailored for the individual.

CONCLUSIONS

It is clear that the future of HIT in behavioral health is wide open. Changes in the ACA and recent work in EHRs and mHealth suggest great potential in this area. These issues also highlight the case for evidence-based policy-making whereby an important subset of this evidence will be derived from a variety of sources including EHRs, ecological observations and mHealth applications. These data should be used to better support screening, diagnosis, and treatment, as well as methods for enhancing the use of HIT by behavioral health practitioners. The ability to use large amounts of data to inform policy-making, however, will require better understanding of the relationship between the metrics of interest pertaining to the physical, physiological, and behavioral targets of interest. In this manner, HIT will be an integral and essential component of evidence-based behavioral health policy-making processes.

ACKNOWLEDGMENTS

The views expressed in this article are those of the authors and do not necessarily reflect the position or policy of the U.S. National Institutes of Health or any other author-affiliated organizations.

REFERENCES

1. Blumenthal D. Launching HITECH. *New England Journal of Medicine* 2010; 362:382–385.
2. Druss BG, Dimitropoulos L. Advancing the adoption, integration and testing of technological advancements within existing care systems. *General Hospital Psychiatry* 2013; 35:345–348.
3. Harvell J, Dougherty M, Millenson M, Williams M. EHR payment incentives for providers ineligible for payment incentives and other funding study. Washington, DC: Office of the Assistant Secretary for Planning and Evaluation (HHS), Office of Disability, Aging, and Long-Term Care Policy; 2013.
4. Steinhubl SR, Muse ED, Topol EJ. Can mobile health technologies transform health care? *Journal of the American Medical Association* 2013; 310:2395–2396.
5. Kumar S, Nilsen WJ, Abernethy A, Atienza A, Patrick K, Pavel M, et al. Mobile health technology evaluation: The mHealth evidence workshop. *American Journal of Preventive Medicine* 2013; 45:228–236.
6. Kellermann AL, Jones SS. What it will take to achieve the as-yet-unfulfilled promises of health information technology. *Health Affairs* 2013; 32(1):63–68.
7. Woolf SF, Aron L (eds.). *Panel on Understanding Cross-National Health Differences Among High-Income Countries* (U.S. Health in International Perspective: Shorter Lives, Poorer Health). Washington, DC; 2013.
8. Strupp HH, Hadley SW. Specific vs. nonspecific factors in psychotherapy. A controlled study of outcome. *Archives of General Psychiatry* 1979;36:1125–1136.
9. Brody DS. The patient's role in clinical decision-making. *Annals of Internal Medicine* 1980; 93:718–722.
10. Chambers DA, Haim A, Mullican CA, Stirratt M. Health information technology and mental health services research: a path forward. *General Hospital Psychiatry* 2013; 35:329–331.
11. Jones SS, Heaton PS, Rudin RS, Schneider EC. Unraveling the IT productivity paradox—lessons for health care. *New England Journal of Medicine* 2012; 366: 2243–2245.
12. Kumar S, Nilsen WJ, Pavel M, Srivastava M. Mobile health: Revolutionizing healthcare through transdisciplinary research in computing. *Computing* 2013; (January): 28–35.
13. Saranummi N, Spruijt-Metz D, Intille S, Korhonen I, Nilsen WJ, Pave M. Moving the science of behavioral change into the 21st century. *IEEE Pulse* 2013;4(5):23–24.
14. Nicolaides C, Cueto-Felgueroso L, Juanes R. The price of anarchy in mobility-driven contagion dynamics. *Journal of the Royal Society Interface* 2013; 10:1742–5662.
15. Hammond D, Fong GT, McNeill A, Borland R, Cummings KM. Effectiveness of cigarette warning labels in informing smokers about the risks of smoking: Findings from the International Tobacco Control (ITC) Four Country Survey. *Tobacco Control* 2006; 15(s3):19–25, 2006.
16. Hsieh C-K, Tangmunarunkit H, Alquaddoomi F, Jenkins J, Kang J, Ketcham C, et al. Lifestreams: A modular sense-making toolset for identifying important patterns from everyday life. Presented at ACM Sensys, November 12–14, 2013, Rome, Italy.
17. Moskowitz DS, Young SN. Ecological momentary assessment: What it is and why it is a method of the

future in clinical psychopharmacology. *Journal of Psychiatry & Neuroscience* 2006; 31:13–20.

18. Stone A, Shiffman S. Ecological momentary assessment (EMA) in behavorial medicine. *Annals of Behavioral Medicine* 1994; 16:199–202.

19. Wheeler L, Reis HT. Self-recording of everyday life events: Origins, types, and uses. *Journal of Personality* 1001; 59:339–354.

20. Jimison HB, Pavel M, Bissell P, McKanna J. A framework for cognitive monitoring using computer game interactions. *Studies in Health Technology Information* 2007; 129:1073–1077.

21. Mahncke HW, Bronstone A, Merzenich MM. Brain plasticity and functional losses in the aged: scientific bases for a novel intervention. *Progress in Brain Research* 2006; 157:81–109.

22. Adams SA. Use of "serious health games" in health care: A review. *Studies Health Technology and Informatics* 2010; 157:160–162.

23. Hilbert M. (2013, April 12). Big data for development: From information to knowledge societies. 2013 (April 12). Retrieved from https://papers.ssrn.com/sol3/papers.cfm?abstract_id=2205145.2

24. Anderson C. The end of theory: The data deluge makes the scientific method obsolete. *Wired Magazine* 2008; 16. Retrieved from http://archive.wired.com/science/discoveries/magazine/16-07/pb_theory

25. M. Graham. Big data and the end of theory? 2012. Retrieved from http://www.theguardian.com/news/datablog/2012/mar/09/big-data-theory

22

Envisioning the Future

Transformation of Healthcare Systems via Technology

LISA A. MARSCH

THE PROMISE OF TECHNOLOGY IN HEALTHCARE

Overview of the Digital Landscape

The digital landscape of Internet and mobile technologies has transformed our society, including in areas of finance, retail, travel, and social relations. By leveraging these technologies, transactions in these sectors can be conducted remotely, securely, and conveniently. These technologies similarly offer tremendous promise for transforming healthcare. They can enable entirely new models of healthcare service delivery both within and outside of formal systems of care, while substantially increasing the quality and reach of care and reducing costs.

Internet access has been rapidly increasing around the world (1) and offers great promise for promoting widespread access at a population level to effective preventative health and behavior change tools. Over 85% of Americans currently have Internet access, an increase from 14% in 1995 (2). And more than half of all Americans report having searched online for health information in the past year (3).

Mobile health (mHealth), defined by the Global Observatory for eHealth within the World Health Organization as "medical and public health practice supported by mobile devices," has particularly exploded in recent years. Mobile health tools include mobile phones, patient monitoring devices, wireless devices, the use of short messaging service (SMS), as well as more complex functions, such as global positioning systems (GPS), 4G systems, and Bluetooth technology (4). The introduction of smartphones in particular has taken the mHealth landscape to an unprecedented level. The tremendous computing capability and connectivity of smartphones, along with the widespread penetration of wireless networks, allows for Internet access anytime and anywhere. And, access to smartphones worldwide is striking. There are over 1.4 billion smartphones in the world, and smartphone access is expected to triple globally to 5.6 billion by 2019 (5).

Behavioral health technologies embedded in Web and mobile devices offer considerable promise to deliver engaging and effective self-monitoring and self-management interventions to promote health and wellness (including preventative health and behavior change). Interactive informational and communication technologies can provide lifestyle education, skills training, and therapeutic support for individuals, families, and clinicians, and they can engage consumers and a care network of their choosing in shared decision-making through use of electronic decision support systems and social media. They can also expand the self-monitoring and coping strategies of patients and the reach of clinicians (6).

Although a great deal of research and development work is being conducted in the mobile medical device space (7), this chapter (as well as this book) largely focuses on the role that technology can play as part of therapeutic tools targeting behavioral health and wellness. Behavioral health includes a constellation of issues including substance use, mental health, medication-taking, and physical inactivity, among others.

State of the Science of Behavioral Health Technology

Harnessing technology in healthcare delivery has also been shown to increase the quality, reach, and personalization of care at an extraordinary rate, and in a manner that is cost-effective (8–11). Prior work has shown that training clinicians to deliver evidence-based behavioral treatment is time consuming, clinicians infrequently deliver evidence-based treatments with fidelity, and intensive ongoing training and supervision are needed. Technology-based tools can ensure the fidelity of intervention delivery, thus assuring the provision of empirically supported treatment.

Technology can also overcome some of the striking disparities in treatment access and treatment quality evident in healthcare settings across the United States and elsewhere around the world. These disparities are evident along racial and ethnic lines, socioeconomic status, and geographic settings, among other factors (12). These lines can become increasingly blurred and disparities reduced via the use of technology. Importantly, if a portion of clinician-delivered care is instead delivered via technology, clinical programs can have a much larger service capacity (ability to treat a much larger number of clients with the same number of behavioral health clinicians). This increase in service capacity has considerable public health significance given the large unmet health needs of persons with behavioral disorders, including wait lists for behavioral healthcare. Additionally, by having on-demand access to "just-in-time" therapeutic support via electronic devices, individuals can prevent costly escalation of health-related problems and unnecessary healthcare utilization. Leveraging technology in this way offers great promise for enabling entirely new models for delivery of science-based approaches to addressing behavioral health (13).

The Critical Role of Behavioral Health in Health and Wellness

Based on the promising data from scientific research summarized above, the application of technology to behavioral health promises to have a marked impact at a population level, for several reasons. First, mental health and substance use disorders are common in the United States In any given year, roughly 1 in 4 adults in the United States is diagnosable with one or more mental health disorders (14), and almost 1 in 10 adults in the United States is diagnosable with one or more substance use disorders (15). Unfortunately, the majority of these individuals (as high as 90% by

some estimates) do not receive treatment for their behavioral health disorders—perhaps because they do not seek treatment for behavioral health problems when they are engaged in the healthcare system and/or do not have access to behavioral health services.

Second, individuals with one or more behavioral health disorders are among the most frequent and costliest utilizers of healthcare services. These individuals typically have little social support, and half of those with multiple behavioral health disorders are hospitalized in a given year. The overall annual economic cost for mental health disorders is estimated at over $300 billion (a dramatic increase from approximately $35 billion in 1996). According to the World Health Organization, mental illness accounts for more disability in developed countries than any other group of illnesses, including cancer and heart disease (16).

Third, behavioral health disorders are also highly prevalent among clinical populations with a wide array of chronic diseases. An estimated 133 million Americans, representing 45% of the U.S. population, are living with one or more chronic diseases. Over 75% of all healthcare costs in the U.S. are due to the management of chronic disease—estimated at about $1.3 trillion annually in 2007 and projected to increase to $4.2 trillion by 2023 (17).

About 34 million American adults, or 17% of the adult population, have co-occurring substance use and/or mental health disorders along with chronic physical health diseases (18); such co-occurrence greatly impairs the effective management of chronic illness. For example, studies have shown that individuals with diabetes have a 40–72% incidence of depression. These behavioral health issues typically complicate and significantly worsen the course and treatment of chronic medical illnesses. Co-occurring chronic illness and behavioral health problems are associated with lower quality of life, poorer response to treatment, worse medical and psychiatric outcomes, higher mortality, and higher costs of care. For example, when depression co-occurs with diabetes, healthcare costs increase by about 50–75% relative to the cost of diabetes care in the absence of depression (19). Similar patterns have been observed when mental health disorders and substance use (e.g., heavy alcohol use, smoking, nonmedical use of prescription drugs, which is considered an epidemic in the U.S.) co-occur with many other chronic diseases, including cardiovascular disease, cancer, and pulmonary disease (20).

Thus, a central focus within behavioral health is the potential to impact the entire spectrum of health and wellness. Using technology to promote widespread reach of effective behavioral healthcare to target prevalent and costly behavioral health problems could have a substantial public health impact.

OPPORTUNITIES FOR SCALING UP SCIENCE-INFORMED TECHNOLOGY TO TRANSFORM HEALTHCARE SYSTEMS

Despite the explosion of interest and promising results to date from leveraging technology in healthcare delivery, much work is still needed in order to effectively "scale-up" the use of science-based technology to transform health and healthcare systems and have a marked public health impact. These opportunities exist in the realms of technology development, evaluation, and implementation. Each of these categories will be discussed here in turn.

Opportunities in Technology Development
Clinical Considerations

Technological devices are being developed at staggering rates. Likewise, innovations in processing speed, memory capacity, transistors on integrated circuits, and sensors are all being developed at exponential rates (21). In this arena of rapid innovation, it is all too easy to become intrigued by the technological gadget of the moment as a driving factor in how technology is applied to areas of health and wellness. However, to stay true to a systematic and organized clinical research agenda for harnessing technology for health applications, it is key that clinical goals instruct how technology is used. That is, the clinical problem that needs solving (e.g., increased personalization of care, access to care, and/or care coordination) should drive the use of technology. A key focus should be on identifying the active ingredients of technology-based tools in solving a clinical challenge—active ingredients that persist despite changes in the technology of the moment. This is not to say that emerging technologies will not

enable new innovations in the health space when new tools and functionality are possible. Rather, in order to enable technology-based innovation that promises to transform health and healthcare, clinical considerations should centrally drive use of the tools and evolution of technology and health.

Consumer-Centric Development

A key benefit of technology-based therapeutic tools is their ability to enable greater consumer-centric models of health promotion and healthcare. Consumer-facing, technology-based tools have been shown to be most effective when consumers are the main influence in the development of the tools (including their functionality and content), to ensure that they bring the greatest value to the targeted consumer audience (22–24). Additionally and importantly, technology-based tools provide unprecedented levels of consumer control over their own health and self-management. That is, these tools enable greater consumer choice and access to care, greater engagement in their own health, and a greater opportunity to engage an extended support network. By leveraging social monitoring and social reinforcement tools (e.g., sharing progress toward goals with an extended support network), consumers may share information about themselves and receive support in reaching their goals in real time from an extended support network that may include significant others and family members, virtual (and optionally anonymous) support communities, and/or clinicians of various types (when integrated into systems of care). Although scientific research is rapidly evolving to inform optimal ways to engage consumers and their support systems via technology-based approaches, there is tremendous opportunity to expand the scope of rigorous research to understand how to best develop systems that have a priority focus on consumer values, needs, and preferences.

Mechanisms of Behavior Change

A growing body of scientific research has demonstrated that a variety of technology-based tools can be acceptable to an array of target audiences, effective in promoting behavior change, and feasible to implement in many contexts. However, limited research has focused on the putative mechanisms of behavior change from these tools (25). An assessment of the mechanisms of behavior change allows one to go beyond understanding that a change has occurred to understanding *how* it has occurred (see Chapter 13, this volume). Technology-based interventions may work by increasing an array of personal and social resources (e.g., coping skills, social reinforcement) and decreasing factors related to self-defeating behavior (e.g., ineffective problem solving). An understanding of the mechanisms of behavior change from technology-based interventions is key to replicating intervention effects and to understanding scenarios where effects are not observed (e.g., when changes in key mechanisms of change were not evident). It is also important to understand if similar mechanisms of change drive effects across an array of technology-based therapeutic tools, thereby illuminating the criteria that need to be achieved for a tool to be effective (when key mechanisms of change are impacted). This information is critical for implementation efforts to help ensure that mechanisms of behavior change are present and affected in the way in which technology-based therapeutic tools are deployed, even when specific devices and technologies change over time.

Breaking Down Disorder-Specific Approaches to Development of Technology-Based Health Systems

Although there has been a recent explosion of interest in leveraging technology in healthcare delivery, much of this work has been siloed, typically focusing on one disease or disorder at a time. For example, in the behavioral health arena, technology-based interventions have typically focused on a single behavioral health topic at a time (e.g., depression, addiction, eating disorders, exercise). Additionally, very few tools in the behavioral health arena are integrated with the many physical health considerations that frequently co-occur and intersect in important ways with behavioral health (e.g., chronic disease management).

This trend is likely driven by many factors, including the way funding streams are often structured in focused priority areas and the way in which developers of technology-based therapeutic tools typically have specialized training in a focused area of health and wellness. Unfortunately, this siloed approach does not fully realize the ability of technology to deliver integrated and personalized care that is responsive to whatever combination of needs and preferences each individual user of the technology may have. In addition, the current model does not consider the high rate at which various types of health-related problems and needs cluster together and impact one another.

To better realize the potential of technology to transform the space of health and wellness, it is important to create and systematically evaluate systems that are not diagnosis- or disorder-specific but rather enable integrated care for any combination of health-related needs and preferences. An integrated, personalized suite of technology-based therapeutic tools may address diverse issues, including chronic physical diseases, mental health, critical care, and health and wellness promotion. An integrated system would provide a large offering of content and tools for different populations, and each end user of the system could access the subset of content relevant to their experience and goals. Research has repeatedly shown that science-based approaches to effectively initiating and maintaining health behavior transcend many areas of health and wellness and are common across a wide array of health conditions (26). Because the need to alter health-related behavior (e.g., smoking, depression, medication adherence, diet, exercise) is ubiquitous across medicine, and because the principles of effective health behavior change are common across health conditions (and include increasing personal and social resources that support and reinforce healthy behavior and promote reduction of self-defeating behavior), an integrated, personalized technology-based therapeutic system can have broad applicability to a wide array of health conditions.

Deployment of technology-based tools focused on integrated behavioral and physical health can meet a tremendous need as the healthcare delivery requirements of the Affordable Care Act (ACA) are implemented nationally in the United States over the next few years. There are a number of reasons why this is the case. First, the ACA *requires* that healthcare settings, which have traditionally focused on the treatment of physical health conditions, must now offer care for substance use and mental health disorders. Second, within the emerging accountable healthcare model, provider groups can no longer refuse to treat or transfer elsewhere individuals with substance use and/ or mental health disorders but must cover the entirety of their care (27). Third, the ACA will expand Medicaid eligibility and provide coverage for the first time to an estimated 32 million individuals who are currently uninsured—many of whom are poor and unemployed, with disproportionately high mental health and substance use problems (28).

As a result of this confluence of factors, there is a tremendous and growing need to care for behavioral health problems in healthcare settings that do not currently have sufficient capacity to meet this need. This creates an unprecedented opportunity to offer cost-effective, integrated technology-based solutions.

Opportunities in Evaluation
Opportunities in Measurement, Experimental Design, and Data Analytics

Emerging methodologies and analytic tools may be particularly useful in understanding the impact of technology-based tools on health behavior. Although traditional randomized, controlled trials offer considerable scientific rigor in evaluation, the time needed to produce conclusive results regarding the effectiveness of technology-based interventions with this research design is typically quite lengthy. Additionally, randomized, controlled trials often do not allow for a clear understanding of the specific components of multicomponent, technology-based therapeutic tools that produce observed effects. Further, they typically do not allow for modification of the intervention during the life of the trial for persons who do not respond to the intervention.

Several novel and underused methodological approaches may be relevant to developing and evaluating technology-based interventions and may greatly supplement the findings from randomized, controlled trials (see Chapter 12, this volume). This may, for example, include novel applications of multiphase optimization strategy (MOST) (29), which starts with a screening phase in which randomized full or fractional factorial designs are applied to efficiently identify the most promising combinations of content and delivery. In a refining phase, intervention components showing promise in the screening phase can be examined in greater detail to determine optimal settings of each component in combination with other components

(by fitting a regression surface and finding a point that maximizes or minimizes a response of interest). Such response surface methods (30) can be useful for identifying optimal doses and combinations of intervention components (see Chapter 12 in this volume).

Another design that may be particularly relevant but has been infrequently applied in the evaluation of technology-based therapeutic tools is the sequential multiple assignment randomized trial (SMART) (29). The key feature of a SMART design is random assignment of individuals to conditions more than once during a study, based on their response to conditions experienced earlier in the study. That is, the nature or dose of an intervention can be varied over time for some participants based on rules developed in advance and depending on some characteristic of the individual, called a tailoring variable. The SMART design fits particularly well with technology-based interventions, because assessment of dynamic tailoring variables and adaptive changes to interventions in response to those variables are facilitated by the technology. This effort may lead to technology-based tools that can be readily tailored to optimally meet the needs of an individual.

Finally, given the considerable financial constraints under which many community-based treatment and other service systems operate, understanding the cost-effectiveness and, thus, the "community-friendliness" of technology-based interventions is critical, along with an understanding of their effectiveness in changing the targeted behavior (see Chapter 14, this volume). That is, although assessing the effectiveness of technology-based therapeutic tools is a critical research activity, assessing the cost-effectiveness of such interventions and the financial consequences of adopting these new therapeutic tools within various systems of care (e.g., specialty addiction or mental health treatment, criminal justice, primary care) is essential to better understanding the potential utility and adoption potential of these programs. Economic analyses can often be conducted in parallel to clinical trials and other types of experimental designs examining effectiveness. Adding an economic aim to such studies often brings little additional cost but offers promise to bring considerable additional value.

Models that Enable Ongoing Evaluation and Rapid Iteration in Real-World Implementation

As reviewed above, a number of experimental research designs can offer new and timely insights into the role of technology in healthcare. Although rigorous experimental designs are critical to identify science-informed models of care, ongoing research evaluations of real-world implementation efforts are important for understanding the ability of this approach to scale up across settings, populations, and time.

Evaluations of practical, real-world trials and demonstration projects may include the models, methods, and metrics of implementation research designed to integrate and promote sustained use of empirically supported practices in routine clinical settings (31). Implementation research leverages community engagement and community collaboration to study methods that can accelerate the dissemination and continued use of new research findings in community populations.

Implementation research goes beyond dissemination (efforts to persuade various groups to adopt an innovation), to instead prioritize the mainstreaming of an innovation within a system and ensuring its sustainability (to make it a routine part of the system). Thus, this approach not only considers a novel intervention strategy (e.g., an effective technology-based therapeutic system) but also prioritizes strategies for its successful implementation and sustained use (e.g., at the levels of the environment, organization, clinician, or client). Important outcomes from this work may include implementation outcomes (e.g., acceptability, adoption, appropriateness, cost, feasibility, fidelity, penetration, and sustainability), service outcomes (e.g., efficiency, safety, effectiveness, equity, client-centeredness, and timeliness), and client and consumer outcomes (e.g., satisfaction, symptoms, and functioning) (31,32). A comprehensive focus on both the novel service delivery model, as well as the accompanying payment model, is also critical. This approach requires that an interdisciplinary team share data in a coordinated effort, including clinicians, program administrators, health economists, finance experts, payers and technologists. Evaluating data from all such relevant stakeholders and on a wide array of dimensions will enable a much broader understanding of the optimal model for implementation and the promise of sustainability of an innovation.

In addition, deployment models in real-world systems of care should be designed to enable rapid iteration to refine the model of implementation and/or the technology-based system being deployed as needed, in response to data collected on an ongoing basis post-deployment. This means that at the launch time of a new implementation effort, the implementation team would be best served by conducting small trials, learning from errors and from opportunities to improve the innovation or deployment strategy, and then being sufficiently flexible to modify strategy in a timely manner to then expand implementation, evaluation, and iterative refinement as an ongoing process (33,34). Many experimental designs used in scientific study follow rather rigid prescriptive models for evaluation. Although these experimental models are essential for establishing rigor during a scientific process, evaluation opportunities in real-world implementation efforts allow much greater flexibility and offer the opportunity for a wealth of clinically rich data. Extending the definition of *evaluation* to encapsulate this full spectrum of measurement opportunities will broaden the scope of data available to inform the way in which technology-based therapeutic systems may bring value—informing a "business model" for transforming healthcare systems.

Evaluating Trajectories of Consumer Engagement

Consumer engagement in technology-based therapeutic tools has been identified as a key factor affecting behavior change. That is, if a technology-based therapeutic tool does not engage the end user and ensure that he or she contacts key content and functionality within the tool, the end-user will not be able to benefit from it (even if it has been shown to be highly effective).

Understanding factors that optimally drive patient engagement with technology-based tools is an important area of research. An array of research activities have focused on the use of persuasive messaging, interactive learning technologies, and multimedia elements that may enhance or detract from engagement and enhance or reduce the effectiveness of multimedia tools (35,36). Among other findings, this work has highlighted essential elements when creating functionality and content (e.g., interactivity, modularity) and indicates that combining too many entertaining multimedia elements in these systems can be distracting to end users and have a negative impact on desired outcomes (35). Furthermore, although at an early stage, other findings have demonstrated that providing incentives to individuals to engage with technology-based therapeutic interventions can increase levels of engagement. For example, monetary or prize incentives have been used to promote module completion in technology-based interventions (37) and "push reminder" systems (e.g., text prompts, e-mails) (38) have been shown to enhance engagement. Social monitoring and social reinforcement models that leverage online social networks to support and reinforce behavior change have also shown promise (39); however, the optimal way to arrange and employ social networks in technology-based therapeutic systems remains a largely unanswered and important scientific question.

An additional important and unanswered question relates to the optimal trajectories of consumer engagement with technology-based therapeutic tools. Many research teams that develop and evaluate Web- and mobile-based behavioral interventions propose that end users in some targeted clinical population (e.g., depressed persons) use the technology support system at a certain frequency (e.g., 30-minute sessions twice weekly), complete a targeted number of modules per week (e.g., two modules per session or a total of four per week), for a certain number of weeks (e.g., 8 weeks). Persons who do not use these tools as indicated by a researcher are often referred to as "partially compliant" or "non-adherent." This reported problem of "non-adherence" or "attrition" is common in evaluations of technology-based interventions for a range of health conditions, such as obesity, smoking, diabetes, and chronic pain, with a 50% attrition rate commonly reported (40–42).

Although some empirical support exists to support decisions about the optimal "dose" of such behavioral interventions for certain types of disorders (26), the optimal patterns of use of technology-based therapeutic systems remain unclear. If indeed, the goal of technology-based therapeutic tools is to aid individuals in initiating and maintaining some change in their health behavior by helping them learn new skills and learn new patterns of behavior that reduce self-defeating behaviors, it may not be the case that continual use at a regular interval is required. Rather, one important outcome of this approach may be that end

users of these systems start to develop skills and initiate new behavior patterns that then become a regular, internalized part of their behavioral repertoire. That is, the technology tools may be most useful in helping individuals reach such a point and then may be used for strategic episodic use thereafter (e.g., as reminders, boosters, "just-in-time" therapeutic support). A systematic line of research to understand optimal patterns of use with technology-based systems, focused on understanding clinical trajectories of client engagement over time, as well as the importance of regular doses of these interventions vs. strategic episodic use, is needed. A key understanding of critical mechanisms of behavior change to target (as discussed earlier) when delivering technology-based interventions will be important in this process. This information will be critical for informing deployment efforts of these systems as they are increasingly made available outside of research studies and offered within real-world settings.

Opportunities for Models of Deployment
Promoting Partnerships among Academic–Foundation–Governmental–Industry Partners

A wide array of funding agencies have supported the recent explosion of research and development in the Web- and mobile-health arena, including federal, local, and international government agencies, private foundations, corporations, and philanthropy organizations. This work has generated a wealth of information about how to best develop tools in various communities and for diverse populations, how these tools work in different contexts, and how to best implement them via various models of deployment.

However, to date, the public health impact of this work has generally been limited to relatively small and specific communities and contexts. A truly transformative approach to reforming healthcare by centrally leveraging new technologies is arguably beyond the scope of a single organization or sector. Rather, well-designed partnerships among academic, foundation, government, and industry sectors offer considerable promise for scaling up the scope and impact of this work. A partnership model that ensures that a scientific process drives the development and evaluation of technology-based systems (e.g., via academic partners) but also ensures that a sustainable and scalable infrastructure is in place for deployment (e.g., via foundation and commercial partners) and helps support policies and regulations that may facilitate successful adoption of effective technology-based systems (via government partners) offers the opportunity for health technology to have a transformative and substantive impact on the entire spectrum of health and wellness. A coordinated structure among these various entities could lead to a new level of innovation in the types of systems that are developed and accelerate their translation into practice.

Scaling Up Evaluations of Various Models of Deployment

As reviewed above, scientific research to date has demonstrated that, when embedded within models of service delivery in various healthcare systems, effective technology-based therapeutic tools can play an important role as a "clinician-extender" of care and enhance patient and organizational-level outcomes. Experimental studies have also demonstrated that when used to replace a portion of standard care, these tools (if developed and tested using scientific approaches) can often produce comparable and sometimes better outcomes than standard models of care. They can alternatively or additionally be provided directly to consumers to enhance the reach of effective therapeutic support to persons for whom current models of care are inaccessible or unacceptable.

There is tremendous opportunity to scale up this work to a population level by conducting an array of demonstration projects to evaluate various models of deployment both within and outside systems of care. One promising model is an expansion of the "clinician-extender" role of technology via a "prescription model." That is, clinicians may "prescribe" certain types of technology support systems to their patients, based on the needs and preferences of the patient. These may be tools to better manage medication adherence, blood glucose testing regimens, activity levels, or anxiety conditions. The possibilities for tools are nearly endless. They can include a wide array of topics, behavioral self-monitoring systems (via self-report and sensor-based data capture of individual behavior), as well as social monitoring and social reinforcement systems (to engage extended support networks). Provider-level endorsement of these tools within this prescription model may promote greater patient engagement with the tools and may aid providers in providing better and more expanded care of their patients. Also, by offering these tools via a prescription model, these tools can bring value without needing to interface directly into the rapidly evolving and highly complex world of interoperable electronic health records.

An additional promising model (that is not necessarily incompatible with a prescription model) is one which leverages centralized technology-support centers. As Web and mobile health tools become increasingly pervasive, they will undoubtedly be increasingly embraced within healthcare systems. However, successful integration of a technology-based care delivery model into existing models of care requires changes in the operation of the care delivery system. That is, although clinicians may wish to recommend technology-based therapeutic support tools to their clients, they may not have the core competencies to support their clients in the use of these tools. For example, as patients use technology-based, self-monitoring and self-management tools, they need some basic support in their use as well as education about privacy and security considerations when using these tools. They may also need additional levels of support beyond what the technology offers when in crisis (e.g., when they feel at risk of self-harm) or when they have an acute health need (e.g., hyperglycemia). Centralized technology-support centers could be established as a resource to any clinical program that seeks to encourage use of technology among their clients. These centers could play a variety of roles, including helping clinical programs initially set up a model for integrating technology into their workflow, providing basic education and support to clinicians and patients, and providing access to higher levels of support for managing crises and acute episodes (in a stepped-model of care). A centralized technology-support bank, which can be accessed by multiple systems of care, will prevent each clinical site from needing to obtain all requisite skill sets and core competencies in-house and can aid in larger scale adoption of technology-based tools. Additionally, such centers may be a valuable resource for individuals who access technology-based therapeutic tools outside of traditional systems of care, via direct-to-consumer models. Although a few early-stage projects have explored the promise of centralized technology support centers (including stepped models of care [43]), the effectiveness and cost-effectiveness of this model of care delivery remain largely unexplored.

Technology as Minimally Disruptive Healthcare

Individuals living with chronic illness experience not only significant burden from their illness but also considerable burden from treatment for their illness. That is, as medical testing and medical responses to illness have become increasingly sophisticated, managing multiple physician visits, tests, treatment regimens, and insurance issues places significant burden on patients. This is particularly the case when individuals are living with multiple chronic diseases, requiring the involvement of multiple specialists and often complex therapeutic regimens. This significant burden of treatment substantially contributes to patients' non-compliance with complex treatment regimens. Non-compliance can lead to worsened health states, increased healthcare costs, and challenges in relationships between providers and patients (44).

May, Montori, and Mair (45) have argued for a new model of "minimally disruptive medicine," designed to reduce the burden on patients, improve the treatment process, improve treatment outcomes, and reduce the cost of care. The central tenets of this approach include understanding the weight of the burden on patients, encouraging coordination in clinical practice, acknowledging comorbidity in clinical evidence, and prioritizing the patient's perspective to provide coordinated, "lean" or "minimally disruptive" treatment.

Technology offers an ideal means to support minimally disruptive medicine at a population level. Technology provides new opportunities for self-care that can be coordinated to respond to the entirety of needs and preferences of each individual (facilitating integrated care) and that can be provided in the privacy of their homes (reducing the need for travel to multiple specialists). It also enables systems for sharing information among providers to facilitate coordinated care. It further offers the opportunity for tracking medication taking and other treatment regimens to decrease tracking burden on patients and increase compliance with therapeutic regimens. Many exciting research possibilities exist to examine the role that technology systems may have in facilitating minimally disruptive medicine and improving treatment process and treatment outcomes while reducing the burden and cost of care.

Opportunities for Global Health

Technology offers great promise to transform models of health and healthcare globally (46,47). Although high-income countries are leading the development of mobile and Web-based health-related tools, the opportunities in low- and middle-income countries are striking. Landline technology is often absent in many low- and middle-income countries, but mobile phone penetration in these countries has exceeded that in wealthier countries. Globally, mobile phones are more accessible than clean water and sanitation.

To date, health-related mobile phone applications in low- and middle-income countries have focused on topics ranging from adherence to HIV antiretroviral therapy, identifying and tracking infectious outbreaks, remote diagnosis, and epidemiological health surveillance research. Given that most mobile phones available in these countries are not (yet) smartphones, most applications have employed voice calling, short message service (SMS), or multimedia messaging (MMS). Most of the research conducted with these applications has been composed of small, uncontrolled pilot studies. Results of this work have revealed some promising results and underscore the importance of larger scale and more systematic research and implementation efforts in these settings.

Additionally, as smartphones become increasingly affordable, smartphone access in these countries is expected to markedly increase, which may allow for new and enhanced functionality available in these contexts. Further, given that these countries often do not have the same level of highly complex, exceptionally costly and systemically problematic healthcare systems with strongly vested and resistant-to-change stakeholders as in many high-income countries (such as the United States), there is potential for effective technology-based tools to be adopted more rapidly and efficiently in low- and middle-income countries. This may create many opportunities for "reverse innovation," where innovation in the use of technology in developing countries may spread to the industrialized world (48).

CONCLUSIONS

As reviewed in this chapter, technology has transformed many sectors of our lives, and we are now on the verge of a major transformation of healthcare systems via technology. The body of research to date evaluating technology-based therapeutic tools has highlighted that, if a scientific process drives the development, evaluation, and implementation of these tools, they can enhance traditional models of care or produce outcomes that are comparable to, and sometimes better than, traditional models of care. The opportunities for deployment are considerable and include the ability for technology to increase service capacity while improving outcomes and reducing costs in a wide variety of healthcare settings as well as the ability to provide therapeutic support via entirely new models outside of formal care settings.

Although there has been rapidly growing interest in leveraging technology in healthcare delivery, much of this work has been siloed (e.g., targeting one disease or disorder at a time) and infrequently grounded in the science of health behavior, informational technologies, and implementation of empirically supported innovations.

As reviewed in this chapter, much work is still needed in the areas of technology development, evaluation, and implementation in order to effectively scale up the use of science-based technology to transform health and healthcare systems and have a substantial population-level impact. A central focus on integrated behavioral and physical health, as well as new models, metrics, and partners for development, evaluation, and implementation efforts, offers great promise for impacting the full spectrum of health and wellness. Collectively, this work can lead to entirely new models for delivering science-based and cost-effective healthcare.

REFERENCES

1. International Telecommunication Union. Statistics 2014. Retrieved from http://www.itu.int/en/ITU-D/Statistics/Pages/stat/default.aspx
2. Pew Internet & American Life Project. Trend data (adults): Internet adoption, 1995–2013. Retrieved from: http://www.pewinternet.org/Static-Pages/Trend-Data-(Adults)/Internet-Adoption.aspx
3. Fox S. Pew Internet: Health 2013 Retrieved from http://www.pewinternet.org/Commentary/2011/November/Pew-Internet-Health.aspx
4. mHealth: New horizons for health through mobile technologies: Second global survey on eHealth: Based on the findings of the second global survey on eHealth. World Health Organization, 2011.
5. Ericsson mobility report on the pulse of the networked society: Ericsson; 2013. Retrieved from http://www.ericsson.com/res/docs/2013/ericsson-mobility-report-november-2013.pdf
6. Marsch LA, Dallery J. Advances in the psychosocial treatment of addiction: the role of technology in the delivery of evidence-based psychosocial treatment. *Psychiatric Clinics of North America* 2012; 35(2):481–493.
7. Barton AJ. The regulation of mobile health applications. *BMC Medicine* 2012; 10:46.
8. Marsch LA, Ben-Zeev D. Technology-based assessments and interventions targeting psychiatric and substance use disorders: Innovations and ppportunities. *Journal of Dual Diagnosis* 2012; 8(4):259–261.
9. Marsch LA, Carroll KM, Kiluk BD. Technology-based interventions for the treatment and recovery management of substance use disorders: A JSAT special issue. *Journal of Substance Abuse Treatment* 2014; 46(1):1–4.
10. Newman MG, Szkodny LE, Llera SJ, Przeworski A. A review of technology-assisted self-help and minimal contact therapies for anxiety and depression: Is human contact necessary for therapeutic efficacy? *Clinical Psychology Review* 2011; 31(1):89–103.
11. Mohr DC, Burns MN, Schueller SM, Clarke G, Klinkman M. Behavioral intervention technologies: Evidence review and recommendations for future research in mental health. *General Hospital Psychiatry* 2013; 35(4):332–338.
12. Gibbons MC, Fleisher L, Slamon RE, Bass S, Kandadai V, Beck JR. Exploring the potential of Web 2.0 to address health disparities. *Journal of Health Communication* 2011; 16(Suppl 1):77–89.
13. Marsch LA. Leveraging technology to enhance addiction treatment and recovery. *Journal of Addictive Diseases* 2012; 31(3):313–318.
14. Substance Abuse and Mental Health Services Administration. Results from the 2012 National Survey on Drug Use and Health: Mental health findings 2013. Retrieved from http://www.samhsa.gov/data/NSDUH/2k12MH_FindingsandDetTables/2K12MHF/NSDUHmhfr2012.htm#ch2
15. Substance Abuse and Mental Health Services Administration. Results from the 2012 National Survey on Drug Use and Health: Summary

of national findings. Rockville, MD. 2013. Retrieved from http://www.samhsa.gov/data/NSDUH/2012SummNatFindDetTables/NationalFindings/NSDUHresults2012.htm#ch7

16. Thornicroft G, Tansella M. What are the arguments for community-based mental health care? 2003. Retrieved from http://www.euro.who.int/__data/assets/pdf_file/0019/74710/E82976.pdf

17. DeVol R, Bedroussian A, Charuworn A, Chatterjee A, Kim IK, Kim S, et al. An unhealth America: The economic burden of chronic disease—charting a new course to save lives and increase productivity and economic growth. Milken Institute; 2007. Retrieved from http://www.milkeninstitute.org/publications/publications.taf?function=detail&ID=38801018&cat=ResRep

18. Druss BG, Walker ER. Mental disorders and medical comorbidity. Princeton, NJ: Robert Wood Johnson Foundation; 2011. Retrieved from http://www.rwjf.org/content/dam/farm/reports/issue_briefs/2011/rwjf69438/subassets/rwjf69438_1

19. Simon GE, Katon WJ, Lin EH, Ludman E, VonKorff M, Ciechanowski P, et al. Diabetes complications and depression as predictors of health service costs. *General Hospital Psychiatry* 2005; 27(5):344–351.

20. Moussas G, Tselebis A, Karkanias A, Stamouli D, Ilias I, Bratis D, et al. A comparative study of anxiety and depression in patients with bronchial asthma, chronic obstructive pulmonary disease and tuberculosis in a general hospital of chest diseases. *Annals of General Psychiatry* 2008; 7:7.

21. Keyes RW. The impact of Moore's Law. *Solid-State Circuits Society Newsletter, IEE.* 2006; 11(5):25–27.

22. Moore SK, Guarino H, Acosta MC, Aronson ID, Marsch LA, Rosenblum A, et al. Patients as collaborators: Using focus groups and feedback sessions to develop an interactive, Web-based self-management intervention for chronic pain. *Pain Medicine* 2013; 14(11):1730–1740.

23. Hilgart MM, Ritterband LM, Thorndike FP, Kinzie MB. Using instructional design process to improve design and development of Internet interventions. *Journal of Medical Internet Research* 2012; 14(3):e89.

24. Noar SM, Benac CN, Harris MS. Does tailoring matter? Meta-analytic review of tailored print health behavior change interventions. *Psychological Bulletin* 2007; 133(4):673–693.

25. Webb TL, Joseph J, Yardley L, Michie S. Using the Internet to promote health behavior change: A systematic review and meta-analysis of the impact of theoretical basis, use of behavior change techniques, and mode of delivery on efficacy. *Journal of Medical Internet Research* 2010; 12(1):e4.

26. Ritterband LM, Thorndike FP, Cox DJ, Kovatchev BP, Gonder-Frederick LA. A behavior change model for internet interventions. *Annals of Behavioral Medicine* 2009; 38(1):18–27.

27. Substance Abuse and Mental Health Services Administration. Health care reform, overview of the Affordable Care Act. What are the implications for behavioral health? *SAMHSA News* 2010; 18(3).

28. Substance Abuse and Mental Health Services Administration. Office of Applied Studies. Substance abuse treatment need among uninsured workers. A report from the National Household Survey on Drug Use and Health. The NSDUH Report. Rockville, MD. February 4, 2010.

29. Collins LM, Murphy SA, Strecher V. The multiphase optimization strategy (MOST) and the sequential multiple assignment randomized trial (SMART): New methods for more potent eHealth interventions. *American Journal of Preventive Medicine* 2007; 32(5 Suppl):S112–S118.

30. Box GEP, Hunter WG, Hunter JS. *Statistics for Experimenters: An Introduction to Design, Data Analysis, and Model Building.* New York: Wiley; 1978.

31. Proctor EK, Landsverk J, Aarons G, Chambers D, Glisson C, Mittman B. Implementation research in mental health services: An emerging science with conceptual, methodological, and training challenges. *Administration and Policy in Mental Health* 2009; 36(1):24–34.

32. Glasgow RE, Vogt TM, Boles SM. Evaluating the public health impact of health promotion interventions: The RE-AIM framework. *American Journal of Public Health* 1999; 89(9):1322–1327.

33. Mohr DC, Cheung K, Schueller SM, Hendricks Brown C, Duan N. Continuous evaluation of evolving behavioral intervention technologies. *American Journal of Preventive Medicine* 2013; 45(4):517–523.

34. Chambers DA, Glasgow RE, Stange KC. The dynamic sustainability framework: Addressing the paradox of sustainment amid ongoing change. *Implementation Acience: IS* 2013; 8:117.

35. Aronson ID, Marsch LA, Acosta MC. Using findings in multimedia learning to inform technology-based behavioral health interventions. *Translational Behavioral Medicine* 2013; 3(3):234–243.

36. Bennett GG, Glasgow RE. The delivery of public health interventions via the Internet: Actualizing their potential. *Annual Review of Public Health* 2009; 30:273–292.

37. Campbell AN, Nunes EV, Miele GM, Matthews A, Polsky D, Ghitza UE, et al. Design and methodological considerations of an effectiveness trial of a computer-assisted intervention: An example from the NIDA Clinical Trials Network. *Contemporary Clinical Trials* 2012; 33(2):386–395.

38. Fenerty SD, West C, Davis SA, Kaplan SG, Feldman SR. The effect of reminder systems on patients' adherence to treatment. *Patient Preference and Adherence* 2012; 6:127–135.

39. Meredith SE, Grabinski MJ, Dallery J. Internet-based group contingency management to promote abstinence from cigarette smoking: A feasibility study. *Drug and Alcohol Dependence* 2011; 118(1):23–30.

40. Donkin L, Glozier N. Motivators and motivations to persist with online psychological interventions: A qualitative study of treatment completers. *Journal of Medical Internet Research* 2012; 14(3):e91.

41. Brindal E, Freyne J, Saunders I, Berkovsky S, Smith G, Noakes M. Features predicting weight loss in overweight or obese participants in a Web-based intervention: Randomized trial. *Jounral of Medical Internet Research* 2012; 14(6):e173.

42. Kelders SM, Kok RN, Ossebaard HC, Van Gemert-Pijnen JE. Persuasive system design does matter: A systematic review of adherence to Web-based interventions. *Journal of Medical Internet Research* 2012; 14(6):e152.

43. McKellar J, Austin J, Moos R. Building the first step: A review of low-intensity interventions for stepped care. *Addiction Science & Clinical Practice* 2012; 7(1):26.

44. Haynes RB, McDonald HP, Garg AX. Helping patients follow prescribed treatment: Clinical applications. *Journal of the American Medical Association* 2002; 288(22):2880–2883.

45. May C, Montori VM, Mair FS. We need minimally disruptive medicine. *British Medical Journal* 2009; 339:b2803.

46. Bastawrous A, Armstrong MJ. Mobile health use in low- and high-income countries: An overview of the peer-reviewed literature. *Journal of the Royal Society of Medicine* 2013; 106(4):130–142.

47. van Velthoven MH, Car J, Zhang Y, Marusic A. mHealth series: New ideas for mHealth data collection implementation in low- and middle-income countries. *Journal of Global Health* 2013; 3(2):20101.

48. Govindarajan V, Trimble C. *Reverse Innovation: Create Far from Home, Win Everywhere*. Boston: Harvard Business Press; 2012.

INDEX

ABOUT THE EDITORS

Lisa A. Marsch, PhD is the Director of the Center for Technology and Behavioral Health at Dartmouth College (www.c4tbh.org), the Director of the Dartmouth Psychiatric Research Center, and a faculty member within the Geisel School of Medicine at Dartmouth College. The Center for Technology and Behavioral Health is a national P30 "Center of Excellence" supported by the National Institutes of Health (NIH), composed of an interdisciplinary research group focused on the systematic application of state of the science technologies to the delivery of behavioral health interventions.

Sarah Lord, PhD is Assistant Professor of Psychiatry and Pediatrics at the Geisel School of Medicine at Dartmouth College. She is Director of the Dissemination and Implementation Core at the Center for Technology and Behavioral Health, and Director of the Center for Supported Employment Technology at Dartmouth Psychiatric Research Center. A clinical-developmental psychologist, Dr. Lord received her Ph.D. from the University of Colorado, Boulder and completed a clinical residency and post-doctoral fellowship in the Department of Psychiatry at the University of Wisconsin-Madison School of Medicine and Public Health.

Jesse Dallery, PhD is a Professor in the Department of Psychology at the University of Florida, and a Licensed Psychologist in the state of Florida. Dr. Dallery received his Ph.D. in Clinical Psychology at Emory University and completed a postdoctoral fellowship at the Johns Hopkins University School of Medicine in Behavioral Pharmacology.